A Textbook of Veterinary Systemic Pathology

Second Revised and Enlarged Edition

J. L. Vegad

Former Professor and Head
Department of Pathology
College of Veterinary Science and Animal Husbandry
Jabalpur - 482001, M.P., India

Madhu Swamy

Associate Professor of Pathology
College of Veterinary Science and Animal Husbandry
Jabalpur - 482001, M.P., India

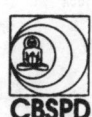

CBSPD

CBS Publishers & Distributors Pvt Ltd

New Delhi • Bengaluru • Chennai • Kochi • Kolkata • Lucknow • Mumbai
Hyderabad • Jharkhand • Nagpur • Patna • Pune • Uttarakhand

A Textbook of Veterinary Systemic Pathology

ISBN: 978-81-239-2689-6

Copyright © Publisher

First CBS Reprint: 2015
Reprint: 2016, 2018, 2020, 2021, 2023

Published by Satish Kumar Jain and produced by Varun Jain for

CBS Publishers & Distributors Pvt Ltd

4819/XI Prahlad Street, 24 Ansari Road, Daryaganj, New Delhi 110 002, India
Ph: 011-23289259, 23266861, 23266867   Website: www.cbspd.com
Fax: 011-23243014   e-mail: delhi@cbspd.com; cbspubs@airtelmail.in.

Corporate Office: 204 FIE, Industrial Area, Patparganj, Delhi 110 092, India
Ph: 011-4934 4934   Fax: 011-4934 4935   e-mail: publishing@cbspd.com;
                                                                              publicity@cbspd.com

Branches

- **Bengaluru:** Seema House 2975, 17th Cross, KR Road, Banasankari 2nd Stage, Bengaluru 560 070, Karnataka, India
  Ph: +91-80-26771678/79   Fax: +91-80-26771680   e-mail: bangalore@cbspd.com
- **Chennai:** 7, Subbaraya Street, Shenoy Nagar, Chennai 600 030, Tamil Nadu, India
  Ph: +91-44-26680620, 26681266   Fax: +91-44-42032115   e-mail: chennai@cbspd.com
- **Kochi:** 42/1325, 1326, Power House Road, Opp KSEB, Power House, Ernakulum Kochi 682 018, Kerala, India
  Ph: +91-484-4059061-65.67   Fax: +91-484-4059065   e-mail: kochi@cbspd.com
- **Kolkata:** 147, Hind Ceramics Compound, 1st Floor, Nilgunj Road, Belghoria, Kolkata-700056, West Bengal, India
  Ph: +91-9096713055/7798394118, 9836841399   e-mail: kolkata@cbspd.com
- **Lucknow:** Basement, Khushnuma Complex, 7 Meerabai Marg (Behind Jawahar Bhawan),Lucknow-226001, UP, India
  Ph: +0522-4000032   e-mail: tiwari.lucknow@cbspd.com
- **Mumbai:** PWD Shed, Gala no 25/26, Ramchandra Bhatt Marg, Next to JJ Hospital Gate no. 2, Opp. Union Bank of India, Noorbaug, Mumbai-400009, Maharashtra, India
  Ph: 022-66661880/89   e-mail: mumbai@cbspd.com

Representatives

• Hyderabad	0-9885175004	• Jharkhand	0-9811541605	• Nagpur	0-9421945513
• Patna	0-9334159340	• Pune	0-9623451994	• Uttarakhand	0-9716462459

Printed at Neekunj Print Process, Sonipat, Haryana, India

PREFACE

The second edition of this book has been revised with the same objective in mind that guided the first edition. That is, to provide the student with a textbook comprehensive enough to meet every need in systemic pathology as per the course outline prescribed by the Veterinary Council of India.

All chapters have been thoroughly updated, but the digestive, endocrine, nervous, and reproductive chapters have been rewritten and the muscle chapter extensively revised. Thirty four new photographs have been added to help understand text discussions, whereas the old illustrations have been either replaced or modified. The total number of figures has thus increased from 25 in the previous edition to 59 in this second edition.

In addition to the inclusion of new discussions and illustrations, another objective of this revision was to increase the clarity of expression and lucidity of the text. We have attempted to highlight the role of pathogenesis as a basis of understanding the sequence for the development of gross and microscopic changes. Also, we have attempted to use the current bacteriological terminology. The names of some bacteria have changed several times in the last decade. We have used the most recent name and placed the commonly known older name within brackets on the initial use of the name of the organism.

The other minor changes to make the book handy and more useful include that important words and certain portions of the text are given in bold type for an easy grasp. Presentation of 'Contents' has been revised, and in the 'Index', the numbers that indicate the main discussion, put in bold for an easy search.

We like to thank Shri Suneel Gomber, Manager, International Book Distributing Co. Lucknow, for publication of the revised edition. We are grateful to Shri Vijay Parmar of Jabalpur Graphics and Amit Vegad who were most generous in extending help relating to computer work. Finally, we extend our profound appreciation to Mrs. Nita Vegad and Dr. Parimal Swamy for their support and patience.

J. L. Vegad
Madhu Swamy

CONTENTS

CHAPTER 4
Urinary System

CHAPTER 5
Endocrine System

CHAPTER 13
Eye and Ear

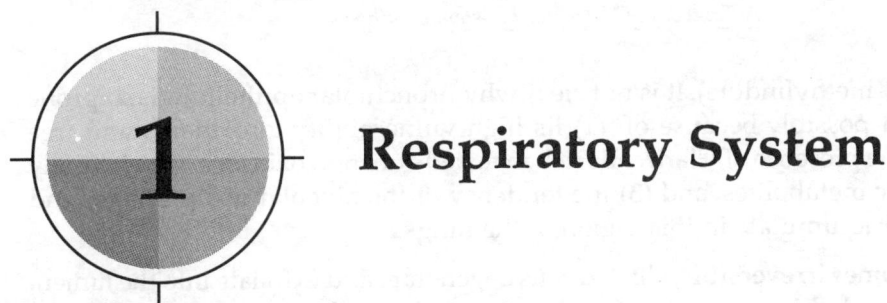

Respiratory System

Introduction

The respiratory system is prone to injury due to constant exposure to countless microbes, particles, fibres, and toxic gases and vapours present in the air. Vulnerability of the system to airborne (aerogenous) injury is mainly due to: (1) the vast area of the contact (interface) between the respiratory system and the inspired air, (2) the large volume of air passing continuously into the lungs, and (3) the high concentration of harmful substances that may be present in the air, such as microbes (viruses, bacteria, fungi, animal products (dander, feathers, mites), toxic gases (ammonia, hydrogen sulphide, sulphur dioxide), and chemicals (herbicides, asbestos, nickel, lead). For example, in humans, the surface of the respiratory tract is about 200 square metres (m^2), roughly the area of a tennis court. And each day the lungs are exposed to around 10,000 litres of air. The surface of the **horse lung** is estimated to be around 2,000 m^2.

Lungs are also susceptible to haematogenously borne microbes, toxins, and emboli. This is not surprising since **the pulmonary capillary bed is the largest in the body,** with a surface area of 70 m^2 in an adult human. This area is equal to 2400 km of capillaries, with 1 ml of blood occupying up to 16 km of capillary bed.

Structure and Function

Bronchioles

The structure of bronchioles differs both from that of the larger bronchi and the alveolus. The bronchiolar surface is covered with cilia, which are surrounded by a water-protein layer rich in lysozyme and immunoglobulins. However, like alveoli, their surface layer contains no surfactant (discussed later) and, like bronchi, no mucus. In fact, bronchioles have no mucus-secreting goblet cells, but in their place they have other types of secretory cells, mainly the **Clara cells** (Fig. 1A). These cells are functionally important in two ways. First, they are actively metabolic, and play an important role in detoxification of foreign substances (xenobiotics). This is similar to the role hepatocytes play in the liver. Second, they give rise to ciliated epithelial and other cells.

The epithelial lining of the bronchioles is extremely susceptible to injury, particularly to that caused by some respiratory viruses (parainfluenza-3, adenoviruses, oxidant gases (nitrogen dioxide), sulphur dioxide, and toxic substances (3-methylindole). It is not clear why bronchiolar epithelium is so prone to injury, but possibly because of: (1) its high vulnerability to oxidants and free radicals, (2) the presence of **Clara cells** rich in mixed-function oxidases, which locally generate toxic metabolites, and (3) the tendency of the alveolar macrophages and leukocytes to accumulate in this region of the lungs.

If injury becomes irreversible, ciliated cells degenerate and exfoliate into the lumen, leaving a denuded basement membrane. Repair in the bronchioles is similar to that in the tracheal or nasal mucosa, but is less effective. Normally, the accumulated phagocytic cells remove exudate and cell debris from the lumen. Thus the basement membrane is prepared to be repopulated with new cells originating from the rapidly dividing **Clara cells.** After several days, these cells differentiate into normal ciliated cells.

In severe injury, exudate cannot be removed from the basement membrane of bronchioles. The exudate becomes infiltrated by fibroblasts. These form small masses of fibrovascular tissue. They eventually become covered by ciliated cells. This lesion is referred to as **bronchiolitis obliterans.**

However, **if the injury is mild but persistent,** goblet cells normally absent in the bronchioles proliferate from basal cells. This results in **goblet cell metaplasia** and causes a change in the properties of bronchiolar secretions. The normal serous fluid released by **Clara cells** becomes a thick and sticky material when mucus produced by goblet cell is added. Due to the increased adhesiveness of the mucus, the secretions cannot be removed effectively by ciliary action. This leads to plugging and obstruction of distal airways. These conditions are grouped as **chronic obstructive pulmonary disease.** Under such conditions, cough is required to clear mucus from the obstructed bronchioles. Further complications could be pulmonary emphysema and atelectasis, depending on the extent of the bronchiolar obstruction. These two abnormalities are present in chronic obstructive pulmonary disease (COPD) of **horses.**

Alveoli

The alveoli have an extremely delicate structure, and are therefore very prone to injury once defence mechanisms are damaged. **The alveolus has a thin, three-layered wall** composed of **vascular endothelium, alveolar interstitium** (basement membrane) and **alveolar epithelium** (pneumocytes). These three layers of cells constitute 'air-blood barrier'. The epithelial side of the alveolus is lined by two types of epithelial cells: **type I and type II pneumocytes** (Fig. 1B). **Type I pneumocyte,** also known as **membranous pneumocyte**, covers 95% of the alveolar surface. These cells are arranged as a very delicate continuous membrane on the alveolar surface (Fig. 1B). Type I pneumocytes are particularly susceptible to harmful agents. Injury to type I pneumocytes causes their swelling and vacuolation. When damage becomes irreversible, type I cells detach. This results in denudation of the

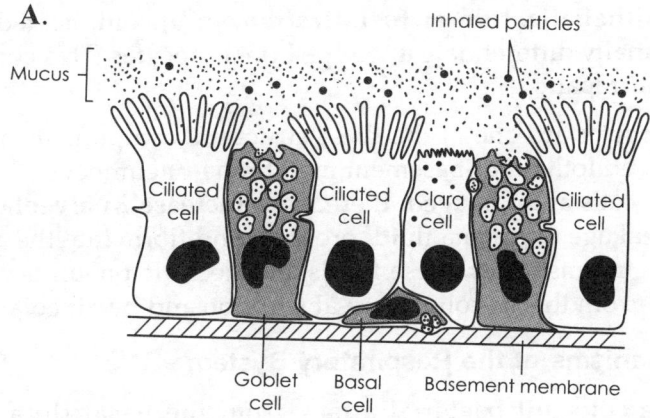

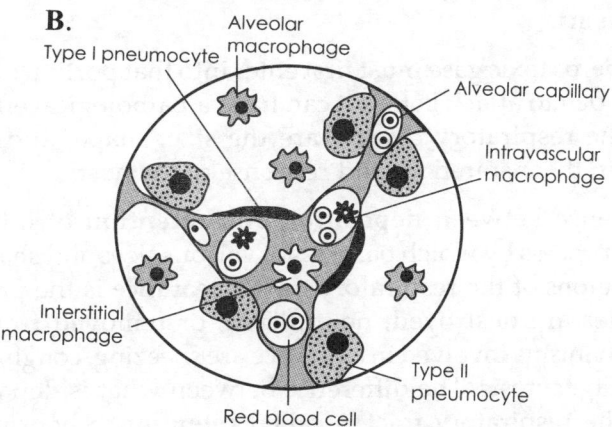

Fig. 1. Schematic representation of the mucociliary escalator. A. The conductive system from nasal cavity to bronchi is lined by the mucociliary escalator, which is made of ciliated and non-ciliated secretory cells and mucus. The large dots (•) indicate particles trapped by mucus. **B.** Particles reaching bronchioles and alveoli are ingested by the pulmonary alveolar macrophages, which leave the lung through the mucociliary escalator. The alveolar wall is composed of capillaries, interstitium, and alveolar lining (type I and type II pneumocytes).

basement membrane and increased alveolar permeability. **Alveolar repair is possible as long as the basement membrane remains intact** and lesions are not complicated by further injury or infection. Within 3 days, cuboidal **type II pneumocytes** (also known as 'granular pneumocytes'), which are the precursor cell and more resistant to injury, undergo mitosis and provide a large number of new cells. These new cells line (cover) the denuded alveolar basement membrane and finally differentiate in type I pneumocytes. When alveolar injury is diffuse, proliferation of type II pneumocytes becomes so striking that the microscopic appearance of the alveolus resembles that of a gland or foetal lung. The lesion has been called **epithelialization** or **foetalization.** In uncomplicated cases, type II pneumocytes finally differentiate into type I pneumocytes. This completes the last stage of alveolar repair.

Type I pneumocytes are one of the three structural components of the **air-blood barrier,** that is, endothelium-basement membrane-pneumocyte. Therefore, when these epithelial cells are damaged, there is **an increase in alveolar permeability** and transient leakage of plasma fluid, proteins, and fibrin into the alveolar lumen. Under normal circumstances, these fluids and necrotic pneumocytes (type I) are rapidly cleared from the alveolus by re-absorption and by alveolar macrophages.

Defence Mechanisms of the Respiratory System

In spite of the constant bacterial attack from the nasal flora and from the contaminated air, **normal lungs remain sterile due to their remarkably effective defence mechanisms.**

A particle, microbe, or toxic gase must first enter into that portion of the respiratory system which is open to attack before it can have a pathological effect. The factors that determine the respiratory disease are the size, shape, and distribution of particles present in the inspired air and response of the host.

There is a difference between **deposition** and **retention** of inhaled particles. **Deposition** is the process by which particles of various sizes and shapes are trapped within specific regions of the respiratory tract. **Clearance** is the process by which deposited particles are destroyed, neutralized, or removed from the mucosal surfaces. The mechanisms involved in clearance are sneezing, coughing, mucociliary transport, and phagocytosis. The difference between what is deposited and what is cleared from the respiratory tract is called **retention.** Abnormal retention of particles from increased deposition, decreased clearance, or a combination of both is the underlying mechanism involved in many pulmonary diseases.

The anatomical configuration of **nasal cavity** and **bronchi** plays an important role in preventing or reducing the penetration of harmful material into the lungs, especially into the alveoli, which are the most vulnerable portion of the respiratory system. The coiled arrangement of the nasal turbinates creates a great turbulence (violent movement) of airflow. As a result, centrifugal forces are created that forcefully strike particles larger than 10 μm on the surface of the nasal mucosa. Therefore, particles larger than 10 μm are trapped in the nasal passages. However, particles smaller than 10 μm escape trapping, but these medium-sized particles meet a second barrier at the bifurcation of the trachea and in the lumen of the bronchi. Here, sudden changes in the direction of air (inertia), which occur at the bifurcation of **major airways,** cause particles between 2-10 μm in size to strike against the surface of bronchial mucosa. On the other hand, velocity of air in the **small bronchi and bronchioles** is somewhat slow. Therefore, here, inertial and centrifugal forces do not play a significant role in the process by which inhaled particles contact the mucosal surface. However, in the bronchiolar and alveolar regions, particles 2 μm or smaller, may come in contact with the mucosa by means of sedimentation due to gravitation, or by diffusion due to Brownian movement (random movement). Infective air containing bacteria and viruses arewithin the size range to gain entry into the bronchioloalveolar region. To conclude, **the anatomical characteristics of the nasal cavity and airways provide an effective barrier and thereby prevent penetration of most large particles into the lungs.**

Once larger particles are trapped in the mucosa, it is important that these foreign materials are removed to prevent or minimize injury to the respiratory system. To enable this, the respiratory system is supplied with several defence mechanisms. These will now be discussed.

Mucociliary Defence Mechanisms

Mucociliary clearance is a physical movement in only one direction. Its purpose is removal of deposited particles and dissolved gases in the mucus from the respiratory tract. This is achieved by the **mucociliary blanket**, also known as **mucociliary escalator** (Fig. 1B). It is the main defence mechanism of the nasal cavity, trachea, and bronchi. **Mucus** is a complex mixture of water, glycoproteins, immunoglobulins, lipids, and electrolytes produced by goblet (mucous) cells, serous cells and sub-mucosal glands. Once serous fluid and mucus are secreted on the mucosa, a thin, double-layer of mucus is formed on top of the cells. The outer layer is thick and sticky, while the inner layer which is fluid is directly in contact with cilia. **A healthy human being** produces about 100 ml of mucus per day. Each ciliated cell in the mucosa has about 250 cilia (6 μm long). These beat spontaneously and harmoniously at about 1000 strokes per minute. **In horse,** they produce movement of up to 20 mm per minute. **Rapid and powerful movement of cilia creates a series of waves. These push forward the mucus, and as a result, any trapped particles and exfoliated cells on the epithelial surface, are thrown out of the respiratory tract.** The mucus is finally swallowed, and if present in large amounts, it is coughed out.

The mucociliary blanket of the nasal cavity, trachea, and bronchi also play an important role in preventing injury from toxic gases. If a soluble gas comes in contact with the mucociliary blanket, it mixes with the mucus. This reduces concentration of the gas reaching deep into the alveolar region. In other words, mucus dissolves gases and then clears them from the respiratory tract through mucociliary transport. If ciliary transport is reduced (from loss of cilia), or mucus production is excessive, coughing becomes an important mechanism for clearing the airways.

The mucociliary escalator provides the physical transport. However, **there are also other cells closely associated with ciliated epithelium that contribute to defence mechanism of the respiratory system.** Among these, the most important are **M cells** ('microfold cells'). These are modified epithelial cells covering the **bronchial associated lymphoid tissue (BALT).** M cells are particularly located at the bifurcation of bronchi and bronchioles, where inhaled particles often strike on the mucosa due to inertial forces. **From here, inhaled particles and soluble antigens are phagocytosed and transported by macrophages, dendritic cells, and other 'antigen-processing cells' (APC) into the BALT.** This provides a unique opportunity for B and T lymphocytes to enter into close contact with potentially pathogenic substances. Lymphocytes in BALT are not stationary but are in continual movement to other organs and contribute to both **cellular** (cytotoxic, helper, suppressed T cells) **and humoral immune responses.** IgA, and to a lesser extent, IgG and IgM play important roles in the local immunity of the respiratory system, especially in preventing attachment of pathogens to the mucociliary blanket. Chronic respiratory diseases, especially those of infectious nature, are often accompanied by **severe hyperplasia of the BALT.**

The mucociliary clearance ends at the pharynx. Here, mucus pushed forcefully from the nasal cavity and tracheo-bronchial tree, is finally swallowed. It is thus removed from the respiratory tract.

Phagocytic Defence Mechanisms

Alveoli have no ciliated and mucus-producing cells. Therefore, the defence against inhaled particles cannot be provided by mucociliary clearance. The alveoli are protected mainly through **phagocytosis** carried out by **pulmonary alveolar macrophages** (see Fig. 1B).

These cells are highly phagocytic. They are derived mostly from blood monocytes and, to a much lesser extent, from a slowly dividing population of interstitial macrophages. The monocytes reduce their glycolytic and increase their oxidative metabolisms to function in aerobic rather than in anaerobic environment. **Pulmonary alveolar macrophages rapidly attack and ingest bacteria and other particles that reach alveoli.** The number of macrophages in the alveoli is almost the same as the number of particles that reach the lungs. The ability to increase the number of macrophages within hours is very important in protecting the lungs against foreign material. Unlike that of tissue macrophages, the life-span of alveolar macrophages is short, only a few days. **Alveolar phagocytosis plays an extremely important role in the defence mechanism against inhaled bacteria without the need of an inflammatory reaction.** Bacteria reaching the alveoli are rapidly ingested. Then, bactericidal enzymes present in the lysosomes are discharged into the phagosome containing bacteria. Except certain organisms that are resistant to intracellular killing (e.g. *Mycobacterium tuberculosis, Listeria monocytogenes*) most bacteria are rapidly destroyed by activated alveolar macrophages. Similarly, inhaled particles such as dust, pollen, spores, carbon, or erythrocytes from intra-alveolar haemorrhage are all phagocytosed and finally removed from the alveoli.

Clearance by alveolar macrophages operates in a well-coordinated manner with other cells and secretions of the lung. These **cell-to-cell interactions** are complex and involve many cells. A **humoral immune response** also plays an important role in protecting the lungs against pathogens. Although IgA is the most abundant antibody in the nasal and tracheal secretions, IgG is the most abundant antibody in the alveolar surface. Here, it acts as an opsonizing antibody to increase engulfment and destruction of inhaled pathogens by alveolar macrophages and neutrophils. Besides antibodies, there are many secretory products locally released into the alveoli that make up the alveolar lining material and contribute to defence mechanisms of the lungs. The most important of these antimicrobial products are transferrin, anionic peptides, and pulmonary surfactants (**Table 1**).

Table 1. Defence mechanisms present in the respiratory system

Cell / Secretory Product	Action
Alveolar macrophages	Phagocytosis. Main line of defence against inhaled particles and pathogenic micro-organisms in the alveoli
Intravascular macrophage	Phagocytosis. Removal of particles, endotoxin, and microbial pathogens in the circulation
Ciliated cells	Expel mucus, inhaled particles, and microbial pathogens by ciliary action
Clara cells	Detoxify foreign substances through mixed function oxidases
Mucus	Traps inhaled particles, microbial pathogens, and neutralizes soluble gases
Surfactant	Protects alveolar wall and increases phagocytosis
Lysozyme	Antimicrobial enzyme
Transferrin and lactoferrin	Suppress bacterial growth
Alpha1-antitrypsin	Protects against the harmful effects of proteolytic enzymes released by phagocytic cells. Also inhibits inflammation
Interferon	Antiviral and modulator of the immune and inflammatory responses
Antibodies	Prevent microbe attachment to cell membranes, opsonization
Complement	Increases chemotaxis and phagocytosis
Antioxidants*	Prevent injury caused by superoxide, hydrogen peroxide, and free radicals generated during phagocytosis, inflammation, or by inhalation of oxidant gases (nitrogen dioxide, sulphur dioxide, ozone)

*Antioxidants include superoxide dismutase, catalase, glutathione peroxidase, free radical scavengers (tocopherol, ascorbic acid)

Alveolar macrophages are supplied with a wide variety of **specific receptors** on their surfaces. These facilitate phagocytosis and enable macrophages to differentiate between 'self' and 'foreign' antigens. The most important are IgG, Fc and complement (C3b, C3a, and C5a), tumour necrosis factor (TNF), and CD40 receptors. **These facilitate phagocytosis of opsonized particles.**

Defence Mechanisms against Blood-Borne Pathogens

Lungs are also susceptible to pathogens, toxins, or emboli coming through the blood. In **dogs, human beings,** and **rodents** (rat, mouse), the Kupffer cells in the liver and splenic macrophages are the main cells responsible for removing circulating bacteria and other particles from the blood. In contrast, removal of circulating pathogenic bacteria and particles from the blood of **ruminants, cats,** and **pigs** mainly depends on **pulmonary intravascular macrophages.** These cells are different from alveolar macrophages, and make a separate population of phagocytes normally residing within pulmonary capillaries. **In pigs,** 16% of the pulmonary capillary surface is lined by intravascular macrophages. **In ruminants,** 95% of intravenously injected tracer particles or bacteria are rapidly phagocytosed by these intravascular macrophages.

Defence Mechanisms against Oxidant Induced Lung Injury

Lungs exist in an oxygen-rich environment. They are also the site of numerous metabolic reactions. Therefore, lungs also require an efficient defence mechanism against oxidant-induced cellular damage. This form of damage can be caused by inhalation of oxidant gases (e.g. nitrogen dioxide, ozone, sulphur dioxide), by foreign toxic metabolites produced locally or reaching the lungs through the bloodstream (e.g. 3-methylindole), or by free radicals released by phagocytic cells during inflammation. Free radical scavengers such as catalase, superoxide dismutase, and vitamin E are largely responsible for protecting pulmonary cells against peroxidation and are present in the intracellular and extracellular spaces of the lung.

In summary, the defence mechanisms are very effective in trapping, destroying, and removing bacteria. They are so effective that under normal conditions animals can be exposed to air containing massive numbers of bacteria without any ill effects. **If defence mechanisms are damaged, inhaled bacteria colonize, multiply, and produce infection, which in some cases results in fatal pneumonia.** Similarly, when air-borne and blood-borne pathogens, inhaled toxic agents, or free radicals overcome the protective defence mechanisms, cells of the respiratory system could be injured, often causing serious respiratory diseases.

Impairment of Defence Mechanisms

Factors that damage defence mechanisms include viral infections, toxic gases, and certain other conditions.

Viral Infections

Viral agents predispose humans and animals to secondary bacterial pneumonias by **viral-bacterial synergism**. In humans, a good example is that of influenza virus in which the mortality rate is significantly increased due to secondary bacterial pneumonia. **In animals,** the most common viruses that predispose to secondary bacterial pneumonia include influenza virus **in pigs** and **horses**; bovine herpesvirus 1 (BHV-1), parainfluenza-3 (PI-3), and bovine respiratory syncytial virus (BRSV) **in cattle**; and canine distemper virus **in dogs**. The **mechanism** of the synergistic effect of viral-bacterial infections is the **destruction of mucociliary blanket** and a simultaneous **reduction of mucociliary clearance.** Five to seven days after a bacterial infection, the phagocytic function of alveolar macrophages is greatly impaired (damaged). However, the mechanisms by which viruses damage defence mechanisms are many and remain poorly understood.

Toxic Gases

Certain gases also damage respiratory defence mechanisms and make animals more susceptible to secondary bacterial infections. For example, hydrogen sulphide and ammonia can damage pulmonary defence mechanisms and increase susceptibility to bacterial pneumonia.

Pathology

Nasal Cavity and Sinuses

Anomalies

Congenital anomalies of the nasal cavity are **rare in domestic animals**. Anomalies such as **choanal atresia** (imperforate bucco-pharyngeal membrane), some types of **chondrodysplasia,** and **osteopetrosis** are incompatible with life. That is, they are fatal. **Non-fatal congenital anomalies** include cystic nasal conchae, nasal and sinus cysts, deviation of nasal septum, cleft upper lip (harelip, **cheiloschisis**), and hypoplastic turbinates, and cleft palate (**palatoschisis**).

Metabolic Disturbances

These are also rare in domestic animals. **Amyloidosis**, which is associated with deposition of amyloid protein (fibrils with beta-pleated configuration) in various tissues, has been reported in the nasal cavity of **horses**. Affected horses have difficulty in breathing, epistaxis, and show large firm, nodules in the nasal septum and floor of nasal cavity. **Microscopic lesions** consist of a deposition of hyaline material (Congo red-positive) in nasal mucosa. Unlike amyloidosis in other organs of domestic animals, where amyloid is of the reactive type (**amyloid AA**), in equine nasal amyloidosis it is of the immunocytic type (**amyloid AL**).

Circulatory Disturbances

The nasal mucosa is highly vascularized. **Active hyperaemia** is associated with early stages of inflammation, whether caused by viral infections, secondary bacterial infections, allergy, trauma, or irritants such as ammonia. **Passive hyperaemia (congestion)** is a non-specific lesion. **Haemorrhage** from the nose (**epistaxis**, nosebleed) may result from local trauma, erosions of sub-mucosal vessels by inflammation, such as in acute septicaemic diseases, or neoplasms. An important cause of epistaxis in **horses** is mycotic infection of the guttural pouches. **Ethmoidal haematomas** are important in **older horses.** They are characterized by chronic, progressive, often unilateral bleeding.

Inflammation

Inflammation of the nasal mucosa is called **rhinitis** and that of the sinuses, **sinusitis.** They usually occur together.

Rhinitis

Rhinitis is very common in domestic animals. The **infectious rhinitis** occurs from a disturbance in the balance of the nasal microbial flora of the nasal cavity. Harmless bacteria present normally protect the host through a process called **competitive exclusion**, by which the number of potential pathogens is kept under control. Disruption of this protective mechanism can be brought about by a number of factors **which then cause rhinitis.** The **causes** of rhinitis include:

1. **Respiratory viruses** such as infectious bovine rhinotracheitis and feline viral rhinotracheitis. Also, as a part of infectious diseases involving other parts of the body, rhinitis may occur in bovine malignant catarrhal fever, equine influenza, swine influenza, canine distemper, and fowl pox and infectious laryngotracheitis in poultry.

2. **Pathogenic bacteria,** such as *Fusobacterium necrophorum, Pseudomonas aeruginosa, Streptococcus equi,* and *Burkholderia mallei (Malleomyces mallei).*

3. **Physical irritants,** such as dust and other foreign bodies.

4. **Chemical agents,** such as irritant gases and smoke.

5. **Parasites,** such as the larvae of *Oestrus ovis* in sheep.

6. Local trauma.

7. Immunosuppression.

8. Stress.

9. Environmental changes.

10. Prolonged antibacterial therapy.

Based on the nature of exudate, rhinitis can be classified into **serous, catarrhal, purulent (suppurative), fibrinous,** or **granulomatous.** Other changes such as

haemorrhage, ulcers, and **mucosal hyperplasia** can also be found in inflamed nasal mucosa. Rhinitis can also be classified according to the age of the lesions as **acute, sub-acute,** or **chronic;** and according to the aetiological agent as **viral, bacterial, allergic, mycotic,** or **toxic.** Microscopic examination of impression smears and bacterial cultures are usually required to establish cause of the exudate.

Serous Rhinitis

This is the **mildest form of inflammation.** It is characterized by hyperaemia and increased production of a **clear fluid** by serous glands present in the sub-mucosa. It is caused by mild irritants or cold air, and occurs during the early stages of viral infections such as the common cold in humans and upper respiratory tract infections in animals, or in mild allergic reactions.

Catarrhal Rhinitis

This is **a slightly more severe inflammation.** In addition to serous fluid, there is a great increase in **mucus** produced by increased activity of goblet cells and mucous glands. The mucosa is hyperaemic, swollen or covered with mucus exudate. The mucous exudate is a thick, translucent, or slightly turbid viscous fluid. Sometimes it contains a few leukocytes and cellular debris. In **chronic cases,** catarrhal rhinitis is characterized **microscopically** by marked hyperplasia of goblet cells. When inflammation is severe, the mucus is infiltrated with neutrophils which have a cloudy appearance. This exudate is referred to as **mucopurulent.**

Purulent (Suppurative) Rhinitis

This inflammation occurs when the **nasal mucosa suffers a more severe injury.** It is usually accompanied by mucosal necrosis and secondary bacterial infection. It is characterized by a **neutrophilic exudate.**

Cytokines, neutrophils, complement activation, and bacterial products cause emigration of leukocytes, **especially neutrophils,** which mix with nasal secretions, and mucus. This type of inflammation occurs in **equine strangles,** and **canine distemper,** and also in *Oestrus ovis* **larvae infestation in sheep. Grossly,** there are collections of creamy, yellow, pus on the mucosa, and in the recesses of the turbinates. The colour may vary from white, green, or brown, depending on the types of bacteria and type of leukocytes present in the exudate. In severe cases, the nasal passages are completely blocked by the exudate. **Microscopically,** neutrophils are seen in the sub-mucosa and mucosa and form plaques (patches) of exudate on the mucosal surface.

Fibrinous Rhinitis

This inflammation occurs when nasal injury causes a **severe vascular damage.** This results in the leakage of plasma fibrinogen, which coagulates into fibrin. **Grossly,** fibrin appears like a yellow, brown, or grey rubbery coating on nasal mucosa. Fibrin accumulates on the surface and forms a characteristic film of exudate known a **pseudomembrane.** If this exudate can be removed, and leaves an intact underlying mucosa, it is **croupous** or **pseudodiphtheritic rhinitis.** But if removal of this pseudomembrane leaves an ulcerated mucosa, it is called as **diphtheritic** or **fibrino-necrotic rhinitis.** The term diphtheritic was derived from human diphtheria, which causes a severe and destructive inflammation of the respiratory mucosa. **Microscopically,** the lesions comprise perivascular oedema with fibrin, a few neutrophils infiltrating the mucosa, and plaques of exudate consisting of fibrin strands mixed with leukocytes and cellular debris covering a necrotic and ulcerated epithelium.

Granulomatous Rhinitis

This type of inflammation is characterized by infiltration of macrophages, lymphocytes, and plasma cells in the mucosa and sub-mucosa. In some cases, inflammation leads to the formation of **polypoid nodules.** In severe cases, these are large enough to cause obstruction of the nasal passages. It occurs in **systemic mycoses, tuberculosis,** and with **foreign bodies.** In some cases, the cause is less specific such as in **allergic rhinitis.** In certain others, causes remain unknown.

Inflammatory processes in the nasal cavity usually resolve completely. However, **some adverse results** in infectious rhinitis include broncho-aspiration of exudate leading to **bronchopneumonia** and **lung abscesses.** Also, nasal inflammation may extend into the sinuses causing **sinusitis,** into facial bones causing **osteomyelitis,** through the cribriform plate causing **meningitis,** along the Eustachian tubes causing **otitis media** and **interna** and **vestibular syndrome** (abnormal head tilt and abnormal gait).

Sinusitis

Sinusitis is sporadic (occasional) in animals and is usually combined with rhinitis. It also occurs as a sequel to septic wounds, improper dehorning in cattle (**frontal sinus**), or tooth infection in horses and dogs (**maxillary sinus**). Paranasal sinuses **have poor drainage.** Therefore, exudate tends to accumulate, causing **mucocele** (accumulation of mucus), or **empyema** (accumulation of pus). **Chronic sinusitis** may extend into the nearby bone (**osteomyelitis**), or through the bone into the meninges and brain (**meningitis** and **encephalitis**).

Specific Diseases of the Nasal Cavity and Sinuses

Diseases of Cattle

Infectious Bovine Rhinotracheitis (IBR or 'Rednose')

IBR is caused by **bovine herpesvirus-1 (BHV-1).** The disease is important in **cattle** because of the synergism of the IBR virus with *Pasteurella haemolytica* in producing pneumonia. It is also associated with abortion in cattle, systemic infection of **calves,** and infectious postural vulvo-vaginitis (IPV). The disease appears as a transient, acute, febrile illness. In very severe cases, it results in dyspnoea (difficult breathing) due to obstruction of airflow by the exudate.

In the **respiratory form,** the **lesions** include severe hyperaemia and focal necrosis of nasal, pharyngeal, laryngeal, tracheal, and bronchial mucosa. Secondary bacterial infection in areas of necrosis results in the formation of a thick layer of fibrino-necrotic material (**diphtheritic**) in the airway. **Intranuclear inclusion bodies** are rarely seen in field cases, because inclusion bodies occur only during the early stages of the disease.

The most important sequel to IBR is **pneumonia.** This is caused either by direct aspiration of exudate from airways, or as a result of damage to lung's defence mechanisms. This predisposes the animal to secondary bacterial infection, usually *P. haemolytica.*

Bovine Malignant Catarrhal Fever (Bovine Malignant Catarrh)

This is the other infection that may involve the upper respiratory tract of **cattle.** It is a highly fatal disease, and is caused by a herpesvirus. It is an acute infectious disease of **cattle, buffalo,** and **other ruminants** including **deer** and **antelope.** The disease is characterized by severe inflammation of the mucous membrane of the upper respiratory tract, the upper digestive tract, conjunctiva, and meninges of brain. The most characteristic clinical sign is profuse mucopurulent discharge from the eyes and nose. When the crusts are removed from the nose, **ulcers are seen.** Sequelae include involvement of the lungs and intestinal tract. In the terminal stages, ulceration or diphtheritic lesions are often found in the mucosa of the nasal passages and digestive tract.

Nasal Granulomas

These occur in **cattle** probably as a result of repeated exposure to certain unidentified inhaled antigens. **Nasal granulomas (atopic rhinitis)** are reported mainly in **cattle** in Australia, South Africa, and the United Kingdom. The affected cattle develop multiple, small, pink or red, polypoid nodules in the nasal passages. These nodules are composed of fibrovascular tissue mixed with lymphocytes (**granulation tissue**).

Diseases of Sheep and Goats

Oestrus ovis (Nasal Bot)

Oestrus ovis is the fly that deposits its first-stage larvae in the nostrils of **sheep.** Larvae mature into large bots that spend most of their larval stages in nasal passages and sinuses, causing irritation and obstruction of airways. Mature larvae drop to the ground and pupate into flies. This type of parasitic infection in which living tissue is invaded by larvae of flies is known as **myiasis.** Besides sheep, *O. ovis* also affects **goats, dogs,** and sometimes **humans** (shepherds). Larvae in the nasal passages cause chronic irritation and mucopurulent rhinitis. Bots (larvae) of *O. ovis* can be found if the head is cut to expose the nasal passages.

Rhinitis is rare in goats. Most cases are associated with infections with *Pasteurella multocida* or *P. haemolytica*. The lesions are that of mild serous to catarrhal or mucopurulent inflammation.

Diseases of Horses

Equine Viral Rhinopneumonitis (EVR)

This disease is caused by **equine herpesvirus** (EHV). In foal and racehorses, it occurs as a mild respiratory disease (EHV- 4), in mares as abortion (EHV- 1). The **respiratory form** of EVR is mild and therefore lesions in the nasal mucosa and lungs are rarely seen at postmortem unless complicated by secondary bacterial rhinitis, pharyngitis, or bronchopneumonia.

Equine Influenza

This disease is common. It is a highly contagious, self-limiting upper respiratory infection of **horses** caused by type A strains of influenza virus. It has high morbidity but low mortality, and is characterized by fever, conjunctivitis, and **nasal discharge**. It usually occurs in 2-3-year-old horses. Equine influenza is mild, but sometimes it can cause severe broncho-interstitial pneumonia with pulmonary oedema. In some horses, equine influenza is complicated by secondary bacterial bronchopneumonia.

Equine rhinopneumonitis virus, adenovirus, rhinovirus and **parainfluenza virus** produce mild and transient upper respiratory infection in **horses**, unless complicated by secondary pathogens. In all, the clinical signs consist of fever, coughing, and a nasal discharge varying from serous to purulent.

Strangles, Glanders, and Melioidosis (Pseudoglanders)

Strangles, glanders and melioidosis (pseudoglanders) of **horses** are grouped as upper respiratory diseases because they all produce **nasal lesions,** and **nasal discharge** is often the most common clinical sign. **Basically,** they are **systemic bacterial diseases** that cause rhinitis and suppuration in various organs.

Strangles

Strangles is **an acute infectious disease** of **young horses, asses,** and **mules**. It is caused by *Streptococcus equi*. The disease is characterized by **suppurative rhinitis** and lymphadenitis (mandibular and retropharyngeal) with occasional spread through blood to internal organs. The animal may suffer from the disease many times in its lifetime, because the resulting immunity lasts only for few months.

Infection occurs when susceptible **horses** come into contact with feed, or air droplets containing the organism. After penetrating through the naso-pharyngeal mucosa,

S. equi goes to mandibular and retropharyngeal lymph nodes through lymphatic vessels. **Clinically**, the disease is characterized by nasal discharge, conjunctivitis, and marked swelling of lymph nodes.

The **gross lesions** include the presence of a large amount of mucopurulent exudate in the nasal passages with marked hyperaemia of nasal mucosa. Affected lymph nodes are enlarged, painful, warm, and contain thick purulent exudate (**purulent lymphadenitis.**) When spread of *S. equi* through blood results in metastatic abscesses in such organs as the lungs, liver, spleen, kidney, brain, or joints, the disease is called '**bastard strangles**'.

Common complications of strangles are: (1) **bronchopneumonia** due to aspiration of exudate, (2) **laryngeal hemiplegia** ('**roaring**') from compression of the recurrent laryngeal nerves by enlarged lymph nodes, (3) **facial paralysis** due to compression of cranial nerves, and (4) **purpura haemorrhagica** as a result of vasculitis caused by deposition of **S. equi** antigen-antibody complexes in arterioles, venules, and capillaries. In severe cases, nasal infection extends into the paranasal sinuses or to the guttural pouches through Eustachian causing inflammation and accumulation of pus (**empyema**). Rupture of abscesses in the mandibular and retropharyngeal lymph nodes leads to suppurative inflammation of adjacent subcutaneous tissue (cellulitis).

Glanders

This infectious disease of **horses, asses**, and **mules** is caused by *Burkholderia mallei* (*Malleomyces mallei*). It can be transmitted to **dogs** by consuming infected horse meat. **Humans** are also susceptible, and the infection is usually fatal. **In India, glanders is a serious problem in army horses.**

The pathogenesis of glanders is not fully understood. The infection occurs through the ingestion of contaminated feed and water, and very rarely, through inhalation of infectious droplets in air. **At the site of entry,** the oropharynx or intestine, bacteria penetrate the mucosa and spread through lymph vessels to lymph nodes. Then they enter into the bloodstream and through blood to internal organs, particularly the **lungs. Gross lesions** in the nasal cavity begin as pyogranulomatous nodules. These nodules afterwards ulcerate and release a large amount of *B. mallei*-containing exudate into the nasal cavity. Finally, ulcerative lesions in the mucosa are replaced by star-shaped fibrous scars. In some cases, the lungs also contain numerous grey, hard, small (2 to 10 mm), miliary (very small) nodules, distributed in one or more pulmonary lobes. **Microscopically,** these nodules are granulomas composed of a necrotic centre, with or without calcification. They are surrounded by a thick band of connective tissue infiltrated with numerous macrophages, some giant cells, lymphocytes and plasma cells. The skin lesions, called **equine farcy**, are characterized by nodular thickening of lymph vessels in the subcutaneous tissue of the legs and ventral abdomen. This thickening is the result of severe suppurative lymphangitis. Ultimately, the affected lymph vessels rupture and release large amounts of purulent exudate through sinuses to the surface of the skin.

Clinically, like strangles, there may be fever and cough, particularly in **mules** and **donkeys. Horses are more prone to chronic form.** The signs vary with the location of lesions, but most common are cough, epistaxis, and dyspnoea caused by pulmonary disease.

Melioidosis

This life-threatening disease of **humans, horses, cattle, sheep, goats, pigs, dogs, cats,** and **rodents** (rat, mouse) is caused by *Burkholderia pseudomallei* (*Pseudomonas pseudomallei, Malleomyces pseudomallei*). The disease in **horses** is clinically and pathologically similar to glanders, hence the name pseudoglanders (G. pseudo = false). In humans, it can be fatal.

Ingestion of contaminated feed and water appears to be the main route of infection. Direct transmission between infected animals and insect bites has also been suggested. After entering into the animal, *B. pseudomallei* is spread by the bloodstream and causes **suppuration** and **abscesses** in most internal organs, nasal mucosa, joints, brain and spinal cord, liver, spleen, and lymphnodes. The exudate is creamy or caseous and yellow to green. The **lung lesions** are those of an embolic bacterial pneumonia with formation of pulmonary abscesses. Where abscesses rupture through the pleura and heal, focal adhesive pleuritis develops.

Diseases of Pigs

Inclusion Body Rhinitis

This disease of **young pigs** is caused by a **porcine cytomegalovirus (herpesvirus).** The disease is characterized by **mild rhinitis** and high morbidity but low mortality. The virus infects the nasal epithelium of **piglets** younger than 5 weeks and causes **nasal discharge**, sneezing and excessive lacrimation. This disease is seldom fatal and therefore lesions are seen only rarely. **Microscopic lesions** consist of necrotizing, non-suppurative rhinitis with **basophilic intranuclear inclusion bodies** in the epithelial cells of the mucosa and glands.

Atrophic Rhinitis

Atrophic rhinitis of **pigs** is clinically characterized by sneezing, coughing, and **nasal discharge** as a result of inflammation and atrophy of nasal turbinates. In severe cases, atrophy of the turbinates may cause a striking facial deformity due to deviation of the nasal bones.

The **aetiology** and **pathogenesis** of atrophic rhinitis is complex and not fully understood. The pathogens include *Bordetella bronchiseptica, Pasteurella multocida, Haemophilus parasuis* and viral infections such as porcine cytomegalovirus (inclusion body rhinitis). In addition, predisposing factors include genetic make-up, environment, and nutritional deficiencies. The disease is characterized by **mild to moderate turbinate atrophy**. However, the degree of turbinate atrophy varies considerably, and in most pigs, the severity of the lesions does not correspond with the severity of symptoms.

The best diagnostic method of evaluating this disease is to make a transverse section of the snout. **In normal pigs**, turbinates are symmetrical and fill most of the cavity. The nasal septum is straight and divides the cavity into two cavities. In contrast, **septum in the affected pigs** is deviated and turbinates are smaller and asymmetrical. In most advanced cases, the turbinates may be missing, **leaving a large, empty space**. Therefore, **morphological diagnosis of atrophic rhinitis is easy.**

Diseases of Dogs

Dogs have no specific viral infections affecting only the nasal cavity or sinuses. **Acute rhinitis** occurs as part of general respiratory disease caused by several viruses such as **canine distemper virus, canine adenovirus 1 and 2, canine parainfluenza virus, reovirus,** and **canine herpesvirus.** The viral lesions in the respiratory tract are mild. Secondary bacterial rhinitis, sinusitis, and pneumonia are possible sequelae of respiratory viral infections as in other species. With bacterial rhinitis, the most common isolates are *Bordetella bronchiseptica, Escherichia coli,* and *Pasteurella multocida.* **Immotile cilia syndrome (ciliary dyskinesia),** a congenital disease, reduces mucociliary clearance and plays an important role in recurrent canine rhinosinusitis, bronchitis, bronchiectasis, and pneumonia.

Other rhinitis in dogs includes **mycotic rhinitis** caused by fungi of **Aspergillus** sp. and **Penicillium** sp. The infection is characterized by mucopurulent **nasal discharge**. At times, *Cryptococcus neoformans* and *Rhinosporidium seeberi* infections of the nasal cavity also occur in dogs. **Lesions** comprise granulomas in the nasal mucosa. **Allergic rhinitis (hay fever),** so common in humans sensitized to pollens or allergens, has been reported only rarely in **dogs** and **cats**. Hay fever in humans and animals is a type I hypersensitivity reaction.

Parasitic rhinitis mainly includes those caused by *Linguatula serrata* (an arthropod) and *Capillaria aerophila* (a nematode). The adult parasite (*L. serrata*) is found throughout the nasal passages. Sometimes it may reach sinuses and middle ear by moving through the Eustachian tubes. It acts as an irritant and causes catarrhal inflammation. *Capillaria aerophila* is a parasite of nasal passages, sinuses, trachea, and bronchi of **dogs.** Usually asymptomatic, some dogs cough because of the local irritation caused by the parasite on the mucosa. The lesions are catarrhal to mucopurulent inflammation of the mucosa. The nasal cavity and sinuses of **dogs** can sometimes be infested with mite *Pneumonyssus caninum,* causing mild rhinitis and sinusitis.

Diseases of Cats

Feline Viral Rhinotracheitis (FVR)

This **common disease of cats** is caused by a **feline herpesvirus** (FHV-1). It is characterized by oculo-nasal discharge, severe rhinitis, and conjunctivitis. The infection damages the pulmonary defence mechanisms, predisposing the **cats** to secondary bacterial pneumonia. Replication of the virus in the nasal, conjunctival, pharyngeal, and tracheal epithelium causes degeneration and exfoliation of cells. **Lesions** are mild and fully reversible, but secondary infection with bacteria such as *Pasteurella multocida, Bordetella bronchiseptica*, **Streptococcus** sp. and *Mycoplasma felis* can cause a chronic, severe suppurative rhinitis and conjunctivitis.

Feline Calicivirus (FCV)

It is an important infection of the respiratory tract of **cats** caused by **different strains of feline calicivirus.** Depending on the virulence of the strain, lesions vary from mild oculo-nasal discharge to severe rhinitis, mucopurulent conjunctivitis, and ulcerative stomatitis. These primary lesions are usually mild, but secondary bacterial infections are a common complication.

Feline Chlamydiosis

This disease is a persistent respiratory infection of **cats**. It is caused by feline strains of *Chlamydia psittaci (felis)*. Infection causes mild conjunctivitis and serous or mucopurulent rhinitis, but in severe cases, can also produce a mild broncho-interstitial pneumonia.

Mycoplasma felis can also cause conjunctivitis and a mild upper respiratory infection.

Mycotic rhinitis

The most common infection is caused by *Cryptococcus neoformans*. The lesions vary from nasal granulomas to large masses of mucopurulent exudate filling the entire nasal cavity.

Allergic rhinitis is also reported in **cats.**

Neoplasms of the Nasal Cavity and Sinuses

These may arise from bone (**osteoma** or **osteosarcoma**), cartilage (**chondroma** or **chondrosarcoma**), connective tissue (**fibroma** or **fibrosarcoma, myxoma** or **myxosarcoma**), blood vessels (**haemangioma** or **haemangiosarcoma**), and from all the different types of cells of glands and lining epithelium (**adenoma** or **adenocarcinoma**). **In general, nasal neoplasms are rare in domestic animals, except for enzootic ethmoidal neoplasms of cattle and sheep.**

Nasal neoplasms are seen most commonly in **dogs**. The **cat** and the **horse** are much less affected. The common sites are the nasal passages in **dogs**, nasal vestibule for **cats**, and maxillary sinus in **horses**.

Nasal neoplasms become secondarily infected by bacteria. Clinical signs often overlap those of infectious rhinitis, including catarrhal or mucopurulent nasal discharge, periodic haemorrhage, and sneezing. Some neoplasms infiltrate adjacent structures and produce significant facial deformations, loss of teeth, exophthalmos (protrusion of the eyeballs), and nervous signs.

Most of the neoplasms in the nasal cavity are malignant. Benign neoplasms (papilloma and adenoma) are rare and small. Carcinomas and sarcomas are usually of larger size. Malignant neoplasms are locally invasive and tend to infiltrate sinuses, brain, nerves, and vessels, resulting in haemorrhage. Because nasal tumours in **dogs** and **cats** are usually large and invasive at the time of diagnosis, survival time is usually short.

Enzootic Ethmoidal Neoplasms

Tumours arising from the mucosa lining the ethmoid bone occur in **cattle, sheep, buffalo, goat, pig,** and **horse. In India, they are seen mainly in cattle in the southern states of Kerala and Tamil Nadu.** Isolated cases have also been reported from other parts of the country such as **Orissa** and **West Bengal.** Their enzootic nature in both **cattle** and **sheep** suggests involvement of an infectious agent. **A retrovirus has been suggested as the oncogenic agent, and tumours have been successfully transmitted with the virus, or infected tissue.**

Adenocarcinoma is the most common type in **sheep**. In **cattle**, the types include squamous-cell carcinoma, adenocarcinoma, and undifferentiated carcinoma. **The tumour arises from the mucosa of the ethmoid** and then spreads. **Cattle** affected with ethmoid carcinoma usually do not show any **clinical signs**, until the tumour assumes a considerable size, fills up the sinuses, and blocks the nasal and pharyngeal passages. The earliest **symptoms** include sudden **epistaxis** (nosebleed)), or blood-tinged **mucus or mucopurulent nasal discharge**, accompanied by sneezing and **dyspnoea** (difficult breathing). As the disease advances, the animal develops respiratory disease, dysphagia (difficulty in swallowing), and later on **exophthalmos** (protrusion of the eyeball) of one or both eyes, with swelling of the submaxillary lymph nodes. Most of the animals go blind, or develop photophobia (intolerance to light), conjunctivitis and keratitis (inflammation of the cornea). **Exophthalmos is considered as a pathognomonic symptom** and is due to the invasion of the tumour into the retrobulbar region. As the condition progresses, the forehead bulges out progressively and the tumour appears in the forehead in the subcutaneous tissue as a frontal swelling – varying in size from lemon to a coconut. Rarely, the tumour may invade the cranial cavity. The animal then exhibits nervous symptoms such as circling movements. **The affected animals eventually**

die in course of time. Symptoms in **sheep** and **goats** resemble those of the cattle. In **pigs**, however, epistaxis is the most common symptom and exophthalmos is rare.

Grossly, the **tumour fills up the nasal cavity and the paranasal sinuses and destroys turbinates.** There is congestion and marked oedema of the ethmo-turbinates, which are covered with copious mucus. It is fleshy, grey-white, and presents a varying degree of necrosis. It may invade the retrobulbar region, pharynx, and sometimes the frontal bone and come out as frontal swelling. The tumour may even perforate the cribriform plate of the ethmoid and penetrate into the lateral ventricles of the brain. **Metastases** usually occur in the regional lymph nodes, and very rarely in the lungs and liver. **Microscopically,** the tumour consists of irregular clusters of anaplastic cells with prominent mitotic figures along with neutrophilic infiltration and stromal fibrosis. Tumour giant cells with multiple nuclei are present. Areas of necrosis and haemorrhage are also observed. **Diagnosis** is based on symptoms and exfoliative cytology.

Nasal Polyps

Polyps are non-neoplastic masses that resemble tumours. They are therefore discussed here. They commonly occur following chronic rhinitis in **horses** and **cats**, and to a lesser extent, in other species such as **sheep**. In **horses**, polyps tend to form in the ethmoidal region, whereas in **cats** polyps are mostly found in the nasopharynx and Eustachian tubes. **Grossly,** polyps appear as firm, pedunculated nodules protruding from the nasal mucosa into the air passages. The surface may be smooth, ulcerated, secondarily infected, and haemorrhagic. **Microscopically,** polyps are characterized by a core of well-vascularized stromal tissue that contains inflammatory cells.

Pharynx, Larynx, and Trachea

Anomalies

Congenital anomalies of this region are rare in all species, and include:

Brachycephalic Airway Syndrome

These abnormalities are seen in brachycephalic breeds of **dogs** (G. brachy = short; cephale = head, i.e. short-headed or broad-headed), such as bulldogs and boxers. The syndrome is characterized by stenotic (narrow) external nostrils and an excessive length of soft palate.

Hypoplastic Epiglottis

This anomaly of **horses** leads to respiratory noise associated with dorsal displacement of the soft palate.

Subepiglottic and Pharyngeal Cysts

These types of anomalous lesions are sometimes seen in **horses**.

Tracheal Hypoplasia

Tracheal hyoplasia has been reported in **English bulldogs**. The tracheal lumen is decreased throughout its length.

Tracheal Collapse

Tracheal collapse occurs in smaller breeds of **dogs**. The defect also occurs in **horses, cattle,** and **goats. Grossly,** there is dorso-ventral flattening of the trachea and widening of the dorsal tracheal membrane, which may then prolapse ventrally into the lumen. The defect usually involves the entire length of the trachea. Tracheal collapse is associated with reduced glycoproteins and loss of elasticity in tracheal cartilages.

Other tracheal anomalies include **scabbard trachea** in **horses**, in which there is lateral flattening. The tracheal lumen is therefore a narrow vertical slit. **Tracheo-oesophageal fistula** has been reported in **dogs** and **cattle.**

Inflammation

Pharyngitis, Laryngitis, and Tracheitis

Inflammations of the pharynx, larynx, and trachea are important. This is because they can obstruct airflow and lead to **aspiration pneumonia.** The pharynx is vulnerable to diseases of both the upper respiratory and upper digestive tracts, and the **trachea** can be involved by extension from both lungs and upper respiratory regions. **Chronic polypoid tracheitis** occurs in **dogs** and **cats,** probably secondary to chronic infection. **Laryngeal abscesses** occur in **calves** and **sheep,** caused by secondary infection with *Arcanobacterium pyogenes* (*Actinomyces pyogenes; Corynebacterium pyogenes*).

Laryngitis

Inflammation of the larynx is common in most inflammatory diseases of the upper respiratory tract. **Causes** include:
1. Diphtheritic laryngitis occurs in calf diphtheria, glanders, tuberculosis, and uraemia in dogs.
2. Mechanical injuries of the throat region produced by kicks and bites, or when objects such as stomach tubes and probangs are inserted into the larynx.
3. Excessive use of the larynx, such as barking in the dog.

Laryngitis may be acute or chronic, and is catarrhal, suppurative, fibrinous, haemorrhagic, ulcerative, or necrotic in type. Catarrhal inflammation is the most common and is associated with most respiratory diseases.

Necrotic Laryngitis (Calf Diphtheria, Laryngeal Necrobacillosis)

Necrotic laryngitis is a common disease of **cattle** affected with other diseases, or nutritional deficiency, or living under unsanitary housing conditions. It also occurs in **sheep**. Necrotic laryngitis is caused by *Fusobacterium necrophorum*. It may produce lesions in tongue, gingiva, cheeks, palate, and pharynx. *F. necrophorum* produces several **exotoxins** and **endotoxins** after gaining entry. It enters either through lesions of viral infections such as infectious bovine rhinotracheitis and papular stomatitis in **cattle** and contagious ecthyma in **sheep**, or after traumatic injury produced by feed or careless use of specula or balling guns.

The **clinical signs** of necrotic laryngitis are fever, anorexia, halitosis (bad breath), moist painful cough, dysphagia (difficult swallowing), dyspnoea (difficult breathing), and respiratory failure due to fatigue of the respiratory muscles. The **gross lesions** consist of well-demarcated, dry, yellow-grey, necrotic areas bounded by a zone of hyperaemia. With time, there is deep ulceration which is followed by healing in non-fatal cases. **Microscopically**, necrotic foci have initially hyperaemic borders. In time, these areas are replaced by granulation tissue and collagen (fibrosis). The lesions can extend deep into the sub-mucosal tissues. The bacteria are seen at the advancing edge. The most important **sequel** of calf diphtheria is **death due to toxaemia or septicaemia.** The exudate may cause asphyxiation, or be aspirated and cause bronchopneumonia.

Degenerative Diseases

Laryngeal Hemiplegia (Paralysis)

Also called **'roaring'**, it is a common but poorly understood disease of **horses**. It is characterized by atrophy of the crico-arytenoid muscles, particularly on the left side. Atrophy is due to denervation as a result of axonal disease or nerve damage caused by compression or inflammation of the left recurrent laryngeal nerve. The **abnormal respiratory sounds (roaring)** during exercise in horses are due to paralysis of the left dorsal and lateral crico-arytenoid muscles, which cause incomplete dilation of the larynx and obstruct airflow. **Therefore, loose vocal cords vibrate.**

Grossly, affected laryngeal muscle is smaller than normal (**muscle atrophy**). **Microscopically**, muscle fibres show lesions of denervation atrophy (see Chapter 10, Muscle).

Circulatory Disturbances

Laryngeal and Tracheal Haemorrhages

Haemorrhages are usually seen as mucosal petechiae in septicaemic diseases such as swine fever (hog cholera) and salmonellosis in **pigs.**

Laryngeal Oedema

It is common in acute inflammation, but is of particular importance as it can obstruct the laryngeal opening and cause **asphyxiation**. Laryngeal oedema occurs in **pigs** with oedema disease, in **horses** with purpura haemorrhagica, in **cattle** with acute interstitial pneumonia, systemic anaphylaxis in **cats**, and in **all species** as a result of trauma, inhalation of irritant gases (smoke), local inflammation and allergic reactions. **Grossly**, the laryngeal mucosa is thickened and swollen.

Tracheal oedema occurs in **cattle**. It is an acute disease of unknown aetiology. **Clinical signs** include dyspnoea that can progress to oral breathing, lying down, and death by asphyxiation in less than 24 hours. Severe oedema and a few haemorrhages are present in the mucosa of the trachea.

Laryngeal Contact Ulcers

These are circular ulcers found in **cattle**. They are deep enough to expose the underlying arytenoid cartilages. The cause is unknown. Viral, bacterial, and traumatic causes have been suggested. Contact ulcers predispose **calves** to diphtheria and laryngeal papillomas.

Pharynx

Equine Pharyngeal Lymphoid Hyperplasia

This lesion is a common cause of partial upper airway obstruction in **horses**. The aetiology is unknown, but chronic bacterial infection may cause excessive antigenic stimulation and lymphoid hyperplasia with clinical signs.

Guttural Pouches

Inflammation

The guttural pouches are present in horses. These are large diverticula of the ventral Eustachian tubes. They are therefore exposed to the same pathogens as is the pharynx and have drainage problems. The lesions mostly seen are **guttural pouch mycosis** and **guttural pouch empyema**.

Guttural Pouch Mycosis

It occurs mainly **in stabled horses**, and is caused by *Aspergillus fumigatus* and other **Aspergillus** species. Infection begins with the inhalation of spores from mouldy hay. **Grossly**, the guttural pouch mucosa is covered by a diphtheritic, fibrino-necrotic exudate. **Microscopically**, the lesion is of severe necrotic inflammation of the mucosa and sub-mucosa.

Empyema of Guttural Pouches

This may occur following suppurative inflammation of the nasal cavities, mostly from *Streptococcus equi* infection (strangles). It is characterized by nasal discharge, enlarged retropharyngeal lymph nodes, dysphagia (difficult swallowing), and respiratory distress. In severe cases, the entire guttural pouch can be filled with purulent exudate.

Trachea

Inflammation

Tracheitis

Inflammation of trachea is usually associated with inflammatory diseases of the upper and lower respiratory tract. The trachea can be involved by extension from both the lungs and upper respiratory regions. The **aetiology** is varied and includes physical injuries, bacterial infections such as pasteurellosis, and viral diseases such as infectious bovine rhinotracheitis, canine distemper, and infectious laryngotracheitis in the chicken. The **lesions** may be **acute** or **chronic**, and the exudate may be **catarrhal, suppurative, fibrinous, necrotic,** or **haemorrhagic.**

Suppurative tracheitis is commonly associated with suppurative pneumonia in all animals, and in strangles in the **horse. Haemorrhagic tracheitis** is commonly observed in pasteurellosis of **cattle**. It is also observed in pneumonia of all animals when severe dyspnoea precedes death for a long time. **Ulcerative tracheitis** is often observed in glanders. With healing, star-shaped scars are observed in the trachea. Tuberculosis of the trachea is quite common in animals having tuberculous pneumonia. The **necrotic and gangrenous form** sometimes occurs from improper medication because of irritant's entry into the trachea.

Canine Infectious Tracheo-bronchitis

Also known as **'kennel cough'**, this highly contagious infection of **dogs** is characterized by an acute attack of coughing, aggravated by exercise. The term is non-specific, much like 'common cold' in humans. The **aetiology** is complex, and many pathogens and environmental factors are involved. These include *Bordetella bronchiseptica*, **canine adenovirus 2**, and **canine parainfluenza virus.** Severity of the disease is increased when more than one agent is involved.

Gross and **microscopic lesions** may be absent, or they vary from catarrhal to mucopurulent tracheo-bronchitis with enlargement of the tonsils and adjacent lymph nodes. Complications include spread into the respiratory tract leading to chronic bronchitis and bronchopneumonia.

Parasite

Oslerus osleri (*Filaroides osleri*) occurs in **dogs** and produces protruding **nodules** into the lumen at the tracheal bifurcation. *O. osleri* is considered the most common respiratory nematode of **dogs**. It usually causes chronic cough which is aggravated by exercise. Severe infestation can result in dyspnoea, exercise intolerance, emaciation, and even death in **young dogs.**

The **gross lesions** include sub-mucosal nodules that extend into the tracheal lumen. **Microscopically,** a mild mononuclear cell reaction is present when parasites are alive. With the death of the parasite, an intense foreign body reaction develops with neutrophils and giant cells.

Besnoitia bennetti

This coccidian can cause **papilloma-like lesions** in the **larynx** and **skin** of **horses.** Besnoitiosis has been reported from Africa, Central and South America, and Britain.

Neoplasms

These are rare in **horses** and are usually squamous-cell carcinomas. Laryngeal neoplasms are rare in **dogs** and they are even rarer in other species, although they have been reported in **cats** and **horses**. The most common laryngeal neoplasm in dogs is squamous-cell carcinoma. When they are large, they cause obstruction, change or loss of voice, cough, or respiratory distress. The **prognosis** is poor, as most lesions recur after excision.

Tracheal neoplasms are even more uncommon than those of the larynx. Giant cell tumour has been reported in the **horse** and adenocarcinoma in the **dog.** **Chondromas** may occur in tracheal cartilages. **Lymphosarcomas** in **cats** can extend from mediastinum to trachea.

Bronchi

Inflammation

Inflammation of the bronchi may be **acute** or **chronic.**

Acute Bronchitis

Depending on the type of exudate, **acute bronchitis** can be **catarrhal, purulent (suppurative), fibrinous, fibrino-necrotic (diphtheritic), haemorrhagic,** and sometimes **granulomatous.** It is usually associated with diseases of the upper and lower respiratory tract, and is always present in pneumonia. The **causes** include:

1. **Viral diseases.** In cases of bovine rhinotracheitis, the pseudo-diphtheritic process can extend to bronchi; canine infectious tracheo-bronchitis (kennel cough) involves bronchi in addition to trachea, and many pneumonias are in fact bronchopneumonia. That is, both bronchi and lung parenchyma are involved. Other viral diseases include Ranikhet disease, infectious bronchitis, and chronic respiratory disease in the chicken.

2. **Bacterial diseases** such as pasteurellosis.

3. **Inhalation of dust, pollen, smoke, toxic gases, and foreign material** such as medicines, or feed (timothy heads in **sheep**). Timothy is a European grass that has long cylindrical spikes and is widely grown for hay.

4. Bronchitis is commonly associated with **parasitic infestations** such as *Dictyocaulus viviparous* (**cattle**), *D. filaria* (**sheep** and **goats**), and *D. arnfieldi* (**horse**); *Muellerius capillaris* (**sheep and goats**); *Metastrongylus apri* (**pigs**).

Complete resolution usually occurs in bronchi of animals that survive the disease process. The pattern of repair in bronchi is similar to that previously described for the nasal and tracheal epithelium. **In brief**, injury in ciliated bronchial epithelium may result in degeneration, detachment, and exfoliation of these cells. Under normal circumstances, this loss is followed by exudative inflammation and repair.

Chronic Bronchitis

When epithelial injury becomes **chronic**, production of mucus is increased due to **goblet cell hyperplasia (chronic catarrhal bronchitis)**. This form of chronic bronchitis is best seen in habitual smokers, who are continuously required to cough out excessive mucous secretions (sputum). In some cases excessive mucus cannot be effectively cleared, and this leads to **chronic obstructive bronchitis**. Chronic bronchial irritation can also cause **squamous metaplasia**, in which highly functional ciliated epithelium is replaced by a poorly functional, but more resistant, squamous epithelium. **Squamous metaplasia has a disastrous effect in mucociliary clearance.**

Feline Allergic Bronchitis

Also known as **'feline asthma'**, this condition is a clinical syndrome in **cats**. It is characterized by recurrent attacks of broncho-constriction, cough, and dyspnoea. The **pathogenesis** is not well understood but, as in human asthma, it appears to be a type I hypersensitivity (IgE-mast cell reaction) to inhaled allergens. Dust, cigarette smoke, plant and household materials, and parasitic proteins have been suspected as possible allergens.

Bronchiectasis

Bronchiectasis is a serious complication of chronic bronchitis. Bronchiectasis is a **permanent dilation of a bronchus** as a result of the accumulation of exudate in the lumen and partial rupture of bronchial walls. Destruction of walls occurs when proteolytic enzymes released from phagocytic cells during chronic inflammation break down and weaken the smooth muscle and cartilage of the wall.

Bronchiectasis may be **saccular** when destruction involves only a small localized portion of the bronchial wall. It may be **cylindrical** when destruction involves a large segment of the bronchus. **Grossly,** bronchiectasis is seen as prominent lumps in the lungs resulting from distension of bronchi and simultaneous obstructive atelectasis of surrounding parenchyma. The cut surfaces of dilated bronchi are filled with purulent exudate. For this reason, bronchiectasis is usually confused with pulmonary abscesses. Microscopic examination reveals that bronchiectatic exudate is surrounded by bronchial wall and not by a pyogenic membrane (connective tissue) as it is in the case of a pulmonary abscess. **Microscopically,** there is destruction of all layers of the bronchial wall. The lumen is filled with debris, leukocytes, mucus and possibly blood. **Complications** of bronchiectasis include bronchopneumonia and metastatic abscessation.

Bronchostenosis

Bronchostenosis is a narrowing of the bronchial lumen. It is due to accumulation of exudate, parasites and other objects in the bronchial lumen, and also from peribronchial pressure. Bronchial stenosis is usually observed in parasitic diseases, when masses of helminths or flukes collect in the bronchi. **Peribronchial stenosis** is caused by pressure from enlarging lymph nodes, tumours, abscesses, cysts, and exudate in the pleural cavity.

Bronchioles, Bronchial Injury, Bronchiolitis

The epithelial lining of the bronchioles is extremely susceptible to injury, particularly to that caused by certain respiratory viruses (parainfluenza-3, adenovirus, and bovine respiratory syncytial virus), oxidant gases (nitrogen dioxide-NO_2, sulphur dioxide-SO_2, and ozone-O_3), and toxic substances (3-methylindole). It is still not clear as to why bronchiolar epithelium is prone to injury, but it is presumed to be due to: (1) its high susceptibility to oxidants and free radicals, (2) the presence of Clara cells rich in mixed-function oxidases, which locally generate toxic metabolites, and (3) the tendency of the alveolar macrophages and leukocytes to accumulate in this region of the lungs.

Once injury becomes irreversible, bronchiolar epithelial cells degenerate and exfoliate into the bronchiolar lumen, leaving behind a denuded basement membrane. Repair in the bronchioles is less effective than that in the tracheal or nasal mucosa. Under normal circumstances, accumulated phagocytic cells remove exudate and cell debris and prepare the basement membrane to be repopulated with new cells originating from the rapidly dividing **Clara cells.**

In severe injury, exudate cannot be removed. It then becomes infiltrated by fibroblasts which form fibrovascular tissue. Their external surface ultimately gets covered by ciliated cells. This lesion is referred to as **bronchiolitis obliterans.**

If bronchial injury is mild but persistent, goblet cells normally absent from bronchioles proliferate from basal cell. This results in **goblet cell metaplasia**. This causes a change in the physico-chemical properties of bronchiolar secretions. The normal serous fluid released by **Clara cells** becomes a thick and sticky material when mucus produced by goblet cells is added. As a result of increased thickness and stickiness of the mucus, bronchial secretions cannot be removed effectively by ciliary action. This leads to plugging and obstruction of distal airways. Such conditions are called **chronic obstructive pulmonary disease.** Coughing is then required to clear mucus from obstructed bronchioles. **Complications** of the obstruction are **emphysema** and **atelectasis**. These two conditions are present in chronic obstructive pulmonary disease of **horses** known as **'heaves'**.

Chronic Obstructive Pulmonary Disease (COPD) of Horses

Also known as **'heaves'** and **'broken wind'**, chronic obstructive pulmonary disease is a common asthma-like syndrome of **horses** and **ponies**. It is characterized by respiratory distress, chronic cough, and poor athletic performance. The pathogenesis is still not clear, but airways exceptionally sensitive to allergens have been suggested as the basic underlying mechanism. Recently it has been suggested that sustained inhalation of dust particles, whether antigenic or not, increases the production of cytokine interleukin-8 (IL-8) and monokine-inducible protein (MPI-2) by alveolar macrophages. These cytokines attract neutrophils into the region and promote leukocyte-induced bronchial injury.

Grossly, lungs appear normal. In extreme cases, alveolar emphysema may be present. **Microscopically,** there is goblet cell metaplasia, plugging of bronchioles with mucus, peribronchiolar infiltration with lymphocytes, plasma cells, eosinophils, and hypertrophy of smooth muscle in bronchi and bronchioles. In severe cases, accumulation of mucus leads to complete obstruction of bronchioles and alveoli, and causes **alveolar emphysema.**

Lungs

Species Differences

Cattle and **pigs** have well-lobated and well-lobulated lungs; **sheep** and **goats** have well-lobated but poorly lobulated lungs; **horses** have both poorly lobated and poorly lobulated lungs and resemble human lungs; and **dogs** and **cats** have well-lobated but not well-lobulated lungs. **The degree of lobulation determines the degree of air movement between the lobules.** In **pigs** and **cattle,** movement of air between lobules is absent because of the thick connective tissue wall separating individual lobules. This movement of air between lobules and between alveoli (pores of Kohn) constitutes **collateral ventilation. This collateral ventilation is poor in cattle and pigs and good in dogs.**

Congenital Anomalies

These are rare in all species, but are commonly reported in **cattle. Accessory lungs** consist of lobulated masses of pulmonary tissue in the thorax, abdominal cavity, or anywhere in the trunk. Large accessory lungs cause dystocia.

Immotile Cilia Syndrome (ciliary dyskinesia) is characterized by lack of ciliary movement due to a defect in the microtubules of cells in the ciliated respiratory epithelium. This condition has been reported in **dogs** having chronic pneumonia.

Pulmonary agenesia, pulmonary hypoplasia, abnormal lobulation, congenital emphysema, and **congenital bronchiectasis** are sometimes seen in domestic animals. **Congenital melanosis** is common in **pigs** and **ruminants** and is usually seen at slaughter. It is characterized by **black spots** in lungs and other organs. **Melanosis has no clinical significance.**

Metabolic Disturbances

Pulmonary Calcification (Calcinosis)

Calcification of the lungs occurs in certain hypercalcaemic states associated with hypervitaminosis D, or from ingestion of toxic plants such as *Solanum malacoxylon* (Manchester wasting disease) that contain vitamin D analogues (i.e. chemicals similar in structure to Vitamin D). Calcified lungs fail to collapse when the thoracic cavity is opened, and have a gritty texture. **Microscopic lesions** vary from mild calcification of the alveolar basement membranes to ossification of lungs. In most cases, **pulmonary calcification has no clinical significance.**

Circulatory Disturbances

Lungs are highly vascular organs having a double blood supply by pulmonary and bronchial arteries. Circulatory disturbances in the lungs can have influence on many organs due to **passive congestion** and **generalized oedema (anasarca).**

Hyperaemia and Congestion

Hyperaemia is an active process and is part of acute inflammation, whereas **congestion** is a passive process resulting from decreased outflow of venous blood. This occurs in congestive heart failure. **In the acute stage of pneumonia,** lungs appear red, and microscopically, blood vessels and capillaries are engorged with blood from hyperaemia. **Pulmonary congestion** is caused by heart failure. It results in stagnation of blood in pulmonary vessels, leading to oedema and escape of red cells in alveolar spaces. Erythrocytes in alveolar spaces are rapidly phagocytosed **(erythrophagocytosis)** by alveolar macrophages. When erythrocytes are more, large number of macrophages may accumulate in the alveolar spaces. Their cytoplasm is brown due to the accumulation of large amounts of **haemosiderin**. These macrophages **(siderophages)** are referred to as **'heart failure cells'.**

Haemorrhage

Haemorrhages in lungs can occur as a result of trauma, coagulopathies, pulmonary thromboembolism, disseminated intravascular coagulation, or septicaemia. **Grossly,** affected lungs have numerous, focal (1 to 10 mm) areas of red discoloration throughout the lobes.

Rupture of a major pulmonary vessel with massive haemorrhage occurs sometimes in **cattle** when a growing abscess in the lung invades and disrupts the wall of a major blood vessel. In most cases, animals die rapidly, often with haemoptysis. On postmortem examination, the airways are filled with blood.

Exercise-Induced Pulmonary Haemorrhage (EIPH)

This is a specific form of pulmonary haemorrhage in **racehorses** following exercise. It is characterized by epistaxis. The pathogenesis is still not clearly understood. EIPH is rarely fatal. Postmortem lesions include large areas of dark brown discoloration in the lung lobes. **Microscopically**, lesions are alveolar haemorrhage, macrophages containing haemosiderin, and mild interstitial fibrosis.

Pulmonary Oedema

In normal lungs, fluid from the vascular space continuously passes into the interstitial tissues where it is rapidly drained by the lymph vessels. Recently it has been demonstrated that alveolar fluid clearance across the alveolar epithelium is also a major mechanism of fluid removal from the lung. Oedema occurs when the rate of fluid escape from pulmonary vessels into the interstitium or alveoli is greater than that of lymph and alveolar removal. **Pulmonary oedema** is of **two types:** (1) **Haemorrhagic**, or (2) **permeability**.

(i) Haemorrhagic Pulmonary Oedema

This type of oedema occurs when there is an increased rate of fluid escape due to increased hydrostatic pressure in the vessels, or decreased osmotic pressure in the blood. Once the lymph drainage has been overcome, fluid accumulates in the perivascular spaces. This causes distension of the broncho-vascular bundles and alveolar interstitium. The fluid eventually leaks into the alveolar spaces. **Causes** include congestive heart failure (increased hydrostatic pressure), disorders in which blood osmotic pressure is reduced such as in hypoalbuminaemia in some hepatic diseases, nephrotic syndrome, and protein-losing enteropathy. The oedema also occurs when lymph drainage is damaged as in neoplastic invasion of lymph vessels.

(ii) Permeability Pulmonary Oedema

This type of oedema occurs when there is increased opening of endothelial gaps, or damage to the air-blood barrier (type I pneumocytes or to endothelial cells). It is a part of the inflammatory response and occurs because of the effect of inflammatory mediators that increase the permeability of pulmonary vessels. It may also result from direct damage to the endothelium and pneumocytes, allowing plasma fluids to escape into the alveolar lumen. Since type I pneumocytes are highly susceptible to some pneumotropic viruses (influenza, bovine respiratory syncytial virus), toxic substances (NO_2, SO_2, H_2S, 3-methylindole), and particularly to **free**

radicals, permeability oedema usually occurs in many viral or toxic pulmonary diseases. Permeability oedema may also occur when endothelial cells in the lung are injured by **bacterial toxins** (endotoxaemia, sepsis, and disseminated intravascular coagulation), anaphylactic shock, milk allergy, and adverse drug reactions.

The concentration of protein in oedematous fluid is more in permeability oedema (**exudate**) than in haemorrhagic oedema (**transudate**). **Microscopically,** oedematous fluid stains more intensely eosinophilic in lungs with inflammation or damage to the air-blood barrier than the fluid present in haemorrhagic oedema.

Pulmonary Embolism

The lungs, with their vast capillary bed and position in the circulation, catch emboli before they reach brain and other tissues. However, this is often to its own disadvantage. The most common emboli in domestic animals include **thromboemboli, septic (bacterial) emboli, fat emboli,** and **tumour cell emboli.**

Thromboemboli usually originate from a thrombus present elsewhere in the venous circulation. Fragments released reach the lungs and get trapped in their blood vessels. Sterile thromboemboli have no pathological significance since they are rapidly degraded and disposed of by the fibrinolytic system. Parasites such as *Dirofilaria immitis* and *Angiostrongylus vasorum,* hyperadrenocorticism and hypothyroidism, glomerulopathies, and hypercoagulable states can cause pulmonary arterial thrombosis and pulmonary thromboembolism in **dogs.**

Septic emboli are pieces of thrombi containing **bacteria**. These are broken free from infected mural thrombi in heart and vessels. Septic thrombi finally get trapped in the pulmonary circulation. These emboli usually originate from bacterial endocarditis (right side) in all species, hepatic abscesses that discharge their contents into vena cava in **cattle**, and septic arthritis and omphalitis in farm animals. If present in large numbers, they may cause sudden death due to massive lung oedema.

Fat emboli occur after bone fractures, but they are not important in animals as they are in human beings. **Brain emboli** have been recently reported in **cattle** following stunning at slaughter. **Hepatic emboli** occur after severe trauma and liver rupture. **Tumour emboli** (e.g. osteosarcoma and haemangiosarcoma in **dogs,** uterine carcinoma in **cattle**) can be numerous and cause death in malignant neoplasms.

Pulmonary Infarction

Pulmonary infarction is rare and usually asymptomatic **because of the double arterial supply to the lung.** However, lung infarcts can also occur when pulmonary thrombosis and embolism are superimposed on an already damaged pulmonary circulation. This may occur in **congestive heart failure.** It also occurs in **dogs** with torsion of a lung lobe.

The **gross appearance** of infarcts varies depending on the stage. It can be red to black, swollen, firm, and cone or wedge shaped. In the acute stage, **microscopic lesions** are severely haemorrhagic with necrosis. In 1-2 days, a border of inflammatory cells develops. If sterile, infarcts heal as fibrotic scars. If septic, an abscess may form.

Abnormalities of Inflation

Atelectasis

Atelectasis means **incomplete distension of alveoli**. It can be **congenital** or **acquired**. If lungs fail to expand with air at the time of birth, it is **congenital atelectasis**, and when lungs collapse after inflation has taken place, it is **acquired atelectasis**.

(i) Congenital Atelectasis

During foetal life, lungs are not fully distended, contain no air, and are partially filled with a fluid called **'foetal lung fluid'**. Therefore, lungs of aborted and stillborn (born dead) fetuses sink when placed in water, whereas those from animals that have breathed float. At the time of birth, foetal lung fluid is reabsorbed and replaced by air. This causes normal distension of alveoli.

Congenital atelectasis occurs in **newborns** who fail to inflate their lungs after taking a few breaths of air. It is caused by obstruction of airways, usually due to aspiration of amniotic fluid and meconium (first faeces of a newborn) (see 'meconium aspiration syndrome').

Congenital atelectasis also occurs when alveoli cannot remain distended after first breathing. This is because of a defect in pulmonary surfactant produced by type II pneumocytes. A pulmonary surfactant is a surface-active agent that lines the alveoli to prevent alveolar walls sticking together. Its deficiency in human newborn children causes a form of congenital atelectasis referred to as **'acute respiratory distress syndrome'** and also as **'hyaline membrane disease'**. It usually occurs in babies who are premature or born to diabetic or alcoholic mothers, and is sometimes found in animals, particularly **foals** and **piglets**.

To determine whether atelectasis is present or not, the suspected portion of the lung is placed in water. **If it sinks, it indicates that atelectasis is present, but if it floats that is an indication that air is present within the lung and that the animal has breathed.** The atelectatic portion of the lung has a deep red colour and is firm in consistency. The areas stand out in sharp contrast to the surrounding pink colour of the lung. Their surface is depressed because of the lack of alveolar distension. Upon incision, it cuts with ease compared with normal lung.

(ii) Acquired Atelectasis

This type of atelectasis occurs in **two forms: Compressive** and **Obstructive.**

Compressive atelectasis occurs from the presence of fluids or masses, or from pressure on the pleura. Examples include pneumothorax, haemothorax, chylothorax (accumulation of chyle - lymph rich in triglycerides - in the thoracic cavity), empyema (pus in the thoracic cavity), neoplasms, and bloat.

Another form of compressive atelectasis occurs when the negative pressure in the thoracic cavity is lost due to pneumothorax. This form is usually massive atelectasis and therefore is also referred to as **lung collapse.**

Obstructive or **absorption atelectasis** occurs when an airway is blocked by exudate, mucosal oedema, aspirated foreign material, parasites, or neoplasms. The trapped air in the lung is reabsorbed. Unlike the compressive type, obstructive atelectasis usually has a lobular pattern and is more common in species with poor collateral ventilation such as **cattle** and **sheep**. Atelectasis also occurs when **large animals** are kept lying down on one side for long periods, such as during anesthesia (**hypostatic atelectasis**).

Grossly, lungs with atelectasis of any type appear dark blue and collapsed and may be soft or firm. They are firm if there is concurrent oedema. Distribution and size differ with the process. For example, it is patchy (multifocal) in congenital atelectasis, lobular in the obstructive type, and of various degrees in between in the compressive type. **Microscopically**, the alveoli are collapsed. Therefore, the interstitial tissues become prominent even without any inflammation.

Emphysema

Emphysema is an extremely important **primary disease in humans, but in animals it is always a secondary lesion** resulting from other types of pulmonary lesions.

Primary emphysema does not occur in animals. It occurs only in human beings. Therefore, no animal disease should be called simply emphysema. In animals, emphysema is always secondary to obstruction of outflow of air. Secondary pulmonary emphysema usually occurs in animals with bronchopneumonia in which exudate that plugs bronchi and bronchioles causes an airflow imbalance. That is, the volume of air entering is greater than the volume leaving the lung.

Classification: Depending on the affected area, emphysema can be classified into **alveolar** or **interstitial. Alveolar emphysema** occurs in **all species**. It is characterized by distension and rupture of the alveolar walls forming air bubbles of various sizes in lungs. **Interstitial emphysema** occurs mainly in **cattle.** Probably this is due to thick interlobular septa and lack of collateral ventilation which does not allow air to move freely into adjacent pulmonary lobules. As a result, accumulated air breaks apart and forces its way into connective tissue, causing **marked distension of the interstitial septa.** It is also possible that forced respiratory movements predispose to interstitial emphysema when air at high pressure breaks into the loose connective tissue of the interlobular septa. Sometimes these bubbles of trapped air merge and form large pockets of air that are called as 'bullae' (singular: bulla). This type of lesion is called 'bullous emphysema'. However, this is not a specific type of emphysema and does not indicate a different disease process. **In fact it is a larger accumulation of air at one place.**

Grossly, emphysematous lung is pale and enlarged. Sometimes, it may even have rib imprints on the lateral surfaces. The **microscopic appearance** is of irregular-sized air spaces.

Important diseases that cause secondary pulmonary emphysema in animals are **small airway obstruction** (such as **heaves**) in **horses** and **pulmonary oedema and emphysema (fog fever)** in **cattle.**

Inflammation

The pulmonary defence mechanisms described earlier deal effectively with harmful stimuli and mild tissue injury without the need for an inflammatory response. However, if normal defence mechanisms are ineffective or insufficient, **the inflammatory process rapidly comes into action as a second line of defence.**

General Aspects of Lung Inflammation

Inflammation of lungs involves a complex interaction between cells derived from the blood (neutrophils, eosinophils, mast cells, lymphocytes) and pulmonary cells (pneumocytes types I and II, endothelial, Clara, and stromal interstitial cells). Leukocytes from blood are brought into the area of inflammation by a large number of **chemical mediators** of the pulmonary inflammation. Communication between pulmonary cells and blood cells is done by **cytokines**. The pulmonary macrophages (alveolar, intravascular, and interstitial) are the main source of cytokines for all stages of lung inflammation. Once in the lungs, accumulated leukocytes communicate with pulmonary and vascular cells through **adhesion and other inflammatory molecules**. Acting together, these and many other molecules initiate, maintain, and resolve the inflammatory process without causing injury to the lung.

There are three important features of lung injury: (1) Leukocytes leave through alveolar capillaries, unlike other tissues, where post-capillary venules are sites of leukocyte emigration. (2) The lung contains within alveolar capillaries a large pool of resident leukocytes (**marginal pool**). (3) Additional neutrophils accumulate in alveolar capillaries within minutes of local or systemic inflammatory response. These three characteristic features of the lung, along with its extremely long capillary network, **explain why emigration of leukocytes into alveolar spaces occurs so rapidly.** In experimental studies, when endotoxin or Gram-negative bacteria were given through a fine spray, within minutes of exposure, there was a marked increase in capillary leukocytes. **By 4 hours the entire alveolar lumen was filled with**

cellular exudate.

Movement of plasma proteins into the alveolar lumen is a poorly understood phenomenon. Apart from the direct physical damage to the air-blood barrier (endothelium and type I pneumocytes), leakage of fibrin and plasma proteins is promoted by **cytokines**. **Excessive exudation of fibrin in the lung is particularly common in ruminants and pigs.** In some cases, plasma proteins in the alveoli mix with pulmonary surfactant and form eosinophilic membranes along the lining of alveolar septa. These membranes are known as **'hyaline membranes'**. They are found in specific types of lung diseases, particularly in **cattle** with acute interstitial pneumonias such as **bovine pulmonary oedema and emphysema** and **extrinsic allergic alveolitis.**

Recently **nitric oxide (NO)** has been found to be a major regulatory molecule of inflammation in the lung. Locally produced by macrophages, pulmonary endothelium, and pneumocytes, nitric oxide regulates the vascular and bronchial tone, modulates the production of cytokines, and the recruitment and regulation of neutrophils in the lung. **Pulmonary surfactant** increases the production of **nitric oxide** in the lung, supporting the view that **pneumocytes** are also very important in increasing and decreasing the inflammatory and immune responses in the lung.

As the inflammatory process becomes chronic, the cells change from mainly neutrophils to mononuclear cells. This change in cellular picture is accompanied by an increase in cytokines such as interleukin-4, gamma-interferon, and interferon-inducible protein. These cytokines are chemotactic for lymphocytes and macrophages. Under different conditions, these cytokines activate T-lymphocytes, regulate granulomatous inflammation, and induce formation of multinucleated giant cells.

If the alveolar injury is mild and the host response normal, the entire process of injury, inflammation, and repair can occur in less than one week. However, if the alveolar injury is persistent or when the host response is damaged, changes can progress to an irreversible stage where repair is no longer possible. **Fibronectins** released from **macrophages** and other mononuclear cells at the site of chronic inflammation regulate the recruitment, attachment, and proliferation of **fibroblasts**. Fibroblasts, in turn, synthesize and release extracellular matrix (collagen, elastic fibres, and proteoglycans). This finally leads to **fibrosis and total destruction and disappearance of normal alveoli. In other words, in diseases in which there is chronic and irreversible alveolar damage, lesions always progress to a stage of terminal alveolar fibrosis.**

Pneumonia

Pneumonia is inflammation of the lungs. The term **pneumonitis** has the same meaning, but is no longer in use.

Classification

Pneumonia in animals have been classified on the basis of: (1) **aetiology**, such as viral pneumonia, bacterial pneumonia, and verminous pneumonia; (2) **type of exudate,** such as suppurative pneumonia, fibrinous pneumonia, and pyogranulomatous pneumonia; (3) **morphological features,** such as gangrenous pneumonia, embolic pneumonia, proliferative pneumonia; (4) **distribution of lesions,** such as focal pneumonia, lobar pneumonia, diffuse pneumonia; (5) **epidemiology,** such as enzootic pneumonia, contagious bovine pleuropneumonia; and finally, (6) **miscellaneous features,** such as atypical pneumonia, cuffing pneumonia, aspiration pneumonia.

Until a systematic nomenclature for animal pneumonia is established, we must be aware that one pneumonia can be known by different names. For example, in **pigs**, enzootic pneumonia, virus pneumonia, and mycoplasma pneumonia all refer to the same disease caused by *Mycoplasma hypopneumoniae.*

Pneumonia in domestic animals can be classified into four distinct types: (1) **bronchopneumonia,** (2) **interstitial pneumonia,** (3) **embolic pneumonia,** and (4) **granulomatous pneumonia.** With this classification, it is possible to indicate the possible **aetiology** (viruses, bacteria, fungi, parasites), **routes of entry** (by air or through blood), and possible **sequelae.** However, overlapping of these four types is possible, and sometimes two types may be present in the same lung.

The criteria used to classify pneumonias are based on morphological changes. These include distribution of lesions, texture (feel, consistency), colour, and appearance of affected lungs (**Table 2**). According to **distribution** of lesions,

Table 2. Classification of pneumonias in domestic animals

Type	Route of entry of pathogen	Distribution of lesions	Texture of lung	Nature of exudate	Example of disease	Common sequelae/complication
Bronchopneumonia Suppurative (or lobular pneumonia)	Aerogenous (bacteria and mycoplasmas)	Cranio-ventral consolidation	Firm	Purulent exudate in bronchi	Enzootic pneumonia	Cranio-ventral abscesses, bronchiectasis,
Fibrinous (or lobar pneumonia)	Aerogenous (bacteria and mycoplasmas)	Cranio-ventral consolidation	Hard	Fibrin in lung and pleura	Pneumonic pasteurellosis	BALT hyperplasia, 'sequestra', pleural adhesions, abscesses
Interstitial pneumonia	Aerogenous or haematogenous (virus, toxins, septicaemias and allergens)	Diffuse	Elastic	Exudate not visible, trapped in alveolar septa	Extrinsic allergic alveolitis, influenza	Oedema, emphysema,
Granulomatous pneumonia	Aerogenous or haematogenous (Mycobacteria, systemic mycoses)	Multifocal	Nodular	Pyogranulomatous, caseous necrosis, calcified nodules	Tuberculosis, blastomycosis, cryptococcosis	Dissemination of infection to lymph nodes and distant organs
Embolic pneumonia	Haematogenous (septic emboli)	Multifocal	Nodular	Purulent foci surrounded by hyperaemia	Vegetative endocarditis, ruptured liver abscess	Abscesses in all pulmonary lobes randomly distributed

Aerogenous means through inspired air
Haematogenous means through blood circulation

pneumonias can be **cranio-ventral** (antero-ventral) as in bronchopneumonias; **focal**, as in embolic pneumonias; **diffuse**, as in interstitial pneumonias; or **locally extensive**, as in granulomatous pneumonias. **Texture** of pneumonic lungs can be **firmer** or **harder** (bronchopneumonias), **more elastic** (rubbery) than normal lungs (interstitial pneumonias), or have a **nodular feeling** (granulomatous pneumonias). **Changes in the appearance include** abnormal colour, presence of nodules or exudate, fibrinous or fibrous adhesions, and presence of rib imprints on serosal surfaces. **On cut surfaces,** pneumonic lungs may have exudate, haemorrhage, oedema, necrosis, abscesses, bronchiectasis, granulomas or pyogranulomas, and fibrosis.

1. Bronchopneumonia

Bronchopneumonia is the most common type of pneumonia seen in domestic animals. It is almost always characterized by cranio-ventral (antero-ventral) consolidation of the lungs. **Causes** include bacteria and mycoplasmas, or by broncho-aspiration of feed or gastric contents. Bacteria arrive in the lungs through inspired contaminated air (**aerogenous**). Before establishing the infection, pathogens must either overcome or avoid the pulmonary defence mechanism. The **first injury** occurs in the mucosa of **bronchioles** and **alveoli**. From here, the inflammatory process can spread **downward** to distant portions of alveoli and **upward** to the bronchi. In bronchopneumonias, the inflammatory exudate collects in the bronchial, bronchiolar, and alveolar lumina leaving the alveolar interstitium unaffected. Through the pores of Kohn, the lesions and exudate spread to neighbouring alveoli until all the alveoli in a lobule are involved. If the inflammatory process cannot control the cause of injury, the lesions spread rapidly from lobule to lobule through alveolar pores and the damaged alveolar walls, **until an entire lobe of a lung is involved.**

In the early stages, the pulmonary vessels are engorged with blood (**active hyperaemia**) and the bronchi, bronchioles, and alveoli contain some fluid (**permeability oedema**). If injury is mild to moderate, cytokines cause rapid recruitment of neutrophils and alveolarmacrophages into bronchioles and alveoli. **When injury is severe,** chemical mediators of inflammation produce pronounced vascular changes. That is, they increase vascular permeability which results in **fibrinous inflammation** or sometimes haemorrhage. The permeability changes can be further aggravated by microbial toxins. The final result is that the blood vessels become severely permeable **and allow substantial leakage of plasma fluid and proteins (fibrinogen) into the alveoli**. Filling of alveoli, bronchioles, and small bronchi with inflammatory exudate destroys airspaces. As a result, **portions of severely affected (consolidated) lungs sink** to the bottom of the container when put in fixative. The replacement of air by exudate also changes the texture of the lungs. **The lung becomes firmer or harder than normal.**

The term '**consolidation**' is used when the texture (consistency) becomes firmer or harder than normal. This results from loss of airspaces due to exudation and atelectasis. **Inflammatory consolidation** of lungs in the past has been referred to as '**hepatization**', because the affected lung had the appearance and texture of liver. It was called as '**red hepatization**' in acute cases because of marked active hyperaemia, whereas it was called as '**grey hepatization**' in those chronic cases in which hyperaemia was no longer present. **This terminology, although correctly applicable and used in human pneumonias, is rarely used in veterinary medicine. This is because development of pneumonia in animals does not in all cases follow the red-to-grey hepatization pattern.**

Bronchopneumonias in domestic animals can be divided into:

(i)   **Suppurative bronchopneumonia** if the exudate is composed mainly of **neutrophils,** and

(ii) **Fibrinous bronchopneumonia** if fibrin is the main component of the exudate (Table 2).

At present the term '**bronchopneumonia**' is used for both suppurative and fibrinous inflammation of the lungs. This is because both forms of inflammation have basically the same pathogenesis. **It is the severity and not the type of injury that determines whether bronchopneumonia becomes suppurative or fibrinous.** In some cases, however, it is difficult to differentiate between suppurative and fibrinous bronchopneumonia since both types can co-exist (fibrino-suppurative bronchopneumonia) **and one type can progress to the other.**

(i) Suppurative Bronchopneumonia

Suppurative bronchopneumonia is characterized by the presence of **purulent or mucopurulent exudate** in the airways and cranio-ventral consolidation of lungs. The exudate can be demonstrated by squeezing intrapulmonary bronchi. This forces the exudate out of the bronchi. The inflammation is usually confined to individual lobules. As a result, **the lobular pattern of the lungs becomes prominent.** This is particularly seen in **cattle** and **pigs**, because these species have prominent lobulation of the lungs. The lobulation is further increased due to widening of the interlobular septa. **Grossly,** the lung presents a pattern of alternating colours **(checker-board appearance)** due to a mixture of normal and abnormal (consolidated) lobules (Fig. 2). Because of this typical lobular distribution, **suppurative bronchopneumonias are also referred to as lobular pneumonias.**

Causes: The most common pathogens that cause suppurative bronchopneumonia in domestic animals include *Pasteurella multocida, Bordetella bronchiseptica, Arcanobacterium (Actinomyces) pyogenes,* **Streptococcus** sp., *E. coli* and several species of mycoplasmas. Most of these organisms are secondary pathogens. They require damage of the lung's defence mechanisms to colonize and establish an infection. Suppurative bronchopneumonia can also result from aspiration of bland (sterile) material (e.g. milk).

The **colour of consolidated lungs** varies depending on the age of the lesion. In **acute cases** (few days), pneumonic lobules are **red** from active hyperaemia. **In longer duration cases,** the purulent exudate and the collapsed alveoli make the lungs grey pink. Finally, in the **most chronic cases,** the lungs become somewhat pale grey in appearance. **Enzootic pneumonias** of

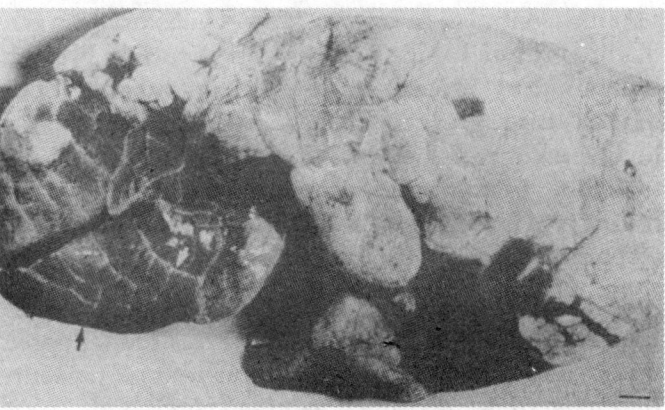

Fig. 2. **Left lung. Pig. Suppurative bronchopneumonia.** Cranioventral consolidation of the lung involves about 40% of lung parenchyma. Note **lobular pattern** is prominent due to widening of the interlobular septa (arrows).

ruminants and **pigs** are examples of chronic suppurative bronchopneumonias.

Microscopically, there is extensive infiltration of **neutrophils** and macrophages and presence of cellular debris within the lumen of bronchi, bronchioles, and alveoli. Accumulation of leukocytes is caused by cytokines, complement, and other chemotactic factors that are released in response to alveolar injury, or by the chemotactic effect of bacterial toxins, particularly **endotoxin**. In most severe cases, purulent or mucopurulent exudate completely obliterates (destroys) the entire lumen of bronchi, bronchioles, and alveoli.

If suppurative bronchopneumonia is a **mild infection**, lesions resolve soon. Within 7-10 days, exudate is removed from the lungs by the mucociliary clearance, and complete resolution occurs within 4 weeks. **If infection is persistent,** suppurative bronchopneumonia can become **chronic** with goblet cell hyperplasia, an important component of the inflammatory process. The exudate in chronic cases varies from mucopurulent to mucoid.

Hyperplasia of bronchial associated lymphoid tissue (BALT) is also commonly seen in chronic cases. **Grossly,** it appears as prominent white nodules (cuffs) around bronchial walls (**cuffing pneumonia**). **Sequelae** of chronic suppurative bronchopneumonia include bronchiectasis, pulmonary abscesses, and pleural adhesions (from pleuritis). Atelectasis and emphysema can also occur from obstructed bronchi or bronchioles (e.g. bronchiectasis).

(ii) Fibrinous Bronchopneumonia

This is similar to suppurative bronchopneumonia except that the **exudate is fibrinous** rather than neutrophilic. Fibrinous bronchopneumonias usually also have a cranio-ventral distribution. However, exudation is not confined to the boundaries of individual lobules as in suppurative bronchopneumonia. Instead, the inflammatory process involves many adjacent lobules and the exudate moves quickly through lung tissue until the entire lobe is affected. Because of the involvement of the entire lobe, **fibrinous bronchopneumonias are also referred to as lobar pneumonia.** Fibrinous bronchopneumonias are the result of **more severe injury,** and therefore are **more life threatening** than suppurative pneumonias. Even when fibrinous bronchopneumonia involves 30% or less of the total area, clinical signs and **death can occur as a result of severe toxaemia.**

Causes: Pathogens that cause fibrinous bronchopneumonias in domestic animals include *Pasteurella haemolytica* (pneumonic pasteurellosis), *Haemophilus somnus,* *Actinobacillus pleuropneumoniae* (porcine pleuropneumonia), and *Mycoplasma mycoides* subsp. **mycoides** small colony (contagious bovine pleuropneumonia). Fibrinous bronchopneumonia can also occur from aspiration into bronchi of irritant materials, such as gastric contents.

The **gross appearance** depends on the age and severity of lesion, and also whether lung is observed externally or on cut surface. **Externally,** early stages are characterized by severe congestion and haemorrhage. This gives the affected lungs a characteristic intense red discoloration. A few hours later, fibrin accumulates on the surface and forms plaques of fibrinous exudate over the red dark lung. At this stage, a yellow fluid starts to accumulate in the thoracic cavity. The **colour** of fibrin deposited on the pleural surface can be **yellow** when the exudate is formed mainly by fibrin, tan (**yellowish brown**) when fibrin is mixed with blood, and **grey** when a large number of leukocytes are part of the fibrinous plaque. Because fibrin has a tendency to deposit on the pleural surface, **sometimes the term pleuropneumonia is used as a synonym for fibrinous bronchopneumonia.**

On the cut surface, early stages appear as red consolidation. In more advanced cases (24 hours), there is marked dilation and thrombosis of lymph vessels and oedema of interlobular septa. Distension of the interlobular septa gives lungs **a typical marbled appearance** (i.e. marked like coloured patterns of a marble). Focal areas of coagulative necrosis are also common. In animals that survive the early stages, necrosis usually develops into 'sequestra'. These are areas of necrotic lung surrounded by connective tissue.

Microscopically, in the early stage there is massive leakage of **plasma proteins** into the bronchioles and alveoli. As a result, most of the airspaces are destroyed by fluid and **fibrin.** Movement of fibrin and fluid into alveolar lumens is due to disruption of the integrity and increased permeability of the blood-air barrier. Since fibrin is chemotactic for **neutrophils,** these cells are always present in fibrinous inflammation. As inflammation progresses (3 to 5 days), fluid exudate is gradually replaced by a fibrino-cellular exudate composed of fibrin, neutrophils, macrophages, and necrotic debris (Fig. 3). **In chronic cases** (after 7 days), there is **marked fibrosis**

of the interlobular septa and pleura.

In contrast to suppurative bronchopneumonia, **fibrinous pneumonia rarely resolves completely.** This leaves **scars** in the form of **fibrosis** and **pleural adhesions.** The most common **sequelae** include bronchiolitis obliterans, gangrene, sequestra, fibrosis, abscesses, and chronic pleuritis with pleural adhesions.

2. Interstitial Pneumonia

Interstitial pneumonia is **a special type of pneumonia** in which injury and the inflammatory process occur mainly in any one of the three layers of the alveolar walls (endothelium, basement membrane, and alveolar epithelium)

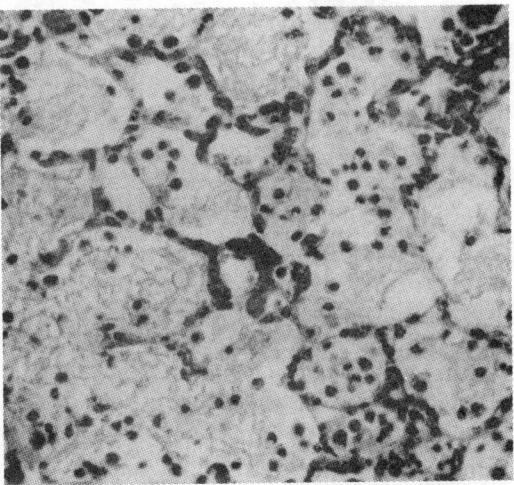

Fig. 3.   Lung; calf. Pneumonic pasteurellosis (*P. haemolytica*). Alveoli contain abundant fibrin mixed with neutrophils and macrophages. H & E stain.

and the adjacent bronchiolar interstitium. **This type of pneumonia is most difficult to diagnose at necropsy and requires microscopic examination.**

The pathogenesis is complex. It can occur from aerogenous injury (through air) to the alveolar epithelium (pneumocytes I and II), or from haematogenous injury (through blood circulation) to the alveolar capillary endothelium or alveolar basement membrane. **Causes:** Inhalation of toxic gases, toxic fumes such as smoke, local generation of toxic metabolites by Clara cells, release of free radicals, and infection with pneumotropic viruses can damage alveolar epithelium. Injury to the vascular endothelium. occurs in **septicaemias,** disseminated intravascular coagulation, circulating larva migrans, toxins absorbed into the alimentary tract, or toxic metabolites locally produced in the lungs, and from infections with endotheliotropic viruses. Also, inhaled antigens such as fungal spores can combine with circulating antibodies and form deposits of antigen-antibody complexes in the alveolar wall. These initiate inflammation, damage alveolar wall, and produce injury (**allergic alveolitis**). As in humans, **interstitial pneumonias** in domestic animals are also divided into **acute** and **chronic**. Not all acute interstitial pneumonias are fatal, or progress into a chronic form.

(i) Acute Interstitial Pneumonia

Acute interstitial pneumonia begins with **injury to either type I pneumocytes or alveolar capillary epithelium.** The injury causes disruption of the air-blood-barrier and exudation of plasma proteins into the alveolar space. The leakage of proteinaceous fluid into the alveolar lumen constitutes the **exudative phase.**

Sometimes exuded plasma proteins mix with lipids and components of pulmonary surfactant and form membranes, which get partially attached to the alveolar and bronchiolar walls. These membranes are referred to as **hyaline membranes** because they have a hyaline appearance (eosinophilic, homogeneous, and amorphous) on microscopic examination. Besides alveolar lumen, the inflammatory exudate and neutrophils accumulate in the alveolar interstitium and cause thickening of the alveolar walls. The exudative phase is followed by the **proliferative phase** characterized by hyperplasia of type II pneumocytes to replace the lost type I alveolar cells. In fact, type II pneumocytes are the ancestor cells (progenitor cells) that differentiate and replace necrotic type I pneumocytes. As a result, **the alveolar walls become thickened.**

Acute interstitial pneumonia is often **mild**, especially that caused by some respiratory viruses. In **severe** cases, animals may die of respiratory failure due to diffuse alveolar damage. The leakage of proteinaceous fluid (exudative phase) into the alveolar spaces, causes   fatal pulmonary oedema. **Examples of this fatal type include** bovine pulmonary oedema, acute respiratory disease syndrome (ARDS) in all species, and massive pulmonary migration of **Ascaris** larvae in **pigs.**

(ii) Chronic Interstitial Pneumonia

When the alveolar injury persists, the proliferative and infiltrative lesions can progress into a stage called **chronic interstitial pneumonia**. The typical feature is **alveolar fibrosis**, and in some cases accumulation of mononuclear inflammatory cells in the interstitium and persistence of hyperplastic type II pneumocytes. Although the lesions are present in the alveolar walls of interstitium, desquamated epithelial cells, macrophages, and mononuclear cells are usually present in the lumen of bronchioles and alveoli. Other changes that may occur are formation of microscopic granulomas and hyperplasia of smooth muscle in airways or blood vessels. Examples of chronic interstitial pneumonia include **ovine** progressive pneumonia, hypersensitivity pneumonitis in **cattle** and **dogs**, silicosis in **horses.**

In contrast to bronchopneumonias, where distribution of lesions is mostly cranio-ventral, in acute or chronic interstitial pneumonias, lesions are more diffusely distributed and involve all pulmonary lobes. **Three important gross features** of interstitial pneumonia are: (1) the failure of lungs to collapse when the thoracic cavity is opened, (2) sometimes presence of rib impressions on the lung's pleural surface, and (3) lack of exudate in airways unless complicated with secondary bacterial pneumonia. The **colour** varies from red to pale grey to a mottled red pale appearance i.e. marked with patches of different colour. **Pale lungs** are due to disappearance of alveolar capillaries (reduced blood/tissue ratio), especially when there is fibrosis. The **texture of lungs** in uncomplicated cases is elastic or rubbery.

The term **'broncho-interstitial pneumonia'** has been introduced to describe cases in which lung lesions share some microscopic features of both bronchopneumonia and interstitial pneumonia. This is seen in many viral infections in which viruses replicate and cause injury in bronchial, bronchiolar, and alveolar cells. Damage to the bronchial and bronchiolar epithelium causes accumulation of neutrophils similar to that of bronchopneumonias, and damage to alveolar walls causes proliferation of type II pneumocytes, similar to that which occurs in the proliferative phase of acute interstitial pneumonias. Examples of broncho-interstitial pneumonias include canine distemper and influenza in **pigs** and **horses.**

(3) Embolic Pneumonia

Embolic pneumonia is characterized by **multifocal lesions randomly distributed in all pulmonary lobes,** caused by the arrest of septic emboli. Lungs act as a biological filter for circulating particulate matter. **Sterile thrombi,** unless very large, are rapidly dissolved and removed from blood vessels by fibrinolysis and cause no harm. However, most types of bacteria in circulation (**bacteraemia**) usually bypass the lungs and are finally trapped in the liver, spleen, joints, or other organs. To cause lung infection, circulating bacteria must first attach to the vascular endothelium and escape phagocytosis by intravascular neutrophils. Once trapped in the pulmonary vessels, usually alveolar capillaries, bacteria spread from the vessels to the interstitium and surrounding lung, forming finally a focus of infection.

Grossly, the early lesions are characterized by the presence of very small (1 mm) **white foci in the lungs, surrounded by a distinct, red, haemorrhagic halo** (Fig. 4).

Unless emboli arrive in great numbers, causing fatal lung oedema, **embolic pneumonia is rarely fatal.** Therefore, these acute lesions are rarely seen at postmortem examination. In most cases, acute lesions if unresolved form **abscesses** that are randomly distributed **in all lobes.** They are not restricted to the cranio-ventral aspects of the lungs, as is the case with abscesses developing from suppurative broncho-pneumonia. The early

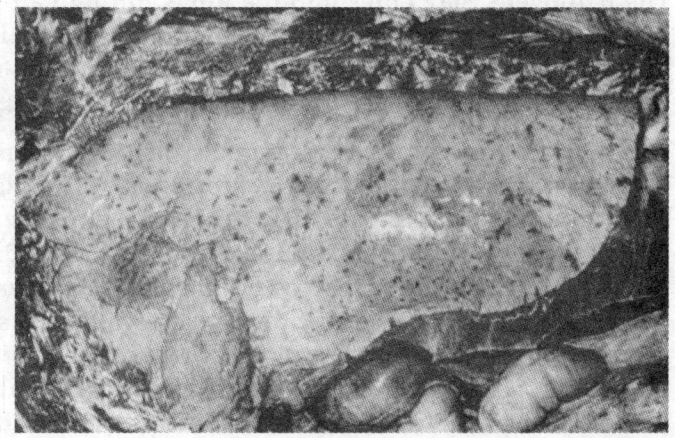

Fig. 4. Left lung; Foal. Acute embolic pneumonia. Note numerous small, dark foci of haemorrhagic and inflammatory exudate randomly distributed in the lung parenchyma.

inflammatory lesions in embolic pneumonias are **always focal.** Thus, they differ from those of endotoxaemia or septicaemia, in which endothelial damage and interstitial reactions (interstitial pneumonia) are **diffusely distributed** in the lungs.

43

When embolic pneumonia or its sequelae (abscesses) are present, careful postmortem examination is required to locate the source of septic emboli. **Most common causes** include rupture of hepatic abscesses into the vena cava in **cattle**, omphalophlebitis in **farm animals**, and chronic bacterial skin or hoof infections. Valvular or mural endocarditis in the right side of the heart is also a usual source of septic emboli and embolic pneumonia in all species. Bacteria commonly isolated from septic pulmonary emboli are *Arcanobacterium* (*Actinomyces*) *pyogenes*, *Fusobacterium necrophorum, Erysipelothrix rhusiopathiae, Streptococcus suis* type II, *Staphylococcus aureus*, and *Streptococcus equi.*

4. Granulomatous Pneumonia

Granulomatous pneumonia is characterized by the **presence of caseous or non-caseous granulomas in the lungs.** On palpation, lungs have a typical nodular character due to nodules of various sizes that usually have a firm texture, especially if calcification has occurred. At postmortem examination, granulomas in the lungs can be mistaken for neoplasms.

The **pathogenesis** of granulomatous pneumonia has some similarities with those of interstitial and embolic pneumonia. What makes granulomatous pneumonia a different type is not the portal of entry or site of initial injury in the lungs, **but the unique type of inflammatory response that results in the formation of granulomas,** which can be easily recognized at gross or microscopic examination. The pathogens may enter into the lungs through air or via blood. **As a rule the pathogens causing granulomatous pneumonia are resistant to intracellular killing by phagocytic cells and to the acute inflammatory response. As a result, they persist in affected tissues for a long time.**

The **most common causes** in animals include systemic fungal diseases such as cryptococcosis (*Cryptococcus neoformans*), coccidioidomycosis (*Coccidioides immitis*), histoplasmosis (*Histoplasma capsulatum*), and blastomycosis (*Blastomyces dermatitidis*). In most of these fungal diseases, the route of entry is through air. From the lungs, the fungi spread to other organs, particularly lymph nodes, liver, and spleen. Some bacterial diseases, such as tuberculosis (*Mycobacterium bovis*) in all species, *Rhodococcus equi* in **foals**, and inhaled foreign material (starch) also cause granulomatous pneumonia. At times, aberrant (wandering) parasites such as *Fasciola hepatica* in **cattle** and aspiration of foreign bodies can also cause granulomatous pneumonia. Feline infectious peritonitis is a viral infection that results in granulomatous pneumonia. **Lesions** are caused by the **deposition of antigen-antibody complexes** in the blood vessels of many organs, including the lungs, and subsequent vasculitis.

Microscopically, granulomas are composed of a centre of necrotic tissue, surrounded by a rim of macrophages (epithelioid cells) and giant cells, and an outer layer of connective tissue infiltrated by lymphocytes and plasma cells. The causative agent in many cases can be identified in sections stained by periodic acid-Schiff stain (PAS), or by silver stains for fungi, or the acid-fast stain for mycobacteria.

Pneumonias in Cattle

Enzootic Pneumonia

Sometimes also called as **'calf pneumonia'**, enzootic pneumonia is a disease caused by several agents and produces a variety of lesions in calves. Enzootic pneumonia is also called **'viral pneumonia'** because it usually begins with an acute respiratory infection with parainfluenza-3 (PI-3) virus, or with adenoviruses, bovine herpesvirus-1 (BHV-1), reoviruses, and rhinoviruses. **Mycoplasmas** and possibly **Chlamydia** may also be primary agents. Following infection with any of these agents, opportunistic bacteria such as *Pasteurella multocida*, *Arcanobacterium* (*Actinomyces*) *pyogenes*, and *Escherichia coli* cause secondary suppurative bronchopneumonia. **This is the most serious stage of enzootic pneumonia.** The **pathogenesis** of the disease is poorly understood. However, it is clear that there is damage to the lung's defence mechanisms. The immune status of the calf plays a role in the development of enzootic pneumonia. **Calves with bovine leukocyte adhesion deficiency (BLAD) are highly susceptible to bronchopneumonia.**

Lesions vary and depend on the agents involved as well as on the duration of the inflammatory process. In the acute stage, lesions caused by **viruses** are those of broncho-interstitial pneumonia. **Microscopically**, the lesions are necrotizing bronchiolitis. The **mycoplasmas** too cause bronchiolitis, but in contrast to virus-induced pneumonia, mycoplasmal lesions tend to progress to a chronic stage characterized by peribronchiolar lymphoid hyperplasia (**cuffing pneumonia**). When complicated by **secondary bacterial infections,** viral or mycoplasmal lesions change from a pure broncho-interstitial to a **suppurative bronchopneumonia.** In late stages, the lungs have abscesses or bronchiectasis.

Pneumonic Pasteurellosis (Shipping Fever)

Pneumonic pasteurellosis is clinically characterized by **acute fibrinous bronchopneumonia** with toxaemia. *Pasteurella haemolytica* (biotype A, serotype 1) is the main aetiological agent. However, *P. multocida* and other serotypes of *P. haemolytica* are also involved.

The **pathogenesis** of the disease is still incompletely understood. It is believed that viruses predispose **cattle** to pneumonic pasteurellosis. These include BHV-1, PI-3, BRSV, and several others. Once established in the lungs, *P. haemolytica* causes lesions by **different virulence factors.** These include endotoxin and outer membrane proteins. However, the most important is production of a **leukotoxin (exotoxin)** that binds and kills bovine macrophages and neutrophils. During *P. haemolytica* infection, alveolar macrophages release pro-inflammatory cytokines, particularly tumour necrosis factor-alpha (TNF-alpha), interleukin-8 (IL-8), and leukotrienes. The bacterial toxins further increase the inflammatory response.

Clinically, cattle usually become depressed, febrile, and anorexic and have a productive cough, encrusted nose, mucopurulent nasal discharge, and shallow respiration.

The **gross lesions** are those of **fibrinous (lobar) bronchopneumonia** with prominent fibrinous pleuritis and pleural effusion. The interlobular septa are distended by yellow, gelatinous oedema and fibrin. The **'marbling'** of the lobules (having mottled appearance like marble) is due to areas of coagulation necrosis, interlobular interstitial oedema, and congestion. The necrotic areas are bordered by a rim of degenerating neutrophils mixed with a few alveolar macrophages. Oedema and fibrin are the major components of the exudate in alveoli and interlobular septa. Because of the necrotizing process, outcome of pneumonic pasteurellosis can be serious and may result in abscesses, sequestra, fibrous pleural adhesions, and bronchiectasis.

Haemorrhagic Septicaemia (HS)

Pneumonic pasteurellosis should not be confused with haemorrhagic septicaemia of ruminants. HS is caused by serotypes B and E of *P. multocida*. Haemorrhagic septicaemia is a very important disease of **cattle** in India. In contrast to pneumonic pasteurellosis in which lesions are always confined to the lower respiratory tract, the bacteria in haemorrhagic septicaemia always spread haematogenously to many organs. The disease is clinically characterized by a severe acute septicaemia, high fever, and rapid death. **Gross lesions** include generalized petechiae on the serosal surfaces of intestine, lungs, and skeletal muscles. Superficial and visceral lymph nodes are swollen and haemorrhagic. Other lesions may include fibrino-haemorrhagic interstitial pneumonia, haemorrhagic enteritis, blood-tinged fluid in the thorax and abdomen, and subcutaneous oedema.

Contagious Bovine Pleuropneumonia (CBPP)

This is an important disease of **cattle** in India, and is caused by *Mycoplasma mycoides* subsp. *mycoides* small colony. **It is the most pathogenic of all mycoplasmas that infect domestic animals.** The **pathogenesis** of the disease is still poorly understood, but involves toxin production, unregulated production of TNF-alpha, ciliary dysfunction, immunosuppression, and immune-mediated vasculitis. Vasculitis and thrombosis of blood vessels lead to lobular infarction.

Grossly, the disease is characterized by **severe, fibrinous bronchopneumonia (pleuropneumonia)** similar to that of pneumonic pasteurellosis, but **has more pronounced 'marbling' of the lobules** (different stages of inflammation) **and larger sequestra** (necrotic lung encapsulated by connective tissue). **Microscopically,** it again resembles pneumonic pasteurellosis, except that vasculitis and thrombosis of pulmonary arterioles and capillaries are much more pronounced and are the major cause of infarction. *M. mycoides* remains viable in the sequestra for many years, and under stress the fibrous capsule may break down and the mycoplasma are released into the airways and become a source of infection to other animals. **Vaccination is highly effective in preventing the disease.**

Tuberculosis

Tuberculosis is a worldwide, chronic disease of human beings and domestic animals. **Cattle** can be infected with *Mycobacterium bovis*, *M. tuberculosis*, and *M. avium-intracellulare* by several routes, **but infection of the lungs by inhalation of *M. bovis* is the most important in adult animals.** However, ingestion of infected milk is more important in young animals.

Respiratory infection starts when inhaled bacilli reach the alveoli and are phagocytosed by pulmonary alveolar macrophages. If these cells are able to destroy the bacteria, infection is prevented. However, *M. bovis* may multiply intracellularly, kill the macrophage, and initiate infection. From here, the bacteria spread through airways within the lungs and eventually to tracheo-bronchiolar and mediastinal lymph nodes through the lymph vessels. The initial focus of infection (lungs) and the involvement of regional lymph nodes are termed the **'primary complex'** of tuberculosis. If the infection is not prevented within the primary complex, bacteria spread through the lymph vessels to distant organs and other lymph nodes. Haematogenous spread occurs rarely when the inflammatory process containing mycobacteria gradually destroys the walls of blood vessels. If the bacterial spread is sudden and massive, numerous small foci of infection develop in many tissues and organs. The condition is referred to as **'miliary tuberculosis'** (small foci like millet seeds). The **animal becomes hypersensitive** to the mycobacteria, which increases the **cell-mediated immune defences** in early or mild infections. But this can result in host-tissue destruction in the form of **caseous necrosis.** The development and spread of lung infection are regulated by **cytokines and TNF-alpha production** by alveolar macrophages.

Clinically, there is debilitation, reduced milk production, and emaciation. In the **pulmonary form**, which is more than 90% of bovine cases, a chronic, moist cough can progress to dyspnoea. Enlarged tracheo-bronchial lymph nodes may increase dyspnoea by pressing on the airways.

Grossly, tuberculosis is characterized by the presence of a few to many caseated granulomas (Fig. 5). The early gross changes are small foci (tubercles). With progression, the lesions enlarge and become confluent (get fused) with the formation of large areas of caseous necrosis. Single nodules or clusters occur on the pleura and peritoneum. This condition has been termed **'pearl disease'**. **Microscopically**, the **tubercle** is composed of mononuclear cells of various types. In young tubercles, which are non-caseous, epithelioid and Langhans' giant cells are in the centre, surrounded by lymphocytes, plasma cells, and macrophages. Later, caseous necrosis is in the centre, enclosed by other cell types and fibrosis at the periphery. Acid-fast organisms may be numerous, but are usually difficult to find in histological sections or smears.

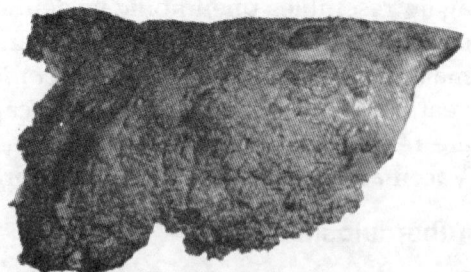

Fig. 5. Lung; aged cow. Pulmonary tuberculosis. Note the presence of

Atypical Interstitial Pneumonia (AIP)

This is a vague clinical term and has led to much confusion. It was first used to describe acute or chronic form of bovine pneumonia that did not fit in any of the 'classical forms' because of the absence of exudate and lack of productive cough.

Most of the syndromes previously grouped under AIP had different aetiology and pathogenesis. It is now proposed that, all those syndromes previously grouped into ATP, should be named according to their specific aetiology and pathogenesis. The most common syndromes include:

(i) Acute bovine pulmonary oedema and emphysema (ABPE), and

(ii) Extrinsic allergic alveolitis (hypersensitivity pneumonitis)

(i) Acute Bovine Pulmonary Odema and Emphysema (ABPE)

Known as **'fog fever'** in Britain, it occurs in **cattle** usually grazing 'fog' pastures. That is, on pastures having a re-growth (a second-growth) after grass/hay/silage has been cut. Usually the disease occurs when there is a change in pasture, from a short dry grass to a lush, green grass. It is believed that **L-tryptophan** present in the pasture is metabolized in the rumen to **3-methylindole.** This is absorbed into the bloodstream and carried to the lungs. Mixed function oxidases present in **Clara cells** (described earlier) metabolize **3-methylindole** into **a highly pneumotoxic compound** that causes extensive necrosis of bronchiolar cells and type I pneumocytes and increases alveolar permeability leading to oedema, interstitial pneumonia, and alveolar and interstitial emphysema.

(ii) Extrinsic Allergic Alveolitis (Hypersensitivity Pneumonitis)

A common allergic disease of cattle, it is seen mainly in **adult dairy cows** in winter. The most common types of inhaled antigens that cause this disease are **fungal spores** commonly found in mouldy hay. **Clinically**, it can be acute or chronic. Weight loss, coughing, and poor exercise tolerance are the clinical features.

Parasitic Pneumonia (Verminous Pneumonia)

The word **'parasitic pneumonia'** is used here to mean **helminth infestations** of the lungs. The lesions in parasitic pneumonia vary from **interstitial** in larvae migration to **chronic bronchitis** caused by some intra-bronchial adult parasites to **granulomatous pneumonia** caused by dead larvae, aberrant (wandering) parasites, or eggs of parasites. In many cases, an **'eosinophilic syndrome'** in the lungs is characterized by infiltration of eosinophils in the lung interstitium (interstitial tissue) and broncho-alveolar spaces, and blood eosinophilia. Atelectasis and emphysema following obstruction of airways are also common findings. The adult parasites are usually seen grossly. The severity of the lesions depends on the numbers and size of the parasites and the nature of the host reaction, which sometimes includes hypersensitivity reactions. A common term for all these diseases is **'verminous pneumonia'**.

Dictyocaulus viviparus is an important pulmonary nematode (**lungworm**) of **cattle**, and causes verminous pneumonia also known as **'verminous bronchitis'**. Adult parasites live in the bronchi and cause severe bronchial irritation, bronchitis and pulmonary oedema, which in turn, produce lobular atelectasis and interstitial emphysema. In addition to the inflammation of bronchial mucosa, broncho-aspiration of larvae and eggs also causes an entry of leukocytes into the broncho-alveolar space (**alveolitis**). Verminous pneumonia is commonly seen in **calves**.

The **clinical signs** (coughing) vary with the severity of infection. Severe cases can be confused with interstitial pneumonia. **Dyspnoea** and **death** can occur with heavy infestations when there is massive obstruction of airways.

At postmortem, lesions appear as large, grey, depressed wedge-shaped areas of alterations. On cutting open, **bronchi contain large amounts of foamy oedematous fluid and numerous slender lungworms.** In most severe cases, huge numbers of lungworms fill the entire bronchial tree. **Microscopically,** the bronchial lumen is filled with parasites mixed with mucus. There is also squamous metaplasia of bronchial and bronchiolar epithelium from chronic irritation. There are also a few eosinophilic granulomas around the eggs and dead larvae. **Grossly,** these granulomas are grey nodules (2 to 4 mm) and may be confused with those caused by tuberculosis.

Reinfection Syndrome

A different form of bovine pneumonia, known as **reinfection syndrome**, occurs when previously sensitized **adult cattle** are exposed to large numbers of larvae of *D. viviparus*. Basically, it is acute allergic reaction. Lesions are those of hypersensitivity pneumonia as described earlier.

Ascaris suum

Ascaris suum is the common intestinal roundworm of **pigs**. The larvae cannot complete their life cycle in **calves**, but they can cause **severe pneumonia and death** within two weeks. **Pigs**, the natural host, also can be killed if exposed to massive larval migration. **Clinical signs** include cough and severe dyspnoea to the point of oral breathing. The **lesions** include diffuse interstitial pneumonia with haemorrhagic foci, atelectasis, and interlobular oedema and emphysema. **Microscopically**, larvae are present in the bronchioles and alveoli. The alveoli have thickened walls and contain oedema fluid and cellular exudate (including eosinophils) in the lumens.

Hydatid Cysts

Hydatid cysts are the intermediate stage of *Echinococcus granulosus*. They can be found in the lungs and other organs of **sheep** and to a lesser extent in **cattle, pigs, goats, horses,** and **humans.** The adult is a tapeworm that occurs in the intestine of **dogs. Hydatidosis** is an important zoonosis and continuation of the parasite's life cycle occurs from close association with **sheep, dogs,** and consumption of un-inspected meat from previously slaughtered **sheep**. Hydatid cysts are 5 to 15 cm in diameter. They have little clinical significance in animals, but are of economic importance due to carcass condemnation.

Aspiration Pneumonia of Cattle

The inhalation of regurgitated ruminal contents or iatrogenic (causedby doctor by mistake) deposition of medicines or milk into the trachea can cause a severe and usually **fatal aspiration pneumonia.** Bland (not irritating) substances, such as mineral oil may cause only a mild or suppurative bronchopneumonia, whereas ruminal contents or medicines may be highly irritating and cause **a fibrinous, necrotizing bronchopneumonia. The right lung is more severely affected** because the right cranial bronchus is closest to the trachea. In some severe cases, necrosis can be complicated by infection with saprophytic organisms present in ruminal contents, causing **fatal gangrenous pneumonia.** Aspiration pneumonia should always be considered in animals whose swallowing has been made difficult because of disorders such as hypocalcaemia (**milk fever**).

Pneumonias of Sheep and Goats

Four main forms of *Pasteurella haemolytica* infection occur in sheep. Two are acute or chronic lung infections and are called as **'ovine pneumonic pasteurellosis'** and **'chronic enzootic pneumonia',** respectively. The third form is a systemic and often severe infection known as **'septic pasteurellosis';** the fourth form affects the mammary gland causing **severe mastitis in ewes.**

Ovine Pneumonic Pasteurellosis

It is caused by *P. haemolytica* biotype A and has lesions similar to those of pneumonic pasteurellosis of cattle. Lesions are characterized by a severe fibrinous bronchopneumonia (lobar) with pleuritis.

Chronic Enzootic Pneumonia,

In contrast to ovine pneumonic pasteurellosis, this condition is multifactorial in origin and causes only mild to moderate pneumonia and it is rarely fatal. It usually affects animals younger than one year of age.

Septicaemic Pasteurellosis

This condition is common and is caused by *P. haemolytica* biotype T in animals 5 months or older, or by biotype A in lambs younger than 2 months of age. Both biotypes are carried in the tonsils and oropharynx of normal **sheep**. Under abnormal circumstances, such as stress caused by dietary or environmental changes, bacteria can invade adjacent tissues, enter the bloodstream and cause septicaemia. **Affected animals die after short illness. Gross changes** include necrotizing pharyngitis and tonsillitis, congestion and oedema of the lungs, focal hepatic necrosis and infarcts in the lungs. **Microscopically,** main lesion is disseminated intravascular thrombosis. *P. haemolytica* is readily isolated from many organs.

Contagious Caprine Pleuropneumonia

This disease occurs in **goats,** and closely resembles contagious bovine pleuropneumonia of cattle. Three mycoplasmas, namely *M. mycoides* sp. *mycoides* large colony, *M. mycoides* sp. *capri* and *Mycoplasma* strain F38 are all associated with respiratory infections in **goats**. Their transmission from goats to sheep or cattle does not occur to any significant degree.

Clinically, the disease is similar to contagious bovine pleuropneumonia. There is high morbidity and mortality, fever, cough, dyspnoea, and increasing debility. The **gross lesions** are **similar to the cattle disease** and consist of a severe fibrinous bronchopneumonia and pleuritis. However, sequestra formation in the lungs and interlobular septal distension are less noticeable than bovine disease.

Maedi (Maedi-Visna)

This is an important, lifelong, persistent viral disease of **sheep** and occurs in India. Maedi is an Icelandic word and means 'shortness of breath'. More recently, the disease has been referred to as **'lymphoid interstitial pneumonia (LIP).**

Maedi is caused by a non-oncogenic retrovirus of the lentivirus subfamily (**ovine lentivirus**). It is antigenically related to the retrovirus causing caprine arthritis-encephalitis (discussed next). Sero-epidemologic studies indicate that infection is widespread in **sheep** population, yet the clinical disease seems to be rare. The

pathogenesis is incompletely understood. Transmission occurs mainly through ingestion of infected colostrum and also by close contact between infected and susceptible sheep. Once in the body, the lentivirus remains for long periods of time within monocytes and macrophages, including alveolar and pulmonary intravascular macrophages. Clinical signs do not develop until after a long incubation period of two years or more (**slow virus infection**).

Clinically, maedi is characterized by dyspnoea, and a slowly progressive emaciation despite good appetite. Death occurs once clinical signs are present, but may take many months.

Gross lesions include severe interstitial pneumonia, and the lungs fail to collapse when the thorax is opened. The lungs are pale and mottled and heavy (2 to 3 times normal weight). The tracheo-bronchial lymph nodes are enlarged. **Microscopically,** the interstitial pneumonia is characterized by marked thickening of inter-alveolar septa due to heavy infiltration of lymphocytes, mainly T-cells, and other mononuclear leukocytes. Recruitment of mononuclear cells is due to the production of **cytokines** by retrovirus-infected pulmonary macrophages and lymphocytes. There is some fibrosis and smooth muscle hypertrophy in bronchioles. Secondary bacterial infections often confuse the microscopic lesions. Enlargement of regional lymph nodes is due to severe lymphoid hyperplasia, mainly B-lymphocytes. The virus can also affect many other tissues, causing non-suppurative encephalitis (**visna**), arthritis, mastitis, or vasculitis.

Caprine Arthritis-Encephalitis (CAE)

This retroviral disease of **goats** (**lentivirus**) has a pathogenesis very similar to that of maedi-visna in **sheep**. **The disease occurs in two forms:** one involves the **central nervous system** of **goat kids** and **young goats**, and the other involves the **joints of adult goats** and is characterized by chronic, non-suppurative arthritis-synovitis. EBV virus can also cause **chronic lymphocytic interstitial pneumonia.**

The lentivirus of CAE is closely related to the maedi-visna virus. Like maedi, CAE infection occurs during the first weeks of life when the doe (female goat) transmits the virus to her offspring through infected colostrum or milk. Horizontal transmission between infected and susceptible goats has also been described. After entering through the mucosa, the virus first replicates in monocytes-macrophages. Infected macrophages are spread to the central nervous system, joints, lungs, and mammary glands. Recruitment of lymphocytic cells results from **cytokine** production by infected macrophages and lymphocytes in affected tissues. **It takes several months before serum antibodies can be detected in infected goats.**

Clinically, goats are active and without fever, but gradually lose weight in spite of normal appetite. **Grossly,** there is **diffuse interstitial pneumonia.** The lungs are grey-pink and firm in texture with numerous 1-2 mm size grey-white foci on the cut surface. The tracheo-bronchial lymph nodes are greatly enlarged. **Microscopically,** thickening of the alveolar walls is due to infiltration of lymphocytes and marked hyperplasia of type II pneumocytes.

Tuberculosis

This disease is uncommon in sheep and goats. However, infection with *Mycobacterium bovis* or *Mycobacterium avium* does occur when the disease is prevalent in other species in the area. The **pulmonary form,** as in cattle, is characterized by a granulomatous pneumonia with multiple, large, caseous, calcified granulomas spread throughout the lungs.

Parasitic Pneumonias of Sheep and Goats

Dictyocaulus filaria occurs in the lungs of mostly lambs and goat kids, but also occurs in adults. The life cycle and lesions are similar to those of *Dictyocaulus viviparus* of cattle. The **clinical signs** include cough, dyspnoea, and loss of condition. **Gross lesions** occur from obstruction of the small bronchi by adult worms and exudate. As in cattle, areas of atelectasis and pneumonia are microscopically characterized by catarrhal, eosinophilic bronchitis with peribronchial lymphoid hyperplasia, thickening of alveolar interstitium, and focal infiltration of leukocytes. Secondary bacterial pneumonia is common in small ruminants with this disease.

Muellerius capillaris, also called the **nodular lungworm,** occurs in **sheep** and **goats**. It requires snails as intermediate host. The lesions in **sheep** are multifocal, subpleural nodules. These nodules are soft in early stages, but later become hard or even calcified. **Microscopically,** a focal, eosinophilic, and granulomatous reaction occurs in the alveoli where adults, eggs, and larvae are present.

Goats differ from sheep. Goats have diffuse interstitial rather than focal lesions, and the reaction against parasites microscopically varies from no lesions to a **severe pneumonia** with some eosinophils.

Protostrongylus rufescens is a parasite of both **sheep** and **goats**. It requires an intermediate snail as a host. Infection is usually sub-clinical, but *P. rufescens* can be pathogenic for **lambs** and **goat kids** and cause diarrhea, weight loss, and mucopurulent nasal discharge. The adult parasite lives in bronchioles like **Dictyocaulus** sp. but causes pulmonary nodules similar to *Muellerius capillaris.*

Pneumonias of Horses

Viral infections of the respiratory tract, particularly **equine influenza** and **equine viral rhinopneumonitis** are important diseases of horses. Effects of respiratory diseases in horses are seen in three ways:

1. As pure viral infections, their severity may range from mild to severe.
2. Superimposed infections by opportunistic bacteria such as **Streptococcus** sp.,

Escherichia coli, Klebsiella pneumoniae, Rhodococcus equi and various anaerobes can cause **fibrinous or suppurative bronchopneumonia.**

3. Viral infections may also predispose **horses** to 'airway hyper-responsiveness' and 'chronic obstructive pulmonary disease'.

Equine Influenza

This is **a contagious disease of horses** and has **high morbidity**, but **low mortality.** Severe outbreaks occur in susceptible populations of horses. Two antigenically different subtypes of equine influenza viruses, **A/equine-1** and **A/equine-2**, have been identified. The course of **the disease is mild and short-lived.** Its importance is mainly due to its economic impact on horse racing. The type of injury and response of the respiratory system are described under 'specific diseases of the nasal cavity and sinuses' (see 'equine influenza under 'equine nasal diseases'). Uncomplicated **lesions in the lungs** are those of mild broncho-interstitial pneumonia. Secondary infection is a common complication of equine influenza.

Equine Viral Rhinopneumonitis (EVR)

This respiratory disease is particularly important in **weaned young horses**

between 4 and 8 months of age, and to some extent also in **young foals** and **adult horses.** It is caused by an **equine herpesvirus** that also causes abortion in pregnant mares and neurological diseases in horses of all ages (see also EVR under Equine Nasal Diseases).

The **respiratory form** of EVR in adult horses is a mild and short-lived **broncho-interstitial pneumonia.** Complications with secondary bacterial infections cause a fatal bronchopneumonia. Uncomplicated lesions in aborted foetuses or in foals consist of focal areas of necrosis in various organs.

Equine Viral Arteritis (EVA)

This disease of **foals** and **horses** is caused by **arterivirus. Clinical signs** include respiratory distress, fever, abortion, diarrhoea, colic, and oedema of the limbs and ventral abdomen. There is mucopurulent rhinitis and conjunctivitis. EVA predisposes horses to secondary bacterial pneumonias. **Gross lesions** consist of haemorrhage in most tissues, lung oedema, hydrothorax and hydropericardium, and enteritis. **Microscopic lesions** include fibrinoid degeneration and inflammation of the vessel walls (**vasculitis**), particularly the small muscular arteries (**arteritis**). These lesions explain most of the clinical and pathological features. Lung lesions are those of the interstitial pneumonia and vasculitis.

African Horse Sickness

This **highly fatal disease of horses, mules, and donkeys** is caused by an **orbivirus.** It is characterized by respiratory distress, or cardiovascular failure. It has a high mortality rate, up to 95% in the native (local) population of horses. The disease was originally present in South Africa, but later it crossed the boundaries and entered into other countries. **At present the disease does not exist in India, but in 1960 India had experienced the worst outbreak of African horse sickness. The disease had then inflicted heavy mortality, reaching up to 90%. Since 1963 no case has been reported.** The virus is transmitted mainly by insects by small mosquito-like insects (**Culicoides**) to horses. **Even goats may be infected.** Other animals such as **dogs** can be infected by eating infected horse flesh.

Clinically, African horse sickness is divided into **four different forms: pulmonary, cardiac, mixed,** and **mild**. The **pulmonary form** is characterized by severe respiratory distress and rapid death due to massive pulmonary oedema. **Grossly,** great amounts of froth are present in the airways, lungs fail to collapse, and the ventral parts of the lungs are particularly oedematous. In the **cardiac form,** recurrent fever occurs, and heart failure results in subcutaneous oedema, mainly in the neck and supra-orbital region. The **mixed form** is a combination of the respiratory and cardiac forms. The mild form is characterized by fever and clinical signs similar to those of equine influenza. In most cases it is followed by complete recovery. This **mild form** is usually seen in **donkeys, mules,** and **zebras** and in **horses. The pathogenesis remains unclear.**

Hendra Virus (Equine Morbillivirus)

A new respiratory disease in horses and **humans** was recorded in 1994 in Hendra, Australia. The **disease was fatal** and was due to a newly recognized virus which is referred to as **Hendra virus,** a new member of the subfamily Paramyxoviridae. Lungs of the affected horses are severely oedematous. Microscopically, the lungs have diffuse alveolar oedema.

Rhodococcosis

Rhodococcus equi (earlier *Corynebacterium equi*) is an important cause of morbidity and mortality in **foals**. It is a facultative (optional) intracellular bacterium that causes **two main forms of disease. One** involves intestine, causing ulcerative enterocolitis, and **other** affects the respiratory tract, resulting in a severe and often **fatal bronchopneumonia.**

Clinical disease is sporadic and usually restricted to **young foals** or to **adult horses** with severe immunosuppression. **Clinically,** *R. equi* infection can be **acute** with rapid death due to **severe bronchopneumonia,** or **chronic** with cough, weight loss, and respiratory distress.

It is still not clear whether natural infection occurs through the respiratory tract from where *R. equi* reaches the intestine via swallowed sputum, or whether the infection occurs through oral route with subsequent bacteraemia into the lungs. **Recent studies suggest that natural infection occurs from inhalation of infected**

dust. Once in the lung, *R. equi* undergoes phagocytosis by alveolar macrophages. However, defective phagosome-lysosome fusion and premature lysosomal degranulation result in the survival of bacteria and their multiplication. This leads to the destruction of macrophages. Surprisingly, *R. equi* are easily killed by neutrophils but not macrophages. Releasedcytokines and lysosomal enzymes and bacterial toxins are responsible for extensive caseous necrosis of the lungs, and the recruitment of large numbers of neutrophils, macrophages, and giant cells containing intracellular Gram-positive organisms in their cytoplasm. These changes eventually lead to **pyogranulomatous pneumonia with abscesses** and **tracheo-bronchial pyogranulomatous lymphadenitis**, the characteristic lesions of *R. equi* infection.

Aspiration Pneumonia of Horses

This usually occurs following improper gastric tubing, particularly **lipid pneumonia** from mineral oil delivered into the trachea in the treatment of colic. **Gross and microscopic lesions** are described under '**Aspiration pneumonia of cattle**'.

Parasitic Pneumonias of Horses

Parascaris equorum is a large nematode (roundworm) of **small intestine** of **horses**. The larval stages migrate through the lungs as ascarid larvae do in pigs. Small necrotic foci and petechiae occur in the liver, hepatic and tracheo-bronchial lymph nodes, and lungs.

Dictyocaulus arnfieldi is not a very pathogenic nematode, but should be considered if there are signs of coughing in **horses** when they go to pasture along with **donkeys**. Mature parasites cause **obstructive bronchitis**, oedema, and atelectasis. The **microscopic lesion** is an **eosinophilic bronchitis**.

Pneumonias of Pigs

Swine Influenza

Swine influenza is caused by **type A influenza virus**. It also infects **human beings** who are in close contact with sick pigs. Infection in pigs occurs mainly through respiratory or oral route. However, the virus can also be transmitted by lungworms and the common earthworm (when ingested). In severe outbreaks there is greater involvement of intrapulmonary airways and secondary infection with *Pasteurella multocida, Arcanobacterium pyogenes*, or **Haemophilus** sp.

Clinically, a sudden onset of coughing is followed by respiratory distress, nasal discharge, high fever, weakness, or even prostration. The outbreak subsides without mortality within a week, unless the pigs have secondary infection with bacteria. The most important effect of most outbreaks is severe weight loss. **The pregnant sows abort or give birth to weak piglets.**

Lung lesions caused by influenza virus alone are rarely seen at postmortem, unless complicated with secondary bacterial infections. **Grossly,** catarrhal to mucopurulent inflammation extends from the nasal passages to the bronchioles. The mucus plugs small airways and causes a lobular or multilobular atelectasis. The appearance is similar grossly, but not microscopically, to that of **Mycoplasma** pneumonia. Fatal cases have severe alveolar and interstitial lung oedema. **Microscopically,** lesions in uncomplicated cases include necrotizing bronchitis-bronchiolitis which in severe cases extends into the alveoli as **broncho-interstitial pneumonia.** It is characterized by thickening and infiltration of the alveolar wall with mononuclear cells, and aggregates of macrophages, neutrophils, mucus, and some necrotic cells within the alveolar lumen.

Mycoplasmal Pneumonia of Swine (Porcine Enzootic Pneumonia)

This is **a highly contagious disease of pigs.** It is caused by *Mycoplasma hyopneumoniae* and is characterized by **suppurative bronchopneumonia**. Although an infectious disease, it is very much influenced by immune status and management factors such as crowding, ventilation, concentration of noxious gases in the air (ammonia, hydrogen sulphide), relative humidity, and temperature fluctuations.

Mortality is low unless complicated by secondary pathogens such as *Pasteurella multocida, Arcanobacterium pyogenes, Bordetella bronchiseptica,* **Haemophilus** sp., *Mycoplasma hyorhinis,* and other mycoplasmas. Pathogenesis is not completely understood. *M. hyopneumoniae* first adheres to the cilia of the bronchi and finally colonizes the respiratory system. Once attached to the respiratory epithelium, it stimulates an accumulation of neutrophils into the tracheo-bronchial mucosa, causes extensive loss of cilia, stimulates hyperplasia of lymphocytes in BALT, and attracts mononuclear cells into the broncho-alveolar interstitium. It also reduces the phagocytic activity of neutrophils in the lung and changes the chemical composition of mucus predisposing the lung to secondary bacterial infections.

Clinically, the disease occurs as a herd problem in **two forms**. A **newly acquired infection** in a clean herd causes disease in all age groups. This results in acute respiratory distress and low mortality. In a **chronically infected herd**, the mature animals are immune, and clinical signs are seen only in growing pigs at times of stress, such as at weaning. In such herds, coughing is the most important symptom unless secondary bacterial infection causes severe bronchopneumonia.

The **lesions** are characterized initially by a **broncho-interstitial pneumonia**. This is rarely seen at postmortem. It then rapidly progresses to **suppurative bronchopneumonia** once secondary pathogens are involved. This is usually seen at postmortem. The affected lungs are dark red in the early stages and have a pale-grey ('fish-flesh') appearance in the more chronic stages of the disease. On cut surface, exudate can easily be squeezed out from airways and depending on the stage the exudate varies from purulent to mucopurulent. **Microscopic lesions** are characterized by an accumulation of macrophages and neutrophils into the broncho-alveolar spaces with marked peribronchial and BALT hyperplasia. The suppurative bronchopneumonia is usually more severe if *M. hyorhinis*, *P. multocida*, or *Actinobacillus pleuropneumoniae* are also involved.

Porcine Pasteurellosis

This disease occurs either as a primary infection caused by *Pasteurella multocida* alone, or more commonly as a secondary infection when it colonizes the lung after its defence mechanisms are damaged (**porcine pneumonic pasteurellosis**). Although *P. multocida* is part of the normal nasal flora, it is also an important secondary pathogen for porcine lungs, especially when defence mechanisms are damaged by viral or mycoplasmal infections, or following stress associated with poor management practices.

The most important role of *P. multocida* in pig pneumonias is its **secondary involvement in swine influenza**, pseudorabies, hog cholera, and porcine pleuropneumonia. Secondary infections with *P. multocida* modify the early and mild reactions into a severe suppurative bronchopneumonia with multiple abscesses. The other important role of *P. multocida* is that it can cause a severe fibrinous bronchopneumonia (pleuropneumonia) in pigs without a previous mycoplasmal infection.

Porcine Pleuropneumonia

This is **a highly contagious disease of pigs** caused by *Actinobacillus pleuropneumoniae (Haemophilus pleuropneumoniae)*. It is characterized by a severe, often fatal, fibrinous pleuropneumonia with extensive pleuritis (**pleuropneumonia**). Survivors become carriers of the organisms. **Infection occurs by the respiratory route**. The pathogenesis of the disease is not yet well understood.

Clinically, the disease can vary from an **acute form** with unexpected death to a **subacute form** characterized by coughing and dyspnoea. A **chronic form** is characterized by decreased growth rate and persistent cough. Animals that survive carry the organisms in the tonsils, shed the organism, and infect susceptible pigs.

The **gross lesions** include a **fibrinous bronchopneumonia**. Both **gross and microscopic lesions** are very similar to those of pneumonic pasteurellosis of cattle.

Haemophilus Pneumonia

Some serotypes of *Haemophilus parasuis* (originally, *H. suis*) in addition to **polyserositis** and **polyarthritis (Glasser's disease)**, can also cause lung infections characterized by a suppurative bronchopneumonia. In some severe cases it can be fatal.

Streptococcal Pneumonia

Streptococcus suis **type II** is carried in the nasal cavity, tonsils, and mandibular lymph nodes of **healthy pigs**, particularly in survivors after an outbreak. **Sows can vertically transmit the infection to their offspring.** Some serotypes of *S. suis* (type I) are associated with neonatal septicaemia. Other serotypes may reach the lung by the respiratory route and cause **suppurative bronchopneumonia**, usually in combination with *Pasteurella multocida* and *Escherichia coli*. It can also produce **fibrinous bronchopneumonia** when *S. suis* infection occurs in combination with *Actinobacillus pleuropneumoniae.*

Streptococcus suis **type II is also a serious zoonosis.** In humans, it is capable of causing death by septic shock or meningitis. **Butchers and pig farmers are particularly at risk.**

Tuberculosis

Tuberculosis is an important disease in pigs. In some countries tuberculosis is more common in pigs than in cattle. Pigs are susceptible to all the three mycobacteria, namely, *Mycobacterium avium, Mycobacterium bovis*, and *Mycobacterium tuberculosis.* Tuberculous granulomas usually involve mandibular and mesenteric lymph nodes, to a lesser extent intestine, liver, and spleen, **and only in rare cases the lungs.** The route of infection to lungs is usually haematogenous after oral exposure and intestinal infection. The **microscopic lesions** are basically those of tubercles. However, the degree of caseation and calcification vary with the type of mycobacterium, age of the lesion, and host immune response.

Other Infectious Pneumonias of Pigs

Porcine reproductive and respiratory syndrome is caused by an **arterivirus**, and is characterized by late-term abortions and stillbirths and respiratory problems in young pigs. The **respiratory form** is characterized by cough, dyspnoea, and occasional death. On postmortem examination lung lesions vary from very mild changes to consolidation in cases complicated with bacterial pneumonia. **Microscopically**, pulmonary changes are those of interstitial pneumonia.

Foreign body granulomatous pneumonia occurs in **pigs** following inhalation of vegetable material (**starch pneumonia**) from dusty (non-pelleted) feed. There are no significant gross lesions. **Microscopically**, lung changes are typical of foreign body granulomatous inflammation in which feed particles are surrounded by macrophages and neutrophils. Usually multinucleated giant cells are also present.

Parasitic Pneumonias of Pigs

Metastrongylus apri (elongatus), M. salmi, and *M. pudendotectus* (lungworms) occur in pigs. They require earthworms as intermediate hosts for transmission. Lungworms may transmit the virus of swine influenza. **The importance of**

lungworms is mainly due to growth retardation of pigs. Clinical signs include coughing due to **parasitic bronchitis**.

Gross lesions consist of **small grey nodules in the lungs.** The adult worms are grossly visible in bronchioles and small bronchi and cause catarrhal inflammation with infiltration of eosinophils and lobular atelectasis.

Ascaris suum

During migration through the lungs of **pigs**, larvae of *Ascaris suum* can cause oedema, focal haemorrhages, and interstitial inflammation. Haemorrhages also occur in the liver, and after fibrosis they become large, white **'milk spots'** seen so commonly as incidental finding at postmortem.

Pneumonias in Dogs

In general, inflammatory diseases of lungs are less common in dogs than in other species. They can be divided into **two groups**: **infectious** and **non-infectious pneumonias.** Of the infectious causes two are important: canine distemper and infectious tracheo-bronchitis (kennel cough), already discussed earlier. Non-infectious causes of lung disease include uraemia and paraquat toxicity.

Canine Distemper

Canine distemper is an important infectious disease of dogs. It is caused by a **morbillivirus** that is antigenically related to the human measles, rinderpest, and 'peste-des- petits-ruminants (PPR)' virus. Distemper virus enters through the respiratory tract, proliferates in the lymphoid tissues, causes viraemia, and infects almost all body tissues (pantropic), particularly the epithelial cells. During viraemia, distemper virus suppresses immune response and decreases cytokine production. The virus may cause pneumonia either directly, or by its immunosuppressive effects which render lungs susceptible to secondary bacterial infections. **Clinical signs** include biphasic fever, diarrhoea, vomiting, weight loss, mucopurulent oculo-nasal discharge, coughing, and respiratory distress. After some weeks, hyperkeratosis of foot pads (**'hard pad'**) and nose are observed, along with nervous signs such as paralysis, convulsions, and muscle twitches (tremors, 'tics').

Gross lesions include catarrhal to mucopurulent naso-pharyngitis and conjunctivitis. The lungs are oedematous and have a diffuse interstitial pneumonia. **Microscopically**, it is characterized by necrotizing bronchiolitis, necrosis, and later by thickening of the alveolar walls due to interstitial infiltration of mononuclear cells and hyperplasia of type II pneumocytes. Secondary infections with *Bordetella bronchiseptica* and mycoplasmas are common and may cause fatal suppurative bronchopneumonia. The thymus may be small. **Eosinophilic inclusions** are present in the epithelial cells of many tissues in the nuclei or cytoplasm, or both. They appear first in the bronchiolar epithelium, but are most prominent in the epithelium of the stomach, renal pelvis, and urinary bladder. **These tissues are good choices for diagnostic examination.**

Of all distemper lesions, **demyelinating encephalitis,** which develops late, is the most serious.

Canine Adenovirus Type 2 Infection

This is a common contagious disease of the respiratory tract of dogs. It causes mild fever, oculo-nasal discharge, coughing, and poor weight gain. **Lung lesions** are those of a broncho-interstitial pneumonia. **Large basophilic intranuclear viral inclusions** are seen in bronchiolar and alveolar epithelial cells. The disease is clinically mild unless complicated with a secondary bacterial infection.

Canine Herpesvirus 1

This viral infection can cause fatal generalized disease in **newborn puppies.** Canine herpesvirus 1 causes necrotizing rhinotracheitis and secondary bronchopneumonia in older animals. The virus remains latent and can be activated following stress. This results in transmission of the virus to offspring through placenta resulting in abortion or stillbirths.

Bacterial Pneumonias of Dogs

Dogs generally have bacterial pneumonias when lung's defence mechanisms are damaged. *Pasteurella multocida,* **Sreptococcus** sp., *Escherichia coli, Klebsiella pneumoniae,* and *Bordetella bronchiseptica* are involved in pneumonia secondary to distemper, or after aspiration of gastric contents. *Streptococcus zooepidemicus* also causes fatal haemorrhagic pleuropneumonia in dogs. **Death** is usually from septic embolism which affects the lungs, liver, brain, and lymph nodes. The role of **mycoplasmas** in canine pneumonia is still not clear.

Tuberculosis is uncommon in dogs. Dogs are quite resistant to infection. Most cases occur in immuno-compromised dogs. Dogs are susceptible to the *Mycobacterium tuberculosis, M. bovis,* and *M. avium* strains. Therefore, infection in dogs indicates their contact with human or animal tuberculosis.

Mycotic Pneumonias of Dogs

These can be serious diseases. There are **two main types:** (1) those caused by **opportunistic fungi,** and (2) those caused by **fungi of systemic or deep mycosis.** All these fungi affect human beings and most domestic animals. But they are not transmitted between species.

Opportunistic fungi, such as *Aspergillus fumigatus,* are important in birds. In domestic animals, they affect immuno-compromised animals, or those which have been on prolonged antibiotic therapy. The lung lesion is a focal, nodular, pyogranulomatous, or granulomatous pneumonia. **Microscopically,** fungal hyphae are present. There is usually necrosis, vasculitis, and infiltration of neutrophils, macrophages, lymphocytes, and fibroblasts. This eventually leads to the formation of **granulomas**.

Systemic (deep) mycoses are caused by *Blastomyces dermatitidis, Histoplasma capsulatum, Coccidioides immitis,* and *Cryptococcus neoformans.* **Blastomycosis** usually affects **dogs** and is discussed here. **Cryptococcosis** is discussed under 'Pneumonias of Cats'. In contrast to opportunistic fungi such as **Aspergillus** sp., fungi of systemic mycoses are all **primary pathogens** of human beings and animals. Therefore, they do not require any earlier immunosuppression in order to cause disease. These fungi contain **virulence factors** which cause haematogenous spread and evasion of immune and phagocytic responses.

Blastomycosis

Blastomycosis is caused by *Blastomyces dermatitidis* and is seen mainly in **young dogs** and sometimes **cats**. Inhalation of spores, present in the soil, is the route of infection. From the lung, infection is spread haematogenously to other organs. Pulmonary effects include cough, decreased exercise tolerance, and respiratory distress. Lung lesions are characterized by granulomatous pneumonia, with multiple firm nodules (**pyogranulomas**) spread throughout the lungs. **Microscopically,** nodules are granulomas with numerous macrophages (epithelioid cells), some neutrophils, multinucleated giant cells, and thick-walled yeasts. Nodules can also be present in other tissues, mainly lymph nodes, skin, spleen, liver, kidneys, bones, testes, prostate, and eyes.

Coccidioidomycosis

This is caused by the fungus *Coccidioides immitis.* It is mainly a respiratory tract (aerogenous) infection seen commonly at slaughter in **cattle.** In **dogs,** it is usually a systemic disease. **Clinical signs** depend on the location of lesions. Lung infection is accompanied by respiratory distress. The lesions are focal granulomas or pyogranulomas having suppurative or caseated centres. The fungi are easily seen in tissue sections.

Histoplasmosis

This is a systemic infection that occurs from the inhalation of fungus *Histoplasma capsulatum.* Histoplasmosis occurs in **dogs** and **human beings,** and to a lesser extent, in **cats** and **horses.** **Lung lesions** are characterized by firm, well-encapsulated **granulomas. Microscopically,** granulomas have many macrophages. Similar nodules may be present in other tissues, mainly lymph nodes, spleen, intestines, and liver.

Aspiration Pneumonia

This is an important pneumonia in **dogs** and occurs when vomited or regurgitated materials are aspirated into the lung, or when drugs or radiographic contrast media are accidentally introduced into the respiratory system. Aspiration pneumonia in **dogs** and **cats** is more severe because of the low pH of the gastric contents. **In severe cases, dogs may die from septic shock,** whereas in **chronic cases** lesions progress into **bronchopneumonia.** Aspiration pneumonia in dogs is also an important anaesthetic complication.

Toxic Pneumonias

Paraquat

Paraquat is a broad-spectrum herbicide widely used in gardening and agriculture. It can cause severe and often fatal toxic interstitial pneumonia in **dogs, cats, human beings,** and other species. Following ingestion or inhalation, paraquat metabolites cause local release of **free radicals.** These cause extensive injury to air-blood barrier, through lipid peroxidation of type I and II pneumocytes and alveolar endothelial cells. **Grossly,** the lungs are pale, fail to collapse when the thorax is opened and have interstitial emphysema. **Microscopic findings** include necrosis of type I pneumocytes, interstitial and alveolar oedema, intra-alveolar haemorrhages, and proliferation of type II pneumocytes. In chronic stages (4 to 8 weeks later) there is severe interstitial and intra-alveolar fibrosis.

Uraemic Pneumonopathy (Pneumonitis)

It is a **non-renal lesion** seen in **dogs** with **chronic uraemia. Lesions** include pulmonary alveolar oedema and calcification of vascular smooth muscle. **Grossly,** lungs appear distended and pink or red in colour. On palpation, the lung parenchyma has a typical 'gritty' texture due to mineralization of the alveolar and vascular walls. Since this is not an inflammatory lesion, the term **pneumonitis** should not be used.

Parasitic Pneumonias of Dogs

Toxoplasmosis

Toxoplasmosis is caused by an obligate intracellular, protozoal parasite *Toxoplasma gondii.* Cats are the definitive host, in which the mature parasite divides sexually in the interstitial mucosa. **Human beings, dogs, cats,** and **many wild animals** can become **intermediate hosts** following ingestion of fertile oocysts shed in cat faeces. Even foetuses can be infected transplacentally.

The parasite infects many cells of different tissues, induces an antibody response (sero-positive animals), but does not cause clinical disease. **Toxoplasmosis is usually triggered by immunosuppression,** such as that caused by canine distemper virus. Toxoplasmosis is characterized by necrosis. Lung lesions are severe and include **necrotizing interstitial pneumonia** with marked proliferation of type II pneumocytes and infiltration of macrophages and neutrophils. **Other lesions include** necrotizing hepatitis, myocarditis, splenitis, myositis, and encephalitis. **Microscopically,** the parasites are seen as small basophilic cysts found free in affected tissues or within the cytoplasm of epithelial cells and macrophages.

Pneumocystis carinii sometimes causes chronic interstitial pneumonia in **dogs.** *Filaroides hirthi* is a lungworm of the alveoli and bronchi of **dogs.** Sometimes it may cause severe and even fatal disease as a result of immunosuppression. **Clinical signs** include coughing and respiratory distress. **Grossly lesions** are subpleural nodules. **Microscopically,** these nodules are **eosinophilic granulomas** with larvae or dead worms. No reaction develops against live adults. *Crenosoma vulpis* is a lungworm of **dogs.** The adults live in small bronchi and bronchioles and cause eosinophilic, catarrhal bronchitis-bronchiolitis. *Paragonimus kellicotti* and *P. westermanii* are asymptomatic fluke infections. **Gross lesions** include pleural haemorrhages when metacercariae migrate into the lungs. *Angiostrongylus vasorum* and *Dirofilaria immitis* are parasites of the vascular system. However, depending on the stage, they produce different forms of lung lesions.

Pneumonias of Cats

Viral Pneumonias

Pneumonias in cats are uncommon except when there is immunosuppression. Viral infections such as feline rhinotracheitis and calcivirus may cause lesions in the lungs. But, unless there is secondary invasion by bacteria, they do not usually create a problem.

Feline Pneumonitis

This mild, sub-clinical broncho-interstitial pneumonia is caused by *Chlamydia psittaci* (*felis*). The term, 'feline pneumonitis', is misnomer. This is because the main lesions are severe conjunctivitis and rhinitis, and pneumonia is only mild.

Bacterial Pneumonias

Pasteurella multocida and **Pasteurella**-like organisms are sometimes associated with secondary bronchopneumonia in **cats. There are reports of** *P. multocida* **pneumonia in older and immunosuppressed human beings acquired through contacts with domestic cats.** Mycoplasmas are commonly isolated from lungs of cats with pulmonary diseases, but are not the primary pathogens of pneumonias in cats.

Cats are susceptible to all three types of mycobacterial infections: classical tuberculosis, feline leprosy, and atypical mycobacteriosis. Classical tuberculosis in cats is caused by *Mycobacterium bovis,* but *M. tuberculosis* and *M. avium* are also involved. The route of infection is oral, through infected milk. Therefore, lesions are mainly in the alimentary organs. From here the organisms spread to other organs. The gross appearance of **tuberculous nodules** is similar to that of neoplasms. Therefore, they must be differentiated from pulmonary neoplasms, such as lymphosarcoma.

Mycotic Pneumonias

Cryptococcosis

This is caused by the fungus *Cryptococcus neoformans*. **It is the most common systemic mycosis in the cats.** Lesions are similar to those discussed under 'mycotic pneumonias of dogs'. Besides cats, the disease also occurs in **horses, dogs,** and **human beings. In cat,** lesions can occur in any tissue, resulting in a wide variety of clinical signs. The lung lesion is a **granulomatous pneumonia. Microscopically,** the lesions contain a large number of fungi and only a few macrophages, lymphocytes, and multi-nucleated giant cells.

Other Pneumonias of Cats

Endogenous Lipid Pneumonia

This condition is a sub-clinical pulmonary disease of **cats** and sometimes of **dogs.** Lipids from pulmonary surfactant and degenerated cells accumulate within alveolar macrophages. The **gross lesions** are white, **firm nodules scattered throughout the lungs. Microscopically,** alveoli are filled with foamy, lipid-laden macrophages along with lymphocytes and plasma cells.

Aspiration Pneumonia

This condition is common in cats as a result of vomiting, regurgitation, dysphagia (difficult swallowing), anaesthetic complication, or following accidental administration of food, oral medicines, or contrast media into the trachea.

Parasitic Pneumonias

Aelurostrongylus abstrusus, known as **'feline lungworm'** occurs in **cats** wherever the necessary snail intermediate hosts are found. It can cause chronic respiratory disease with coughing and weight loss, and sometimes, severe dyspnoea and death. The **gross lesions** are **sub-pleural nodules throughout the lungs.** These granulomatous nodules contain eggs, larvae, and turbid exudate. **Microscopically,** the parasites and their eggs and larvae are present in the bronchioles and alveoli where they cause catarrhal bronchiolitis and granulomatous alveolitis.

Toxoplasma gondii, Paragonimus kellicotti and *Dirofilaria immitis* can also affect cats.

Foetal and Perinatal Pneumonias

Foetal Pneumonias

Pneumonia is one of the most common lesions found in fetuses submitted for postmortem examination, particularly in **foals** and **food-producing animals.**

Aspiration of amniotic fluid contaminated with meconium (the first faeces of newborn) and bacteria is the most common route by which microbial pathogens reach the foetal lungs. **Gross lesions** are rare. **Microscopic changes** are those of **bronchopneumonia.**

In **cattle**, *Brucella abortus* and *Arcanobacterium pyogenes* are the two most common bacteria isolated from the lungs of aborted fetuses. Aspiration of amniotic fluid carries the organisms into the foetal lungs, causing a **suppurative bronchopneumonia** *Aspergillus* sp. (mycotic abortion) causes placentitis, which result in foetal pneumonia and abortion.

In addition to aspiration pneumonia, pathogens can also reach the lungs through foetal blood and cause **interstitial pneumonia.** Listeriosis (*Listeria monocytogenes*), salmonellosis (**Salmonella** sp.) and chlamydiosis (*Chlamydia psittaci*) are the best known examples of blood-borne diseases causing foetal pneumonia. Foetal broncho-interstitial pneumonia occurs also in some viral abortions, such as with infectious bovine rhinotracheitis virus and parainfluenza-3 virus in **cattle** and equine viral rhinopneumonitis in **horses.** Foetal pneumonias in dogs and cats are rare.

Meconium Aspiration Syndrome (MAS)

This is an important condition in **human babies.** It originates when amniotic fluid contaminated with meconium is aspirated during labour, or immediately after birth. The pathogenesis is the same as in foetal bronchopneumonia and abortion. Foetal hypoxia, a common event in delivery, causes the foetus to expel meconium into amniotic fluid. Aspiration can occur from aspirating contaminated amniotic fluid before delivery, or immediately after delivery. **MAS is well known in human babies, but its occurrence and significance in animals remain largely unknown.**

Neoplasms of the Lungs

Lung cancers in animals are rare, unlike in human beings. A standard nomenclature of pulmonary neoplasms is not universally accepted. As a result, a large number of names and synonyms occur in the literature. The most common types of pulmonary neoplasms in domestic animals are given in **Table 3.**

Primary Neoplasms

These arise from cells normally present in the lung and can be **epithelial** or **mesenchymal. Mesenchymal are rare.** Primary benign neoplasms, such as **adenoma,** are **extremely rare** in domestic animals. **Most neoplasms are malignant**

Table 3. Classification of pulmonary neoplasms

Primary
Epithelial origin
    Benign
        Bronchial papilloma
        Bronchial gland adenoma
        Bronchiolar-alveolar adenoma
    Malignant
        Carcinomas
            Squamous-cell (epidermoid) carcinoma
            Adenocarcinoma
            Adenosquamous carcinoma
            Anaplastic (undifferentiated) carcinoma
                Small cell
                Large cell
            Bronchiolar-alveolar carcinoma
            Alveolar carcinoma
            Bronchial gland carcinoma
            Carcinoid tumour (neuroendocrine)
Mesenchymal origin
        Benign, e.g., haemangioma, granular cell tumour (myoblastoma) of horses
        Malignant, e.g., haemangiosarcoma
Secondary (metastatic)
  Any malignant tumour, metastatic from another body location, for example,
  osteogenic sarcoma in dogs, uterine carcinoma in cows, malignant melanoma in horses.

and appear as solitary (single) masses of different size. With time, they can metastasize to other areas of the lungs and to different organs.

It is often difficult to determine the exact origin of neoplasm, as to whether it has originated in the conductive system (**bronchogenic carcinoma**), transitional system (**bronchiolar carcinoma**), exchange system (**alveolar carcinoma**), or bronchial glands (**bronchial gland carcinoma**). However, lung carcinomas in animals appear to originate usually from the bronchiolo-alveolar region (Clara cells or type II pneumocytes), **in contrast to humans, which are mostly bronchogenic.**

Dogs and cats are the **species mostly affected with primary lung neoplasms.** They are usually **carcinomas** and occur in animals 6 years of age or older (Fig. 6). **Carcinomas in other animals are less common.** These neoplasms can be invasive or extensive. They have varying colour and texture (soft or firm) and usually have areas of necrosis and haemorrhage.

Ovine Pulmonary Carcinoma (Pulmonary Adenomatosis)

Also known as **pulmonary adenomatosis and jaagsiekte,** this condition is **a transmissible, retrovirus-induced neoplasm of sheep lung.** This carcinoma is very much like a chronic pneumonia, and it shares many similarities with the sheep lentivirus responsible for maedi.

The disease affects usually mature sheep. Clinical signs are a gradual loss of condition, coughing, and respiratory distress, especially after exercise. Appetite and temperature are normal, unless there are secondary bacterial infections. If the animals are raised by the hind limbs, copious fluid produced by the neoplastic cells in the lungs, pours from the nostrils of some animals. **This is an important differentiating feature from maedi.**

Grossly, in the early stages of the disease, the **lungs** are enlarged and **have several firm, grey nodules.** In the later stages, the nodules become confluent and large portions of both lungs are diffusely infiltrated by neoplastic cells. On cross section, airways show copious mucoid fluid.

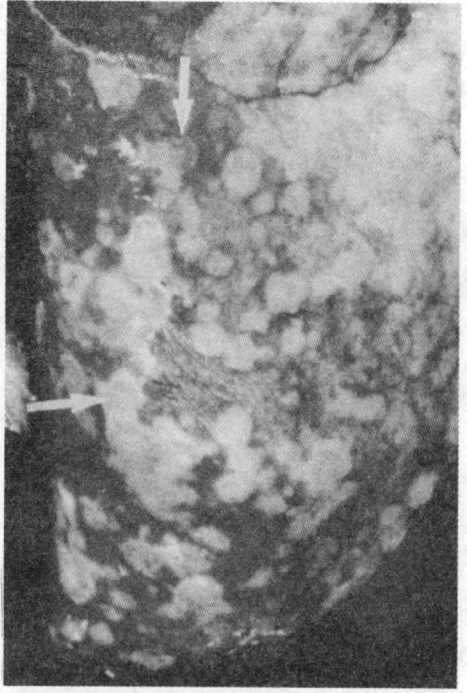

Fig. 6. Lungs, right caudal lobe. Dog. Pulmonary adenocarcinoma. Note metastases are present widely within the lung. Some of the tumourous nodules are **'umbilicated'** (arrows) due to central necrosis. That is, they show a central depression.

Microscopically, the nodules are composed of cuboidal or columnar epithelial cells lining airways and alveoli, **and form papillary structures in adenomatous (gland-like) patterns.** These cells originate from type II alveolar epithelial cells and the non-ciliated bronchiolar epithelial (Clara) cells. Therefore, the neoplasm is considered a **'bronchiolo-alveolar' carcinoma. Sequelae** include secondary bronchopneumonia, abscesses, and pleural adhesions. Metastases occur in regional lymph nodes, and to a lesser extent in pleura, muscle, liver, and kidneys. **Death occurs after several months.** Differential diagnosis between maedi and pulmonary adenomatosis is difficult, because both diseases may co-exist in the same flock or in the same animal.

Secondary Neoplasms

These are all malignant because they are the result of metastases to the lungs from malignant neoplasms elsewhere. They also can be of **epithelial** or **mesenchymal**

origin. Common sources include uterine carcinoma in **cows**, mammary and thyroid carcinomas in **cats**, haemangiosarcoma, osteogenic sarcoma, and malignant melanoma in **dogs**, and malignant lymphoma in **dogs** and **pigs**. **Secondary neoplasms are relatively uncommon in comparison to primary neoplasms.** Usually, they are multiple and spread to all lobes (haematogenous spread), or are of different sizes as nodular, diffuse, or radiating.

Diseases of the Pleura and Thoracic Cavity

Anomalies

Congenital anomalies are **rare.**

Degenerative Disturbances

Pleural Calcification

This disorder is usually found in **dogs** with chronic uraemia. **Lesions** are seen as linear white streaks in parietal pleura, mainly over the intercostal muscles. The lesions indicate severe renal problem. **Vitamin D toxicity** (hypervitaminosis D) can cause a similar pleural lesion.

Pneumothorax

Pneumothorax is presence of **air in the thoracic cavity** where there should normally be negative pressure to facilitate inspiration. Human beings have a complete and strong mediastinum. Therefore, pneumothorax in humans is not a serious problem. In **dogs**, it is less complete; therefore some communication exists between left and right sides.

Causes of pneumothorax include penetrating wound (from accident) and spontaneous rupture of emphysematous bullae or parasitic cysts that communicate with airways (**Paragonimus** sp.). **Clinical signs** of pneumothorax include respiratory distress. The **lesion** is a collapsed, atelectatic lung. The air is readily reabsorbed from the thoracic cavity if the site of entry is sealed.

Circulatory Disturbances

Pleural Effusion

This is accumulation of any fluid, such as transudate, exudate, blood, lymph, or chyle **in the thoracic cavity.**

Hydrothorax

When the **fluid is serous, clear,** and without smell, and fails to coagulate when exposed to air, the condition is called as **hydrothorax (transudate). Causes** of hydrothorax are the same as those involved in oedema formation in other organs. These include increased hydrostatic pressure (heart failure), decreased oncotic pressure (hypoproteinaemia, as in liver disease), alterations in vascular permeability (ANTU toxicity), or obstruction of lymph drainage (neoplasia). If the leakage of transudate is corrected, fluid is rapidly reabsorbed. If the fluid persists, it irritates pleura and causes mesothelial hyperplasia and fibrosis. **This thickens the pleura.**

In severe cases, the amount of fluid can be considerable. For example, a medium size dog can have 2 litres of fluid, and **a cow may accumulate 25 litres or more.** Excessive fluid in the thorax causes **compressive atelectasis** of the ventral portions of the lungs and respiratory distress. Hydrothorax is most commonly seen in **cattle** with right-sided heart failure or cor pulmonale, **dogs** with congestive heart failure or nephritic syndrome, **pigs** with mulberry heart disease, and **horses** with African horse sickness.

Haemothorax

Haemothorax is presence of **blood in the thoracic cavity**, but the term has been used for exudates with a blood component. **Causes** include rupture of a major blood vessel as a result of severe trauma (e.g., hit by a car), erosion of a vascular wall by malignant cells or inflammation (e.g., arteritis caused by *Spirocerca lupi*), or ruptured aortic aneurysm, clotting defects, disseminated intravascular coagulation (consumption coagulopathy), and bone marrow suppression. **Haemothorax is usually acute and fatal. Grossly,** the thoracic cavity is filled with blood and lungs are partially or completely atelectatic.

Chylothorax

Chylothorax is **accumulation of chyle** (lymph rich in triglycerides) **in the thoracic cavity.** It is due to rupture of major lymph vessels, usually the thoracic duct or the right lymph duct. The clinical and pathological effects of chylothorax are similar to those of other pleural effusions. **Causes** include neoplasia, trauma, congenital lymph vessel anomalies, and iatrogenic (physician-induced) rupture of thoracic duct during surgery. The source of the leakage of chyle is rarely found at postmortem.

Inflammation of the Pleura

Inflammation of the pleura is called **pleuritis** or **pleurisy.** According to the type of exudate, pleuritis can be **fibrinous, suppurative, granulomatous, haemorrhagic, or a combination of exudates.** When suppurative pleuritis causes accumulation of purulent exudate in the cavity, the condition is called **pyothorax** or **thoracic empyema. Clinically,** pleuritis causes pain, and empyema can result in severe toxaemia. **Pleural adhesions** and **fibrosis** are the most common sequelae of chronic pleuritis and interfere with inflation of the lungs.

Pleuritis can occur as part of pneumonia, particularly in fibrinous bronchopneumonia (pleuropneumonia), **or it can occur alone without lung involvement.** For example, bovine and ovine pasteurellosis and porcine and bovine pleuropneumonia are examples of pleuritis associated with fibrinous bronchopneumonias. On the other hand, polyserositis in pigs and pleural empyema in cats and horses are examples in which pleuritis occurs alone and is not associated with involvement of the lungs. **Pleuritis is mostly caused by bacteria.** These may reach the pleural surface haematogenously, as in bacteraemia causing polyserositis. This type of **polyserositis** is caused by *Haemophilus parasuis* (Glasser's disease), *Streotococcus suis* type II and *Pasteurella multocida* in **pigs**, *Streprococcus equi* and *Streptococcus zooepidemicus* in **horses**, *Escherichia coli* in **calves**, and **Mycoplasma** sp. and **Haemophilus** sp. in **sheep** and **goats**. Deposition of bacteria on the pleural surface can be the result of an extension of a septic process, for example, puncture wounds of the thoracic wall, traumatic reticulo-pericarditis, and ruptured pulmonary abscesses (e.g., *Arcanobacterium pyogenes* in **cattle**

In **dogs** and **cats**, bacteria such as **Nocardia, Actinomyces,** and **Bacteroides,** can cause **pyogranulomatous pleuritis** which is characterized by accumulation of blood-stained pus ('tomato soup') in the thoracic cavity. This exudate usually contains yellow flecks called **'sulphur granules'**. Many bacteria such as *E. coli, A. pyogenes, P. multocida,* and *Fusobacterium necrophorum* may be present in **pyothorax** of **dogs** and **cats**. Pyogranulomatous pleuritis with empyema occur sometimes in **dogs**.

Cats with **non-effusive ('dry') form of feline infectious peritonitis** have pyogranulomatous pleuritis, whereas in cats with **'effusive' ('wet') form**, the thoracic involvement is of a pleural effusion.

Pleuritis is also important in **horses**. *Nocardia asteroides* and *Nocardia brasiliensis* can cause fibrino-purulent pneumonia and pyothorax with characteristic sulphur granules.

Neoplasms

Pleura is often involved in neoplasms that have metastasized from other organs to the lungs. **Mesothelioma** is the only primary neoplasm of the pleura.

Mesothelioma

This is a rare neoplasm of the thoracic, pericardial, and peritoneal mesothelium **in the domestic animals.** It is mostly seen in **calves**, in which it can be congenital. No association with inhalation of asbestos fibres has been established in animals, unlike human beings. The **cause** in animals remains unknown. **Clinically**, in animals there may be pleural effusion with resulting respiratory distress, cough, and weight loss.

Grossly, mesothelioma appears as **multiple nodules** on the pleural surface. **Microscopically,** neoplasms can appear as a carcinoma or as a fibrosarcoma. **Although considered malignant, mesotheliomas rarely metastasize.**

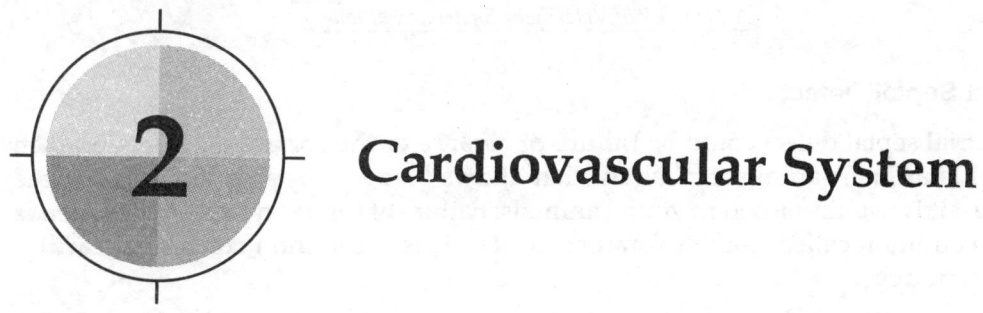

Cardiovascular System

Heart

Congenital Anomalies

Animals with extreme defects are unable to survive in uterus. Those with mild lesions have no clinical signs of disease during life. But animals with defects of intermediate severity come to veterinarian because they gradually develop signs of cardiac failure. The most commonly observed cardiovascular anomalies in domestic animals are presented in **Table 4.**

Table 4. Most common cardiovascular anomalies in domestic animals

Dog	Cow
Patent ductus arteriosus	Atrial septal defect
Pulmonic stenosis	Ventricular septal defect
Subaortic stenosis	Transposition of aorta
Persistent right aortic arch	Pulmonary artery valvular haematomas
Cat	Pig
Endocardial cushion defects	Subaortic stenosis
Mitral malformation	Endocardial cushion defect

Anomalies from Failure of Closure of Foetal Cardiovascular Shunts

Patent Ductus Arteriosus

Ductus arteriosus is a blood vessel in the foetus that connects pulmonary artery directly to aorta, thus bypassing the pulmonary circulation. It normally closes after birth. Failure of the ductus to close leads to a condition called '**patent ductus arteriosus**'. That is, lumen of the ductus arteriosus remains open and blood continues to be shunted from aorta to the pulmonary artery. Generally, blood is shunted from the left to the right ventricle (**left-to-right shunt**). This leads to pulmonary hypertension and congestive heart failure. It is a congenital cardiac defect of man and animals, **particularly dogs. Female dogs have a greater incidence.**

Atrial Septal Defect

An atrial septal defect could be **failure of closure of the foramen ovale.** Foramen ovale is an inter-atrial septal shunt that allows blood to bypass the lungs of the foetus. It is usually closed in young animals. Failure of foramen ovale to close leads to a condition called **'patent foramen ovale'.** It is a common congenital cardiac defect in **dogs.**

Atrial septal defects are tolerated well if they are less than 1 cm in diameter. Small defects in the septum may persist into adult life without significant defect on the health of the animal. Even larger defects do not constitute serious problems during the first years of life, when the low pressure flow is from left to right. Eventually, however, the defect produces continued overload of the right side of the heart due to blood flowing through the foramen ovale into the right atrium. Hypertrophy of the right heart and pulmonary hypertension may result. Should pressure in the right side of the heart exceed that of the left, mixture of venous blood into the aorta may lead to **cyanosis,** and possibly **cardiac failure.**

Ventricular Septal Defect

A ventricular septal defect is failure of complete development of the inter-ventricular septum. This allows shunting of the blood between the ventricles. The defect occurs in many species, **particularly dogs.** The **clinical significance** of a ventricular septal defect depends on its size. Small openings connecting the two ventricles are of no consequence, since defects smaller than 0.5 cm in diameter tend to close spontaneously, or are well tolerated for years. Larger defects remain patent (open) and permit a significant **left-to-right flow.** In some cases, continued overload of the right heart and pulmonary hypertension may lead to reversed flow of blood from the right into left ventricle, resulting in cyanosis.

Tetralogy of Fallot

Fallot, a French physician, described a complicated congenital anomaly of the heart in children ('blue babies') known as **'Tetralogy of Fallot'.** The anomaly is characterized by four defects and include: (1) inter-ventricular septal defect, (2) pulmonic stenosis (see below), and (3) dextroposition of the aorta. The fourth defect develops secondarily and is hypertrophy of the right ventricle. The condition is reported in **dogs** as an inherited disease. It results in severe cyanosis. The basic defect has been found to be hypoplasia and malposition of the conotruncal septum (i.e., septum relating to the conus arteriosus and truncus arteriosus).

Anomalies from Failure of Normal Valvular Development

Pulmonic Stenosis

Stenosis (G. narrowing) is constriction or narrowing of a passage or orifice, and is usually caused by fusion of the cusps. When occlusion of the lumen is partial it is called 'stenosis'; when complete 'atresia'.

Several types of valvular lesions have been described. These include formation of a band of fibrous or muscular tissue beneath the valve (**sub-valvular stenosis**) or malformation of the valve (**valvular stenosis**), with a small central orifice in the thickened valvular tissue. The resulting pressure overload leads to marked hypertrophy of the right ventricle. **Pulmonic stenosis is mostly seen in dogs.**

Subaortic Stenosis

This cardiac anomaly is mostly seen in **pigs** and **dogs. In dogs**, it appears to be an inherited condition. The stenosis is produced by the presence of a thick zone of endocardial fibrous tissue, which forms a circle around the left outflow tract below the valve. Other cardiac lesions develop as a result of the altered left ventricular outflow, such as ventricular hypertrophy and foci of myocardial necrosis.

Valvular Haematomas (Haematocysts)

These lesions are usually seen on the atrio-ventricular valves of **young ruminants.** They generally regress spontaneously when animals are several months of age and do not produce any functional abnormalities. Lesions are blood-filled cysts on the edge of the atrio-ventricular valves.

Other valvular developmental anomalies include **endocardial cushion defects** (persistent atrio-ventricular canal) in **pigs** and **cats**, **mitral dysplasia** in **cats** and **dogs**, and **tricuspid dysplasia** in **cats** and **dogs**.

Anomalies from Malposition of Great Vessels

Persistent Right Aortic Arch

This condition occurs in **dogs**. The defect occurs because the right fourth aortic arch, rather than the left, develops and goes up on the right side of the midline so that the ligamentum arteriosum forms a vascular ring over the oesophagus and trachea. This arrangement finally leads to oesophageal obstruction and proximal dilatation (megaoesophagus) as the animal matures and consumes solid feed.

Transposition of the Aorta and Pulmonary Artery

Transpositions (displacements) are a group of several malformations, in which the aorta and pulmonary artery may be displaced. The aorta may arise from the right ventricle, and the pulmonary artery from the left (ventricle). This may simply be a shift in position. That is, the right ventricle becomes the arterial side of the heart, receiving blood from the left atrium, and the left ventricle becomes the venous side, receiving blood from the right atrium. The right ventricle becomes hypertrophic, but in the absence of other anomalies, functionally normal circulation is maintained. In another form of displacement, the aorta arises from the right ventricle and the pulmonary artery from the left ventricle. However, the right ventricle remains the venous side and the left ventricle the arterial side. This results in two separate and unconnected circulations which are not compatible with life. During foetal life the foramen ovale and ductus arteriosus allow mixing of two circulations.

Sometimes the aorta and pulmonary artery fail to divide, resulting in a single large vessel receiving blood from both the right and left ventricles. The condition is known as **persistent truncus arteriosus.** Less commonly, the aorta and pulmonary artery may both arise from the right ventricle – **double outlet right ventricle. Transposition of aorta and pulmonary arteries are among the most common cardiac anomalies in cattle.**

Other Cardiac Anomalies

Acardia is congenital absence of the heart.

Diplocardia is having a double heart.

Ectopia Cordis

This is a rare condition in which the entire heart lies outside the thoracic cavity. Usually the heart is found in the neck region, or in the abdominal cavity. In **cattle**, cases in the healthy adult animals have been described. The heart was found located subcutaneously in the caudo-ventral neck area. The anomaly in cattle is always fatal.

Endocardial Fibroelastosis

This condition has been described in **cats** as a primary cardiac defect. In this heritable disease, the heart has white, thickened endocardium due to proliferation of fibroelastic tissue. Usually the left ventricle is affected.

Peritoneo-Pericardial Diaphragmatic Hernias

These occur in **dogs** due to incomplete development of the diaphragm. Abdominal viscera can be found in the pericardial sac.

Circulatory Disturbances

Haemorrhage

This is the most common lesion of the epicardium, endocardium, and myocardium. Haemorrhages vary in size, and may be petechiae, ecchymoses, or suffusion. **Animals** dying from septicaemia, endotoxaemia, or anoxia have prominent epicardial and endocardial haemorrhages. **Horses** dying from any cause usually have agonal haemorrhages on the epicardial and endocardial surfaces. **In growing pigs,** cardiac haemorrhages are seen in **mulberry heart disease** associated with selenium-vitamin E deficiency. In these **pigs,** hydropericardium is associated with severe myocardial haemorrhage which causes a red, mottled (mulberry-like) appearance of the heart.

Cardiac Failure

The heart has a remarkable ability to accommodate itself to pathological changes. This ability to maintain circulation under diseased conditions is known as **compensation**. When there is a slowly developing continuous hindrance to circulation, or to heart's action, the myocardium hypertrophies in order to maintain adequate circulation. When the organ becomes fatigued and compensation can no longer occur, **decompensation**, that is, failure of compensation results.

Cardiac failure is the inability of the heart to maintain adequate circulation. It is a leading cause of deaths in humans, owing to the high incidence of coronary vascular disease, particularly atherosclerosis and resultant myocardial infarction. Although domestic animals may develop coronary vascular disease, **the frequency and severity do not approach the proportions seen in man.** Other mechanisms also lead to heart failure in man and domestic animals. Heart failure is the usual immediate cause of death in many acute infectious diseases and poisonings.

Acute Cardiac Failure

Acute cardiac failure results from a sudden stoppage of effective cardiac contraction, and may cause death even within minutes. It may result from anoxia, the action of certain drugs or poisons, myocardial necrosis (especially of the conducting system), shock, cardiac tamponade, or sudden occlusions of the pulmonary artery or aorta. It may also follow repeated chronic injury to the myocardium. In the absence of a primary lesion such as cardiac tamponade, or an occlusive thrombus, the lesions of acute failure are minimal. Pulmonary and/or systemic congestion may be prominent. Oedema is not a feature because of the acute failure of the circulation.

The right and/or left ventricles may be acutely dilated, that is, **acute dilatation of the heart.** This is a pathological enlargement of one or more of the cardiac chambers, mostly of the **right ventricle**. The left ventricle, because of its thicker wall, offers more resistance to dilatation, the atria expand less noticeably. Cardiac dilatation is recognized by a rounded bulging of one or both ventricles. The line from the atrio-ventricular level to the apex, which normally is almost straight, assumes an outward curvature. The muscular wall is flabby and flexible.

Chronic Heart Failure (Congestive Heart Failure, CHF)

Chronic heart failure, more commonly referred to as **congestive heart failure,** occurs when the heart cannot maintain an output adequate for the metabolic needs of the tissues and organs of the body. Serious heart diseases lead to failure either because they decrease the capacity of the myocardium to contract owing to some intrinsic damage to myocytes, or because they damage the ability of the heart to accommodate the volume of venous return. Whatever its basis, **CHF is characterized** by **diminished cardiac output** (**systolic** or **forward failure**), or damming back (i.e. holding back or blocking) of the blood in the venous system (**diastolic** or **backward failure**), or both.

Although diminished myocardial contraction is the cause of heart failure, there is no clear understanding at the biomolecular level of the basis for the contractile failure. A variety of compensatory mechanisms come into operation. Decreased cardiac output and failure of the ventricles to empty lead to dilatation and stretching of the myofibres. Although these changes increase contractility of the heart, **they ultimately lead to myocardial hypertrophy**, and impose new burdens. **Eventually failure occurs.** Thus, **at necropsy** the heart is often dilated and usually hypertrophied. But these changes also may be present in a **'compensated heart'**. It is therefore impossible from examination of the heart alone to differentiate the damaged organ from one that has compensated. The definitive (conclusive) morphological changes of CHF are found away from the heart, and are produced by the hypoxic and congestive effect of the failing circulation upon other organs and tissues.

Although the heart is a single organ, to some extent it acts as two distinct anatomical and functional units. Under various pathological stresses one side may fail before the other, so that from the clinical point of view, **left-sided and right-sided failure may occur separately.** Because the vascular system is a closed circuit, failure of one side cannot exist for long without eventually producing excessive strain upon the other, **terminating in total heart failure.** It is helpful to consider failure of each side separately.

Left-Sided Heart Failure

Left-sided heart failure is usually caused by: (1) myocardial diseases, (2) aortic and mitral valve disease, (3) various congenital defects, or (4) hypertension. Hypertension is particularly common in man, but is much less frequent in animals. Apart from the primary myocardial disease, **the most striking pathological changes are in the lungs.**

Lungs

As the left ventricle fails to keep pace with the venous return from the lungs, pressure in the pulmonary veins increases and is ultimately transmitted to the alveolar capillaries. **Pulmonary congestion and oedema result.** The congestion first leads to the development of a perivascular transudate. In time, it overflows into the alveoli (**pulmonary oedema**). As a result of alveolar haemorrhages, haemosiderin-laden macrophages, termed as **'heart failure cells'** appear in the alveolar spaces. Long persistence of septal oedema often induces fibrosis within the alveolar walls, which together with the accumulation of haemosiderin produce **brown induration of the lungs.**

These anatomical changes account for the major manifestations of left-sided failure, namely, dyspnoea (difficult breathing) and short of breath. Cough is common in left-sided failure.

Right-Sided Heart Failure

Right-sided heart failure is usually a consequence of left-sided failure, because any increase in pulmonary circulation following left-sided failure produces an increased burden on the right side of the heart. The causes of right-sided failure therefore include all those that create left-sided heart failure, particularly **mitral stenosis** or **congenital left-to-right shunts**, which produces great increases in pulmonary pressure. However, right-sided failure may occur in relatively **'pure'** form with primary disease of the lung or pulmonary vasculature that increases resistance to the pulmonary circulation – **cor pulmonale.** In such a case the right ventricle is burdened by increased resistance within the pulmonary circulation. **Dilatation of the heart is confined to the right ventricle. Cor pulmonale** is hypertrophy or failure of right ventricle resulting from intrinsic disease of the lungs or pulmonary vasculature. Emphysema (**'heaves'** in **horses**) and chronic interstitial pneumonia also cause pure form of right-sided failure.

The lesions of pure right-sided failure differ from those of left-sided failure in that pulmonary congestion is minimal, whereas engorgement of the systemic venous and portal circulation is more pronounced. **The major organs affected are the liver, kidneys, spleen, and the entire portal area of venous drainage.** The lungs do not become congested or develop the lesions described in left-sided failure.

Liver

The liver is slightly increased in size and weight, and on sectioning displays a characteristic **'nutmeg pattern'** (**'nutmeg liver'**). The nutmeg liver is the result of **chronic passive congestion**, which leads to persistent hypoxia in centrilobular areas. Because of the oxygen and nutrient deficiency, the centrilobular hepatocytes atrophy, degenerate, and finally undergo necrosis. As a result, sinusoids in these areas are dilated and congested and grossly appearred. In contrast, the peripheral hepatocytes usually undergo fatty change (lipidosis) because of hypoxia. Therefore, this area of the lobule appears **yellow**. The result is markedly increased lobular pattern of the liver, which is especially noticeable on its cut surface. This increased lobular pattern, which occurs following chronic passive congestion, strikingly resembles the cut surface of a nutmeg and is therefore called **'nutmeg liver'**. If the patient does not die of the cardiac failure, chronic passive congestion of the liver ultimately leads to **fibrosis**, creating so-called **cardiac cirrhosis** or **cardiac sclerosis**.

Kidneys

Congestion and hypoxia of the kidneys are more marked with right-sided heart failure than with left, leading to greater fluid retention and peripheral oedema.

Spleen

Acute congestion produces an enlarged spleen that is tense and cyanotic, following marked sinusoidal dilatation and foci of haemorrhage. With chronic congestion there is greater enlargement caused by fibrous thickening of the distended sinusoidal wall – **congestive splenomegaly.** The areas of previous haemorrhage now change to haemosiderin deposits.

Clinically, the increased venous pressure causes some degree of peripheral oedema of dependent portions of the body. It may be severe enough to produce **anasarca**. Right-sided failure may eventually lead to portal hypertension with splenic congestion. This causes abnormal accumulation of transudate in the peritoneal cavity (**ascites**), and congestion of the gut. Oedema is seen mainly as ventral subcutaneous oedema in **horses** and **ruminants**, ascites in **dogs**, and hydrothorax in **cats**.

In summary, right-sided heart failure presents essentially as a venous congestive syndrome with hepatic and splenic enlargement, peripheral oedema, and ascites. **In contrast to left-sided failure, respiratory symptoms may be absent or quite insignificant.**

Pericardial Diseases

Accumulations of Fluid in the Pericardial Sac

Hydropericardium

Hydropericardium is the accumulation of clear to light yellow, watery, **serous fluid in the pericardial sac,** which gets distended. The amount of fluid may be increased from 100 to 200 times. The term **'pericardial effusion'** is used mostly in **man**. In cases associated with vascular injury, such as **'mulberry heart disease'** of **pigs** a few fibrin strands are present and the fluid may clot following exposure to air (Fig. 7).

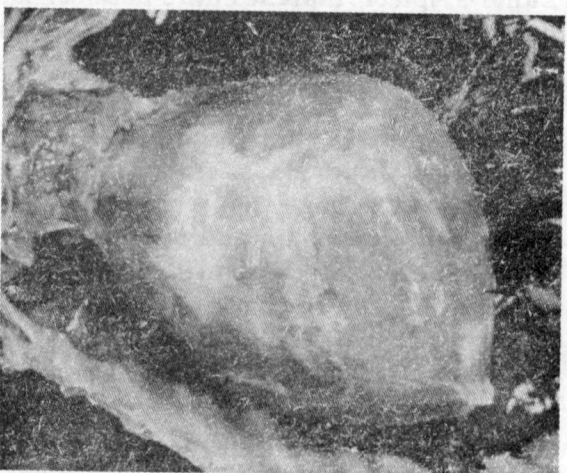

Fig. 7. **Pericardial sac, hydropericardium. Pig. 'Mulberry heart disease'.** The thin-walled pericardial sac (black arrowheads) is distended by serous fluid that has strands of fibrin.

Causes of hydropericardium include those diseases that have generalized oedema; cardiac and nutritional oedema being more important than renal oedema. The effect is to interfere with flow of venous blood returning to the heart. Thus, ascites and hydrothorax often occur together with hydropericardium. Congestive heart failure is an important cause. In animals, it is usually due to primary myocardial, valvular, congenital, or neoplastic diseases. Common specific disease examples include dilated cardiopathy of **dogs** and **cats**, and **'ascites syndrome'** of **poultry**. Hydropericardium may also accompany pulmonary hypertension (e.g. **'brisket disease'** or **'high altitude disease'** of **cattle**), chronic diffuse pulmonary alveolar emphysema (**'heaves'** of **horses**), renal failure, and hypoproteinaemia from various chronic debilitating diseases, including parasitic infestations such as stomach worms in sheep. It may also occur in various systemic diseases with vascular injury, such as septicaemia in **pigs**, **'heartwater'** (rickettsial *Cowdria ruminantium* infection) in **small ruminants**, African horse sickness, and bovine ephemeral fever.

The serosal surfaces are smooth and glistening in acute cases. In chronic cases, the epicardium becomes opaque because of mild fibrous thickening. It appears roughened and granular when there is villous proliferation of fibrous tissue.

Hydropericardium of rapid onset and of sufficient volume leads to the development of **cardiac tamponade** or compression, which interferes with cardiac filling (especially of the atria) and venous return to the heart. In cases with slow development, stretching of the pericardium allows accumulation of a large volume of fluid **without tamponade**. Hydropericardium can be reversible if the underlying cause is removed. **But many cases are associated with progressive cardiac diseases, and death is the outcome.**

Haemopericardium

Haemopericardium is accumulation of **blood** in the pericardial sac. It is caused by trauma (foreign bodies), spontaneous rupture, and dilatation and rupture of the coronary artery. Bleeding in **dogs** may be the result of spontaneous rupture of an atrial or myocardial wall, or from rupture of the intrapericardial aorta in **horses** and **cattle**, or may be a complication of intra-cardiac injections. The blood that escapes fills the sac rapidly under greatly increased pressure and produces **cardiac tamponade. Cardiac tamponade often causes death.** The sudden accumulation of blood in large amounts will so compress the heart it prevents diastole, **and cardiac failure results.** As little as 200-300 ml of blood may be sufficient to cause death. However, if the blood accumulates gradually, the heart gets time to compensate and great amounts of blood may collect before death occurs.

Pyopericardium

Pyopericardium is accumulation of **pus** in the pericardial sac. It is commonly observed in **cattle** affected with **traumatic pericarditis**. Sometimes in cattle, gas produced by bacteria in the exudate accumulates causing distension of the pericardial sac and compression of the heart.

Pneumopericadium

Pneumopericardium is the presence of **air** in the pericardial sac, and is rare.

Metabolic Alterations

Serous Atrophy of Fat

This condition is easily identified by the grey gelatinous appearance of epicardial fat deposits. Healthy animals normally have white or yellow epicardial fat deposits. **Microscopically**, lipocytes are atrophic and oedema fluid is present in interstitial tissues. Serous atrophy of fat occurs rapidly during anorexia, starvation, or cachexia.

Urate Deposits

Urate deposits on the **pericardium** occur **in birds with visceral gout.** The affected serosal surface appears thickened and white.

Inflammation

Pericarditis is inflammation of the pericardium. It includes inflammation of both parietal and visceral surfaces of the pericardial cavity. The exudate formed accumulates in the pericardial sac. Pericarditis is almost always infectious and exudative. The source of infection is nearly always haematogenous except when it enters by direct extension, as in **'traumatic pericarditis'** of **cattle.**

The **causes** include: (1) trauma (foreign bodies penetrating from the reticulum), and (2) infection. The origin of the latter is either (a) haematogenous, or (b) by extension from the myocardium, pleura, bronchial and mediastinal lymph nodes, or stomach. The **classification** of pericarditis is usually based on the character of the exudate: **fibrinous** or **suppurative.**

Fibrinous Pericarditis

Fibrinous pericarditis, the most common type of pericardial inflammation in animals is usually the result of haematogenous infection. Specific diseases include pasteurellosis, blackquarter, coliform septicaemia, and bovine encephalomyelitis in the **cattle**; streptococcal infections, pasteurellosis, enzootic mycoplasmal pneumonia, salmonellosis, and Glasser's disease (*Haemophilus parasuis* infection) in the **pig**; streptococcal infections in the **horse**; and psittacosis in **birds.**

Grossly, the pericardial surfaces are covered by variable amounts of yellow fibrin deposits. This can result in the adherence of parietal and visceral layers. **At necropsy,** when the pericardial sac is opened, these attachments are torn away (so-called **'bread-and-butter pericarditis'** or **'bread-and-butter heart'**). **Microscopically,** an eosinophilic layer of fibrin containing neutrophils lies over a congested pericardium.

The **outcome** varies. Early death is common because many of these cases result from infection by highly virulent bacteria and concurrent septicaemia. When the animal survives, in time, fibrous adhesions form between the pericardial surfaces after fibrous organization of the exudate.

Suppurative Pericarditis

Suppurative pericarditis is seen mainly in **cattle** as a complication of traumatic reticulo-peritonitis (**'hardware disease'**), that is, **traumatic pericarditis.** Foreign bodies, such as nails or pieces of wire that accumulate in the reticulum, sometimes penetrate reticulum and diaphragm, and enter into the pericardial sac and introduce infection. Some affected **cattle** survive for weeks to months until death occurs from congestive heart failure and septicaemia. If the animal survives, organization of exudate occurs. **Adhesions** are then present between the epicardium and pericardium.

Grossly, the pericardial surfaces are greatly thickened by white, rough masses of fibrous connective tissue, which enclose white to grey thick, foul-smelling, purulent exudate. Organization is the usual **outcome.** Resolution is uncommon. The organization produces **constrictive pericarditis.**

Traumatic Pericarditis

This is a disease of cattle and buffaloes. Cattle may swallow nails, bits of wire, and similar hardware as a result of their feeding habits. Many of these sharp metallic objects penetrate the wall of the reticulum and slowly move forward. The direction that the foreign body travels is usually antero-ventral, through the diaphragm and pleura, into the pericardium and heart. Carrying common pathogenic bacteria with them, they initiate acute infectious pericarditis. The **exudate** is mostly **fibrinous** or **fibrino-purulent** in nature and in large amounts. **Cattle** usually live for a number of days or weeks. Therefore, exudate has time to become organized. Rarely the foreign body perforates a coronary artery or the heart, leading to fatal haemorrhage known as **cardiac tamponade** (see 'haemopericardium'). If the foreign body travels in a different direction, **peritonitis** surrounding the reticulum, the adjacent forestomachs, and abomasums occurs (see 'traumatic reticulitis').

A common finding at postmortem examination is **cor rugosum** (L. cor = heart; rugosum = wrinkled, corrugated), or **'shaggy heart'** (i. e. having a rough surface). Such a heart is covered with a layer of white or blood-tinged fibrin, the deeper part of which is organized into vascular fibrous tissue. The organizing fibrin, in time, reaches from the epicardial to the outer pericardial surface, joining the two surfaces firmly - **adhesive pericarditis.** Such an exudate exerts pressure, and if adhesive, it tends to immobilize the heart. In spite of attempts at compensatory hypertrophy, the mechanical interference and toxic effect of the pathogenic organisms and their products **eventually bring about heart failure and death.**

Lesions are those of chronic venous congestion or of toxaemia. The granulation tissue, with its fistulous tract extending from the reticulum and diaphragm, may be extensive or thin. The wire or similar object may still be present, extending into or through the wall of the pericardial sac and at times penetrating into the myocardium itself at time of death. On the other hand, iron may rust and dissolve into body fluids and disintegrate completely before death occurs. Only the narrow sinus tract, its lining blackened by iron sulphide, may remain as evidence.

Constrictive Pericarditis

Constrictive pericarditis is a chronic inflammatory lesion of the pericardium. It is associated with extensive fibrous proliferation and ultimately formation of fibrous adhesions between the surfaces of the visceral and parietal pericardium. Severe lesions destroy the pericardial sac and constrict the heart by fibrous tissue, and can interfere with cardiac filling. Compensatory myocardial hypertrophy can result in reduced volume of the ventricular chambers and lead to congestive cardiac failure.

Myocardial Diseases

Growth Disturbances

Hypertrophy

Hypertrophy of the myocardium is **an increase in muscle mass.** This is due to an increase in the size of cardiac muscle cells. Hypertrophy is **generally secondary,** and occurs as a compensatory response to increased workload. It is usually reversible on removal of the cause. However, primary hypertrophy also occurs in **cats** and **dogs** with idiopathic cardiomyopathy, and is not **reversible.**

Two forms of hypertrophy are recognized. **Eccentric hypertrophy** results in a heart having enlarged ventricular chambers and walls of normal or decreased thickness. It is produced by lesions that increase blood volume load, such as valvular insufficiencies and septal defects. In **concentric hypertrophy** the heart has small ventricular chambers that have thick walls. It results from lesions that increase pressure load, such as valvular stenosis, systemic hypertension, and pulmonary disease.

There are three stages of myocardial hypertrophy: (1) initiation, (2) stable hyperfunction, and (3) deterioration of function associated with degeneration of hypertrophied myocytes. **Microscopically,** in myocardial hypertrophy the myocytes are enlarged and have large nuclei.

Diseases that can cause right ventricular hypertrophy include dirofilariasis (Fig. 8)

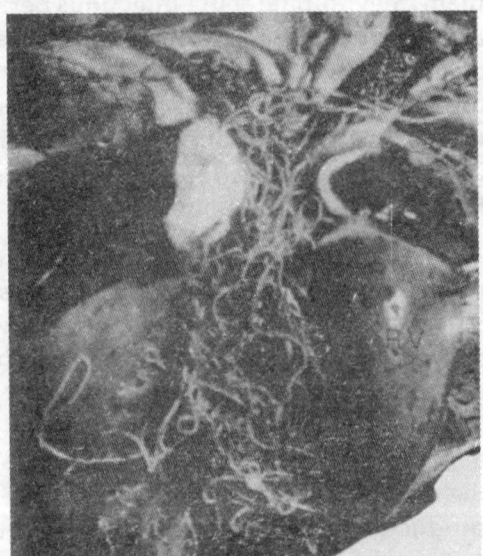

Fig. 8. Heart, opened; Dog. Dirofilariasis. Numerous adult *Dirofilaria immitis* are present in clotted blood in the right ventricle (RV) and pulmonary artery.

and congenital pneumonic stenosis in **dogs**, 'brisket disease' ('high altitude disease') in **cattle**, and chronic alveolar emphysema ('heaves') in **horses. Cattle** kept under hypoxic conditions which exist at altitudes above 700 feet sea level develop pulmonary hypertension and right heart failure with subcutaneous oedema, chronic passive congestion of the liver ('nutmeg liver'), and right ventricular hypertrophy.

Left ventricular hypertrophy occurs in **dogs** with congenital subaortic stenosis.

Infiltration

Fatty Infiltration

Fatty infiltration is the presence of increased numbers of lipocytes (fat cells) between myocardial fibres. The lesion is associated with obesity, and is seen as epicardial and myocardial deposits of adipose tissue in large quantities.

Degeneration

Fatty Change (Fatty Degeneration)

Fatty change is the accumulation of lipid droplets in the myocytes (muscle fibres). **Grossly**, the myocardium is pale and flabby. Moderate hypoxia (e.g. anaemia) produces a **'thrush breast'** (**'thrush breast heart'**) or **'tigered effect'**. Here, the intracellular deposits of fat create bands of yellow myocardium, which alternate with bands of darker, red-brown, uninvolved myocardium. **Microscopically**, affected myocytes have numerous spherical droplets of various sizes which appear as empty vacuoles in paraffin sections, but stain positively for lipids with lipid-soluble stains in frozen sections. Fatty change occurs with systemic disorders such as severe anaemia, toxaemia, and copper deficiency, but is less common in the heart than in the liver and kidneys. The damaged myocardium may lose its ability to contract, and cardiac dilatation is the result. The dilatation may lead to cardiac rupture.

Lipofuscinosis (Brown Atrophy)

This occurs in aged animals and in animals with severe cachexia. It has also been described as a hereditary lesion in certain healthy **cattle.** Affected hearts appear brown (**brown atrophy**), and **microscopically** they show clusters of yellow-brown granules at the nuclear poles of myocytes. These granules are intra-lysosomal accumulation of membranous and amorphous debris (**residual bodies**).

Necrosis

Myocardial necrosis can occur from a number of **causes**. These include nutritional deficiencies, chemical and plant toxins, ischaemia, metabolic disorders, and physical injuries.

Grossly, affected areas appear pale in the beginning. Some progress to prominent yellow to white dry areas made gritty by dystrophic mineralization (calcification). The lesions are focal, multifocal, or diffuse. The most common sites are the left ventricular papillary muscles and the sub-endocardial myocardium. In diseases with diffuse cardiac necrosis, such as **white muscle disease** of **calves** and **lambs** due to selenium-vitamin E deficiency, the pale lesions can be easily seen on the epicardial and endothelial surfaces.

Microscopically, fibres in areas of recent necrosis appear swollen and hyper-eosinophilic (**hyaline necrosis**). Striations are indistinct, and nuclei are pyknotic. Necrotic fibres contain basophilic granules which are calcified mitochondria. This can be confirmed by electron microscopy.

Within 24 to 48 hours after injury, necrotic areas are infiltrated by inflammatory cells, mainly macrophages and a few neutrophils. These phagocytose and lyse the necrotic cellular debris. **Healing** is characterized by proliferation of connective tissue cells (fibroblasts and capillary endothelial cells) and by deposition of connective tissue (collagen and elastic tissue, and acid mucopolysaccharides). **Grossly**, these areas appear as white, firm, contracted scars.

The **outcome** of myocardial necrosis varies depending on the extent of the damage: (1) Animals may die of acute cardiac failure if the damage is extensive, (2) Early deaths from necrosis-related arrhythmias also occur when cardiac conduction is disrupted, and (3) Some animals develop cardiac decompensation and die with cardiac dilatation and lesions of chronic congestive failure.

Mineralization

Myocardial mineralization (**calcification**) is an important feature in several diseases, such as vitamin E-selenium deficiency in **sheep** and **cattle**, vitamin D toxicity in several species, calcinogenic plant toxicosis in **cattle** ('**Manchester wasting disease'**), and spontaneous calcification in **aged rats** and **guinea pigs.**

Calcification occurs in epicardium, myocardium, and endocardium, and is most common in the wall of the left ventricle. The calcium appears as yellow to white, dry, gritty masses. For calcification to occur there must first be necrotic or degenerating tissue. It is therefore observed following coagulative necrosis of the myocardium. **Electron microscopically**, scattered basophilic granules within the necrotic fibres represent mitochondrial accumulations of calcium salts.

Inflammation

Myocarditis

Myocarditis is usually the result of infections spread haematogenously to the myocardium, and occurs in various systemic diseases. Types of inflammation caused by infectious agents that produce myocarditis include **suppurative, necrotizing, haemorrhagic, lymphocytic,** and **eosinophilic**.

Suppurative myocarditis occurs from localization of pyogenic bacteria in the myocardium. These usually originate from the vegetations of vegetative valvular endocarditis on the mitral and aortic valves. **Grossly,** pale, disseminated lesions are present in the myocardium. These foci consist of neutrophils and necrotic myocytes that form abscesses.

Necrotizing myocarditis is a common lesion of toxoplasmosis, a common disease of **cats** and **dogs. Haemorrhagic myocarditis** occurs along with the haemorrhagic inflammation found in skeletal muscle of **cattle** with **blackquarter** (blackleg) caused by *Clostridium chauvoei.* **Lymphocytic myocarditis** is usually seen in viral infections, such as parvoviral myocarditis of **puppies. Dogs** with parvoviral myocarditis die unexpectedly and show lesions of acute congestive heart failure. However, there are no lesions in the intestine, the primary site of viral damage in about 95% of clinical cases. The heart is pale and flabby and has interstitial lymphocytic infiltrations, myocytes with large basophilic, intranuclear viral inclusion bodies, and in **dogs** that survive **fibrosis. Eosinophilic myocarditis** is the result of some parasitic infections, such as sarcocystosis. The various infectious diseases that cause myocarditis in animals are presented in **Table 5.**

Table 5. Diseases that cause myocarditis in animals

Viral

Canine parvovirus, encephlomyocarditis, foot-and-mouth disease, pseudorabies, canine distemper, cytomegalovirus, Newcastle disease (Ranikhet disease), avian encephalomyelitis, Eastern and Western equine encephalomyelitis

Bacterial

Blackquarter (*Clostridium chauvoei*), listeriosis (*Listeria monocytogenes*), necro-bacillosis (*Fusobacterium necrophorum*), tuberculosis (**Mycobacterium** sp.), caseous lymphadenitis (*Corynebacterium pseudotuberculosis*), disseminated infections by *Actinobacillus equuli,* **Staphylococcus** sp., *Pseudomonas aeruginosa,* and *Streptococcus pneumoniae*

Protozoan

Toxoplasmosis (*Toxoplasma gondii*), sarcocystosis (**Sarcocystis** sp.), trypanosomiasis (Chagas' disease (*Trypanosoma cruzi*)

Parasitic

Cysticercosis (*Cysticercus cellulosae*),Trichinosis (**Trichinella** sp.)

Idiopathic

Eosinophilic myocarditis

The outcome of myocarditis include: (1) complete resolution of lesions, (2) randomly spread residual myocardial scars, or (3) more myocardial damage with cardiac failure.

Endocardial Diseases

Endocardial Mineralization and Endocardial Fibrosis

These occur singly or together. Mineralization (**calcification**) occurs from excessive intake of vitamin D and from intoxication by calcinogenic plants that contain vitamin D analogues. These plants induce syndromes in **cattle**, which have been called by different names in different parts of the world. Multiple, large, white, rough, firm plaques of mineralized fibroelastic tissue are present in the endocardium and intima of large elastic arteries.

Valvular Endocardiosis

This disease occurs in **old dogs** and is associated with degeneration of valvular collagen. It is the most common cause of congestive heart failure in old dogs and may have a genetic basis. Lesions usually occur on the mitral valve. **Affected valves are shortened and thickened.** These lesions result in valvular insufficiency. **Microscopically,** the thickened valves have greatly increased fibroelastic proliferation and deposition of acid mucopolysaccharides.

Circulatory Disturbances

Endocardial haemorrhages are the only important circulatory disturbances. They are more common than epicardial, and occur more often in the left ventricle than in other heart chambers. They may exert pressure on the impulse-conducting system (bundle of His) and may induce a disturbance of the rhythmic beating of the heart. **Atrial thrombosis** may be present in the failing hearts of **dogs** and **cats** with idiopathic cardiomyopathies.

Inflammation

Endocarditis

Endocarditis is inflammation of the endocardium. It is usually the result of bacterial infections, exceptions being migrating *Strongylus vulgaris* larvae in **horses** and sometimes of mycotic infection. The lesions are mostly present on the valves (**valvular endocarditis**), or may even extend to the adjacent wall (**mural endocarditis**). Grossly, the affected valves have large, adhering, friable, yellow to grey masses of fibrin called **'vegetations'** that obstruct the valvular orifice. **In chronic cases,** the fibrin deposits are organized by fibrous connective tissue to produce irregular nodular masses called **'verrucae'** (wart-like lesions). **Microscopically,** the lesions consist of layers of fibrin and numerous bacterial colonies. Below the bacterial colonies, is a zone of leukocytes and granulation tissue. The relative frequency of valvular involvement with endocarditis **in animals** is mitral, aortic, tricuspid, and pulmonary.

The **pathogenesis** of endocarditis is complicated and mostly not clearly understood. Affected animals usually have pre-existing infections outside the heart that have already caused one or more bouts of bacteraemia. Focal endocardial damage on the surface of the normally avascular valves allows bacteria to stick, proliferate, and initiate an inflammatory reaction which results in deposition of masses of fibrin. Bacteria usually involved in the vegetative lesions are *Actinomyces pyogenes* in **cattle**, **Streptococcus** sp. and *Erysipelothrix rhusiopathiae* in **pigs**, and **Streptococcus** sp. and *E. coli* in **dogs** and **cats**. **Death** occurs from cardiac failure from valvular dysfunction or the effects of bacteraemia. In some animals, septic emboli lodge in organs such as heart and kidneys leading to infarction.

Ulcerative endocarditis of the left atrium is a lesion associated with acute renal insufficiency in **dogs**. **Grossly**, after the ulcer heals, the area is replaced by white plaques of fibrous and mineralized tissue.

Cardiomyopathies

Cardiomyopathy is a disorder affecting the muscle of the heart. It is of **two types**: (1) primary or idiopathic, and (2) secondary cardiomyopathy.

Primary or Idiopathic Cardiomyopathies

These are progressive cardiac diseases that affect **cats** and **dogs**, and resemble some diseases of human beings. These diseases are divided into three morphologic types: hypertrophic, dilated, and restrictive.

(i) Hypertrophic Cardiomyopathy

This is usually seen in middle-aged **male cats** and sometimes **male dogs**. **Cats** usually have congestive heart failure, and some may show posterior paresis from thrombo-embolism of the caudal abdominal aorta ('saddle thrombosis') due to left atrial thrombosis. Some dogs die unexpectedly as the first clinical sign of the disease. In both **cats** and **dogs**, the hearts are enlarged and have hypertrophy of the left ventricle. **Microscopically**, lesions show prominent disorganization of myocytes.

(ii) Dilated or Congestive Cardiomyopathy

This is an important cause of congestive heart failure in **cats** and **dogs**. Affected cats are usually middle-aged males and dogs are males of large breeds. **At necropsy**, lesions of congestive heart failure are present and the hearts are rounded.

(iii) Restrictive Cardiomyopathy

This is rare and occurs in **cats** as two types of endocardial lesions that cause defective ventricular filling. In one type, the left ventricular endocardium has diffuse fibrosis, whereas in the other numerous bands extend across the left ventricular cavity.

Secondary Cardiomyopathies

Also known as **'specific heart muscle diseases', secondary cardiomyopathies are generalized myocardial diseases of known cause.** The causes include hereditary, nutritional deficiencies, toxic, physical injuries and shock, endocrine disorders, infections, neoplastic infiltration, and systemic hypertension in **cats**. Many are discussed either under degeneration and necrosis of the myocardium, or under myocarditis.

Neoplastic Diseases

Various **primary** and **secondary** neoplasms develop either in or near the heart. The primary neoplasms include rhabdomyoma, rhabdomyosarcoma, schwannoma, and haemangiosarcoma. **Rhabdomyoma** and **rhabdomyosarcomas** are rare in animals and form grey nodules in the myocardium. **Congenital rhabdomyomatosis** in **pigs** is a non-neoplastic hamartoma. **Schwannomas** involve cardiac nerves in **cattle** and appear as single or multiple white nodules.

Cardiac haemangiosarcoma is an important neoplasm of **dogs** and **cats**. They originate either in the heart (**primary**) or by metastasis (**secondary**) from sites such as the spleen. It is usually seen in the right atrium and rarely also involves right ventricle. **Grossly**, red to red-black blood-containing masses are present on the epicardial surface. Rupture produces fatal haemopericardium and cardiac tamponade. **Microscopically**, the neoplasm is composed of scattered, elongated, neoplastic endothelial cells.

Malignant lymphoma (lymphosarcoma) usually occurs in the heart of **cattle**. It can be severe enough to cause death from cardiac failure. Cardiac lesions may also be present in the **dogs** and **cats** with malignant lymphoma. The neoplastic cell infiltration can be diffuse or nodular and involves the myocardium and pericardium. Lymphomatous tissue appears as white masses that resemble deposits of fat (Fig. 9). **Microscopically**, extensive infiltrations of neoplastic lymphocytes are present between myocytes.

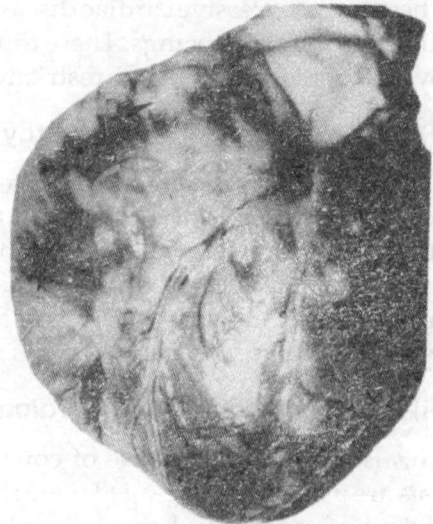

Fig. 9. Heart, myocardium; dog. Lymphosarcoma. Neoplastic infiltration of the ventricular myocardium is seen as numerous white areas.

Heart base tumours are primary neoplasms of extra-cardiac tissue in dogs, but originate at the base of the heart and can produce cardiac obstruction and cardiac failure. The most common neoplasm originating at this location is the aortic **body tumour** or **chemodectoma** (paraganglioma). Certain breeds of **dogs** are commonly affected.

Vascular System

Arterial Diseases

Hyaline Change, Fibrinoid Necrosis and Amyloidosis

These are vascular lesions of small muscular arteries and arterioles and occur in all species. **These lesions are not detected grossly. Microscopically,** in all these lesions there is formation of **a homogeneous eosinophilic area in the wall of vessel.** Special stains reveal three types of deposits: (1) amyloid confirmed by Congo red and methyl violet, (2) **fibrinoid deposits,** positive by the periodic acid-Schiff method, and (3) negative staining of **hyaline deposits** by these stains. **Amyloidosis** and **hyaline degeneration** are observed in small muscular arteries of the myocardium, lungs, and spleen of **old dogs.**

Fibrinoid Necrosis

Fibrinoid necrosis of arteries is associated with endothelial damage. It is characterized by entry and accumulation of serum proteins followed by fibrin deposition in the vessel wall. These materials form an intensely eosinophilic band which destroys cell detail. This lesion is common in many acute degenerative and inflammatory diseases of small arteries and arterioles. It is particularly seen in **pigs** and is an important diagnostic feature in cases of selenium-vitamin E deficiency (heart) and oedema disease (gastric sub-mucosa). Fibrinoid necrosis is seen commonly in **dogs** with uraemia and in **dogs** with hypertension.

In pigs with selenium-vitamin deficiency the vascular lesions produce haemorrhage (**'mulberry heart disease'**) and massive haemorrhagic hepatic necrosis (**'hepatosis dietetica'**). In both, **fibrinoid necrosis** of small muscular arteries and arterioles is widespread and is accompanied by fibrin thrombi in capillaries, especially of the myocardium. The vascular lesions have been called **'dietary microangiopathy'.** Similar capillary lesions and occlusion by fibrin thrombi are seen in the cerebellum of vitamin E-deficient chicks as ischaemia-induced **encephalomalacia** and in the skin and skeletal muscles of selenium-vitamin E-deficient **chicks** with **exudative diathesis.**

Circulatory Disturbances

Thrombosis

Thrombosis is the product of intravascular coagulation during life. Predisposing factors include: (1) endothelial damage, (2) turbulence or stasis of blood flow, and (3) hypercoagulative states. **Endothelial damage** can occur in many arterial diseases. It is present in arteritis, but is not common in degenerative diseases, except fibrinoid necrosis and atherosclerosis. Alterations in blood flow occur in vascular or cardiac valvular lesions that cause **turbulence**, and **stasis** of blood flow in congestive cardiac failure or cardiovascular collapse, as occurs in systemic shock. Hypercoagulative states have occurred in **dogs** with amyloidosis and some types of renal disease.

Examples of arterial thrombosis commonly observed **in animals include** caudal aortic thromboembolism in **cats** and **dogs** with primary cardiomyopathy, thrombosis of mesenteric and intestinal arteries in **horses** with verminous arteritis from strongylosis, thrombosis of the pulmonary arteries in **dogs** with dirofilariasis, and aorto-iliac thrombosis in **horses**. Recently formed mural thrombi appear as yellow, firm masses of fibrin adhered to the arterial intima. Fibroblastic proliferation and organization soon develop in the thrombi.

Thrombosis or **embolism** of the coronary arteries can result in **myocardial infarction** and **cardiac failure**. **These lesions are much less common in animals than in human beings.** Affected animals usually have coronary arterial disease which may be atherosclerosis, arteriosclerosis, or periarteritis. In **atherosclerosis** associated with **hypothyroidism**, severe lesions are present in the epicardial coronary arteries of **dogs**, but this only rarely leads to thrombosis and myocardial infarction. In contrast, severe arteriosclerosis of intramural cardiac arteries in **aged dogs** can cause small multifocal myocardial infarcts.

Disseminated intravascular coagulation (DIC) brought about by several causes, results in formation of widespread clotting within arterioles and blood capillaries. **This clotting is due to:** (1) endothelial damage with exposure of sub-endothelial collagen and subsequent platelet aggregation, and (2) activation of the coagulation process. Diseases associated with DIC include bacterial endotoxaemias, certain viral infections, dirofilariasis, certain neoplastic diseases, shock, and extensive tissue necrosis, such as occurs in animals with burns. **Microscopically**, organs in cases of DIC have **numerous fibrin thrombi** in arterioles and capillaries.

Embolism

Embolism is the occlusion of arteries by lodgment of foreign material, such as broken fragments of thrombi (thromboemboli), neoplastic cells and bacteria. Thromboemboli may be either bland (sterile) or septic. Septic emboli usually originate from lesions of vegetative endocarditis.

Right-sided lesions are spread into the lungs and left-sided lesions to the myocardium, kidneys, spleen, joints, and leptomeninges. Other types of emboli include air bubbles or hair fragments forced into the circulation during intravenous injections, release of fat into the blood vessels from fractures, and release of fragments of dead intravascular parasites, such as *Dirofilaria immitis* into the pulmonary circulation of **dogs** following administration of drugs.

Aneurysms

An aneurysm is a localized dilatation or outpouching of a thinned and weakened portion of a vessel. Usually arteries are affected; especially large elastic arteries, but the lesions can also affect veins. The **causes** of aneurysms are damage done by inflammatory, or arteriosclerotic and degenerative disease. **Known causes include:** (1) infection with *Spirocerca lupi* in the **dog**. Aneurysm usually occurs in the anterior mesenteric artery of the **horse** due to the injury caused by the larvae of *Strongylus vulgaris*. Aneurysms may be sacculated, large ones being fusiform or spherical. Worm larvae are in the thrombus and project from it, (2) copper deficiency in **pigs**, because copper is needed for normal elastic tissue development, (3) aneurysms of the pulmonary artery in **cattle** may result from infectious emboli lodging at this site and weakening the wall, and (4) most cases are idiopathic (i.e. cause remains unknown).

Classification is based on the shape and size of the aneurysm. A **berry aneurysm** refers to a small, spherical dilatation rarely exceeding a diameter of 1-1.5 cm. A **saccular aneurysm** is spherical and varies in size from 5-20 cm in diameter. In fusiform aneurysm there is gradual, progressive dilatation of the vessel lumen. These aneurysms then take on a spindle shape. They vary in diameter and length.

Dissecting aneurysms are rare and have been reported in **birds**. They result from disruption of the intima which allows entry of blood into the media, and this dissects along the wall. **Aneurysms can rupture.** Usually the **outcome** is a rapid fatal haemorrhage. This is because often large arteries are involved.

Growth Disturbances

Arterial Hypertrophy

This is a response to sustained increases in pressure or volume loads. **Affected vessels are usually muscular arteries.** The increase in the thickness of the wall is mainly due to hypertrophy, and to some degree, hyperplasia of smooth muscle cells of the tunica media.

Muscular pulmonary arteries of **cats** are commonly affected. The lesion is associated with infection by several parasites. These include *Aelurostrongylus abstrusus* (the lungworm of **cats**), **Toxocara** sp. and *Dirofilaria immitis*. However, the lesions commonly occur in the absence of parasitic infections. Similar hypertrophy of muscular pulmonary arteries occurs in **cattle** exposed to high altitudes (so-called **'high-altitude disease'** or **'brisket disease'**). Also, animals with cardiovascular anomalies that shunt blood have pulmonary hypertension, and as a result, hypertrophy of the muscular pulmonary arteries. Uterine arteries in pregnant animals also are hypertrophic.

Generalized Vascular Degenerative Diseases

Generalized vascular degenerative diseases in animals are: (1) **Arteriosclerosis**: This is characterized by **intimal fibrosis** of large elastic arteries, (2) **Atherosclerosis**: This is characterized by intimal and medial **lipid deposits** in elastic and muscular arteries, and (3) **Medial calcification**: This is characterized by **mineralization (calcification)** of the walls of elastic and muscular arteries.

Arteriosclerosis

This is an age-related disease. It is common in many species, but rarely causes clinical signs. The disease develops as a chronic degenerative and proliferative response in the arterial wall and results in loss of elasticity, that is, **hardening of the arteries** and **luminal narrowing**. The **abdominal aorta** is usually affected, but other elastic arteries and peripheral large muscular vessels may be involved. **Lesions** are localized around the orifices of arterial branches. **Causes** of arteriosclerosis are not well understood, but role of haemodynamic influences has been suggested because of its frequent occurrence at the arterial branching sites, where blood flow is turbulent.

Grossly, the lesions are seen as slightly raised, firm, white, plaques. **Microscopically,** at first the intima is thickened by accumulation of mucopolysaccharides, and later by the proliferation of smooth muscle cells in the tunica media and fibrous tissue infiltration into the intima. Splitting and fragmentation of the internal elastic lamina are common.

Atherosclerosis

This vascular disease is of the greatest importance in human beings. **It is not common in animals and rarely causes clinical disease,** such as infarction of the heart or brain. The main alteration is the accumulation of deposits (**atheroma**) of lipid, fibrous tissue, and calcium in vessel walls, which ultimately results in narrowing of the lumen. Many studies have shown that the **pig, rabbit,** and **chicken** are susceptible to the experimental disease produced by the feeding of a high-cholesterol diet. The **dog, cat, cow, goat,** and **rat** are resistant.

Lesions of the naturally occurring disease have been found in **aged pigs** and **birds** and in **dogs with hypothyroidism** which is associated with hypercholesterolaemia. Arteries of the heart, mesentery, and kidneys are markedly thickened, firm, and yellow-white. **Microscopically,** lipid globules accumulate in the cytoplasm of smooth muscles cells and macrophages, often called **'foam cells'** in the media and intima. Necrosis and fibrosis develop in some arteries.

Arterial Medial Calcification

This is a common lesion in animals. It is usually associated with endocardial mineralization and involves both elastic and muscular arteries. The **causes** include calcinogenic plant toxicosis, vitamin D toxicosis, renal insufficiency, and severe debilitation, as seen in **cattle** with Johne's disease. Medial calcification occurs naturally in **rabbits** and in **aged guinea pigs** and **rats** with chronic renal disease.

Grossly, affected arteries, such as the **aorta**, appear as solid, dense, pipe-like structures with raised, white, solid intimal plaques. **Microscopically,** in elastic arteries basophilic granular mineral deposits are present on elastic fibres of the media, but in muscular arteries they form a complete ring of mineralization in the tunica media. **Siderocalcinosis (iron rings),** which occur from deposition of both iron and calcium salts, occurs in the cerebral arteries of **aged horses.** These lesions are incidental.

Arterial intimal calcification (intimal bodies) are small, mineralized masses within the sub-endothelium in small muscular arteries and arterioles of **horses.** They have no harmful effect.

Inflammation

Arteritis

Arteritis occurs in many infectious and immune-mediated diseases. These include: (1) **viral**: equine viral arteritis, malignant catarrhal fever, swine fever (hog cholera), bluetongue, equine infectious anaemia, bovine virus diarrhoea, and feline infectious peritonitis, (2) **bacterial**: salmonellosis, erysipelas (*Erysipelothrix rhusiopathiae*), **Haemophilus** sp. infections (*H. suis, H. somnus, H. parasuis*), (3) **mycotic**: aspergillosis, phycomycosis, (4) parasitic: equine strongylosis (*Strongylus vulgaris*), dirofilariasis (*Dirofilaria immitis*), spirocercosis (*Spirocerca lupi*), onchocerciasis, aelurostrongylosis, angiostrongylosis, and (5) **immune-mediated:** canine systemic lupus erythematosus, rheumatoid arthritis, polyarteritis nodosa, drug-induced hypersensitivity, and lymphocytic choriomeningitis.

Usually all types of vessels are affected rather than the arteries. When this happens, the term **vasculitis** or **angiitis** is applied. In inflamed vessels, leukocytes are present within and surrounding the walls. Damage to the vessel wall is seen as fibrin deposits or necrotic endothelial and smooth muscle cells. These changes are accompanied by thrombosis, which can result in ischaemic injury or infarction in the circulating field. The **'diamond skin'** lesions in erysipelas in **pigs** caused by *Erysipelothrix rhusiopathiae* is an example of **cutaneous infarction.**

Arteritis and **vasculitis** can occur from endothelial injury. This may be caused by infectious agents or immune-mediated mechanisms, or from local extension of suppurative and necrotizing inflammatory processes. **Equine viral arteritis** is a systemic infection and has a tropism for endothelial cells. In this disease, small muscular arteries show lesions of fibrinoid necrosis, extensive oedema and leukocytic infiltration. **Grossly,** there is severe oedema of the interstitial wall and mesentery accompanied by marked accumulation of serous fluids in the body cavities.

Arteritis is an important feature of several parasitic diseases. In **dirofilariasis** in **dogs** (heartworm infection), maturation of adult parasites occurs in the pulmonary arteries and right atrium and ventricle. The pulmonary arteries containing parasites have at first an eosinophilic infiltration of the intima (**endoarteritis**) and later on fibromuscular proliferation of the intima, seen grossly as rough granular luminal surface. Live and dead parasites are present within these vascular lesions and cause thromboembolism and pulmonary infarction. Infection of **horses** by *Strongylus vulgaris* is very common. During its larval development, the parasites migrate through the intestinal arteries. Most severe lesions are usually found in the cranial mesenteric artery. The affected vessel is enlarged and its wall is firm and fibrotic. The intimal surface has a thrombus containing larvae. **Microscopically**, the vessel has extensive infiltration of inflammatory cells and proliferation of fibroblasts through the wall.

Polyarteritis occurs in many species, but is more common in **dogs**. The lesions are due to an immune-mediated vascular injury. Medium-sized muscular arteries are selectively involved and grossly appear thick and tortuous. **Microscopically**, the early lesions include fibrinoid necrosis and leukocytic infiltration of the intima and media.

Neoplasms

Neoplasms originating from vascular endothelial cells occur in many different organs. **Haemangiomas** are benign neoplasms usually found in the skin of **dogs**. These are red, blood-filled masses. The malignant neoplasm, **haemangiosarcoma**, occurs in the spleen and the right atrium of **dogs**. This neoplasm is also a red mass, but microscopically the neoplastic cells are pleomorphic and do not form distinct vascular spaces. Another neoplasm of vascular origin is **haemangiopericytoma** of the **dog** skin. **Microscopically**, it reveals laminated arrangement of neoplastic pericytes around small blood vessels.

Venous Diseases

Congenital Anomalies

Portocaval Shunts

These occur in **dogs**, and because blood bypasses the liver, can result in signs of nervous system disease. The resulting nervous system syndrome is called **hepatic encephalopathy**.

Dilatation

A venous dilatation from weakened vascular walls is called a **varicosity** (localized involvement) or **phlebectasia** (generalized alteration). Although a common lesion in humans, it is uncommon in animals.

Inflammation

Phlebitis

Phlebitis is inflammation of the wall of a vein. It is a common vascular lesion and is usually accompanied by thrombosis. **Phlebitis occurs from:** (1) systemic infections, (2) local extension of infection, and (3) faulty intravenous injection procedure. Systemic infections with phlebitis include salmonellosis in several species and feline infectious peritonitis. **In pigs** with various septicaemias, the gastric mucosa is often severely congested and haemorrhagic because of **venous** endothelial damage and thrombosis. In severe local infections, such as metritis or hepatic abscesses, inflammation extends into the walls of adjacent veins and produces phlebitis, with or without thrombosis. Intravenous injections of irritant solutions, injecting solutions into the vascular wall, or intimal trauma produced by indwelling venous catheters, result in vascular damage and phlebitis. **Animals with phlebitis complicated by thrombosis have the risk of septic embolism and development of endocarditis and pulmonary abscesses.**

Omphalophlebitis

Omphalophlebitis or **navel ill** is inflammation of the umbilical vein and usually occurs in neonatal farm animals due to bacterial contamination of the umbilicus following parturition. Bacteria from this site can cause septicaemia, suppurative polyarteritis, hepatic abscesses (the umbilical vein drains into the liver), and umbilical abscesses.

Cats with feline infectious peritonitis often develop phlebitis in various abdominal organs. Several parasitic diseases are characterized by the presence of parasites in the lumen of veins, such as schistosomiasis (blood fluke infection). In schistosomiasis, adult parasites are present in the mesenteric and portal veins. The resulting phlebitis is characterized by intimal proliferation and thrombosis.

Lymph Vessel Diseases

Congenital Anomalies

Hereditary lymphoedema has been described in **dogs, calves**, and **pigs**. Affected animals have subcutaneous oedema. Interference with drainage results from defective development of the lymph vessels.

Dilatation and Rupture

Lymphangiectasis is dilatation of lymph vessels. One important cause is obstruction of lymphatic drainage by invading masses of malignant neoplasms. Another example is intestinal lymphangiectasis of **dogs.**

Rupture of the thoracic duct may occur either as a result of trauma or from spontaneous disruption causing chylothorax in **dogs** and **cats.**

Inflammation

Lymphangitis occurs in many diseases. These include: (1) **bacterial:** anthrax in pigs (*Bacillus anthracis*), Johne's disease (*Mycobacterium paratuberculosis*), actinobacillosis (*Actinobacillus lignieresii*), glanders ('**farcy**') (*Burkholderia mallei*), bovine farcy, ulcerative lymphangitis of horses, sporadic lymphangitis of horses, and (2) mycotic: epizootic lymphangitis of horses (*Histoplasma farciminosum*) sporotrichosis (*Sporothrix schenckii*).

The affected vessels are usually in the distal limbs and are thick, cord-like structures. Lymphoedema can also be present. Nodular suppurative lesions often ulcerate and discharge pus on the surface of the skin. In Johne's disease, the mesenteric lymph vessels are prominent due to granulomatous lymphangitis.

Neoplasms

Lymphangioma is a rare benign neoplasm of lymph channels. **Lymphosarcoma** is more common than the benign neoplasm. Vascular spaces contain lymph rather than blood. Lymph vessels are usually invaded by primary carcinomas and are a common route of metastasis.

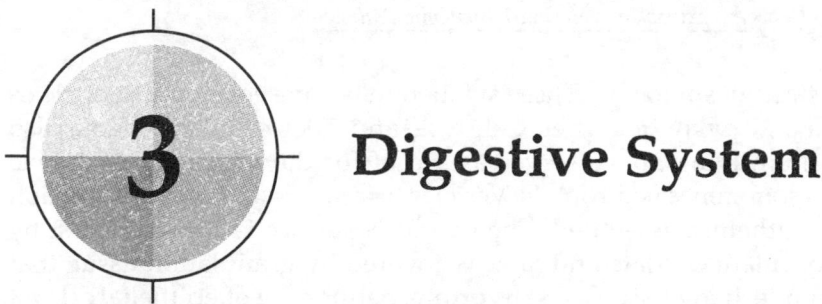

Digestive System

Oral Cavity

Developmental Anomalies

Palatoschisis or **cleft palate** and **cheiloschisis** or **cleft lip** are the common developmental abnormalities of the oral cavity. **Palatoschisis** results from a failure of fusion of the lateral palatine processes. It can be genetic or toxic in origin.

Cheiloschisis is also called **'hare lip'**, since this is as normal feature of the rabbit. It is due to a failure of fusion of the upper lip along the midline or philtrum. (Philtrum is the vertical groove in the median portion of the upper lip.)

Inflammation

Inflammation of the mouth is known as **stomatitis** and pharynx as **pharyngitis**. Inflammation of the lips is called **cheilitis**, of gums **gingivitis**, of tongue **glossitis**, and of the tonsils as **tonsillitis**. Among these, stomatitis is the most common and its common **causes** include viral and bacterial infections.

1. Vesicular Stomatitis

All vesicular stomatitides ('stomatitides' is plural of 'stomatitis') are caused by viruses and on gross and histopathological examination, all have a similar appearance. Examples of vesicular stomatitides include **foot-and-mouth disease** in cloven-footed animals, **vesicular stomatitis** of calves, and **vesicular exanthema** of pigs. They are all characterized in their early stages by the formation of **vesicles** or **blisters** of the oral mucosa. None is fatal. However, secondary bacterial infection of these lesions can result in endotoxaemia.

The **gross lesions** in vesicular stomatitis begin as small, clear, fluid-filled vesicles of the lips, the buccal mucosa, and the surface and margins of the tongue. These lesions enlarge and fuse to create **bullae**, which afterwards break and cause ulcers, exposing irregular patches of red, denuded sub-mucosa. Similar lesions occur in the nasal mucosa, particularly in **pigs** with **vesicular exanthema**, and in the oesophagus and rumen of **cattle** with **foot-and-mouth disease.**

Microscopically, the lesions of these three diseases (foot-and-mouth disease, vesicular stomatitis, and vesicular exanthema) are similar. Each lesion begins as intracellular oedema in the epithelium, which results in **ballooning degeneration**

of the cells of the **stratum spinosum**. These swollen cells have eosinophilic or clear, watery cytoplasm and pyknotic nuclei. Cell lysis and inter-cellular oedema also occur. The epithelium lying above serves as a roof for the **vesicle.** The vesicle contains blood and sometimes neutrophils. Vesicles fuse and from **bullae.** Ulceration occurs when the epithelium is eroded. The denuded surface is coated at first by fibrin or fibrino-purulent exudate and later is covered by granulation tissue that proliferates from underlying tissues. The **hydropic ballooning** of epithelial cells of the stratum spinosum is characteristic of the disease.

Clinical signs include vesicles, bullae, raw ulcerated areas on the tongue and lips, salivation, lameness, fever, and anorexia. The **diagnosis** is based on characteristic gross and microscopic lesions, species affected, serology, and virus isolation.

Foot-and-mouth disease is an extremely important disease in India. It occurs in cloven-footed animals, which include **cattle, sheep, goat,** and **pig,** but not horses. It is characterized in its early stages by vesicle in the nose, oral cavity, and tongue. The coronary bands of the hooves can also be affected, which ultimately can lead to sloughing of the hoof. Although the disease is not fatal, the pain and loss of appetite lead to weight loss. Young animals with foot-and-mouth disease usually have a viral myocarditis.

Vesicular stomatitis is common in **calves,** but does not occur in sheep and goats. It is characterized by the formation of **vesicles in the oral cavity. Clinically,** the disease is usually diagnosed by loss of appetite in the affected animals, accompanied by hyper-salivation.

Vesicular exanthema is a disease of **pigs**. It is not possible in pigs to differentiate clinically and pathologically vesicular exanthema from foot-and-mouth disease.

2. Erosive and Ulcerative Stomatitis

Erosive and ulcerative stomatitis has a number of causes. **Erosion** is loss of a portion of the surface epithelium, whereas an **ulcer** is full-thickness epithelial loss exposing the basement membrane. Causative agents include the **viruses** of rinderpest, malignant catarrhal fever, bovine viral diarrhea, bluetongue, equine viral rhinotracheitis, and feline calicivirus.

3. Papular Stomatitis

Parapox viruses cause the papular stomatitides. The two important diseases of this category are: **bovine papular stomatitis** and **contagious ecthyma.**

Bovine papular stomatitis is characterized by papules on the nares, muzzle, gingival, buccal cavity, palate, and tongue. **Lesions** also occur in the oesophagus, rumen, and omasum. Sometimes, eosinophilic cytoplasmic inclusion bodies are seen microscopically. In humans, the disease is called **'milker's nodules'** and is characterized by papules of the hands and arms.

Contagious ecthyma (**contagious pustular dermatitis, sore mouth, scabby mouth**) occurs in **sheep** and **goats**. It is characterized by macules, papules, vesicles, pustules, scabs, scars, and nodules in areas of skin abrasions. Such areas include corners of the mouth, udder, teats, coronary bands, and anus. Sometimes, mucosa of the oesophagus and rumen are also affected. **Eosinophilic cytoplasmic inclusion bodies** are seen on microscopic examination of lesions early in the course of disease. The condition **in humans** is called **orf**.

4. Necrotizing Stomatitis

Necrotizing stomatitis occurs in **cattle, sheep,** and **pigs. In cattle,** it is called **calf diphtheria.** Necrotizing stomatitis is characterized by yellow-grey round foci surrounded by a rim of hyperaemic tissue in the oral cavity, larynx or pharynx, or both. This stomatitis is the end stage of all other forms of stomatitis when they are complicated by infection with *Fusobacterium necrophorum*, a Gram-negative anaerobe. Animals with oral necrobacillosis have swollen cheeks, anorexia, fever, and a characteristic unpleasant breath. The **gross lesions** consist of a raised core of grey necrotic material, which is readily separated. **Microscopically,** the lesion is characterized by coagulative necrosis surrounded by a zone of granulation tissue and hyperaemia.

Ulcerative Gingivitis

Also known as **'Vincent's gingivitis'** and **'trench mouth'**, ulcerative gingivitis is a fuso-spirochaetal disease (fusiform bacillus+spirochaete) that affects humans, chimpanzees, monkeys, and **rarely puppies**. The acute inflammation and necrosis cause **painful gums**, a foul mouth smell, haemorrhages, and increased salivation.

Two anaerobes, *Borrelia vincentii,* a spirochaete, and **Fusobacterium** sp. **cause** the disease. They cause the disease because of underlying nutritional deficiencies and debilitating conditions. The **lesion** is an acute, necrotizing inflammation of the gingiva. Punched-out ulcers occur in the gingiva, and are sometimes covered by a grey membrane. Large numbers of spirochaetes and fusiform bacteria are present in the smears of the lesions.

Noma

Noma is an **acute gangrenous stomatitis** that occurs in humans, **monkeys,** and **dogs**. Spirochaetes and fusiform bacteria cause this disease, along with other organisms in the mouth. It is similar to necrobacillosis, except that the lesions are more severe and may cause gangrenous perforation of the cheeks, lysis of bone, and death.

5. Eosinophilic Stomatitis

A focal granuloma or ulcer (**rodent ulcer**) of oral tissues occurs in **young dogs** and **cats** and is called **'oral eosinophilic granuloma'**. The cause is not known, but the lesions suggest an immune-mediated mechanism. In both **dogs** and **cats**, a peripheral eosinophilia occurs in most of the cases.

6. Lympho-plasmacytic Stomatitis

This is an idiopathic condition of the **cat** named on the basis of the histological appearance of the lesions. It is characterized by red inflamed gums, foul breath, and loss of appetite. The presence of plasma cells in the sub-mucosa suggests an immune-mediated aetiology.

Hyperplasia and Neoplasia

In the dog, 70% neoplasms of the digestive tract are in the oral cavity.

Hyperplastic Diseases

Gingival hyperplasia is a simple outgrowth of gum tissues. It is most common in **dogs**.

Grossly, it is not possible to differentiate gingival hyperplasia from an **epulis**. **Epulis** is a non-specific term that indicates **a growth of the gingiva.** The several kinds of epulides can only be differentiated by histopathological examination. All epulides are benign. However, one form, **acanthomatous epulis**, involves bone and can be quite destructive. Whether the epulides are fibrous and epithelial hyperplasia or benign neoplasm of tooth germ remains controversial.

Neoplasms

Canine Oral Papillomatosis

It is a papovavirus-induced transmissible condition and occurs in animals younger than one year. The **lesions** are papilliform or cauliflower-like, white, and occur on the mouth, tongue, palate, larynx, and epiglottis. The lesions usually regress spontaneously. Immunity is long lasting.

Grossly, these multiple tumours appear white or grey, are flat or raised, and pedunculated. **Microscopically**, papillomas consist of hyperplastic, stratified squamous epithelium and a proliferated connective tissue stroma. Cells of the stratum spinosum enlarge and have vesicular cytoplasm, so-called **ballooning degeneration**. At some stages, intranuclear inclusion bodies that contain virus particles are present.

Melanomas

Ninety percent of melanomas of the oral cavity of the dogs are malignant. A breed predilection exists. Some melanomas without pigment, called **amelanotic melanomas**, are difficult to diagnose.

Melanomas are composed of melanocytes and are of neural crest origin. Melanoma

102

begins as a black macule (spot) and develops into a firm mass. It may be smooth or have an ulcerated, red, and bleeding surface. The inside of the mass is grey, dark brown, or black, depending on the amount of the pigment present. **Microscopically,** the neoplasm consists of spindle-shaped melanocytes.

Squamous-cell Carcinoma

Squamous-cell carcinomas occur **in the oral cavity,** particularly in the **aged cat** where they account for 6% of oral neoplasms. They usually occur on the ventro-lateral surface of the **tongue** and **tonsils.** Squamous-cell carcinomas of the tongue are more common in **cats** and of tonsils in **dogs.**

About 5% to 10% of **gingival squamous-cell carcinomas** metastasize to regional lymph nodes and about 3% to distant sites. Squamous-cell carcinomas of the tonsil metastasize to regional lymph nodes.

Squamous-cell carcinomas, when small, are granular. With increased size, they become cauliflower-like masses. **Microscopically,** irregular masses and cords of stratified squamous cells invade the sub-mucosa. Well-differentiated neoplasms have numerous keratin pearls, but poorly differentiated neoplasms have only a few keratinized cells and numerous mitotic figures. A characteristic feature is the presence of intercellular bridges (**desmosomes**) between adjacent epithelial cells. The amount of fibrous tissue varies. Some carcinomas are scirrhous (i.e. hard or indurated), whereas others have areas of necrosis caused by rapid tumour growth, and loss of contact with the blood supply.

Fibrosarcomas originate from the fibroblasts of the oral cavity. They are most common in the **cat,** accounting for 20% of the oral neoplasms.

Teeth

Malocclusions

Malocclusion is failure of the upper and lower incisors to inter-digitate properly. This is normal in some **dogs.** When malocclusions are extreme, they can lead to difficulty in prehension (grasping) and mastication of food. Malocclusions are named according to the position of the mandible. Protrusion of the lower jaw is called **prognathia,** whereas a short lower jaw with resultant protrusion of the upper jaw is called **brachygnathia.** Malocclusions result from poor jaw conformation, or from abnormal tooth eruption patterns.

Anomalies of Tooth Development

Tooth agenesis (absence or incomplete development) is common, but is of little clinical significance in animals with simple teeth.

Dentigerous Cysts

These result from abnormal tooth development, which gives rise to cystic structures in the bone or soft tissues of the jaw. **This lesion is rare**, can remain asymptomatic or lead to painful or destructive diseases of the jaw.

Segmental Enamel Hypoplasia

This condition occurs in the permanent teeth of **dogs** infected with the **canine distemper virus** during odontogenesis (development of teeth). The epithelium of the enamel organ during virus infection has necrosis and disorganization. After recovery from canine distemper virus infection, the function and organization of the enamel organ return, and this is followed by re-establishment of normal enamel formation.

Abnormal Coloration of Teeth

Abnormal coloration of teeth can result from the incorporation of chemical agents, typically **tetracyclines**, during mineralization. Incorporation of **porphyrins** into dentin in animals with congenital porphyria can cause pink discoloration of the teeth.

Excessive fluoride incorporation into the enamel and dentin occurs in **fluoride toxicosis**, seen partially in **cattle** and **sheep**. The discolored enamel is usually yellow, dark brown, or black.

Infundibular Impaction

Impaction of infundibulum causes serious dental disease in **ruminants** and also occurs in **horses**. It is similar in pathogenic mechanism to **dental caries** in simple-toothed animals. Impaction of infundibulum has been also called **infundibular necrosis** and **infundibular caries**. Incomplete cementum formation in the infundibulum before the tooth erupts predisposes to infundibular impaction. Bacteria present in the feed material accumulated in the infundibulum, metabolize feed to form acid, which causes **demineralization**. Also bacterial enzymes digest the organic matrix of enamel and dentin. As a result, the pulp cavity is penetrated resulting in **pulpitis** and **periodontitis**. Dental abscesses and formation of fistulous tracks lead to serious dental disease.

Periodontal Disease

In addition to its destructive effect on dental matrices, bacteria on the tooth surface (dental plaques) have a destructive effect on the supporting soft tissues of the gingival and periodontal ligament. Bacterial toxins and the irritation of mineralized plaques (**tartar** and **dental calculi**) lead to inflammation of the gingival epithelium. As inflammation invades the connective tissues of the periodontal ligament, the suspensory apparatus is destroyed, and the tooth loosens. Periodontal disease is common in **dogs, cats,** and **humans.**

Dental Neoplasms

Odontomas

Odontomas are hamartomas of enamel origin and contain fully differentiated dentin and enamel. (A hamartoma is a benign tumour-like nodule composed of an overgrowth of mature tissue in which the elements show disordered arrangement and proportion in comparison to normal.) Odontomas are almost always found in **young animals,** usually **dogs** and **horses,**

Ameloblastoma

This is a generic name used for the epithelial neoplasms of enamel organ origin. **Histologically,** there are several subtypes.

Ameloblastoma occurs anywhere in the dental tissue, usually in **adult dogs**. It can be either superficial or deep. Ameloblastoma is locally invasive, and results in destruction of alveolar bone. **Microscopically,** ameloblastoma includes inter-branching sheets of epithelial cells, intense keratinization and the presence of extracellular hyaline bodies. These hyaline bodies often stain for amyloid.

Salivary Glands

Inflammatory Diseases

Sialoadenitis

Sialoadenitis is inflammation of a salivary gland. **It is relatively rare in veterinary medicine. Rabies** and **canine distemper** are two important diseases that cause inflammation of the salivary glands. *Salmonella typhisuis* has caused parotid sialoadenitis in **pigs.**

Miscellaneous Diseases/Conditions

Changes in the salivary glands are uncommon in domestic animals.

A **ranula** is a cystic distension of the duct of the sublingual or submaxillary gland that occurs on the floor of the mouth by the site of the tongue. The cause is unknown.

A **salivary mucocoele** is a pseudocyst. It is not lined by epithelium and is filled with saliva. The cause is unknown.

Sialoliths are **rare in domestic animals.** When they do occur, they are due to inflammation of the salivary gland with sloughed cells, or inflammatory exudate forming a nidus for mineral accumulation. Thus, they can cause **ranula** formation.

Neoplasms

Salivary gland neoplasms, both benign and malignant **are uncommon** but occur in all species. They are composed of glandular or ductular elements, or a combination of epithelial and mesenchymal components similar to those in mixed mammary neoplasms.

Tongue

Systemic Disease: Primary Involvement of the Tongue

Disease agents that mainly affect the tongue are rare. The exception is *Actinobacillus lignieresii,* a normal inhabitant of the oral cavity. It involves the damaged lingual tissue in **cattle** and sometimes **small ruminants** and **horses.** The **granulomas** resulting from infection have colonies of Gram-negative bacilli at their centres. The colonies are surrounded by a zone of eosinophilic, club-shaped structure composed of immunoglobulin products of host inflammatory cells. Granulocytes, macrophages, epithelioid cells and multinucleated Langhans' type giant cells surround these rosettes. Within and surrounding this granulomatous band are lymphocytes and plasma cells. Regional lymph nodes may have similar granulomas or have abscesses that drain to the surface. The resulting lingual disease called **'wooden tongue' (actinobacillosis).** The name **'wooden tongue'** is derived from the swelling, inflammation, and fibrosis that enlarge and harden the tongue.

Systemic Disease: Secondary Involvement of the Tongue

Thrush is a *Candida albicans* (fungus) infection of the tongue and oesophagus. It occurs in hoofed animals, but has been seen also in carnivores. Thrush shows as a grey-green pseudomembrane that is easily peeled off from the intact underlying mucosal surface. It occurs as a result of antibiotic treatment that kills normal flora.

Parasites

Parasites of the tongue are uncommon, except those that reside in muscles such as **Sarcocystis** sp. and *Trichinella spiralis* in **pigs. Gongylonema** sp. can be present in the lumen of **pigs** and **ruminants** and are of no clinical importance.

Oesophagus

Developmental Anomalies

Cricopharyngeal Achalasia

This is a **congenital disorder** of the upper oesophageal sphincter seen in **dogs.** It is characterized by failure of the upper oesophageal sphincter to relax. Dysphagia (difficulty in swallowing) and regurgitation characterize the disorder. **Acquired cricopharyngeal achalasia** occurs rarely in the **dog.** The cause is unknown in both congenital and acquired forms.

Megaoesophagus

Megaoesophagus or **oesophageal ectasia** is dilation of the oesophagus. This is due to insufficient or un-coordinated peristalsis in the mid and cervical oesophagus. It has been described in **dogs, cats, and horses**

Congenital megaoesophagus is due to partial blockage of the lumen of the oesophagus by a persistent right fourth aortic arch. It has been described in dogs, and **Siamese cats.**

Acquired megaoesophagus or **oesophageal achalasia** is due to failure of relaxation of the cardiac sphincter of the stomach in humans. Although the gross appearance of acquired megaoesophagus **in animals** is similar to that of humans, in animals it does not involve the cardiac sphincter.

Clinically, megaoesophagus is recognized by regurgitation after ingestion of solid food and weight loss. Aspiration pneumonia may occur in some animals. **Grossly,** oesophagus is greatly dilated, about two to three times its normal diameter. The dilated portions usually contain a foul-smelling fluid residue of ingesta.

Oesophageal Parasites

Gongylonema sp.

Gongylonema sp. affects **ruminants, pigs, horses, monkeys,** and sometimes **rodents.** These nematodes live under the mucosa and are thin, red, and winding like a snake. They may be 10-15 cm long. **The parasites are not pathogenic** and produce no local host response.

Hypoderma lineatum

This is the larvae of the warble fly of ruminants. It is commonly observed in the oesophageal sub-mucosa. They are 5-10 mm long, white, and resemble grains of rice. **They are of no clinical importance.**

Gastrophilus sp.

These occur in **horses.** These fly larvae lay their eggs on the skin at different locations. The warmth and moisture from licking activate them. The larvae burrow into the oral mucosa, moult, and then migrate down the oesophagus. They occur both in the distal oesophagus and stomach where they attach to the mucosa through oral hooks. They ultimately detach, **leaving craters (eroded lesions) at the site of attachment,** and pass in the faeces.

Spirocerca lupi

This is the most pathogenic of the oesophageal parasites and causes spirocercosis in dogs. These nematodes reach the oesophageal sub-mucosa after migrating through the aortic wall. A passage forms between the oesophageal lumen and the granuloma containing the parasite. This passage allows discharge of ova into the digestive system and ultimately into the faeces. **Clinical symptoms** include dysphagia (difficult swallowing), aortic aneurysms, and rarely **oesophageal fibrosarcomas** or **osteosarcomas**. *S. lupi* infestations occur in warmer climates. The intermediate hosts are dung beetles, chickens, and reptiles.

Miscellaneous Oesophageal Lesions/ Conditions

Idiopathic muscular hypertrophy of the distal oesophagus occurs in **horses**, but usually is of no clinical importance.

Similarly, **dilation of oesophageal glands of aged dogs** has no clinical significance.

Oesophageal erosions and ulcers are common and have a variety of causes. One of the most common causes is reflux of stomach acid. This reflux causes chemical burning of the lower oesophagus and is called **reflux oesophagitis** or **heartburn in humans**. Other causes include improper use of stomach tubes and infectious diseases such as bovine viral diarrhoea.

Leukoplakia of the oesophagus and stomach is characterized by separate, flat, white mucosal elevations (epithelial plaques) of no clinical significance.

Choke

Choke is a clinical term. It refers to oesophageal obstruction following **stenosis** (narrowing) which has a variety of causes. Choke usually occurs in those anatomical locations where the oesophagus cannot fully expand. These locations are dorsal to the larynx at the thoracic inlet, base of the heart, and at the diaphragmatic hiatus. **Choke** occurs usually from ingestion of large bodies such as potatoes, apples, bones, or medicines such as large gelatin-filled capsules or tablets (**dry boluses**). If these bodies are lodged against the epithelium for longer than 2 days, the interaction often results in pressure necrosis of the oesophageal mucosa, which forms **strictures** during healing. These strictures then can cause **reflex regurgitation** after ingestion of food.

In older horses, poor dentition causes food to be incompletely masticated, resulting in impaction in the oesophagus. Neoplastic or inflammatory lesions of the oesophagus also cause obstruction.

Neoplasms

Neoplasms of the oesophagus are rare in animals.

Squamous-cell Carcinoma

These have been described in **cats** and **horses,** and in **cattle** in Brazil and Great Britain, where consumption of bracken fern is believed to be the cause. **Clinically,** the condition is accompanied by dysphagia, regurgitation, dilation of the oesophagus proximal to the mass, weight loss, and a palpable cervical mass.

Oesophageal squamous-cell carcinomas are usually not detected early because the neoplastic mass grows into the oesophageal lumen. The surface is cauliflower-like and ulcerated. With time, the mass obstructs the oesophagus and produces a **stenosis** (narrowing) of the lumen. Spread to adjacent tissue occurs readily and the neoplasm metastasizes to regional lymph nodes, liver, and lungs.

Rumen, Reticulum and Omasum

Ruminal tympany or **bloat** is overdistension of the rumen and reticulum by gases produced during fermentation. Bloat can be divided into **primary tympany** or **secondary tympany.**

Primary tympany is also known as **frothy bloat**. It usually occurs 1-3 days after animals begin a new diet. Certain legumes and grain concentrates increase the formation of foam. The non-volatile acids of legume and those of rumen origin lower the rumen pH to 5-6, which is most favourable for development of bloat. Foam, mixed with rumen contents, blocks the cardia causing the rumen to distend with the gases of fermentation. **Clinical signs** include a distended abdomen, increased respiratory and heart rates, and decreased ruminal movements. **Death**, when it occurs, is due to distension of abdomen and compression of the diaphragm leading to increased intra-abdominal and intra-thoracic pressure. This, in turn, results in decreased venous return to the heart, which leads to generalized congestion. At postmortem, the most important indication of ante-mortem bloat is the sharp line of demarcation between the pale, bloodless distal oesophagus and the congested proximal oesophagus at the thoracic inlet. This division is known as a **bloat line.**

Secondary tympany is caused by a physical or functional obstruction or stenosis of the oesophagus resulting in failure to eructate. Oesophageal papilloma, lymphosarcoma, and oesophageal foreign bodies are potential causes of secondary tympany.

Foreign Bodies

Foreign bodies can collect or lodge in the rumen. These include **trichobezoars (hairballs)** and **phytobezoars (plant balls)**.

Ingestion of nails and wire can result in perforation of the wall of the reticulum and cause reticulitis (discussed next), peritonitis, and pericarditis (**hardware disease**)

Inflammatory Diseases

Inflammation of the rumen is called **rumenitis** and reticulum **reticulitis.**

Bacterial Rumenitis

Bacterial rumenitis usually occurs from mechanical injury of rumen. Bacteria that colonize the damaged rumen can enter into the portal circulation and to the **liver** resulting in **multiple abscesses.** *Actinomyces pyogenes* is the common cause of bacterial abscess in the liver. *Fusobacterium necrophorum* from rumen may also enter into the liver and cause characteristic liver lesions called **'necrobacillosis'**.

Mycotic Rumenitis

Mycotic infections of the rumen also occur from mechanical injury of rumen. Mycotic rumenitis also occurs from the administration of antibiotics, usually in **calves** but also in **adult cattle. The antibiotics reduce the number of normal flora and allow fungi to proliferate. Lesions** are usually circular and well defined and are mainly due to infarction from thrombosis secondary to fungal vasculitis. The fungi usually include **Aspergillus, Mucor,** and **Rhizopus** sp. Certain fungi can spread to the placenta haematogenously and cause **mycotic placentitis,** which leads to **abortions**.

Traumatic Reticulitis

Cattle do not have highly sensitive prehensile organs (lips and tongue), nor a discriminating sense of taste. As a result, cattle kept at farms, stables, or at other sites close to human mechanical activities are prone to swallow metallic objects such as nails, screws, and pieces of wire that have been carelessly left in their feeding areas. Some of these objects are even picked up from the pasture when the **cow** moves its tongue around a clump of grass.

Most foreign bodies remain in the reticulum. They are retained there by the folds of the reticulum's lining. No harm occurs from the presence of smooth foreign bodies, but **sharp ones** either become **trapped in the perforations** they have made in one or more of the mucosal folds or penetrate the wall of the organ. The perforation of the fold alone is not a very harmful event. This is shown by the fact that many healthy cattle slaughtered have nails or pieces of wire embedded in the reticulum's mucosal folds with small, white, scarred areas around them. **Those that penetrate the wall** are gradually forced through it by the recurrent peristaltic contraction of the organ.

Migration of the foreign body in any direction is possible, but most of them move anterio-ventrally. They pass through the diaphragm into the pericardium and heart muscle, carrying ingesta and contaminating bacteria with them, and cause **traumatic pericarditis** (see 'traumatic pericarditis'), also known as **'hardware disease'**. There may also be a **purulent pleuritis** or **pneumonia** associated with this condition. Movement of the foreign body is usually gradual, so that a dense fibrous wall encircles the path of the wire or penetrating object. Sometimes the foreign body is drawn into the rumen through the peristaltic movement of this organ and is not found at postmortem.

Usually the iron-containing pieces of wire or nail are completely rusted out by the time pericardial infection causes death of the animal. In such cases, diagnosis can still be made in the absence of a foreign body in the lesion by finding the dense fibrous encapsulating mass of variable size and shape. It contains a thin, blackened tract, present along the path created by the penetrating foreign body. The anterior surface of the reticulum is adherent to the diaphragm, and therefore in every postmortem **adhesions** in this region should be examined. Usually, there are also encapsulated abscesses in this area.

Complications of traumatic reticulitis: If the foreign body penetrates the reticulum in a different direction, there is **localized (rarely generalized) peritonitis** with intra-abdominal abscesses that may also be present in the liver or spleen. Bacteria contaminating the foreign body and causing **peritonitis, pleuritis,** or **peritonitis** include the pyogenic organisms *Actinomyces pyogenes* and *Fusobacterium necrophorum*. If the penetrating foreign body happens to involve the vagus nerves, ruminal atony (lack of normal tone or strength) may lead to failure of reticulo-ruminal emptying. This has been termed **'vagal indigestion'.**

Stomach and Abomasum

Gastric Dilatation and Volvulus Syndrome

This condition has been reported in **dogs**. This lesion is life threatening. It should not be confused with simple gastric dilation, which is common in **young puppies** after overeating. Predisposing factors include a source of distending gas, fluid, or feed, and obstruction of the cardia and pylorus.

Abomasal Displacement

Abomasal displacement is usually on the **left side**, although right-sided displacements also occur. **Left-sided displacement** of the abomasum is usually not fatal and is observed in **dairy cattle** during the 6 months following parturition. Fifteen percent of the abomasal displacements are **right-sided**. The abomasums may over-distend and twist on its mesenteric axis. Twenty percent of such cases lead to **abomasal volvulus.** Right-sided displacements occur in post-parturient dairy cows and in calves.

Clinical features include anorexia, weight loss, dehydration, scant faeces, and ketonuria.

Gastric Dilation and Rupture

This condition occurs in the **horses**, usually as a terminal event in intestinal obstruction and displacement.

Acute gastric dilation occurs spontaneously in **monkeys.**

Chronic gastric dilation is always **a secondary event.** In the **dog,** it is due to gastric ulcer, lymphoma of the gastric wall, uraemia, pyloric stenosis or acute gastric dilation. In the **horse,** chronic gastric dilation occurs as a result of consuming non-nutritious feed. It occurs more frequently in **horses** with the vice of cribbing and air swallowing. In **cows,** chronic abomasal dilation occurs with abomasal ulcers, malignant lymphoma, and vagal indigestion.

Clinically, animals with chronic gastric dilation show partial or complete anorexia and distended abdomen.

Inflammation

Gastritis

Inflammation of the simple stomach is called **gastritis** and abomasum as **abomasitis.** Gastritis is often associated clinically with vomiting, dehydration, and metabolic acidosis.

1. Acute Phlegmonous Gastritis

This type of gastritis occurs in the **dog** and is due to infection of the gastric wall by **bacteria.** These bacteria include *Escherichia coli, Proteus vulgaris,* or *Clostridium perfringens.* **Clinically,** phlegmonous gastritis is characterized by sudden onset of epigastric pain, nausea, and vomiting accompanied by fever and prostration. **Death** usually occurs from circulatory collapse.

Grossly, the stomach is dilated and has thickened walls, and a deep red to purple mucosa.

2. Emphysematous Gastritis

This is **due to gas-forming organisms** such as *C. perfringens,* and sometimes occurs with gastric dilation with volvulus. **Microscopically,** the mucosa and submucosa are thickened and distended by oedema. The mucosa has haemorrhage, congestion, and foci of coagulative necrosis. The causative bacteria are usually seen embedded in fibrino-purulent exudate in the gastric wall.

Clostridium septicum causes **haemorrhagic abomasitis** with sub-mucosal emphysema in **sheep** and **cattle** known as **braxy.** The lesions are produced by the exotoxin of the bacteria, and therefore death occurs from an exotoxaemia.

In many septicaemias of **pigs,** bacterial emboli lodge in the vessels of the sub-mucosa and cause thrombosis resulting in infarction and ulceration. This occurs in salmonellosis, swine dysentery, Glasser's disease, and colibacillosis.

3. Granulomatous Gastritis

Microorganisms that invade the deeper tissues of the gastric wall rather than just the mucosa cause a **granulomatous gastritis.** The microorganisms include

Histoplasma capsulatum (a fungus) and rarely *Mycobacterium tuberculosis*. Organisms enter into the deeper tissues (sub-mucosa, muscle layers, lymphatics, sub-serosa, and adjacent lymph nodes) and **cause a granulomatous inflammation.**

The wall of the stomach is thickened and the stomach becomes less functional. **Clinical features** include vomiting, weight loss, weakness, and haematemesis (vomiting of blood). **Microscopically**, macrophages are the main cells. Plasma cells, lymphocytes, fibroblasts, and some neutrophils, eosinophils, and multinucleate giant cells are also present.

4. Eosinophilic Gastritis

This gastritis is rare, but occurs in **dogs, cats,** and humans. In all three species, two forms are recognized: (1) **a focal form** caused by infiltrating eosinophils. This is in response to trapped nematode larvae. (2) **a diffuse form** believed to be allergic in nature. It affects a large portion of the stomach.

In the **dog,** focal eosinophilic gastritis occurs in response to the migration of larval *Toxocara canis*. **Puppies** are infected with *T. canis* larvae through the milk of the bitch, or from eating feed contaminated by the eggs or larvae from the faeces of the bitch. These larvae can remain in the tissues for years, and attract eosinophils because of their waste products, saliva, and sheath. The **lesion** is a nodular mass on the gastric mucosa consisting of an embedded parasite surrounded by eosinophils. **Microscopically**, the lesion is characterized by infiltrates of eosinophils in the mucosa, sub-mucosa, and muscle layers of the stomach, and sometimes in the small intestine and colon.

5. Hypertrophic Gastritis

A long-term chronic gastritis may lead to **hypertrophic gastritis.** This is characterized by thickened rugae (folds of the mucosa) due to hyperplasia of the gastric glands. Hypertrophic gastritis has also been described in **horses**. It occurs in response to infection with **Habronema** sp. and *Trichostrongylus axei*.

6. Parasitic Gastritis

In Ruminants

Haemonchosis

A common gastric parasite of **sheep** and **other ruminants is** *Haemonchus contortus*, the **barberpole worm**. These parasites are acquired on pasture when the third-stage larvae are consumed with grasses. The ingested larvae enter the **abomasum,** where they live within the **gastric glands.** Here they undergo development to adults and move to the surface. Eggs of the nematode pass out in the faeces, thereby completing the cycle.

Haemonchus is a serious problem when **lambs** on pasture ingest large numbers of larvae. **These parasites feed on blood** and cause **severe anaemia** as well as **oedema** and **hypoproteinaemia**, seen clinically as **'bottle jaw'** (marked sub-mandibular oedema). At postmortem, lesions are subcutaneous oedema of the inter-mandibular space, pale conjunctiva and oral membranes, stunted growth, and liquid faeces. The organs are pale because of severe anaemia, blood is watery, and the abomasal contents are fluid and brown. Parasites are seen in the abomasal contents.

Ostertagiosis

In **cattle** and **ruminants**, ostertagiosis is an important disease. Affected animals are unthrifty. In **sheep** and **goats**, the most common species is *Ostertagia circumcinta*, and in **cattle** *O. ostertagia*. The nematodes are 1.5 cm long, and have a direct life cycle. They reside as third, fourth, and fifth-stage larvae in the gastric glands of the abomasum. **Clinical features** include failure to achieve adequate weight gains, anorexia, diarrhoea, and in the later stages, hypoproteinaemia and ventral oedema.

Abomasitis produced by **Ostertagia** sp. is characterized by an infiltration of chronic inflammatory cells (lymphocytes and plasma cell), some eosinophils, and hyperplasia of mucous cells in the abomasum. **Ostertagia** sp. can be demonstrated at the postmortem. The worms are brown, smaller than *Haemonchus contortus*, and more difficult to see without magnification. The parasites occur within the gastric glands and in areas of chronic inflammation.

Horses

Equine bots, *Gastrophilus intestinalis* and *Gastrophilus nasalis* occur in **horses**. *G. intestinalis* colonizes the stratified portion of the stomach. The adult fly lays eggs on the hairs of the distal limbs of the horse. *G. nasalis* lays eggs around the nose of the horse and the larvae hatch after being licked. The larvae live in the glandular portion of the stomach. **Both species attach to the mucosa of the stomach.** The larvae pass in the faeces, pupate, and develop into the flies.

Draschia megastoma is found in the glandular mucosa of the stomach. The infection is sometimes also referred to as **habronemiasis**, based on old nomenclature of the parasite as **Habronema** sp . The adults in the sub-mucosal nodules release eggs through a pore. The eggs pass out in the faeces and are eaten by larvae of a fly that serves as the intermediate host. **Both Draschia sp. and Gastrophilus sp. cause gastric ulcers.**

Dogs and Cats

Ollulaniasis and **gnathostomiasis** rarely produce **gastritis**. *Ollulanus tricuspis*, a minute nematode, is transmitted through the food vomited from the stomach of an infected **cat**, and rarely causes **mild gastritis** and sometimes **chronic fibrosing**

gastritis. This is seen as mucosal nodularity or hypertrophy of the folds of gastric mucosa (gastric rugal hypertrophy). **Gnathostoma** sp. has tooth-like spines that cause sub-mucosal granulomatous masses.

Neoplasms

Neoplasms of stomach are uncommon in domestic animals. Leiomyoma and more rarely **leiomyosarcoma** originate from the tunica muscularis. **Lymphosarcoma** can be primary or metastatic in origin. **In cattle,** it is often caused by the bovine leukaemia virus and has a predilection for the abomasum as well as the right atrium and uterus. **Squamous-cell carcinoma** of the stratified squamous (oesophageal) portion of the stomach is relatively common in **horse. Glandular neoplasms,** adenomas and adenocarcinomas occur in all species, but are usually seen in **dogs** and **cats.**

Intestine

Developmental Anomalies

Atresia is occlusion of the intestinal lumen due to anomalous development of the intestinal wall. It is generally named for the part of the intestine which is occluded, such as **atresia ani** or **atresia coli.** The **causes** of atresia in domestic animals are not completely understood.

Meckel's diverticulum is a remnant of the omphalo-mesenteric duct. It is near the termination of the ileum and represents the stalk of the yolk sac. Usually, it disappears after the first trimester of gestation. However, it can persist in all domestic animals.

Megacolon is a large, usually faeces filled colon. It occurs in **pigs, dogs, foals,** and **human beings. Affected foals** appear normal at birth but fail to pass meconium, develop colic, and die. Such affected animals lack normal peristalsis.

Intestinal Obstruction

Mechanical obstruction of the infected tract occurs in all species of domestic animals.

Enteroliths

Enteroliths are rare in species other than the **horse.** Generally, the affected animals are older than 4 years. The **stones** are made of ammonium magnesium phosphate **(struvite)** and form around the central nidus or foreign body. They vary in size from several centimeters in diameter to greater than 20 cm and can weigh several kilograms. They usually lodge at the pelvic flexure or transverse colon.

Impaction of the intestine occurs in all species. However, it **is especially common in horses** following administration of anthelmintic drugs and is the result of rapid deaths of large numbers of nematodes, particularly ascarids.

Strictures and Obstruction

Intussusception

Intussusception is the invagination of one segment of intestine into another. It occurs in all species. The **cause** is often unknown, but is thought to be associated with intestinal irritability and hypermotility. Foreign bodies, neoplasms, and some parasites such as the nodular worm of **sheep, Oesophagostomum** sp., may cause the intestine to telescope (invaginate) into itself. In the **dog,** intussusception of the intestine is caused by the granulomas of visceral larva migrans and histoplasmosis, surgical exposure and manipulation of the small intestine. In the **cat,** causes include foreign bodies and adenocarcinomas of the intestine. In **cattle,** papillomas, abscesses, fibromas, and lipomas are causes; in the **horse,** ascarids, parasitic granulomas, verminous arteritis, and leiomyoma are identified as causes.

As peristalsis continues even after death, intussusception can occur after death. Before death is diagnosed to be due to intussusception, it is important to determine whether intussusception took place before or after death. Since inflammation occurs only in the living organism, postmortem intussusceptions are easily diagnosed **because there are no adhesions** and they are not accompanied by hyperaemia or fibrin on the peritoneal surfaces, which remain smooth and glistening.

Clinical features are those of intestinal obstruction and include abdominal distension, dilated intestinal loops, palpable abdominal mass, signs of abdominal pain, complete anorexia, and vomiting. The intussusception is an enlarged, thickened segment of intestine. The segment is grossly swollen, distended, dark red or black because of congestion and haemorrhage. **Microscopically,** ischaemic necrosis involves the mucosa, with congestion and oedema of the sub-mucosa, muscularis, and sub-serosa.

Paralytic Ileus

Paralytic ileus is a hypomotility which results in functional obstruction of the intestine. It can be due to paralysis of the intestinal wall, which may result from peritonitis, shock, and several other causes. Paralytic ileus can also occur from manipulation and handling of the intestine at surgery. In such cases the gut is not paralyzed, but is adynamic (lack of muscle tone and peristaltic movement) because of sympathetic nerve inhibition. The stomach and intestines fail to respond to the presence of ingesta. **Adynamic ileus** is a disease with a biochemical rather than a morphological lesion. **Clinical signs** of adynamic ileus are anorexia, abdominal distension, absence of intestinal sounds, failure to pass faeces, and vomiting. Adynamic ileus occurs in **humans, dogs, cats, cattle,** and **horses.**

Intestinal Displacements

Intestinal displacements include herniations that finally lead to strangulation.

Herniations can be **internal** or **external**.

Internal hernias are displacements of intestine through a normal or pathological foramen in the abdominal cavity. It is common in **horses. External hernias** occur when a hernial sac, formed by a pouch of parietal peritoneum, penetrates outside the abdominal cavity. **Sites of external hernias** include umbilical, ventral, diaphragmatic, inguinal, scrotal, and perineal. Perineal hernia is seen in **old male dogs** with prostate gland enlargement. Umbilical hernias are usually caused by a defect in the abdominal wall. **Strangulated hernias** (usually umbilical or scrotal) cause complete obstruction in any species, but are most common in **horses** and **pigs**. The long intestine of the horse is prone to obstruction because of accidents caused by its tortuosity and the length of mesentery which suspends it. These are **torsions**, or twisting upon itself, or **volvulus**, in which a loop of intestine passes through a tear in the mesentery or similar abnormality (discussed next).

Volvulus and Torsion

Volvulus is a twisting of the intestine on its mesenteric axis. **Torsion** is a rotation of a tubular organ along its long axis. Torsion is common in the caecum of **cattle** and **horses** and sometimes in the abomasum of **calves**. Both volvulus and torsion result in intestinal obstruction and ischaemic injury. First, veins of the mesentery are occluded, while the arteries allow blood flow into the affected segment. The mesentery is thickened, congested, and dark red.

At postmortem, volvulus is a twisted segment of small intestine, which is distended with gas and fluid, and dark red or black. There is a sharp line of demarcation between the affected and normal intestine. Oedema and severe congestion thicken the entire wall of the affected segment. **Microscopically,** the affected intestine shows necrosis, congestion, and haemorrhage. **Finally, the process leads to gangrene, intestinal rupture, peritonitis, and death.**

The most common site of large intestine volvulus in the **horse** is the **left colon**.

Miscellaneous Diseases/Conditions

Rupture of the caeca or large intestine is common in **post-parturient mares,** but can also result from impaction. The sites of rupture vary, and the mechanisms are unknown.

Diverticula (singular 'diverticulum') are epithelium-lined cavities which are derived from mucosal epithelium. The cavities extend through the muscularis mucosa, submucosa and muscularis and reach the serosa, where they sometimes rupture and cause **peritonitis.**

Muscular hypertrophy of the distal ileum: This condition has been described in **horses** and **pigs**. The cause is unknown. Although usually an incidental finding, it can lead to impaction and rupture of the ileum. **Horses** with muscular hypertrophy of the intestine have intermittent or subacute colic. In some species, diarrhoea is a feature. An intestinal mass can be palpated, caused by the thickened ileum. In small animals, vomiting is a feature. Muscular hypertrophy of the ileum in **pigs** occurs either with regional enteritis, or as an independent disorder. **Cats** can have severe hypertrophy of the inner, circular layer of the tunica muscularis. Hypertrophy of the muscularis of the gastric antrum and segments of the small intestine occurs in **cats** with **hypereosinophilic syndrome**. It is a disease characterized by intramural eosinophilic infiltrates. Muscular hypertrophy of the intestine and medial hyperplasia of the pulmonary arteries occur in **cats** given large oral doses of *Toxocara cati* larvae.

Intestinal lipofuscinosis or **leiomyometaplasia** is also called 'brown dog gut'. The brown, discolored small intestine occurs in bile duct occlusion, chronic enteritis, pancreatic insufficiency, vitamin deficiency, or excess dietary lipids. **Brown pigmentation** of smooth muscle is a lesion of vitamin E deficiency in laboratory animals. In **dog** and **human,** intestinal pigmentation is also the result of vitamin E deficiency. Intestinal lipofuscinosis does not cause intestinal signs. The small intestine is brown. In severely affected **dogs,** portions of the stomach, caecum or colon are also pigmented.

Microscopically, the brown colour is due to the perinuclear lysosomal accumulation of **lipofuscin granules** in the cytoplasm of the smooth muscle cells of the intestine. These granules vary from basophilic to brown with haematoxylin-eosin (H & E) stain and stain variably periodic acid-Schiff (PAS) positive and Sudan black positive depending on the age of the lesion. Older granules are acid-fast when stained by the special acid-fast technique for lipofuscin. Younger lesions have proportionally more carbohydrate and are thus PAS positive. Acid-fast granules are called **ceroid pigment.**

Vascular Diseases of the Intestine

Parasites

In **horses,** *Strongylus vulgaris* fourth-stage larvae are present in the wall of the cranial mesenteric artery, resulting in **arteritis**. As a result, aneurysms and mural thrombosis develop. But in many cases, even complete occlusion of the cranial mesenteric artery does not result in intestinal infarction. This is because collateral circulation develops if the vascular occlusion develops slowly.

Eggs produced by *S. vulgaris* in the colon are discharged with the faeces, embryonate in the pasture, and within 2 weeks, develop into third-stage infective larvae. These larvae, ingested with feed, penetrate small and large intestinal mucosa, go to sub-mucosa, where they moult and enter into the sub-mucosal arteries. In these arteries, they migrate under the intima to the cranial mesenteric artery. After 3-4 months, larvae ex-sheath and migrate as young adults to the sub-mucosa of the caecum and colon. Afterwards, young adults are trapped in intramural nodules **which ultimately rupture into the intestinal lumen.** Larvae that travel beyond the cranial mesenteric artery reside in the aorta or its major abdominal branches.

Wherever the larvae reside, they cause **arteritis** that damages the intima causing **mural thrombosis, mural thickening** and **aneurysms.** Larvae, 1 cm in length, penetrate the intima. They number from a few to several hundred. **Clinical signs** include recurrent bouts of colic, weight loss, variable appetite, and poor hair coat. **Death** occurs when strongyle-induced thrombi or emboli occlude branches of major arteries in the caecum, colon, or small intestine, with resultant infarction. At postmortem, the intestine is black and blood-engorged. Often perforation may have occurred and caused a terminal peritonitis.

Lymphangiectasia

Lymphangiectasia, or **lacteal dilation** is the most common cause of protein-losing enteropathy in the **dog. Clinical signs** include diarrhoea, hypoproteinaemia, and ascites. **Microscopically,** intestinal lymph vessels and lacteals are markedly dilated.

Inflammation

Inflammation of the intestine is known as **enteritis.**

1. Viral Enteritis

Rinderpest

Also known as **'cattle plague',** rinderpest is a serious disease of **cattle**. It is caused by a **morbillivirus**. The mortality in **cattle** varies from 25-90%, depending on the strains of virus involved and resistance of the animals. The **incubation period** is from 6-9 days after infection by contact. Besides **cattle, buffaloes, sheep, pigs, goats, deer,** and **camels** are also susceptible. The virus is antigenically related to viruses of canine distemper, peste-des-petits-ruminants (PPR), and human measles. Once the most serious viral disease of cattle in India inflicting very heavy mortality and ruining cattle farmers' economy, rinderpest has been effectively controlled and has not been reported since June 1995.

The onset is characterized by a sharp rise in temperature to 104^0-105^0F, accompanied by restlessness, dryness of the muzzle, and constipation. Within a day or two nasal and lachrymal discharges appear. Other signs include photophobia (fear of light), depression, excessive thirst, retarded rumination, anorexia, lymphopaenia, necrotic stomatitis and excessive salivation. The fever usually reaches its peak between 3rd to 5th day, **and drops suddenly with the onset of diarrhoea.** Lesions in the oral mucosa appear by the 2nd and 3rd day of fever, but become prominent only after the onset of diarrhoea. As the diarrhoea increases in severity, it is accompanied by abdominal pain, increased respiration, severe dehydration, emaciation, prostration, subnormal temperature and death, usually after a course of 6-12 days.

Lesions

The rinderpest virus has a particular affinity for lymphoid tissue and for epithelial tissues of the gastrointestinal tract, in which it produces severe and characteristic lesions. In the **lymphoid tissue**, the virus causes necrosis of lymphocytes. This is striking in microscopic sections of lymph nodes, spleen, and Peyer's patches. The destruction of lymphocytes is first seen by fragmentation of nuclei in the germinal centres. Multi-nucleated giant cells containing eosinophilic cytoplasmic inclusion bodies are often present in the lymph nodes. The Peyer's patches are darkened with haemorrhage and slough out, leaving **deep craters in the intestinal wall.**

In the **digestive system** of **cattle**, the rinderpest virus produces typical lesions in the epithelium. The virus is conveyed to the oral mucosa by the bloodstream. It first produces necrosis of epithelial cells in the deep layers of the stratum Malpighii of squamous epithelium of the oral cavity. As the necrotic areas increase in size and extend towards the surface, the cornified layer above gets elevated and appears as tiny, greyish-white, slightly raised puncta (points). **Eosinophilic cytoplasmic inclusion bodies** form in the mucosal epithelial cells and giant cells. **Vesicles are not formed in this disease.** The foci of necrosis later coalesce to form large areas of erosion. Since the basal layer of the squamous epithelium is rarely penetrated, **ulcers seldom form.** The erosions are shallow, with a red, raw floor bounded by normal epithelium. Lesions have selective distribution and occur on the inside of the lower lip, the adjacent gum, the cheeks, near the commissures, and the ventral surface of the free portion of the tongue.

The **abomasum** is a common site of the lesions. Necrotic foci of microscopic size in the epithelium are accompanied by congestion and haemorrhage of the lamina propria. **Grossly,** they appear as superficial streaks of bright red to dark brown in colour. Oedema may be extensive. As the necrosis progresses, the infected areas slough away, leaving sharply outlined irregular erosions with freshly oozing blood.

In the **small intestine,** severe lesions are less common than in the mouth, abomasum, or large intestine. **Lesions** include streaks of haemorrhage, and sometimes erosions, along the crest of the folds of mucous membrane, particularly in the initial part of the duodenum and terminal ileum. **Peyers' patches are exceptionally vulnerable.** The lymphoid tissue may become so necrotic that patches slough out, **leaving deep, raw craters,** (bowl-shaped deep eroded lesions) **in the intestinal wall.**

The **large intestine** is more seriously damaged than the small intestine, with prominent lesions around the ileo-caecal valve, at the caeco-colic junction, and the rectum. In the caecum, the crests of the folds of mucous membrane are bright red from numerous petechiae. **Microscopically,** capillaries in the lamina propria are greatly distended and packed with erythrocytes. The **rectum** is always affected and shows parallel bands of congestion known as 'zebra markings', or 'zebra-striped' appearance. As the disease progresses and the mucosa becomes eroded, diffuse congestion and bleeding from the raw surfaces may occur over large areas.

The **respiratory system** is susceptible to the virus. Petechiae appear on the turbinates and in the larynx. Trachea presents streaks of haemorrhage in the mucosa; most common being longitudinal streaks of rusty haemorrhage in the anterior third of the trachea.

The clinical, gross, and microscopic features of the disease are adequate for a **presumptive diagnosis**, which should be confirmed by serological methods and other tests. These include isolation of the virus and its identification, agar gel precipitation test (AGPT), complement fixation test (CFT), immunocapture sandwich ELISA, and the use of specific cDNA probes.

Peste-Des-Petits-Ruminants (Goat Plague)

'Peste-des-petits-ruminants (PPR)' is a French name and means **'plague of the small ruminants'**, that is, **goats** and **sheep**. PPR is therefore also known as **'goat plague'.** The other names for the disease include **erosive stomatitis and enteritis of goats, goat catarrhal fever,** and **stomatitis-pneumoenteritis complex.** PPR is a severe infectious and contagious disease of **goats** and **sheep**, and is caused by a **morbillivirus (ssRNA).** PPR was first recognized in 1942 in Ivory Coast, in French West Africa. In India, it was first reported in 1989 in native sheep flocks in Villupuram district of Tamil Nadu. PPR is characterized by fever, lymphopaenia, erosive stomatitis, enteritis, pneumonia, and death. **It thus closely resembles rinderpest (cattle plague). In India, the disease every year takes a heavy toll of lives, mostly in goats, and less so in sheep.** PPR virus is antigenically and immunologically closely related to the viruses of rinderpest, canine distemper, and measles (in humans). All these are also morbillivirus. In particular, PPR and rinderpest (RP) viruses cross-immunize and cross-protect, so much so that tissue culture rinderpest vaccine has been found to be an effective prophylactic against PPR.

The disease is particularly severe in goats, and is usually fatal. The virus is shed by sick animals in body excretions and secretions, especially in diarrhoeic faeces, and they initiate new infections when inhaled. **The virus enters through the cells of the upper respiratory tract**, but could also enter through the conjunctiva and oral mucosa. The disease can be acute or subacute. The **acute form** is seen mainly in **goats** and is similar to rinderpest in cattle. **Clinically,** short fever follows an incubation period of 2-6 days and is accompanied by serous nasal discharge, depression, and anorexia. Mucosal erosions soon appear and diarrhoea develops 2-3 days later. Terminal stages are complicated by bronchopneumonia, mostly caused by pasteurella. **Mortality rate in goats** ranges from 55%-90%, and death usually occurs within a week of the onset of illness. In pregnant animals abortions occur. **Subacute form** is more common in **sheep** and is manifested by catarrh, low-grade fever, and intermittent diarrhoea. Most recover after a course of 10-15 days.

Gross lesions in the **acute disease** include necrotic stomatitis and pronounced hyperaemia of the abomasum, ileo-caecal region, and along the course of the colon and rectum as **'zebra stripes'**. Lymph nodes are enlarged. An important postmortem finding is a **purulent** or **fibrinous bronchopneumonia.** Intra-cytoplasmic inclusion bodies may be abundant in necrotic glands of the small and large intestines. Both intra-cytoplasmic and intra-nuclear eosinophilic **inclusion bodies** are common in the epithelial cells of the airways and in the type II pneumocytes and multinucleated giant (syncytial) cells.

Presumptive diagnosis can be made from the clinical signs and postmortem findings. **Pneumonia is usually a feature of PPR, but not rinderpest.** Confirmation may be made by isolation of the virus and its identification. Blood at the height of the fever is the best source of the virus. Virus has been successfully isolated in primary lamb or kidney cultures. For provisional diagnosis antigen in lymph nodes can be detected by agar gel precipitation test (AGPT), or by counter-immunoelectrophoresis. Unlike rinderpest, cases of PPR usually contain high levels of antigen at death. **Since PPR and rinderpest in goats are indistinguishable both clinically and pathologically,** it is important to ascertain by other means that it is PPR virus and not rinderpest virus that caused the disease. For this, immunocapture sandwich ELISA has been developed which employs specific PPRV and RPV detector MABs (monoclonal antibodies). Also, specific cDNA probes for selected segments of N genes of the two viruses are useful in differentiating PPR and RP, on postmortem materials. Differential diagnosis is also possible by complement fixation and virus neutralization tests. Recently a PCR test (polymerase chain reaction test) has been found to be valuable in confirmatory diagnosis in tissues otherwise unsuitable for standard techniques. **Surviving goats and sheep develop a life-long active immunity, as in rinderpest, associated with the presence of humoral neutralizing antibodies.**

Rotavirus Enteritis

Rotaviruses are present everywhere in the environment, including air and water. **Each species of animal has its specific rotavirus.** These viruses are important pathogens. However, in all species these viruses cause disease along with other enteropathogens. **In calves,** the disease is most important during the first week of life and **in piglets** in the first 7 weeks of life. These ages correspond with a decrease in the colostral and milk-associated anti-rotavirus antibody titres that occur after weaning.

Affected **calves and piglets** have yellow fluid diarrhoea, appear depressed, are unwilling to stand and nurse, and sometimes have a few strings of thick saliva hanging from their lips. **Grossly,** intestines are distended with yellow fluid. **Microscopically,** there is sloughing of villus cells. This is followed by blunting and fusion of villi. The infection extends to the epithelial cells of the middle and distal small intestine.

Coronavirus Enteritis

Coronaviruses cause **calfhood enteritis** and are composed of single-stranded RNA. Calves up to 21 days of age (usually 4 to 6 days old) are susceptible. The incubation period is 36 to 60 hours. **Clinically**, the disease is characterized by yellow fluid, sometimes bloody diarrhoea, depression, unwillingness to suckle, dehydration, and weakness. **Lesions** include enterocyte loss, blunting, and fusion of villi similar to rotavirus enteritis.

The **course of infection, clinical signs, and tissue damage** last longer in coronavirus enteritis than in rotavirus-induced disease, and **death** occurs after 2 to 4 days of diarrhoea. The **gross lesions** are similar to those of rotavirus enteritis or enterotoxigenic colibacillosis. The small and large intestines are distended with yellow fluid. **Microscopically**, changes are first seen in villus epithelial cells of the proximal small intestine and, afterwards, in the distal small intestine and epithelial cells lining the colon. Virus is present in all the cells lining the villi at the onset of diarrhoea. In the colon, virus is present in surface cells and cells of the crypts.

In the colon, surface cells are lost and replaced by less mature cuboidal and squamous cells. Crypts lumens contain degenerate and necrotic cells. A haemorrhagic form of coronavirus enterocolitis also occurs in which all colonic crypts are damaged. A bloody fibrino-necrotic pseudomembrane covers the denuded colonic lamina propria.

Bovine Viral Diarrhoea

Also known as **'mucosal disease'**, bovine viral diarrhoea (BVD) affects **cattle of all ages**, but is more important in animals 8 months to 2 years of age. BVD is caused by a **pestivirus** related to the virus of swine fever. Animals infected early in life with noncytopathic BVD virus develop a persistent infection. Later in life, if exposed to cytopathic virus, they develop disease. **Clinical signs** include anorexia, depression, profuse diarrhoea, stoppage of milk production, fever, rumen atony, lacrimation, and mucopurulent nasal discharge. **Lesions** include erosions and ulcers in the tongue, gingiva, palate, oesophagus, rumen, abomasum, and coronary bands of the hooves. **In the intestine**, lesions include areas of necrosis in the epithelium over the gut-associated lymphoid tissue. Abortions, stillbirths, and mummified foetuses can also result from an in utero infection. Mortality in a herd varies from 20% to 50%. **All affected animals die.**

Microscopically, the lesions in the stratified squamous epithelium begin as focal hydropic degeneration and necrosis of the stratum spinosum. This is followed by erosion and ulceration, with hyperaemia and infiltration of granulocytes. In the abomasum, small intestine, caecum, and colon, the villus and crypt epithelium is necrotic. Loss of epithelium is extensive. The lamina propria is infiltrated by a variety of acute and chronic inflammatory cells. Peyer's patches show extensive necrosis of lymphocytes. A fibrino-necrotic or fibrino-haemorrhagic pseudomembrane may cover Peyer's patches, ileum, and large intestine.

Adenovirus Enteritis

Adenovirus infection occurs in **cattle, sheep, pigs,** and **horses**. Each species-specific virus causes sub-clinical respiratory disease and under some circumstances clinical disease. **In horses, adenovirus enteritis** occurs in immunologically suppressed horses.

Swine Fever (Hog Cholera, Swine Plague)

Swine fever is an acute, febrile, highly contagious and often fatal disease of **pigs,** caused by a **pestivirus**. The tonsil is the primary site of virus invasion following oral exposure. The virus then spreads through lymphatics and enters blood capillaries, resulting in an initial viraemia. After 24 hours, the virus can be found in the spleen and other sites such as lymph nodes, bone marrow, and Peyer's patches. The virus exerts its pathogenic effect on endothelial cells, macrophages, and epithelial cells. **The basic lesions in swine fever are injury to the endothelial cells and suppression of bone marrow activity.** Most of the lesions are produced by hydropic degeneration and proliferation of vascular endothelium, which result in the occlusion of blood vessels. **Clinical signs** initially are depression and high fever (106^0F). These are accompanied by severe leukopaenia, weakness, loss of appetite, nervous symptoms such as lethargy, convulsions, grinding of the teeth, and difficulty in locomotion. In pigs with light skin, erythematous lesions appear on the skin. **Most animals die within 10 days after the onset of symptoms.**

As stated, **the virus of swine fever exerts a direct effect on the vascular system,** and signs and lesions result from changes in the capillaries, arteries, and veins. For this reason, the **gross changes** appear as areas of congestion, haemorrhage, or infarction mainly in the kidneys, lymph nodes, urinary bladder, spleen, lungs, and **large intestine**. In the kidney, sharply demarcated petechiae give a characteristic appearance known as **'turkey egg kidney'**. In the spleen, infarction occurs in about 50% of cases. Infarcts are sharply outlined, irregular or wedge-shaped, and elevated. In the skin, erythematous areas resulting from cyanosis are the most common gross lesions. The characteristic lesion in the **large intestine**, particularly **colon**, is a **spherical ulcer** in the mucosa. These ulcers are sharply circumscribed, and are either single or multiple. The ulcers eventually develop into encrusted button-shaped foci (**'button ulcers'**), a few millimetres in diameter. The lesion develops after occlusion of a small artery by swelling and hydropic changes in its endothelium. Thus, the **button ulcer** is the result of infarction.

Transmissible Gastroenteritis

Transmissible gastroenteritis (TGE) is **an important disease in pigs, younger than 10 days**. It is caused by a **coronavirus**. The virus is inactivated by sunlight. Therefore, this virus occurs mostly in winter. Piglets suffer from acute diarrhoea, weight loss, vomiting, and dehydration. **Morbidity and mortality approach 100% in susceptible herds.** Virus specifically affects the villus enterocytes. Therefore, lesions consist of marked atrophy of villi of the small intestine. Sows are susceptible to the virus. Morbidity among the sows is 100%, but they do not suffer much clinically (vomiting, loss of appetite, agalactia), and mortality is not seen. Immunity is complete.

Like rotavirus, the TGE coronavirus is lytic and sloughed enterocytes carry the virus into the faeces. In TGE most of the villus enterocytes are destroyed, and therefore the clinical disease is more severe. TGE is characterized by sudden onset of vomiting and diarrhoea. The diarrhoea is profuse and contains white, undigested milk, and has an offensive odour. Dehydration is pronounced. Weakness and emaciation progress to **death** from the 2nd to the 5th day of illness. Pigs that survive grow poorly because of continued intestinal malabsorption.

Young pigs that have died are dehydrated. The small intestine is ballooned, gas-filled, and contains copious yellow fluid. Piglets may have empty stomachs caused by vomiting. **Microscopically**, the **diagnosis** to some extent is based on the presence of **villus atrophy. The villus height:crypt depth ratio is reduced from 7:1 in normal to 1:1 in infected pigs.** The atrophy is not accompanied by infiltration of inflammatory cells. **Epithelial cell necrosis** and **villus atrophy** are the main lesions of TGE, but are not pathognomonic.

Parvovirus Enteritis of Dogs and Cats

Parvovirus enteritis of **dogs** and **cats** is **a severe, usually fatal disease.** This is because the **parvovirus** specifically attacks the rapidly dividing crypt cells in the intestine. In the beginning virus replication occurs in the lymphoid tissue. Although there is much common between the disease syndrome in **dogs** and **cats**, the differences require separate discussion for each species.

Canine parvovirus enteritis was first reported from Europe and the United States in 1978. **It was described as occurring in three distinct syndromes: (1) Puppies younger than 2 weeks** had generalized disease with focal areas of necrosis in those tissues with rapidly dividing cells. **(2) Puppies 3 to 8 weeks of age** may develop myocarditis. These animals would die unexpectedly 5 months later because of myocardial scarring and conduction failure. **(3) In puppies 8 weeks or older,** the disease is similar to that in the cat.

At postmortem, the small intestine is dilated, fluid-filled and flaccid. This is quite characteristic. Its contents are brown to red-brown coloured fluid and fibrinous exudate, with or without haemorrhage. Mesenteric lymph nodes are enlarged. The bone marrow is semi-liquid and yellow-grey.

Microscopically, lesion in the intestine is characterized by necrosis of crypt epithelial cells, with necrotic cell fragments in the crypts. The surviving epithelial cells become cuboidal, or squamoid to cover the surface of the denuded crypt. The colon also · has lesions, but these are usually focal and less severe.

Dogs with **haemorrhagic form** of parvovirus enteritis have bloody diarrhoea and die within 24 hours. **Canine parvovirus enteritis has many similarities to feline panleukopaenia, and the sequence of tissue events is almost the same.** The **gross lesion** in the canine disease is segmental or diffuse haemorrhagic enteritis. The affected segment is hyperaemic, congested, and blood-filled. Coagulative necrosis of the lymphoid tissue of Peyer's patches and regional lymph nodes is present in canine parvovirus enteritis, **but these lesions are not seen in panleukopaenia.** This latter change can be diagnostic, even when the intestinal mucosa has been affected by autolysis.

Feline panleukopaenia is an important disease of **cat**, and is caused by **parvovirus**. It is also known by other names such as **cat distemper** and **feline enteritis**. **Clinically,** the disease is characterized by dehydration, depression, and vomiting.

Early lesions are lymphoid depletion and thymic involution. Afterwards, **lesions** include reddened intestine with serositis. Lesions are usually limited to the small intestine, but colitis occurs in some cats. **Microscopically,** villus atrophy occurs following crypt cell destruction. **Basophilic intranuclear inclusion bodies** are present in enterocytes and lymphocytes early in infection. Intrauterine infection causes congenital cerebellar hypoplasia in **kittens.**

Feline Infectious Peritonitis

Feline infectious peritonitis (FIP) is **a fatal disease of cats**. The disease occurs mainly in young and old cats. Twelve percent of deaths in cats are due to FIP. The **cause** of the disease is a **coronavirus**. It forms immune complexes that localize in the blood vessels. **Lesions** are therefore multifocal and most organs have lesions. The **disease occurs in two forms:** (1) The **'wet form'** is characterized by fibrinous polyserositis, and (2) **'dry form'** is without the effusive process. Why one form develops rather than the other is not completely understood. **The virus spreads among cats by saliva.**

During a strong immune response, phlebitis, thrombophlebitis, and thrombosis occur in several organs, including the intestine. Thus the disease is basically an immune-mediated vasculitis with necrosis and pyogranulomas that occur following deposition of immune complexes in vessels.

The **'wet form'** is characterized by large volumes of thick, yellow peritoneal transudate that contains flecks or strands of fibrin, and by multiple granulomas on the serosa of abdominal viscera. The **'dry form'** of the disease, on the other hand, consists of vasocentric, firm, grey towhite masses. The localized **'dry form'** causes granulomatous disease of the ileum, caecum, or colon. The affected intestinal wall is thickened, firm, and fibrotic. **Clinical signs** include weight loss, constipation, obstipation (severe constipation), vomiting, and palpable abdominal masses.

Microscopically, the deeper layers of the colon are thickened by granulomas, accompanied by an intense mononuclear infiltration. The sub-mucosa contains focal granulomatous nodules with areas of intense mononuclear reaction in the mucosa.

2. Bacterial Enteritis

Colibacillosis (*Escherichia coli* Diseases)

E. coli bacteria are among the first to enter intestine after birth and are present there in virtually all animals. Various serotypes induce disease by various means, especially in the young of each species. *E. coli* infections usually occur along with rotavirus, coronavirus, or cryptosporidia. Colibacillosis occurs in various forms:

(i) Enterotoxic Colibacillosis

This is common in animals of 2 days to 3 weeks of age. The faeces of affected animals are profuse, yellow to white, and watery to pasty. Affected animals are dehydrated, their abdomen 'tucked up' and eyeballs sunken. Animals that die are severely dehydrated, emaciated, and have diarrhoeic faeces pasted over and around their perineum.

Gross lesions include dilated small intestine, filled with fluid. Chyle (milky liquid) is present in the mesenteric lymphatic vessels similar to normal animals. **Microscopically,** the intestine is also normal. **Diagnosis** can be made by microscopic examination of small intestine of freshly dead animals and noting the presence of bacteria lining the luminal surface of the enterocytes.

(ii) Septicaemic Colibacillosis

This is a disease of **newborn calves, lambs,** and sometimes **foals** that have not received sufficient colostral immunity. Although the lesions produced are generally those of septicaemia, infection can localize in the intestine causing **enteritis.** The bacteria enter into the body through the respiratory system, oral cavity, or umbilicus and become septicaemic. Fibrinous arthritis, ophthalmitis, serositis, meningitis, and white-spotted kidneys (cortical abscesses) characterize the septicaemia. Mixed bacterial infections usually occur with enterotoxic *E. coli.*

(iii) Enterotoxaemic Colibacillosis

Also known as **'oedema disease',** this is an *E. coli* infection that is specific for **pigs.** It is caused by a bacterial **enterotoxin** produced in the **small intestine** that spreads through blood. It is a disease of pigs of 6 to 14 weeks of age and affects usually the best pigs in a group. The disease is characterized by incoordination of hind legs, difficulty in rising, muscle tremors, aimless wandering, and clonic convulsions.

Haemolytic *E. coli* proliferates in the small intestine following dietary changes, and produces a heat-labile exotoxin. This systemic toxin (**angiotoxin**) causes **generalized vascular endothelial injury of arterioles and arteries** resulting in fluid loss and oedema. The **oedema** is prominent in gastric sub-mucosa, eyelids, gallbladder, and mesentery of the colon. Death is due to an endotoxic shock-like syndrome.

Clostridial Enteritis

All types of clostridial enteritis are **enterotoxaemias. An enterotoxaemia** is a condition characterized by the presence in the blood of toxins produced in the intestine. *Clostridium perfringens* is a Gram-positive, anaerobic rod which is a normal inhabitant of the gastrointestinal tract. These bacilli form spores under adverse conditions and produce toxins in the presence of large quantities of nutrients that favour bacterial proliferation. *C. perfringens* is divided into **five types: A, B, C, D, and E.** This division is based on the production of one or more of the four lethal toxins. *C. perfringens* **type A** produces **alpha toxin; type B** produces **alpha, beta,** and **epsilon toxins; type C** produces **alpha** and **beta toxins; type D** produces **epsilon toxin;** and **type E** produces **alpha** and **iota** toxins.

Enterotoxaemia

Enterotoxaemia is produced by any one of the five *C. perfringens.* Usually it is the *C. perfringens* **type D** that is involved. Clostridial enterotoxaemia usually affects **young fat animals.** Outbreaks usually follow a change in feed or an increase in its carbohydrate content. A change in feed or overfeeding precipitates an alteration in the balance in the bacterial flora of the intestine. This altered condition provides an opportunity for *C. perfringens* to proliferate and produce abundant toxin. **Clinical signs** of enterotoxaemia include diarrhoea, loss of appetite, lethargy, distended abdomen, dehydration, prostration, and death. Affected **lambs** have glucosuria, a feature not seen in other species.

Small intestine is the target organ. **Lesions** include petechiae, ecchymoses, and diffuse haemorrhage of the serosa and mucosa. The intestines are thin-walled, dilated and gas-filled. The intestine can rupture as a result of the thinning of the wall and accumulation of gas. The **spleen** is enlarged and pulpy because of congestion. The toxins produced by *C. perfringens* damage intestinal villi. This is followed by sloughing of cells and haemorrhage. The intestinal sub-mucosa can be oedematous, haemorrhagic, or filled with leukocytes. **Death occurs within 24 hours after the onset of clinical signs.**

Clostridium perfringens Type C

Enterotoxic haemorrhagic enteritis affects **calves, lambs,** and **foals** during the first few days of life, and **piglets** during the first 8 hours of life. **Clinical signs** vary from no signs to bloody diarrhoea. **When piglets are affected, the whole litter dies. Lesions** include haemorrhagic or nectrotizing enteritis of the small intestine, sometimes with gas in the lumen. **Struck** is a disease that affects **adult sheep** and **goats** and **cattle** in winter and early spring. It is also caused by *C. perfringens* **type** C and is characterized by haemorrhagic enteritis with ulceration, ascites, and peritonitis.

Clostridium perfringens Type D

This type affects **fattening sheep, goats,** and **calves**. It is diet related and is associated with overeating. The disease is therefore also called **'overeating disease'**. The sudden change in diet promotes growth of organisms in the small intestine. The disease is characterized by unexpected death, sometimes preceded by nervous signs or **'blind staggers'**. The bacterial toxin (**angiotoxin**) causes endothelial cell damage. The damage can result in bilateral symmetrical encephalomalacia. Lesions of *C. perfringens* type D infection include haemorrhages in many organs, particularly of serosal surfaces. The angiotoxin produces **'pulpy kidney disease' of sheep.**

Salmonellosis

Salmonellosis is an important cause of **acute and chronic diarrhoea** and **death** in **many animal species** and in **humans**. In animals the important species include *Salmonella typhimurium, S. enteritidis, S. dublin, S. cholerasuis,* and *S. typhosa.* The salmonellae are Gram-negative, motile bacilli. In carrier animals, salmonellae reside in the gallbladder, intestinal tract, and mesenteric lymph nodes. Some recovered animals become carriers and shed the organism in their faeces, particularly after stress. **Dogs** and **cats** rarely get clinical salmonellosis, but 10% are carriers and can infect humans.

Salmonella infections occur through ingestion. Contaminated feed and water are important sources of infection in all species. The tonsils and Peyer's patches are portals of entry for some species of salmonellae. The other species colonize the intestine, are invasive, and enter epithelial cells. Salmonellae produce disease through **enterotoxins, cytotoxins (Verotoxins),** and **endotoxins**. Once in contact with macrophages of the lamina propria or Peyer's patches, salmonellae are phagocytosed and transported to regional lymphnodes, or by portal circulation to the liver. The organisms colonize the small intestine, colon, mesenteric lymph nodes, and the gallbladder. **Salmonellosis mostly infects the young.** The young are more severely affected than adults, and they are also more likely to succumb to septicaemia.

The **clinical signs** vary from species to species and with age. The **horse** develops an acute fatal colitis. The **cow** has lingering diarrhoea with the passage of pseudomembranes, and **calves** have acute diarrhoea. **Dogs** develop sudden bouts of acute diarrhoea. **Cats** succumb to enterocolitis. **Pigs** die of septicaemia and enterocolitis.

Salmonellosis is usually an enterocolitis. Lesions occur in the villa of the small intestine, lymphoid tissues, and colonic mucosa. The invasive salmonellae have a cytotoxic effect on epithelial cells, cause their sloughing, and induce a granulocytic cellular infiltration of the lamina propria. Later, diphtheritic pseudomembranes form on the mucosal surface. Macrophages of the mucosa have organisms in their cytoplasm and are accompanied by plasma cells and lymphocytes. In the submucosa, lesions include perivasculitis and vasculitis that can cause thrombosis. The characteristic **gross and microscopic changes** of salmonellosis are the enlargement of Peyer's patches and the lymphoid nodules of the caecum and colon with necrosis of surface epithelium. In the **pig**, Peyer's patches are ulcerated and coated with necrotic pseudomembrane. In the colon, lymphoid nodules are ulcerated, creating so-called **'button ulcers'**.

Mesenteric lymph nodes are enlarged, swollen, oedematous and have foci of necrosis. The **hepatic lesions** are focal necrosis that progress to microgranulomas. **Microgranulomas** are small clusters of macrophages (**'paratyphoid nodules** or **granules'**) that occur following lodgment of **Salmonella** emboli. In the **septicaemic form**, salmonellae spread to other tissues and may produce focal meningoencephalitis, suppurative bacterial arthritis, or renal infarction. In **pigs**, septicaemic salmonellosis is usually accompanied by violet discoloration of the skin and extensive capsular petechiae of the kidneys (**'turkey egg kidney'**).

Peracute Salmonella Septicaemia

This is a disease of **calves, foals,** and **pigs. In foals,** the faeces of affected animals are green. The species often involved in septicaemic salmonellosis is *Salmonella cholerasuis.* **Gross lesions** are due to fibrinoid necrosis of blood vessels. Necrosis of blood vessels causes a widespread petechiation and cyanosis (a blue discoloration) of the extremities. Peracute **Salmonella** septicaemia is usually fatal.

Acute Enteric Salmonellosis

This disease is usually caused by *Salmonella typhimurium* and occurs in **cattle, pigs,** and **horses.** Carnivores are rarely affected. The disease is characterized by **diffuse catarrhal enteritis.** Intestinal contents contain mucus, fibrin, and sometimes, blood. Multiple foci of hepatocellular necrosis and hyperplasia of Kupffer cells (**paratyphoid nodules**) are characteristic of acute enteric salmonellosis. **Fibrinous cholecystitis** at postmortem is pathognomonic for acute enteric salmonellosis in **calves.**

Chronic Enteric Salmonellosis

This disease occurs in **pigs, cattle,** and **horses.**
Lesions are mainly seen in **pigs** and include foci
of necrosis and ulceration in ·caecum and colon.
These are termed **button ulcers** (Fig. 10).

Mycobacterial Enteritis

Intestinal Tuberculosis

Mycobacterium tuberculosis and *Mycobacterium
bovis* enter by the respiratory and gastrointestinal
routes. Intestinal tuberculosis occurs rarely in
cattle, in **calves** sucking infected mammary
glands, monkeys, and human beings ingesting
un-pasteurized milk. **The mycobacteria enter by
ingestion.** They are then phagocytosed by M cells
which cover Peyer's patches and enter into these
patches. The most common site of disease is the
distant ileum and lesions occur at Peyer's patches.
Clinically, animals with intestinal tuberculosis

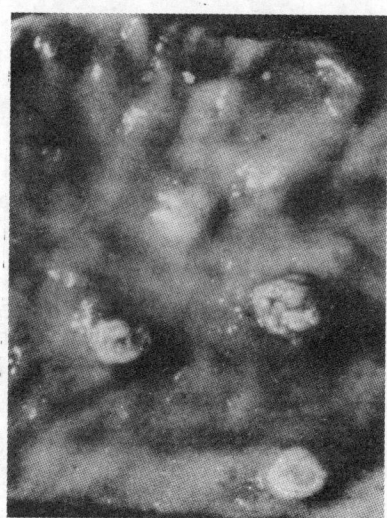

Fig. 10. Colon; pig. Salmonellosis.
Note raised necrotic **'button
ulcers'** on the mucosal
surface.

suffer from chronic diarrhoea, lower abdominal pain, and chronic weight loss. If a
portion of the small intestine has become stenotic (narrow), vomiting is the clinical
sign.

In **some species,** such as the **dog,** a thickened, firm, segment of intestine can be
palpated through the abdominal wall. **In large animals,** thickened, firm loops of
intestine are found at rectal examination. The affected segment of intestine is
thickened, and the mucosa is corrugated or ulcerated. Regional lymph nodes have
granulomas and **calcification.** The **tuberculous lesion** consists of many epithelioid
granulomas with necrotic centres. Epithelioid and giant cells infiltrate the lamina
propria and the sub-mucosa. The affected mucosa and sub-mucosa are distended
by the caseating tuberculoid granulomatous lesion and have prominent infiltrates
of lymphocytes and plasma cells. In some animals, *Mycobacterium avium* infections
result in lesions similar to those of *M. tuberculosis,* with caseation, necrosis, and
calcification. However, in most spontaneous *Mycobacterium avium intracellulare-*
induced diseases, a lepromatous (non-caseating) granulomatous inflammation
occurs, **similar to that of Johne's disease** (see 'Johne's disease', 'paratuberculosis').
Such lesions are described in **dogs, pigs, horses, rhesus monkeys,** and **AIDS
patients:**

Pigs ingest the organisms along with the avian litter sometimes fed as a cheaper
source of dietary protein. In these cases, lesions also develop in the retropharyngeal
lymph nodes. The **lesion** consists of macrophages in the mucosa and sub-mucosa,

and occurs over a large segment of the small intestine, colon, or both. Ziehl-Neelsen staining of these tissues shows large numbers of intracellular acid-fast bacilli.

Johne's Disease (Paratuberculosis)

Johne's disease or paratuberculosis occurs in **many ruminant species**. It is one of the most important diseases facing the dairy industry. In **cattle**, the disease is characterized by diarrhoea, emaciation, and hypoproteinaemia **in animals older than 19 months**. In the average infected herd, 32% to 42% of animals are infected. In small ruminants (**sheep** and **goats**) the clinical disease is similar to that observed in cattle **except that diarrhoea does not occur**. The disease has long course and is considered a wasting disease due to the loss of body mass. **Ruminants** are infected with *Mycobacterium paratuberculosis* (*M. johnii*) from faeces-contaminated soil. Recently it has been suggested that *M. johnii* is closely related to *Mycobacterium avium*.

The **causative organisms** are **very resistant** to environmental changes. **After ingestion** the bacilli penetrate the gastrointestinal mucosa and are taken up by macrophages. **Lesions** in the lamina propria of the intestines, particularly in the **ileum**, include accumulation of **macrophages**.

There is not much correlation between the severity of the gross lesions and the severity of clinical disease. **An age-related immune resistance to infection and disease** occurs in animals older than 2 months. **Foetuses** can be affected, but disease is not seen until the animals are much older. Isolation of newborns from faecal contamination is useful in reducing the incidence of infection in a herd. **Diagnosis** is made by observing clinical signs and by considering characteristic features of the disease. The **gross lesion** is a chronic, segmented thickening of the distal small intestine, caecum, and proximal colon (Fig. 11). Affected segments have a corrugated mucosa which is focally ulcerated. Mesenteric lymph nodes are greatly enlarged.

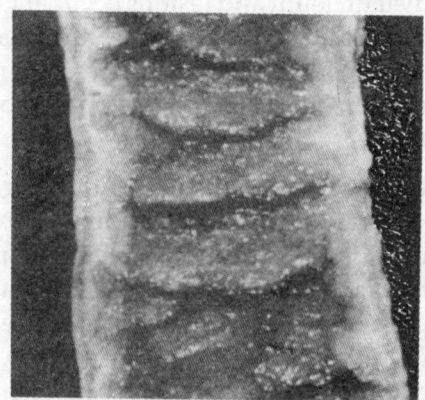

Fig. 11. Ileum mucosa; sheep. Johne's disease. There is marked thickening of the lamina propria from macrophage infiltration.

Microscopically, in cattle, non-caseating granulomas consist of **macrophages** with foamy cytoplasm and large numbers of acid-fast organisms (Fig. 12). In contrast, **sheep, goats**, and **deer** have tuberculoid (caseating) granulomas in the intestines, lymphatics, and lymph nodes, sometimes with central mineralization (calcification). These lesions are composed of epithelioid cells and Langhans-type giant cells (Fig. 13). Organisms are few. Granulomas of either type occur in regional lymph nodes (Fig. 14).

M. paratuberculosis can be isolated from faeces of affected animals, from diseased intestines and regional lymph nodes, and sometimes from other tissues and fluids, including liver, uterus, foetus, milk, urine, and semen. Acid-fast bacteria in rectal mucosal scrapings are found in 60% of the cases. Hepatic microgranulomas occur in about 25% of affected animals. **Aortic mineralization (arteriosclerosis),** when it occurs, **is specific for Johne's disease in cattle.** It is associated with the severe cachexia that occurs in the disease.

Rhodococcus equi Enteritis

Rhodococcus equi (previously *Corynebacterium equi*) is a soil saprophyte and a normal inhabitant of the equine intestine. The disease caused by this Gram-positive rod is characterized by pulmonary pyogranulomas. The common occurrence of helminths and *R. equi* infection together suggests that migrating larvae participate in distributing the bacterium through the body of the **foal.** Helminth control brings about great reduction or elimination of *R. equi* infection. When coughed up and swallowed in large numbers, bacteria enter into the M cells of the intestine and cause pyogranulomas in the gut-associated

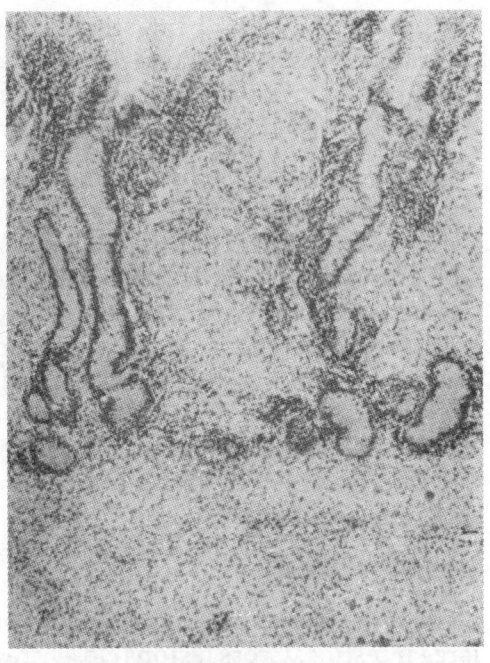

Fig. 12. Small intestine; cow. Johne's disease. Note macrophages distend the lamina propria of the villi and sub-mucosa - a non-caseating granulomatous response.

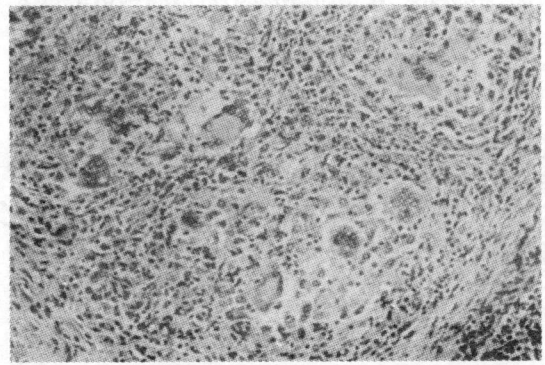

Fig. 13. Small intestine; goat. Johne's disease. Note **epithelioid** and **giant cell granulomas** with collars of lymphocytes, in a Peyer's patch.

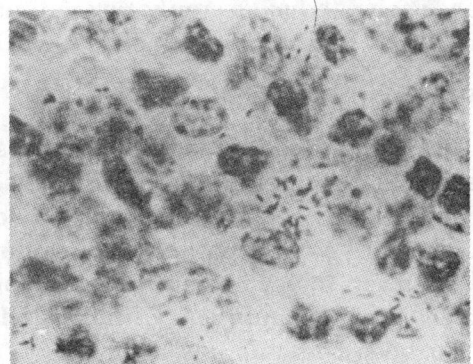

Fig. 14. Mesenteric lymph node; cow. Johne's disease. Note the presence of acid-fast mycobacteria within macrophages.

lymphoid tissues and intestinal lymph nodes. This leads to **pyogranulomas, ulcerative enteritis of the caecum and colon,** and sometimes, segments of the small intestine. About half of the cases of *R. equi* infection involve the intestine. *R. equi* is zoonotic, especially in immuno-compromised human beings.

Affected intestinal segments have greatly thickened, corrugated mucosa, 2 to 5 cm thick, which is mottled red and white. Multiple, irregularly shaped, well-defined, necrotic foci occur in the mucosal surface of the colon along with multiple, small ulcers. Mesenteric, caecal, and colonic lymph nodes are enlarged and firm. On incision, lymph nodes have abscesses. The mucosa of the **small intestine, colon, and caecum** is infiltrated by large macrophages filled with Gram-positive bacilli. The accumulation of large, bacteria-filled macrophages and multinucleated giant cells in the lamina propria distort the shapes of villi in the small intestine. Sharply demarcated foci of coagulative necrosis occur, and the mucosal surface is ulcerated. Affected lymph nodes have masses of the bacteria-filled macrophages, as well as multinucleated giant cells.

Swine Dysentery

Swine dysentery, unlike most of the other diseases of the pigs, is confined to the **large intestine. Gross lesions** closely resemble those of acute intestinal salmonellosis except that blood in faeces is more common in dysentery. Weaned **pigs 8 to 14 weeks old** are usually affected and the disease spreads rapidly through a herd. Morbidity approaches 90% and mortality is around 30%. **Gross lesions** include **muco-haemorrhagic colitis. Lesions** are present in the colon, caecum, and rectum. The intestine usually has a fibrino-necrotic pseudomembrane. **Clinically,** this correlates with severe diarrhoeic faeces containing blood, mucus, and fibrin.

The causative bacterium, *Brachyspira hyodysenteriae* (previously known as **Treponema** and **Serpulina**) acts synergistically with anaerobic colonic flora such as *Fusobacterium necrophorum* to produce disease. *B. hyodysenteriae* produces a **cytotoxic haemolysin,** which is a virulence determinant.

Proliferative Enteritis

This zoonotic condition occurs **in all species of mammals.** It is characterized by segmental proliferation of the intestinal epithelium of the ileum and large intestine. The **cause** is related to **Campylobacter** sp. infection. **Diagnosis** depends on characteristic histopathological findings and demonstration of comma-shaped bacteria in the cytoplasm of intestinal crypt epithelium. In the **dog,** majority of cases occur in **puppies. Clinically,** diarrhoea is of 5 to 15 days' duration. The diarrhoea contains lots of mucus or is watery, with or without blood, and is accompanied by anorexia, vomiting, and slight fever.

Histiocytic Ulcerative Colitis

This condition occurs in **dogs**. Dogs have soft faeces, but usually no diarrhea or weight loss. In some cases, mucus and blood appear in the stool. **Lesions** include raised ulcerative nodules. **Microscopically,** the colon is ulcerated and has marked infiltration of macrophages. The macrophages in granulomatous colitis are filled with *E. coli* antigen.

Lymph nodes that drain the colon, caecum, or rectum are enlarged and have lymphoid hyperplasia.

Chlamydial Enteritis

The chlamydiae are small, 200-1500 nm coccoid bacteria which are obligate intracellular parasites. Their cell envelopes resemble those of Gram-negative bacteria. There are two species: (1) *Chlamydia psittaci*, which occurs mostly in mammals and birds, and (2) *Chlamydia trachomatis*, which affects human beings. Chlamydia can be demonstrated by light microscopy in cells stained by the **Giemsa method**. *C. trachomatis* are clumped in the form of a cytoplasmic inclusion body, which contains glycogen. *C. trachomatis* inclusions (organisms) stain with iodine, whereas *C. psittaci* inclusions do not.

Bovine chlamydias (strains of *C. psittaci*) cause **enteritis in young calves.** Affected calves have diarrhoea, fever, anorexia, and depression. **Grossly, the ileum** is most severely affected, but the jejunum and large intestine also have lesions. The mucosa is congested and shows petechiae. The intestinal wall and mesentery are oedematous. The lumen contains watery, yellow fluid mixed with yellow, fibrin-rich material attached to the surface. Colonic ridges are hyperaemic and have small erosions. Regional lymph nodes are enlarged.

Microscopically, villus epithelial cells, macrophages, and fibroblasts of the lamina propria and endothelial cells of lacteals contain chlamydia. The chlamydiae are adsorbed to the brush border, taken up by endocytosis, and multiply in epithelial cells. They are afterwards released into the lamina propria. Villi are enlarged by dilated lacteals and infiltrates of mononuclear cells and neutrophils. Crypts of both small and large intestine are dilated and have sloughed epithelial cells and inflammatory cells (colitis cystica superficialis). The centres of lymphoid follicles of Peyer's patches are necrotic. The mucosa and submucosa of the intestine are thickened by a diffuse granulomatous reaction.

Rickettsial Enteritis

Potomac Horse Fever

Potomac horse fever is a disease of the horse which **is pathologically and clinically similar to intestinal salmonellosis and colitis X.** First described in the Potomac River Valley of Maryland, Virginia, and Pennsylvania, USA, the disease has since been reported from other places. It is characterized by fever, severe diarrhoea, depression, dehydration, and laminitis.

Affected horses have mild **necrotizing enterocolitis** similar in distribution to colitis X and intestinal salmonellosis. The causative agent, a rickettsia, *Ehrlichia risticii* is an intra-cytoplasmic rickettsial pathogen of epithelial cells, macrophages, and monocytes. Without treatment, one third of cases with diarrhoea die from dehydration. The **gross lesions** occur mainly in the **caecum** and **colon**. The affected mucosa is pink and has petechiae. Intestinal contents are fluid, pale brown, and foetid. **Microscopically,** the mucosa is reduced in thickness by loss of surface epithelium, decrease in the number of crypts, and disappearance of the lamina propria. Capillaries and veins are engorged with blood. Pseudomembranes are focal and consist of fibrin, necrotic cells, and bacteria covering the denuded surface. Clusters of the ehrlichia are easily demonstrated in macrophages of the deep lamina propria and sub-mucosa in sections.

Parasitic Enteritis

Ascariasis

Ascarids are long, smooth, white nematodes. They vary in length from 3 to 4 cm in **small animals** up to 40 to 50 cm in **pigs** and **horses**. They reside in the upper small intestine. Common species include *Ascaris suum* of **pigs**, *Parascaris equorum* of **horses**, *Toxocara canis* of **dogs**, *Toxocara cati* of **cats**, and *Toxocara lumbricoides* of **human beings**. Young animals acquire ascarids from several routes. Intrauterine transmission of larvae occurs during the last 7 to 10 days of gestation. Larvae can be transmitted by the milk of dam, and later in life, embryonated eggs are ingested as a result of faecal contamination of the mammary gland, through feed, or via coprophagy (eating dung). Transmission can also occur through paretenic host. **Infective larvae** penetrate the intestine and migrate to the liver through portal circulation. From the liver, larvae travel through the caudal vena cava to the lungs, where they break out of alveolar capillaries into the alveoli, undergo development, and migrate up the trachea or are coughed up, swallowed, and pass to the intestine for development to adults. **Ova are passed in the faeces.**

Toxascaris leonina, another ascarid of **dogs**, is transmitted through ingestion and through an intermediate host. Hepato-pulmonary migration does not occur. The larvae of ascarids produce **eosinophilic gastroenteritis** when trapped in the sub-mucosa of the stomach or intestine. They cause eosinophilic granulomas of mesenteric lymph nodes, kidneys, and rarely retina or other tissues. **Larvae** produce tracts, granulomas, and portal inflammatory infiltrations containing a large number of eosinophils, as well as focal fibrosis in the liver. The **larvae** also cause focal haemorrhages, infiltrations of eosinophils, and granulomas of the lungs. In aberrant hosts, larvae produce larval migration tracts (necrosis) in the brain, visceral larva migrans, and acute interstitial pneumonia.

Adult ascarids produce **clinical disease** by their physical presence and by inducing malabsorption. Affected animals have poor weight gains, partial loss of appetite, pendulous abdomen, and intermittent vomiting or diarrhoea. Coughing and laboured respiration are signs of **pulmonary larva migrans.** Eosinophilia occurs during the larval migration.

At postmortem, adult ascarids are easily seen in the upper small intestine (Fig. 15). **They produce no gross lesions except an occasional perforation or intussusception. However, large masses can occlude the lumen.** Sometimes, the ascarids enter into the bile duct or pancreas, where

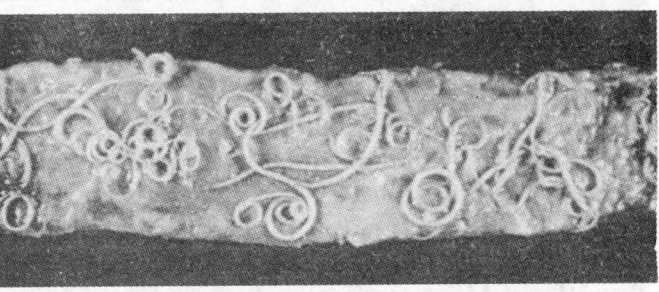

Fig. 15. Upper jejunum; dog. Ascariasis. Note a large number of ascarids in the lumen.

they can cause obstruction and inflammation. **Microscopically,** parasites in the lumen of the intestine produce no lesions. They also do not increase the numbers of mucosal eosinophils or globule leukocytes.

Ancylostomiasis (Hookworm Disease)

Hookworms are short worms, 1 to 1.5 cm long. They reside in the proximal small intestine in several species. Some of the common species include *Ancylostoma caninum* of **dogs, Bunostomum** sp. of **ruminants** and *Necator americanus* of human beings. The canine hookworm, *A. caninum* is transmissible to human beings, causing **eosinophilic enteritis** and abdominal pain. **Hookworm eggs,** discharged from females living in the small intestine, are passed in the faeces. Under suitable environmental conditions, development outside the host progresses to third-stage infective larvae which enter the host by cutaneous penetration or by ingestion. Depending on species and route of entry, the larvae move directly to the intestine, or they follow a route through the lung. Development continues into fourth and fifth-stage larvae to adults that attach to the intestinal mucosa. Larvae of the canine hookworm, *A. canium,* are transmitted in utero and through mammary secretion. These routes of transmission are responsible for the unusual occurrence of hookworm larvae in premature or stillborn puppies and the presence of hookworm eggs in the faeces of puppies.

Hookworm disease affects mainly the young of all species. The young are at risk from intrauterine or mammary transmission. They are also most likely to encounter oral or cutaneous contact with faeces. The house fly, *Musca domestica,* can spread the canine hookworm *A. caninum.* Once larval migration has been completed, adult hookworms reside in the **small intestine.** However, in a few species, adults are found in the colon and rectum. In the colon, caecum, and rectum, ulcerations with haemorrhages, usually 2 to 3 mm, occur focally or in rows on mucosal folds.

Microscopically, the colonic mucosa is hyperplastic and the lamina propria contains a few aggregates of lymphocytes and plasma cells and sometimes a few eosinophils, and haemorrhages. Hookworms first attach and then thrust their heads into the villus. The worm penetrates the epithelium and sucks up a portion of the villus core. It makes sucking movements and ingests tissue fluid, mucus, mucosa, and blood. The worm then shifts from one point of attachment to another. The wound left by the bite continues to ooze blood for as long as 30 minutes. The blood loss that occurs is due to ingestion of blood by the parasites and multifocal intestinal ulceration. **The extent of blood loss varies from 0.07 ml per worm per day for *A. caninum* up to 0.2 ml per worm per day for *A. duodenale.*** Boring and twisting movements help the worm to thrust its head deeper into the villus toward the crypts. **Grossly,** the points of attachment are seen as **punctiform haemorrhages** or **ulcerations. Microscopically,** lymphocytes in the mucosa are increased in the vicinity of hookworms, and granulocytes occur at the site of attachment.

Clinically, canine hookworm disease is characterized by unthriftiness, lethargy, weight loss, poor hair coat, anaemia, diarrhoea, variable appetite, and dehydration. **Death usually occurs in heavy infections in puppies.** The faeces are dark brown or black and variable in consistency. Sometimes, dogs pass red blood. **Laboratory findings** include hyperchromic, microcytic anaemia, eosinophilia, hypoalbuminaemia, occult faecal blood, and characteristic ova. **Cats, cattle, sheep,** and **pigs** have lethargy, weight loss, poor hair coat, diarrhoea, and weakness.

Trichostrongylosis

Trichostrongyles are small nematodes that **parasitize the duodenum** and **jejunum** of **sheep, goats, cattle,** and **other ruminants.** Three genera are important: (1) **Nematodirus,** which are 2 to 3 cm long, (2) **Cooperia,** 1 cm long, and (3) **Trichostrongylus,** 5 to 8 mm long. All these nematodes have a direct life cycle. Eggs are passed in the faeces and larvae are acquired by ingestion. **Young animals are more susceptible.** Crowding, poor sanitation, and inadequate nutrition increase susceptibility. **Clinically,** trichostrongylosis is characterized by weight loss, diarrhoea, poor hair coat, dehydration, sunken eyeballs, anorexia, anaemia, intermandibular oedema, and recumbency (lying down). The faeces can be formed but are usually fluid and dark. **Laboratory findings** include decreased haemoglobin concentration and hypoalbuminaemia. Parasite eggs can be identified in the faeces. Animal heavily parasitized has pendulous abdomen, and faecal staining of the hair or wool at the perineum.

Postmortem findings include intermandibular oedema, pale tissues, and serous atrophy of fat. The intestines have hyperaemia, dark brown or green fluid contents and a grey-white film of exfoliated cells, albumin, and fibrin on the mucosal surface. The parasites can be seen on the mucosal surface. **Microscopically,** adults of the

Trichostrongylus species are found in shallow epithelium-lined tunnels, whereas the adults of **Nematodirus** and **Cooperia** are twisted and wound around the villa. How the parasites cause damage is not quite clear. They cause tunnels in the margins of villa, damage microvilli, and reduce activity of brush border enzymes in electrolytes. Erosions may develop. Lymphocytes, plasma cells, and eosinophils infiltrate the lamina propria.

Strongyloidosis

Strongyloides enteritis can be severe. Infected animals have larvae or larvated eggs in the faeces. The **canine** parasite, *Strongyloides stercoralis*, is transmissible to humans. Other species of **Strongyloides** infect **horses, pigs,** and **cats.** Parasites occur in the upper small intestine, where females reside in shallow epithelium tunnels at the base of villi. In the case of *S. stercoralis* 'autoinfection' is possible. Eggs discharged from females develop into larvae without leaving the host and re-infect the intestine of their host. Larvae (**rhabditiform**) that leave the host with the faeces develop into males and females. Their offspring become parasitic (**filariform**), or they develop into infective (**filariform**) larvae directly. Infective larvae penetrate the skin or are ingested and penetrate the gastrointestinal mucosa. The larvae travel through the blood circulation to the lungs, enter the alveoli, are coughed up and then swallowed. Thus, they come to reside in the small intestine.

Some species of **Strongyloides** are transmitted in the uterus and through mammary secretions for several weeks after parturition. **Clinically,** affected animals have diarrhoea, weight loss, dehydration, hypoproteinaemia, eosinophilia, anorexia, and debility. Larvae or eggs can be seen in the faeces. **Grossly,** the affected intestine may be hyperaemic and fluid filled. **Microscopically,** the nematodes occur in the epithelium near the base of the villa or in the upper crypts, which is ulcerated or hyperplastic. Villi are atrophied and the lamina propria has increased numbers of lymphocytes, plasma cells, and eosinophils.

Oesophagostomiasis

Oesophagostomiasis occurs in **sheep, cattle,** and **pigs.** The important species of **Oesophagostomum** include: *Oesophagostomum columbianum, O. radiatum,* and *O. dentatum.* These are the **nodular worms** of **sheep, cattle,** and **pigs,** and cause sub-serosal mineralized (calcified) nodules that are quite characteristic of the disease. **These nodules generally are of no clinical importance.** Sometimes, they are associated with, and can be the cause of **intussusception.**

Third-stage larvae are ingested, penetrate the mucosa of the distal small intestine or caecum and colon, stay there for a time and then develop into adults. The adults live on the mucosal surface of the caecum and colon. Here, they stimulate a response of eosinophils and globule leukocytes. **Clinically, Oesophagostomum** sp. are responsible for electrolyte and protein loss, diarrhoea, anaemia, and unthriftiness.

The **lesion** usually seen at postmortem is a **granulomatous nodule,** 0.5 to 1.5 cm in diameter, produced by fourth-stage larvae penetrating the caecal and colonic walls. **Very few sheep are free of these lesions.** The nodules protrude from the serosal surface of the intestines. **On incision,** they contain a gritty, yellow to green necrotic centre. Nodules number 50 to 100. Some occur in the mesentery, mesenteric lymph nodes, liver, and lungs. **Microscopically,** the nodules contain parasite fragments and central, caseous, necrotic debris, and eosinophils that are surrounded by granulomatous inflammation, including Langhans' giant cells.

Trichuriasis

Trichuriasis occurs among **several species of animals** and in **human beings.** The parasites usually involved are *Trichurus vulpis* of the **dog,** *Trichuris suis* of the **pigs,** and *Trichuris trichiura* of human beings. The trichurids, 3 to 5 cm in length, are whip-shaped. The life cycle is direct. Eggs discharged in the faeces, embryonate in damp environments, and infection is acquired by ingestion. In the digestive tract, larvae emerge from the eggs and penetrate the small intestinal mucosa. They emerge after a short time, undergo several stages of development, and then attach to the mucosa of caecum and colon.

The trichurids damage the mucosa of caecum, colon, and rectum by producing tunnels as the parasites burrow into the superficial lamina propria. When few parasites are present, the animal has no clinical signs. When great numbers are present, **diarrhoea occurs.**

Trichuris infection in the **dog** causes chronic diarrhoea, which is usually without blood. Less commonly, the faeces contain blood and mucus. Weight loss is not much, but some dehydration occurs. **Laboratory findings** include hypoalbuminaemia, hyperglobulinaemia, anaemia, and electrolyte disturbances.

The eggs of **Trichuris** sp. are lemon shaped with an operculum on both ends. **Dogs** sometimes have clinical signs of typhlitis (inflammation of caecum). They turn in circles trying to bite at their flank. In the **pig,** signs include anorexia, diarrhoea, mucus and blood in the faeces, anaemia, fever, emaciation, laboured respiration, and death.

At postmortem, the entire surface of the caecum can be covered by these parasites (Fig. 16). When parasites are numerous, they cover colon, and in the **dog** even extend to the rectum. **Microscopically,** little tissue damage is

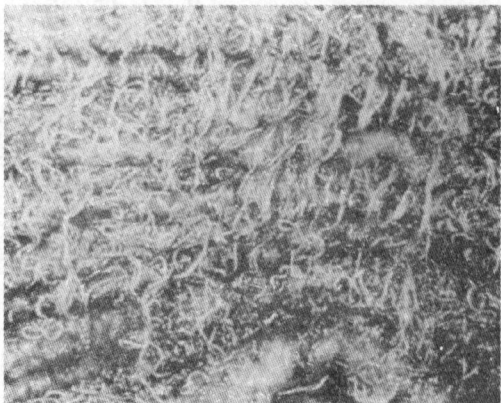

Fig. 16. Colon; dog. Trichuriasis. Note that trichurids (*Trichuris vulpis*) coat the entire mucosal surface.

seen. The parasites cause little leukocytic infiltration and no necrosis. In heavy infections, some parasites migrate into the deeper layers of the intestine and incite a granulomatous inflammation.

Pinworms

Oxyuris equi is the most common pinworm of domestic animals. The parasites occur in the lumen of the distal intestine of **horses**, and cause rectal pruritus by laying their eggs on the perineal region.

Cestodes

Tapeworms, although usually found in the alimentary system, **are of not much clinical importance.** They require two or sometimes three hosts to complete their life cycles. Tapeworms attach to the intestine by means of their anterior scolex, which may have hooks in addition to four suckers. Although they can cause some damage at the site of attachment, usually they compete with the host for nutrients. Since they have no alimentary system, they absorb nutrients through their surface. Examples of tapeworms are **Moniezia** sp. in **ruminants, Anoplocephala** sp. in the **horse,** and **Diphyllobothrium** and **Dipylidium** sp. in **dogs** and **cats. Mesocestoides** sp. can infect **dogs.** This parasite can perforate through the intestine and proliferate in the peritoneal cavity.

Taenia and **Echinococcus** sp. are the **most destructive** of the cestodes. Carnivores are the definitive host, but the larval forms reside in the viscera and body cavities of the **intermediate hosts,** usually **ruminants, pigs, horses,** or **rodents. Human beings** can also become infected, sometimes taking 20 or 30 years for clinical disease to appear. **The damage in the intermediate hosts can be quite severe.**

Trematodes

Trematodes are uncommon parasites of the alimentary tract. Paramphistomiasis is a fluke infestation of ruminant forestomachs. Although adults that live in the forestomachs are of no clinical importance, **heavy infestations of larvae in the small intestine,** before migration to the rumen and reticulum, can cause hypoproteinaemia, anaemia, and death. Larvae burrow deeply into and even through the wall of the small intestine and can be found in the peritoneal cavity. The intermediate host is a snail. Cercariae encyst on aquatic vegetation eaten by the ruminant.

Schistosomiasis of **ruminants, pigs, horses,** and **dogs** can cause granulomatous lesions in the intestine with protein loss, following the parasite's presence in mesenteric veins after migration through the liver. Parasites are acquired by direct penetration of the skin by cercariae.

The thorny-headed worm of **pigs,** *Macracanthorhynchus hirudinaceus,* is a parasite of the small intestine. It is sometimes wrongly identified as a tapeworm, which it resembles. However, it is not truly a segmented parasite. It sometimes penetrates the intestinal wall at the site of its attachment, causing **peritonitis.**

Amoebiasis

Amoebiasis is an acute or chronic disease caused by protozoan parasite *Entamoeba histolytica*. **Dogs, monkeys,** and **human beings** develop **colitis** and **amoebic abscesses.**

Amoebae invade intact mucosa by means of lysozymes. With cellular destruction, a punctiform (pinpoint) **ulcer** is formed. Eventually, a flask-shaped ulcer extends into the sub-mucosa, and sometimes, into the muscle layers. In the mucosa, amoebae do not stimulate an inflammatory response. **Ulcers** are covered by a small amount of yellow, fibrinopurulent exudate or have a bleeding surface. The amoebae that enter the portal circulation spread systemically. The organ most often affected is **liver**, and has **abscesses** and **granulomas.**

Clinically, abdominal pain, intermittent diarrhoea and anorexia characterize amoebiasis. Diarrhoea is the most common feature, and the faeces often contain blood and mucus. **Grossly,** the affected **colon** has numerous, randomly scattered punctate ulcers. **Microscopically,** punctiform ulcers with colonies of amoebae are **diagnostic.** Amoebae are numerous in these areas and are accompanied by eosinophils or granuloma formation. Amoebae are seen in H and E-stained sections, but they are easily recognized in Giemsa-stained sections.

Coccidiosis

Coccidia are extremely host and tissue-specific. They are obligate intracellular pathogens. **Lesions** vary from proliferative in **sheep** and **goats,** to haemorrhagic in **dogs, cats,** and **cattle.** In **pigs**, a fibrino-necrotic pseudomembrane without blood in 5 to 7-day-old animals is characteristic of enteric coccidiosis. Most species of **Eimeria** and **Isospora** infect villus and crypt epithelial cells. Some species reside in the epithelium of lacteals, other species occur in the lamina propria. Sometimes, some organisms reach the regional lymph nodes.

When a small number of coccidia parasitize the intestine of healthy young growing animals, disease does not occur. However, when animals are in crowded conditions and poor sanitation, faecal-oral intake of large numbers of organisms can occur. When such an intake occurs, clinical disease can result. **With each cycle, sexual and asexual, epithelial cell lysis occurs. Total damage is proportional to the environmentally acquired dose of oocysts and the numbers of various stages generated in the body. Young animals are more susceptible.**

Clinically, unthriftiness and diarrhoea characterize coccidiosis. When the large intestine is infected, **blood is present in the faeces** and the animal has tenesmus. **Diagnosis** is made by demonstrating oocysts in the faeces. The size and internal features of the oocysts enable identification of the species.

The **gross lesions** include hyperaemia and fluid distension of affected interstitial segments, often small intestine and/or caecum and colon. If the infecting coccidia (**Eimeria**) produce large schizonts, 300 μm in size, pinpoint white foci are visible from both serosal and mucosal surfaces. The mucosa may be eroded, with or without a fibrino-necrotic pseudomembrane. Erosion and fissuring of the mucosa of the large intestine is accompanied by bleeding. **Microscopically,** coccidiosis is characterized by necrosis of villus or crypt epithelium, hyperaemia, and inflammatory response in the lamina propria. The infiltration usually consists of lymphocytes and plasma cells, but sometimes eosinophils are numerous. The loss of epithelial cells results in villus atrophy or pseudomembrane formation. In some chronic infections, particularly in **sheep** and **goats**, the epithelium is hyperplastic and proliferation produces an adenomatous mucosal surface. The coccidia are easily seen. The schizonts are oval and filled with basophilic, banana-shaped merozoites. Oocysts are oval, macrogametes are large cells, and gamonts are round to oval.

Giardiasis

Giardiasis occurs in many species, including human beings, **dogs, cats, horses, cattle,** rabbit, guinea pigs, rats, mice, and hamsters. In veterinary medicine, giardiasis is usually seen in **puppies** and **kittens**. Giardiasis is caused by a unicellular flagellated protozoan, *Giardia lamblia*. It inhabits the **small intestine**, particularly the duodenum, where it attaches to the microvillus border of epithelial cells producing membrane damage. When Giardia organisms are present in small numbers, they produce no clinical illness. However, when present in great numbers or in immunologically deficient individuals **diarrhoea occurs.**

Clinically, animals with giardiasis have fluid diarrhoea, signs of abdominal discomfort without fever, weight loss, melena (dark faeces due to the presence of partly digested blood), or steatorrhoea (excess of fat in faeces). The **diagnosis** is made by demonstrating **Giardia** in preparations of fresh faeces.

Cryptosporidiosis

Cryptosporidium parvum is a zoonotic protozoan pathogen of mammals. It causes a self-limiting infection in immuno-competent animals, the young and other immuno-compromised individuals, such as AIDS patients, suffer from intractable diarrhoea. **Veterinarians and veterinary students are at particular risk when treating cattle.** Cryptosporidia attach to the surface of epithelial cells of the stomach, small intestine, or colon. The protozoa attach to the epithelial cells, displace the microvilli, and are enclosed by surface cell membranes.

In faecal smears stained by the Giemsa method, oocysts containing 2-5 dense red granules in a blue to blue-green cytoplasm are seen. Cryptosporidiosis causes **subacute or chronic watery diarrhoea**, sometimes tinged with blood and associated with dehydration and weakness.

Grossly, affected portions of the gastrointestinal tract are red and have fluid contents. **Microscopically,** in H and E-stained sections, organisms appear as tiny blue (haematoxylinophilic) dots attached to the epithelial cells of affected portions. The **lesions** of **enteritis** or **colitis** consist of irregular mucosal thickness, crypt necrosis, and an increase in lymphocytes and plasma cells in the lamina propria.

Canine Multifocal Eosinophilic Gastroenteritis

This is a disease of **young dogs.** It is caused by migrating larvae of the ascarid, *Toxocara canis.* The incidence of this disease is low. **Clinically,** chronic diarrhoea, weight loss and eosinophilia characterize the disease.

T. canis larvae enter by the oral route and invade the mucosa of the **stomach** and **small intestine.** Then they become trapped and localized by the inflammation they induce. Larvae migrate into the uterus and fetuses during late pregnancy. Soon after birth, larvae go to the mammary gland, where they are **secreted into the milk of the bitch.** Larvae also can be acquired from faecal contamination of the teats. Larvae that are ingested by the **puppies** usually pass through the mucosa of the stomach and small intestine and travel via intestinal lymph vessels or portal vein to the **liver** and then to the **lungs.** Here they develop into third-stage larvae, which are then coughed up and swallowed. **In the gastrointestinal tract, these larvae mature into adult roundworms.** Usually larvae pass through tissues and complete their life cycle, or the larvae are trapped and killed by granuloma formation, which results in **necrosis of the parasite and calcification. Dogs** with **multifocal eosinophilic gastroenteritis** have *T. canis* larvae trapped in the gastrointestinal wall by an immune reaction and are surrounded by eosinophils, but are still alive. These larvae can remain trapped and alive in the wall of the stomach and small intestine **for as long as 4 years. Waste products of the parasite are chemotactic for eosinophils.** Multiple aggregates of eosinophils occur in the pathways travelled by the larvae in the sub-mcosa and sub mucosa of the stomach and small intestine, in the mesenteric lymph nodes, connective tissue of the pancreas, portal areas of the liver, and kidneys and lungs.

Focal eosinophilic lesions may be grossly visible. **In some dogs,** as many as 40 to 80 white, firm **nodules** can be seen in the intestine from the serosa. Fewer nodules occur in the stomach and colon. **Gross lesions** occur in the renal cortex, pancreas, liver, and under pleura. **Microscopically,** lesions are composed of eosinophils. Some lesions have plasma cells and macrophages, and some of the lesions are granulomas. Larvae can often be demonstrated in these aggregates.

Inflammatory Conditions of Unknown Aetiology

Colitis X of Horses

The **severe diarrhoea** seen in colitis X contains no blood and **is rapidly fatal. The aetiology is unknown.** However, the disease is associated with overgrowth of

Clostridium perfringens type A (**antibiotic enteritis**), or anaphylaxis. **Lesions** are confined to the mucosa of the caecum and colon and include oedema, congestion, and haemorrhage. The location and nature of these lesions resemble with those of acute intestinal salmonellosis and Potomac horse fever. Therefore, elimination of **Salmonella** sp. and *Ehrlichia risticii* as causes is necessary before a diagnosis of colitis X can be made.

Canine Mucosal Colitis

This condition is rare. **Adult dogs,** 3 to 6 years of age, are affected and males are more prone to the disease. **The cause is unknown.** Affected dogs have chronic diarrhoea, and pass fresh blood. The **gross lesions** of the **colon** include hyperaemia and multifocal mucosal ulceration. In some cases, lesions have a diffuse distribution affecting the entire colon and rectum. **Microscopic lesions** include degeneration and necrosis of the colonic epithelial cells. A variety of inflammatory cells infiltrate the lamina propria between the crypts. The epithelium often undergoes regenerative hyperplasia. Ulcers may occur and coalesce with each other.

Diffuse Eosinophilic Gastroenteritis

This type of eosinophilic gastroenteritis occurs in **dogs** and **cats.** It is characterized by recurrent episodes of diarrhoea associated with tissue and circulating eosinophilia. The greatly increased number of eosinophils in the circulation and within lesions suggests a hypersensitivity reaction to some ingested substance or to parasites. **The cause has not been identified.** There are **no gross lesions. Histologically,** eosinophils heavily infiltrate all layers of the stomach and intestine.

Inflammatory Bowel Disease

In **dogs** and **cats** this disease has been identified microscopically as **lympho-plasmacytic enteritis. Diagnosis** can be made by biopsy. **The cause is unknown.** However, the presence of numerous lymphocytes and plasma cells suggests an immune response problem. Malabsorption and chronic protein-losing enteropathy (disease of the intestine) can be the result of marked infiltration of lymphocytes and plasmacytes in the lamina propria. **In cats, but not dogs,** dietary antigens cause some cases of inflammatory bowel disease. Therefore, control of the disease can be achieved by regulation of the diet.

Feline Ulcerative Colitis

Feline ulcerative colitis is grossly and histologically similar to histiocytic ulcerative colitis of dogs (discussed under bacterial disease). **The causative agent is unknown.**

Intestinal Neoplasms

Neoplasms of various types occur in the intestinal tract of domestic animals. Intestinal neoplasms are usually diagnosed in **dogs** and **cats** due to their longer life-span. Also, pets live in close association with humans and thus it is possible that some of the same environmental factors that cause human cancer could also cause similar problems in animals.

In dogs, the common benign neoplasms of the intestine are adenomas or polyps, and their malignant counterparts adenocarcinomas. Smooth muscle neoplasms leiomyomas and leiomyosarcomas originate from muscular layers. **In cats,** the most common neoplasms include alimentary lymphosarcoma, mastocytomas which are associated with ulceration, adenomas, adenocarcinomas, and carcinoids. **In sheep,** adenocarcinomas of the intestine are quite common and are virus induced. **In cows,** alimentary lymphosarcoma is most common. **Horses** rarely develop intestinal neoplasms.

Liver

Hepatic Dysfunction and Failure

Hepatic dysfunction or failure can occur only after severe injury. This is because **liver has a great amount of functional reserve and regenerative capacity.** In healthy animals, more than two thirds of the liver can be removed without significant damage to liver function. Normal liver mass is regenerated by proliferation of hepatocytes, bile duct epithelium, and endothelial cells in the remaining liver lobes within 5 to 7 days. This process of tissue removal and regeneration can be repeated more than five times, and normal function is retained. **In all species, clinical signs** from liver derangement, including jaundice (icterus) and clotting disorders, are similar **regardless of their cause.** However, these signs are seen only when liver's great reserve and regenerative capacity are exhausted, or when biliary outflow is obstructed. **Only those lesions that involve most of the parenchyma may produce the signs of hepatic failure because focal lesions rarely destroy sufficient parenchyma to exhaust liver's reserve.** The term **hepatic failure** means loss of adequate liver function as a result of either acute or chronic liver damage. However, all liver functions are not lost at the same time. **The consequences of liver dysfunction and failure include:**

1. Disturbances of bile flow resulting in hyperbilirubinaemia and **jaundice**
2. Hepatic encephalopathy
3. A number of metabolic disturbances including hyperammonaemia, hypogly-caemia, and acidosis
4. Vascular and haemorrhagic alterations such as shunting of portal blood into the systemic circulation, thus bypassing the hepatocytes, and
5. Cutaneous manifestations such as epidermal necrosis syndrome in dogs and **photosensitization** in **herbivores.**

These will now be discussed.

1. Disturbances of Bile Flow and Jaundice (Icterus)

Bile is composed of water, bile acids, **bilirubin**, cholesterol, inorganic ions, and other constituents.

Bilirubin is produced from the breakdown of haemoglobin, and to a lesser extent, other haeme proteins including myoglobin and the hepatic haemoproteins such as cytochromes. Most of the bilirubin is derived from the haemoglobin in senescent (old) erythrocytes after they have been phagocytosed by the mononuclear phagocytic system of the spleen, bone marrow, and liver. Within the phagocyte, the globin portion is broken down and the constituent amino acids are returned to the amino acid pool. The **haeme iron** is transferred to iron-binding proteins such as transferrin for recycling. The remaining portion of the **haeme molecule** is oxidized by haeme oxygenase to **biliverdin**. In the next step, biliverdin reductase converts biliverdin to bilirubin. Afterwards, bilirubin is released from phagocytes into the blood. However, bilirubin is poorly soluble in plasma. Therefore, before bilirubin is conjugated in the liver, it is bound to albumin to make it more soluble in plasma. The process of elimination of bilirubin from the liver occurs in three phases: **uptake, conjugation,** and **secretion. Uptake** is the process by which hepatocytes remove bilirubin bound to albumin from the circulation. Once in the hepatocyte, the lipid soluble bilirubin undergoes **conjugation.** It is combined with a polar molecule such as glucuronic acid to make bilirubin diglucuronide, which is water soluble and easily secreted into the bile. In the final phase, **secretion,** conjugated bilirubin is transported into the bile canalicules for delivery into the bile duct system.

Within the gastrointestinal tract, conjugated bilirubin is converted to **urobilinogen** by bacteria. A very small amount of urobilinogen is reabsorbed from the ileum into the portal blood and returned to the liver by the entero-hepatic circulation. Most of the urobilinogen that is absorbed from the gastrointestinal tract is secreted again into bile. Urobilinogen has a low molecular weight and is easily filtered through the glomerulus. Low concentrations are normally found in the urine. Urobilinogen that is not absorbed from the intestine gets oxidized to **stercobilin,** which is responsible for the colour of the faeces.

Increased level of conjugated or unconjugated bilirubin in blood is called **hyperbilirubinaemia.** High levels of bilirubin can produce **jaundice (icterus), a yellow discoloration of tissues especially seen in those tissues rich in elastin such as the aorta and sclera.**

The causes of hyperbilirubinaemia are:

1. **Intravascular haemolysis (prehepatic jaundice):** Overproduction of bilirubin as a result of haemolysis, particularly severe intravascular haemolysis. This overpowers liver's capacity to remove bilirubin from the plasma and to secrete conjugated bilirubin into bile.

2. **Extravascular haemolysis (prehepatic jaundice):** The destruction of damaged

red blood cells by extrtavascular haemolysis can also increase the amount of bilirubin presented to the liver. Secretion of conjugated bilirubin into the bile canaliculi is an energy-dependent process.

3. **Severe hepatic disease (hepatic jaundice):** Decreased uptake, conjugation, or secretion of bilirubin by hepatocytes as a result of severe, diffuse hepatic disease, whether acute or chronic.

4. **Biliary obstruction (posthepatic jaundice):** Reduced outflow of bile **(cholestasis)**. Cholestasis means reduced canalicular flow of bile, which occurs as a result of either obstruction of the biliary ducts **(extrahepatic cholestasis)** or impairment of bile flow within canaliculi **(intrahepatic cholestasis)**.

Intrahepatic Cholestasis

This is associated with several disorders of hepatocytes (liver cells), because cytoplasm of the liver cells forms the walls of the canaliculus. Intrahepatic cholestasis starts where bile flow originates, that is, centrilobular areas. As bile accumulates, the canaliculi become distended and bile pigments discolour the cytoplasm of adjacent hepatocytes. **In domestic animals,** intrahepatic cholestasis can occur as a result of **a variety of insults (hepatotoxins,** such as endotoxin or toxic chemicals, viral or bacterial infections, and ischaemia). All of these can inhibit membrane-bound and cytoplasmic enzymes that facilitate metabolism of either bile acids or bilirubin and secretion of bile across the hepatocyte's membrane into the bile canaliculus.

Extrahepatic Cholestasis

This cholestasis is the **result of mechanical obstruction of bile flow.** It can occur from choleliths or foreign body obstructions (such as parasite within the bile duct), neoplasms that compress or constrict the common bile duct, or inflammatory or reparative processes that result in fibrosis which afterwards constricts the lumen of the duct and reduces or prevents outflow of bile. Extrahepatic obstruction first causes distension of the bile ducts, and progressive backward distension of the intrahepatic bile duct system. Within the lobule, changes are seen within the portal areas, and only later plugging of canaliculi and stasis of bile occur within the cytoplasm of liver cells. **Chronic extrahepatic cholestasis** may result in extensive hepatic fibrosis **(biliary fibrosis)** mainly in the portal areas. Sometimes, distension of canaliculi may lead to rupture and extravasation of bile, thereby resulting in focal hepatocellular necrosis.

To conclude, hepatic dysfunction is not the only cause of hyperbilirubinaemia and jaundice. In fact, **jaundice in ruminants,** is usually a result of severe intravascular haemolysis, and less often, an outcome of hepatic damage. **Horses** usually manifest jaundice with an acute hepatic dysfunction, but jaundice may or may not occur in horses with chronic hepatic disease. 'Physiological jaundice' is also common in the **horse**, and horses deprived of feed for several days can become jaundiced because uptake of bilirubin from the plasma by liver cells is decreased. **Jaundice in carnivores** occurs as a result of either haemolysis or hepatic dysfunction. Complete obstruction of bile flow in any species can lead to extrahepatic cholestasis and jaundice. However, in the **dog**, obstruction of the common duct does not always lead to jaundice because supernumerary ducts allow the bile to flow into the duodenum.

2. Hepatic Encephalopathy

Hepatic failure can result in a metabolic disorder of the central nervous system known as **hepatic encephalopathy (hepatic coma)**. The main feature of this disorder is abnormal neurotransmission in the central nervous system and the neuromuscular system. It is believed that **increased levels of plasma ammonia** derived from **amines** absorbed from the gastrointestinal tract are responsible. Normally, amines are absorbed from intestines into the portal blood and metabolized by the liver. If they bypass the liver and enter into the systemic circulation, they can exert toxic effects on the brain. **Hepatic encephalopathy is common in ruminants and horses with hepatic failure, dogs and cats** with congenital porto-systemic shunts, and animals with end-stage liver disease (hepatic fibrosis and nodular regeneration) that leads to shunting of blood within regenerative nodules.

3. Metabolic Disturbances of Hepatic Failure

Animals with **hepatic failure** can suffer from a variety of metabolic disturbances.

Bleeding tendencies: Bleeding tendencies (**haemorrhagic diathesis**) sometimes occur in hepatic failure. Impaired synthesis of **clotting factors** and metabolic abnormalities affecting **platelet function** can affect normal clotting, **All clotting factors, except factor VIII, are synthesized in the liver.** Metabolic disturbances that result from hepatic failure can affect platelet function and lead to the synthesis of abnormal fibrinogen, called **dysfibrinogenaemia**. Obstruction of the biliary system prevents the release of bile into the intestinal tract. The resulting deranged fat absorption restricts vitamin K absorption from the intestine, which leads to an inactivity of factors II, VII, IX, and X. Acute hepatic failure may also cause disseminated intravascular coagulation which can itself cause haemorrhagic diathesis.

Hypoalbuminaemia: Hypoalbuminaemia, a result of liver dysfunction occurs in severe chronic hepatic disease, because of the long half-life of plasma albumin (which ranges from 8 days in the dog to 21 days in cattle), and the time necessary for portal hypertension to develop. Hypoalbuminaemia can occur as a result of severe, diffuse chronic hepatic disease which causes both decreased production of albumin, and because of portal hypertension, increased loss of albumin in ascitic fluid or into intestinal tract.

4. Vascular and Haemodynamic Alterations of Hepatic Failure

Chronic liver injury is accompanied by **extensive diffuse fibrosis of the liver**, which increases resistance to blood flow through the liver. This, in turn, increases pressure within the portal vein (**portal hypertension**). With time, collateral vascular channels open to allow blood in the portal vein to bypass the abnormal liver. In addition, the increased pressure within the hepatic vasculature causes transudation of fluid (modified transudate) into the peritoneal cavity to produce **ascites in several species, except**, in most cases, **horses.** Transudation of fluid into the peritoneal cavity is increased by hypoalbuminaemia because colloid osmotic pressure of plasma is decreased. Hypoalbuminaemia and reduced plasma colloid osmotic pressure occur as a result of increased albumin loss into the lumen of the intestines and reduced synthesis of albumin and other plasma proteins in the liver. **Ascites** associated with hepatic fibrosis in chronic liver disease (end-stage liver) or other causes of portal hypertension, such as right-sided heart failure, occurs usually in **dogs** and **cats**, sometimes in **sheep**, and is unusual in **horses** and **cattle**

Cutaneous Manifestations

1. Epidermal Necrosis Syndrome

This occurs in **dogs** with severe hepatic disease. It is characterized by crusting, ulceration, and full-thickness necrosis of the epidermis of the skin. The mechanism of cutaneous injury is not understood. Probably it results from abnormal hepatic metabolism.

2. Photosensitization

Photosensitization is an injury to the cutaneous tissues. It results from activation of **photodynamic pigments** by ultraviolet light present in the sun's rays. **Photodynamic pigments cause injury through the production of oxygen radicals.** Cutaneous lesions include hairless skin, particularly in the lightly or non-pigmented areas of skin. Photodynamic pigments that induce photosensitization are from plants and certain drugs. It is only in hepatogenous or secondary photosensitization (of the three discussed below) that hepatic dysfunction is responsible for photosensitization.

(i) Primary Photosensitization:

This occurs when some **primary (preformed) photodynamic agent** is deposited in tissues following its absorption into the blood after ingestion. Certain plants, such as St. John's wort, buckwheat, and spring parsley contain compounds that are photodynamic. Certain drugs, such as phenothiazine, tetracyclines, and sulphonamides can cause photosensitization through their photodynamic activity. **Lesions** are described in Chapter 12.

(ii) Hepatogenous or Secondary Photosensitization

This occurs in **herbivores** when liver dysfunction or biliary obstruction interferes with the normal excretion of phylloerythrin in bile. **Phylloerythrin, a photodynamic agent,** is produced from chlorophyll present in the ingested plants by microflora of the gastrointestinal tract of herbivores. Phylloerythrin is normally absorbed from the intestines and excreted in bile, using the same pathway as bilirubin. Therefore, liver dysfunction or biliary obstruction prevents normal excretion **and leads to high concentrations of phylloerythrin in blood and skin.** Hepatic photosensitivity is a result of the increased serum concentration of **phylloerythrin.** This may occur in either acute or chronic liver disease.

(iii) Inherited Photosensitization

This occurs in a variety species which include **cattle, sheep,** and **cats** as a result of metabolic disorders that lead to an accumulation of photodynamic substances. **Cattle** and **cats** have inherited abnormalities of porphyrin metabolism (e.g. **congenital porphyria**), and accumulated porphyrins lead to skin injury.

Developmental Anomalies and Incidental Findings

Developmental anomalies of the liver occur in domestic animals, but most are of little importance.

Congenital Cysts

These cysts can be found within the livers of all domestic animals. They are usually an incidental finding. They may originate from the intrahepatic bile ducts and the hepatic capsule. Although these cysts are considered congenital anomalies, they can be found in animals of any age. It is not clear whether cysts that occur in the liver of **adult cats** are developmental anomalies or benign cystic neoplasms. **Congenital polycystic hepatic disease,** characterized by cysts in the liver and kidneys, occur in the **dog.** Congenital cysts must be differentiated from parasitic cysts, particularly cysticerci.

Hepatic Displacement

Displacement of the liver into the thoracic cavity is called **diaphragmatic hernia**. It occurs when there is a defect in the diaphragm. A congenital malformation that causes an opening in the diaphragm, or trauma that ruptures the diaphragm, can result in herniation of liver into the thoracic cavity.

Incidental Findings

Tension Lipidosis

Distinct, pale areas of parenchyma at the liver margins are common in **cattle** and **horses**. Affected liver cells accumulate fat within their cytoplasm (**lipidosis**) as a result of hypoxia. These lesions are of no functional importance.

Capsular Fibrosis

Distinct fibrous plaques are commonly seen on the diaphragmatic surface of the liver and on the adjacent diaphragm of the **horse**. Resolution of the non-specific peritonitis is believed to be the cause.

Postmortem Changes

Autolysis of the liver occurs rapidly and can be advanced before it is seen in most other tissues. Bacteria released from the gastrointestinal tract into the portal circulation during death reach liver, where they proliferate rapidly after death. This process is especially rapid in **large animals** during hot weather, particularly **cattle,** in which fermentation in the adjacent rumen produces heat, and **pigs,** which are often well-insulated by fat.

Pale areas appear on the surface as bacterial degradation begins. In time, the organ becomes green-blue as bacteria degrade blood pigments to **hydrogen sulphide.** The liver in contact with the gallbladder is rapidly discoloured by bile pigment which has passed through the wall of the gallbladder. The consistency of the organ becomes putty-like (i.e. like soft paste), and gas bubbles my form under the capsule and in the parenchyma from bacterial fermentation.

Haemodynamic and Vascular Disorders

The **centrilobular (periacinar) region** of the lobule receives the blood last. Therefore, it is least oxygenated and the effects of hypoxia are usually seen first in this area. **Acute** and **severe anaemia,** regardless of the cause, can cause centrilobular degeneration and even necrosis of liver cells. This usually occurs in severe anaemias of sudden onset. **Chronic anaemia** can cause atrophy of centrilobular liver cells, which results in dilation and congestion of sinusoids. Livers from animals with severe anaemia, whether acute or chronic, show a prominent lobular pattern on both capsular and cut surface (Fig. 17).

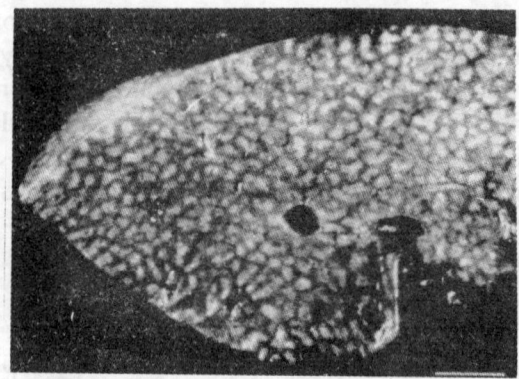

Fig. 17. Liver, cut surface; cat. Note prominent lobular pattern.

Congenital Porto-Systemic Shunts

Congenital porto-systemic shunts are abnormal vascular channels which allow blood within the portal venous system to bypass the liver and to drain into the systemic circulation. Congenital shunts can be either within or outside the liver and are usually limited to a single vessel. **A number of shunts have been described.** One important type involves **failure of closure of the ductus venosus,** a normal vessel during foetal development that carries blood from the portal vein to the vena cava. This occurs mostly in the **large breed dogs.** Shunts have been described in several species, but usually occur in the **dog** and **cat.**

The affected animals are stunted and usually have signs of hepatic encephalopathy (see 'hepatic encephalopathy'). The liver is small and has a characteristic microscopic appearance. Affected livers have lobular atrophy, and portal areas are characterized by reduplication of arterioles, and portal veins may be small or absent. **Typically, the portal vein pressure is normal in congenital shunts and ascites is not associated with these lesions.**

Portal Hypertension

Increased pressure within the portal vein can originate from disturbances of venous blood flow in any of three sites: (1) Increased resistance to venous outflow in the hepatic vein is termed **post-hepatic. Chronic passive congestion** is the most common post-hepatic cause of portal hypertension. Much less common is portal hypertension occurring as a result of portal partial or complete occlusion of the hepatic veins, or the adjacent vena cava. (2) **Intra-hepatic portal hypertension** originates from increased resistance to blood flow within the sinusoids. Chronic hepatic disease which results in increased collagen and loss of normal lobular architecture is the most common intra-hepatic cause of portal hypertension. (3) **Post-hepatic portal hypertension** occurs when blood flow through the portal vein is damaged. This may occur from thrombosis, invasion by neoplasms, or other causes.

Regardless of the cause, persistent portal hypertension can lead to **acquired porto-systemic shunts.** These shunts are usually numerous and connect the mesenteric veins and the vena cava. **Ascites** is common with these types of shunts because of the accompanying portal hypertension.

Passive Congestion

Right-sided heart failure increases the pressure within vena cava, which later extends to the hepatic vein and its tributaries. **Passive congestion** may be either **acute** or **chronic**, and appearance of the liver differs with the duration and severity of the congestion. Passive congestion at the beginning is seen as distension of central veins and centrilobular sinusoids. Persistent centrilobular hypoxia leads to atrophy or loss of hepatocytes, and eventually, to fibrosis around central veins. Fibrosis of the central vein (**phlebosclerosis**) may also occur.

Acute congestion produces slight enlargement of the liver, and blood flows freely when the liver is cut.

Chronic passive congestion leads to persistent hypoxia in centrilobular areas, and because of oxygen and nutrient deficiency, the centrilobular hepatocytes atrophy, degenerate, or undergo necrosis. As a result, sinusoids in these areas are dilated and congested and grossly appear red, whereas periportal hepatocytes usually undergo **lipidosis (fatty change)** because of hypoxia. Therefore, hypoxia causes this area of the lobule to appear yellow. The result is a prominent lobular pattern of the liver called **'enhanced lobular or reticular pattern'**. This pattern is especially seen on the cut surface of the liver. The increased lobular pattern which occurs in severe chronic passive congestion closely resembles the appearance of the cut surface of a nutmeg, and therefore is called the

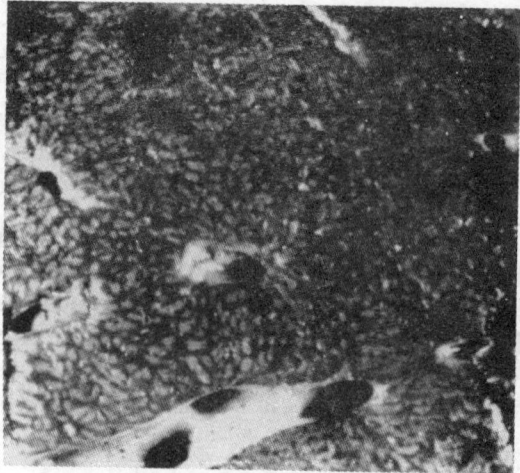

Fig. 18. **Liver, cut surface; cow.** Chronic passive hepatic congestion secondary to severe fibrinous pericarditis. **Note increased lobular (nutmeg) pattern.** The irregular light grey foci are portal tracts. The liver parenchyma between the portal tracts is congested.

'nutmeg liver' (Fig. 18). However, this pattern is not unique to passive congestion. It also occurs in other processes, such as zonal hepatic necrosis. In addition to increased lobular pattern, chronic passive congestion is characterized by focal fibrous thickening of Glisson's capsule, and in severe cases, widespread hepatic fibrosis, particularly around central veins. Central veins are also fibrosed, which reduces their luminal diameters.

Passive congestion of the liver can occur in any species and is the result of cardiac dysfunction. Chronic passive congestion is **particularly common in aged dogs** and usually occurs as a result of valvular insufficiency from endocardiosis (mucoid degeneration) of the right atrio-ventricular valve. Acute passive congestion, on the other hand, can occur as a result of acute right heart failure, which has a number of causes.

Arterio-Portal Shunts (Anastomoses)

Arterio-portal shunts occur in the **dog** and **cat**. They are direct communications between the hepatic artery and branches of the portal vein, and occur anywhere within the liver. Shunting of the blood may lead to portal hypertension and development of acquired porto-caval shunts and **ascites**.

Hepatic Veno-occlusive Disease

This is characterized by intimal thickening and occlusion of the central vein by fibrous connective tissue. It results in passive hepatic congestion and hepatic injury, which may progress to hepatic failure. The cause is unknown. An extremely high incidence is observed in captive exotic **cats** such as **cheetahs**, possibly because of the ingestion of large amounts of vitamin A.

Telangiectasis

Telangiectasis is **marked dilatation of sinusoids** in areas where liver cells have been lost. **Grossly**, these areas appear as dark blue (from un-oxygenated blood) foci of different sizes within the liver. Telangiectasis is particularly seen in **cattle**, but is of no clinical importance. It also occurs in **old cats** where it can be mistaken for vascular neoplasms, such as haemangioma or haemangiosarcoma.

Infarction

Infarction of the liver is rare because of the organ's dual blood supply from the hepatic artery and portal vein. **Infarcts are** usually sharply demarcated and may be either dark red or pale. They mostly occur at the margin of the liver.

Metabolic Disturbances and Hepatic Accumulations

Hepatic Lipidosis or Fatty Liver

The presence of excessive lipid (triglycerides, that is, neutral fat)within the liver is called **hepatic lipidosis** or **fatty liver.** This occurs when the rate of triglyceride accumulation within the hepatocytes exceeds either their rate of metabolic breakdown or their release as lipoproteins. Hepatic lipidosis is not a specific disease entity, but can occur following several disturbances of normal lipid metabolism. **The mechanisms which cause excessive accumulation of lipids within the liver are:**

1. **Excessive entry of fatty acids into the liver,** as a result of excessive dietary intake of fat or increased metabolism of **triglycerides** from adipose tissue as a result of increased demand, for example, lactation, starvation, and endocrine abnormalities.

2. **Abnormal hepatocyte function** leads to accumulation of triglycerides within hepatocytes, as a result of decreased energy for oxidation of fatty acids within hepatocytes.

3. **Excessive dietary intake of carbohydrate** results in the synthesis of increased amounts of fatty acids with formation of excessive triglycerides within hepatocytes.

4. **Increased esterification of fatty acids to triglycerides** in response to increased amounts of glucose and insulin, which stimulate the rate of **triglyceride** synthesis from glucose.

5. **Decreased apoprotein synthesis** and subsequent decreased production and export of lipoprotein from hepatocytes.

6.   **Impaired secretion of lipoprotein** from the liver caused by secretory defects produced by hepatotoxins or drugs.

It is emphasized that some mechanisms may be more important than others depending on the condition of the animal, and that more than one defect may occur in any given hepatic disorder. Regardless of the cause, the **gross appearance** of hepatic lipidosis is very characteristic. With the accumulation of lipid, the liver enlarges and becomes yellow. **In mild cases,** lipids may accumulate only in specific portions of each lobule, such as centrilobular regions. This gives an increased lobular pattern to the liver. **In extreme cases,** the entire liver is affected and the organ becomes greatly enlarged and has a very greasy texture. The parenchyma of severely affected livers bulges from the cut surface when incised and liver sections float in formalin. Lipid vacuoles are easily seen within the cytoplasm of hepatocytes.

Specific causes and syndromes of hepatic lipidosis in domestic animals include:

1.   **Dietary causes** of hepatic lipidosis include simple dietary excess, such as high-fat or high-cholesterol diet. Hepatic lipidosis is particularly common in **ruminants** with high-energy demands, such as in peak lactation or late gestation. This is due to increased entry of lipid into the liver as a result of increased metabolism of lipids from adipose tissue. Very fat animals are particularly prone to hepatic lipidosis when dietary intake is restricted.

2.   **Toxic and anoxic (oxygen deficiency) causes of** hepatic lipidosis are common. Sublethal (reversible) injury to hpatocytes usually results in accumulation of lipids within the affected cell. Injury to hepatocytes can lead to accumulation of lipids because of decreasedformation of or export of lipoproteins by hepatocytes and   decreased oxidation of fatty acids within hepatocytes.

3.   **Ketosis** is a metabolic disorder that results from impaired metabolism of carbohydrate and volatile fatty acids. **In pregnant and lactating animals,** there is a continuous demand for glucose and amino acids, and ketosis occurs when fat metabolism which occurs in response to the increased energy demands, becomes excessive. **Ketosis is characterized by increased concentrations of ketone bodies in blood (hyperketonaemia), hypoglycaemia, and low concentrations of liver glycogen. Ketosis is common in ruminants and usually occurs during peak lactation,** whereas **ketosis of sheep** usually occurs in late lactation, particularly in ewes carrying twins. This disease in sheep is known as **pregnancy toxaemia.**

4.   **Bovine fatty liver syndrome (fatty liver disease):** This is similar to ketosis. **In dairy cattle,** the disease is usually seen in very fat animals within a few days after parturition, and is often precipitated by events that cause anorexia such as retained placenta, metritis, mastitis, abomasal displacement, or parturient paresis. Accumulation of lipid within the liver is due to both increased metabolism of lipids from adipose tissue which results in increased entry of fatty

acids into the liver and **defective liver cell function,** which results in decreased export of lipoprotein from the liver.

5. **Feline fatty liver syndrome:** This is a distinct syndrome of idiopathic hepatic lipidosis seen in **cats.** Affected cats are very fat and anorectic, and usually develop hepatic failure, jaundice, and later hepatic encephalopathy.

6. **Hepatic lipidosis** occurs in **ponies** and **horses.** The condition usually occurs in **pregnant or lactating mares,** after an event that causes anorexia.

7. **White liver disease** is a syndrome of **sheep** and **goats.** It is caused by dietary deficiencies of vitamin B_{12} and cobalt. Affected animals suffer liver damage, but the characteristic lipid accumulation is secondary to anorexia and anaemia.

8. **Endocrine disorders,** such as diabetes mellitus and hypothyroidism, can produce hepatic lipidosis in **several species.** The accumulation of lipids in the liver in the diabetic animal is the result of increased fat mobilization and decreased utilization of lipids by injured liver cells.

Glycogen Accumulation

Glucose is stored within liver cells as glycogen and is usually present in large amounts after feeding. Excessive hepatic accumulation of glycogen occurs with metabolic disturbances associated with diseases such as diabetes mellitus and the glycogen storage diseases. In these cases, hepatic involvement is only one manifestation of a systemic disease process.

Glucocorticoid-Induced Hepatocellular Degeneration

This is a specific disorder characterized by excessive accumulation of glycogen in liver. Excessive amounts of endogenous or exogenous glucocorticoids cause extensive swelling of hepatocytes from the accumulation of glycogen. The swelling is pronounced and may be up to 10 times the normal value. In severe cases, often referred to as **steroid-induced hepatopathy,** the liver is enlarged and pale. The disorder occurs in **dogs. Diagnosis** can be confirmed on the basis of the characteristic microscopic appearance of the liver and identification of the source of the excess glucocorticoids.

Amyloidosis

Hepatic amyloidosis occurs in most species of domestic animals. Amyloidosis is not a single disease entity, but is term used for various diseases that lead to deposition of proteins that are composed of **beta-pleated sheets** of non-branching fibrils. The physical properties of amyloid are responsible for its birefringence and characteristic apple green appearance in Congo red-stained sections seen under polarized light. As many as 15 distinct amyloid proteins have been identified, but hepatic amyloid is usually derived from one of three types. **In primary amyloidosis,**

the amyloid protein AL (amyloid light chain) is derived from immunoglobulin light chains synthesized by plasma cell neoplasms. **In secondary amyloidosis, the most common type seen in animals,** a serum protein synthesized by the liver, called serum amyloid-associated (SAA) protein is the precursor to AA (amyloid-associated) fibrils. Secondary amyloidosis occurs as a result of prolonged inflammation such as chronic infection or tissue destruction. **The third type, inherited or familial amyloidosis,** is uncommon in animals, but occurs in certain breeds of **dogs** and **cats.**

Regardless of the cause, amyloid usually accumulates in the space of Disse and damages the normal entry of plasma into hepatocytes. Amyloid deposits produce **hepatomegaly,** and excessive accumulations cause the liver to appear pale. **In severe cases,** affected animals may have **clinical signs** of either **hepatic dysfunction or failure,** and because the liver is more fragile, **liver rupture** may occur, especially in the **horse.** Often, amyloid is also deposited in the kidneys, particularly the glomeruli. Renal failure usually occurs before signs of liver dysfunction are seen.

Copper Accumulation

Copper poisoning is considered as a metabolic disorder because **liver injury** in copper poisoning in **domestic animals** is usually the result of progressive accumulation of copper in the liver. This occurs particularly in **sheep,** in which storage of copper is poorly regulated. Also, hereditary disorders of copper metabolism have been described in **dogs.**

Copper is an essential trace element of all cells, but even a very slight excess of copper can be life threatening because copper must be properly sequestered to avoid toxicosis. Normally, serum copper is bound to **ceruloplasmin** and hepatic copper is bound to **metallothionein.** In cases of excess, it is concentrated within lysosomes. Excess copper, like excess iron, causes production of **reactive oxygen species (free radicals)** that initiate destructive lipid peroxidation reactions that affect the mitochondrial as well as other cellular membranes. **In domestic animals, causes of copper toxicosis include:**

1. **Dietary excess in ruminants.** This may occur from excessive dietary supplementation to correct copper deficiency or from contamination of pasture with copper from fertilizers or sprays.

2. Animals grazing on pastures with normal concentrations of copper but **inadequate concentrations of molybdenum in soil.**

3. Grazing animals on fields with plants that contain **hepatotoxic phyotoxins,** usually pyrrolizidine alkaloids. **Crotalaria** and **Senecio** species are common examples of such plants. Copper is excreted in the bile. Hepatic diseases that cause cholestasis produce excessive accumulation of copper within the liver, even when dietary intake of copper is not excessive.

4. Hereditary disorders of copper metabolism occur in certain breeds of **dogs.**

The **results** of excessive accumulation of copper in the liver of domestic animals are species-dependent. **In ruminants,** particularly **sheep,** copper accumulates in the liver over a period of time, but some event triggers sudden release of copper, which is followed by **acute, severe intravascular haemorrhages** and **hepatocellular necrosis.** Necrosis of the liver is extensive and affects centrilobular and midzonal regions, but massive necrosis can occur. Despite the acute nature, this process is referred to as **chronic copper poisoning** to differentiate it from disease associated with simple copper intoxication, which causes gastroenteritis. **In contrast, in the dogs** in the hereditary metabolic disorders of copper metabolism, copper continues to accumulate and causes necrosis of liver cells, chronic inflammation, replacement fibrosis, and finally to an end-stage liver (cirrhosis) and signs of hepatic failure.

Pigment Accumulation

Pigments are coloured substances. Some of these are normal cellular constituents, while others accumulate only in abnormal circumstances.

1. **Bile pigments:** These accumulate in excessive amounts as a result of either extra-hepatic or intra-hepatic cholestasis and produce **jaundice** and yellow to green discoloration of the liver.

2. **Haemosiderin:** This is an iron-containing, golden-brown granular pigment. In macrophages, haemosiderin is derived from the breakdown of red cells that have been phagocytosed. Iron bound to plasma glycoprotein **transferrin** is the main source of haemosiderin in liver cells. Within liver cells, iron combines with apoferritin to form **ferritin,** the iron storage protein. As iron accumulates within the liver cells, aggregation of ferritin molecules form **haemosiderin.** Most of the haemosiderin in Kupffer cells and other macrophages in tissues throughout the body is derived from breakdown of red cells, whereas most of the hepatocellular haemosiderin is derived from iron present in **transferrin.**

   Haemosiderin forms in the liver when there is local or systemic excess of iron, such as when red cell breakdown is excessive (e.g. haemolytic anaemia), and within areas of hepatic necrosis. An excessive systemic load of iron in a variety of tissues without damage to organ function is called **haemosiderosis.** In contrast, **haemochromatosis** is an abnormal storage of iron within the body associated with **hepatic dysfunction.** Marked accumulation of iron can produce a dark brown or even a black liver.

3. **Lipofuscin:** This is **an insoluble pigment.** It is yellow brown to dark brown and is derived from incomplete oxidation of lipids such as those in cell membranes. With time, lipofuscin is oxidized. **Therefore, lipofuscin is a group of lipid pigments,** all of which consist of polymers of lipid, phospholipids, and protein. **Ceroid** is the earliest form of lipofuscin and the least oxidized.

Amounts of lipofuscin present in the liver tend to increase with age, hence the name **'wear and tear'** pigment.

4. **Melanin:** This is an endogenous pigment which is dark brown or black. Benign disorders of melanin pigmentation are called **'melanosis'**. **Congenital melanosis of the liver occurs in pigs** and **ruminants** and produces areas of discoloration. **Acquired 'melanosis' of sheep** has been described in Australia and occurs following ingestion of certain plants.

5. **Liver flukes:** These produce very dark excreta that contain a mixture of iron and porphyrin. These excreta produce the characteristic discoloration of bile which occurs in fascioliasis (*Fasciola hepatica*).

Hepatic Injury

Hepatocytes have a high metabolic rate. This renders them highly susceptible to metabolic disturbances which lead to **degeneration** and **necrosis**.

Patterns of Hepatocellular Degeneration and Necrosis

Despite a wide variety of insults the liver is subjected to, degeneration and necrosis occur in only one of three morphological patterns.

(i) Random hepatocellular degeneration or necrosis

This pattern is characterized by the presence of either single-cell necrosis throughout the liver or multifocal aggregates of necrotic hepatocytes. These areas are scattered **randomly** throughout the liver. This pattern is typical of many infectious agents, including viruses, bacteria, and certain protozoa, that come to liver through blood. **Gross lesions** are distinct pale or dark red foci that are sharply demarcated from the adjacent parenchyma. **Liver cells in affected areas either degenerate or become necrotic as a result of the injurious effects of the infectious agents.**

(ii) Zonal hepatocellular degeneration or necrosis

Also known as **zonal change,** this pattern affects liver cells within certain defined areas of the hepatic lobule. The zones are **centrilobular** (periacinar), **midzonal** (between centrilobular and periportal areas), or **periportal** (centroacinar) areas. Regardless of the location within the lobule, zonal change produces a liver which is pale and enlarged with rounded margins, and has an increased lobular pattern on the capsular and cut surface. **Degenerated liver cells swell,** and when most of the liver cells in a zone are affected, that portion of the lobule appears **pale.** In contrast, **necrosis** of liver cells in a particular zone of the lobule results in loss of liver cells and the consequent dilation and congestion of sinusoids so that the affected zone appears **red. Specific forms of the zonal change include:**

1. **Centrilobular degeneration and necrosis of liver cells is most common.** This is because this portion of the lobule receives the least oxygenated blood and is therefore susceptible to hypoxia. Centrilobular necrosis can result from a sud-

den and severe anaemia or right-sided heart failure. Similarly, passive congestion of the liver results in hypoxia due to stasis of blood and produces atrophy of centrilobular liver cells.

2. **Paracentral (periacinar) degeneration** involves only a small area around the central vein because only the periphery of one acinus is affected.

3. **Midzonal degeneration and necrosis** are rare lesions in domestic animals but have been reported in **pigs** and **horses** with aflatoxicosis.

4. **Periportal degeneration and necrosis** are also rare, but may occur following exposure to toxins, such as phosphorus.

5. **Bridging necrosis** is the result of merging of areas of necrosis. Bridging may link centrilobular areas (central bridging), or centrilobular areas to periportal areas.

(iii) Massive Necrosis

Massive necrosis is necrosis of an entire liver lobule or adjacent lobules. All cells within the affected lobules are necrotic. **Grossly**, in acute cases, the liver is slightly enlarged and has a dark parenchyma because of extensive congestion. **Microscopically**, affected areas consist of blood-filled spaces within a connective tissue stroma devoid of liver cells. With time, necrotic liver cells lyse without regeneration. The final result is collapse of the lobule and replacement of the lost liver parenchyma with a scar. **Grossly**, the liver is small with a wrinkled capsule.

Response of the Liver to Injury

After destruction, regeneration of liver parenchyma, replacement by fibrosis, and biliary hyperplasia may occur.

(i) Regeneration

An important feature of the liver is its ability to regenerate lost hepatic mass. Experimentally, two thirds of the liver can be excised from a healthy animal without the signs of hepatic dysfunction, and the liver is rapidly regenerated. Besides regeneration of liver cells, there is regeneration in bile duct epithelium, endothelium, and sinusoidal lining cells which is coordinated with liver cell regeneration.

Regeneration does not involve the production of new lobules. Following removal of liver lobes, the remaining liver responds by increasing the size of the lobules to replace the lost mass. Body carefully controls liver regeneration to replace the lost hepatocyte mass along with bile ducts and vessels **without producing excess liver**. A variety of growth factors stimulate liver cells regeneration. Once normal liver mass has been restored, macrophages release transforming growth factor-beta, which stops liver parenchymal cell proliferation.

Extensive hepatic necrosis is followed by parenchymal regeneration without scarring. However, repeated injury or massive necrosis can disrupt the normal lobular architecture through parenchymal collapse on removal of the dead liver cells.

(ii) Fibrosis

Fibrosis is a common manifestation of chronic injury. The importance of fibrosis depends on its effect on liver function and its reversibility. More advanced fibrosis is usually irreversible. Despite the great regenerative capacity of liver, **fibrosis, when sufficiently severe, can be fatal.**

Widespread (usually centrilobular to massive) **hepatocellular necrosis,** is sometimes **followed** not by the usual regenerative response, but **by fibrosis.** This results in the formation of bands of dense connective tissue. This process is referred to as **post-necrotic scarring.** Other patterns of hepatic fibrosis include **biliary fibrosis** (centred on bile ducts in the portal areas), **focal** or **multifocal hepatic fibrosis** (randomly scattered throughout the liver parenchyma), and **diffuse hepatic fibrosis** (affects all regions of the lobule and is present throughout the liver). **Marked diffuse fibrosis with hyperplastic nodule formation is cirrhosis.**

(iii) Biliary Hyperplasia

Biliary hyperplasia is proliferation of new biliary ducts within the portal areas and periportal regions. The mechanism responsible for this proliferation is unknown.

Cirrhosis (End-Stage Liver)

The **cirrhotic** or **end-stage liver** is characterized by loss of normal liver architecture due to **nodular regeneration of parenchyma, fibrosis,** and often **biliary duct hyperplasia.** Because it is the **final, irreversible result** of several different liver diseases, the term 'end-stage liver' is applied. The term **cirrhosis** is neither descriptive nor accurate in meaning. Originally, it meant brownish-yellow (G. kirrhos=brownish-yellow). However, 'cirrhosis' is still widely used. It is defined as a diffuse process characterized by fibrosis and conversion of normal liver architecture into structurally abnormal lobes. Another view is that its characteristic feature is the total absence of any normal lobular architecture. The architecture of the liver is changed due to: (1) loss of liver parenchyma, (2) condensation of reticulin framework, and (3) formation of tracts of fibrous connective tissue. Regeneration of liver tissue between fibrous bands leads to the formation of **regenerative nodules.** **The entire liver is therefore distorted and consists of nodules of regenerating parenchyma separated by fibrous bands that appear as depression on the surface.** The **causes** of end-stage (cirrhotic) liver are many.

Causes: Chronic toxic injuries from the ingestion of hepatotoxins, for example, **herbivores** ingesting toxic plants that contain pyrrolizidine alkaloids. In **dogs,** it can occur from long-term administration of anticonvulsant drugs such as primidone.

Following chronic toxic injury, fibrosis can occur in portal and centrilobular areas. Chronic **extra-hepatic biliary obstruction** and **cholestasis** lead to extensive portal fibrosis that mainly affects the portal triads, but fibrosis can finally extend into the liver parenchyma. Chronic inflammation of the liver (**hepatitis**) or biliary tract (**cholangitis**) may lead to **end-stage liver.** Although infection of the liver is focal or multifocal, diffuse hepatitis and fibrosis occur in diseases such as **canine chronic (chronic-active) hepatitis. Chronic passive congestion** ultimately leads to fibrosis around central veins, which can progress to **cardiac cirrhosis**. However, the actual amount of fibrosis is small. Abnormal storage or metabolism of metals such as copper as occurs in certain breeds of **dogs** with hereditary copper accumulation, may produce an **end-stage liver.** A number of more poorly defined diseases can lead to progressive hepatocellular injury and fibrosis resulting in end-stage liver disease.

Result: The **end-stage liver cannot perform its normal functions.** Therefore, clinical signs of **liver failure** always occur in affected animals.

Hepatitis

Hepatitis is inflammation of the liver and **cholangitis** inflammation of the bile ducts. Inflammation that affects the bile ducts and adjacent liver parenchyma is called **cholangio-hepatitis. Pericholangitis** is inflammation that surrounds the bile ducts, but does not encroach on them. **Portal hepatitis** refers to accumulation of inflammatory cells within the portal areas.

Routes of infection are haematogenous, direct penetration, and ascending through the biliary system. **The most common route is haematogenous** because liver receives both **arterial blood** through the hepatic artery and **venous blood** from the gastrointestinal tract through the portal vein. Ascending biliary infections and direct penetration are les common. The nature and distribution of lesions usually depend on the nature of infectious agent (e.g. virus, bacterium, and fungus), the route of entry, and any affinity for a cell type in the liver. **The pattern of inflammation usually indicates the route of infection.** Haematogenous infection, viral, bacterial, fungal, or protozoal, causes a random multifocal distribution of lesions. Infections that climb the biliary tract, usually bacterial, such as **Salmonella** sp., produce cholangitis first, but ultimately develop as cholangio-hepatitis because severe infections extend into the adjacent parenchyma. Penetrating wounds or foreign bodies in the digestive tract (reticulum) can cause distinct areas of inflammation with or without necrosis. These foci develop into abscesses that are visible on the capsule and extend into the liver parenchyma.

Acute Hepatitis

Acute hepatitis is characterized by inflammatory cells. At the beginning there are neutrophils, afterwards, lymphocytes and plasma cells, particularly if an infectious agent is present. Especially bacteria and protozoa supply chemotactic stimuli for inflammatory cells, causing them to accumulate. In time, areas of acute hepatitis in which liver cells are killed are replaced by regenerating liver cells or fibrous tissue. If antigen persists, as occurs in some infectious agents, chronic inflammatory lesions, such as an **abscess** or **granuloma**, may form. Usually, toxin-induced necrosis does not produce much inflammatory response other than phagocytes to remove cell debris and a mononuclear cell infiltration in the portal areas. Similarly, acute viral infections in animals usually produce multifocal necrosis, but little inflammation.

Grossly, small foci of acute inflammation are detected only if accompanied by necrosis. A variety of patterns occur. Viral infection produces a random pattern of necrosis with little inflammation. Random foci of neutrophilic hepatitis, as a result of localization of bacterial emboli, are common in all species. In neonates (newborns), especially **calves, lambs,** and **foals**, bacteria usually localize in the liver through the umbilical veins or the portal venous or hepatic arterial systems. **Neutrophilic cholangitis** and **cholangio-hepatitis** occur from ascending bacterial infection of the biliary system, usually as a result of biliary obstruction by parasites or compression of the duct by fibrous tissue or a neoplasm.

Chronic Hepatitis

Chronic hepatitis occurs when there is continued inflammation due to persistence of an **antigenic stimulus.** In the absence of such a stimulus, inflammation rapidly subsides. Certain bacteria (e.g. **Mycobacteria, Salmonella**) and fungi (e.g. *Histoplasma capsulatum*) are particularly resistant to killing by phagocytic cells and produce chronic inflammation and granuloma formation. **Other causes** of chronic inflammation of the liver include chronic cholangio-hepatitis from persistent infection of the biliary system, and chronic (chronic-active) hepatitis of the **dog** (see 'canine chronic hepatitis'). Chronic inflammation is visible grossly if it produces a distinct **granuloma** or **abscess.** Also, when chronic inflammation occurs throughout the liver, loss of parenchyma produces architectural distortion of the liver as a result of fibrosis and nodular parenchymal regeneration.

Whereas acute hepatitis is usually characterized by accumulation of neutrophils, chronic inflammation is characterized by fibrosis and accumulation of mononuclear inflammatory cells including lymphocytes, macrophages, and plasma cells. Neutrophils are usually present in chronic unresolved hepatic inflammation such as that occurs in canine chronic hepatitis. Focal lesions such as abscesses or granulomas are so localized that they do not alter liver function. In contrast, diffuse and severe chronic hepatitis usually leads to end-stage hepatic disease with hepatic failure and its associated clinical signs.

Viral Hepatitis

Infectious Canine Hepatitis

Infectious canine hepatitis is caused by **canine adenovirus 1,** and is now relatively less common because of widespread vaccination. Most of the infections are asymptomatic, and infections that produce disease may not be fatal. **The virus has a predilection for vascular endothelium and liver cells**. Severe disease is characterized by hepatic necrosis and widespread haemorrhage that can affect many organs. Virus-induced endothelial damage can lead to disseminated intravascular coagulation and haemorrhagic diathesis (predisposition towards haemorrhage).

Gross lesions include widespread petechiae and ecchymoses, accumulation of clear fluid in the peritoneal and other serous cavities, presence of fibrous strands on the liver, and enlargement and reddening of the tonsils and lymph nodes. The liver is moderately enlarged, friable, and contains small foci of hepatocellular necrosis around centrilobular areas. The centrilobular necrosis is due to virus's affinity for infection and necrosis of endothelial cells. This leads to vascular stasis and local hypoxia. An increased lobular pattern is sometimes seen as a result of centrilobular hepatic necrosis. The wall of the gallbladder is thickened by oedema.

The severity of **microscopic lesions** in **dogs** indicates the duration of disease. Susceptible **puppies** rapidly succumb to infection and have only scattered foci of hepatocellular necrosis, whereas severe disease in **older dogs** often produces both scattered foci of hepatocellular necrosis and widespread centrilobular necrosis. Large amphophilic inclusions (i.e., staining with either acid or basic dyes) are found in vascular endothelium and liver cells.

Rift Valley Fever

This is an acute, arthropod-transmitted zoonotic viral disease that mainly affects **ruminants**, causing extensive mortality among **calves** and **lambs,** and abortion of **pregnant ewes** and **cows.** The causative virus is a **phlebovirus.** The disease occurs mainly in Africa. Liver is involved in severe cases and is characterized by its enlargement and orange-brown discoloration. Pale foci of hepatocellular necrosis that are scattered throughout the parenchyma give a mottled appearance, and sometimes the lobular pattern is increased because of the centrilobular hepatic necrosis. Diffuse petechiae and ecchymoses are also characteristic of the disease, as are oedema and haemorrhages of the wall of the gallbladder.

Microscopic lesions are characterized by the presence of both randomly distributed foci of hepatocellular necrosis and more widespread zonal necrosis. These lesions are more severe and widespread in young animals and aborted fetuses. **Eosinophilic intranuclear inclusion bodies** may be present in degenerated liver cells in areas of necrosis.

Herpesvirus Infections

A number of herpesviruses that produce **abortion** have been described. Each animal species is affected by a specific virus. These abortogenic herpesviruses cause multifocal, small areas of necrosis in several foetal organs,**including liver.** Similar lesions are sometimes seen in neonates. **Examples of these viruses include** the abortogenic equine herpesvirus (equine herpesvirus 1), infectious bovine rhinotracheitis virus (bovine herpesvirus 1), caprine herpesvirus, feline viral rhinotracheitis virus, and pseudorabies virus. Canine herpesvirus can produce multifocal liver necrosis in **neonatal pups,** but foci are more consistently present in the kidneys, lungs, and spleen.

Other Viral Infections

Certain viral diseases may involve **liver.** Such diseases include feline infectious peritonitis, which is characterized by foci of pyogranulomatous vasculitis or perivascular accumulations of lymphocytes and plasma cells in many organs, **sometimes including the liver.** Subacute and chronic forms of equine infectious anaemia are characterized by cellular infiltration, particularly lymphocytes, **in portal areas of the liver.** Systemic adenoviral infection of **lambs, calves,** and **goat kids** may produce multifocal areas of hepatocellular necrosis, cholangitis, and necrosis of biliary epithelium.

Bacterial Hepatitis

Liver Abscess

Bacteria can reach liver through a number of different routes and produce abscesses. These routes include portal vein and umbilical veins from umbilical infections in newborn animals. This occurs as part of a generalized bacteraemia, bacteria reaching the **liver** through the hepatic artery, as an ascending infection of the biliary system, by parasitic migration, and as a direct extension of an inflammatory process from tissues such as reticulum, immediately adjacent to the liver.

Bacterial infections of the liver and formation of liver abscesses are particularly common in cattle. Liver abscesses usually follow toxic rumenitis because damage to the ruminal mucosa allows ruminal microflora, particularly *Fusobacterium necrophorum,* to enter the portal circulation. After localizing in the liver, bacteria proliferate and produce focal areas of hepatocellular necrosis and **hepatitis**, which in time, develop into liver abscess. Liver abscesses of **cattle** are usually incidental lesions, but affected cattle show loss of weight and decreased milk production. Sometimes, an abscess can encroach on a hepatic vein or vena cava and cause phlebitis which may result in mural thrombosis and, because of the obstruction of the outflow to the venous drainage of the liver, passive congestion of the liver and portal hypertension. Detachment of portions of mural thrombi can produce septic thrombo-emboli that lodge in the lungs. Rupture of liver abscesses directly into the hepatic vein or into the vena cava occurs rarely in cattle and may result in death of the affected animal because of fatal septicaemic embolization of the lungs. Sometimes death can be sudden from the blockage of large areas of pulmonary capillaries by the exudate. Sometimes, fungi such as **Mucor** which proliferate in areas of ruminal ulceration invade the portal circulation and are carried to the liver and there cause extensive areas of necrosis.

Bacillary Haemoglobinuria

This is **an acute and highly fatal disease** of **cattle** and **sheep**. It occurs particularly in those regions where liver fluke (*Fasciola hepatica*) infection also occurs. The cause is spores of *Clostridium haemolyticum,* which are ingested and they come to reside in the Kupffer cells. But they proliferate only in areas of low oxygen tension. Migration of immature liver flukes, or sometimes other parasites, produces a focus of necrotic liver parenchyma in which spores germinate. Bacteria proliferate and **release toxins**, the most important being **phospholipase C**. This toxin produces hepatocellular necrosis and intravascular haemolysisthat characterize the disease.

Clinical signs include jaundice, haemoglobinaemia, and haemoglobinuria. The liver contains one or more distinct foci of hepatic necrosis in which causative organisms are visible in tissue sections. **Grossly,** these foci are sharply demarcated from the adjacent parenchyma and are usually pale and surrounded by a hyperaemic zone. Migration tracts of the immature liver flukes that precipitate the disease are present. Serous cavities (pleura, peritoneum, and pericardium) usually contain excessive amount of red or straw-coloured fluid, sometimes flecked with fibrin.

Infectious Necrotic Hepatitis

Also known as **'black disease'**, it is more common in **sheep** and **cattle**, but also occurs in **pigs** and **horses.** This disease is somewhat similar to bacillary haemoglobinuria in that dormant spores of *Clostridium novyi* (usually type B) germinate in areas of lowered oxygen tension and **release toxins** that produce distinct foci of coagulative necrosis within the liver and ultimately death of the animal. Generation of the spores is brought about by liver necrosis caused by the migration of immature liver flukes.

Affected animals have one or more areas of hepatocellular necrosis, which **grossly** appear as distinct, pale areas of variable size. A zone of hyperaemia usually surrounds these foci. Parasitic migration tracts are also usually present. The **other lesions** include accumulation of fluid within the pericardial sac and pleural and peritoneal cavities. The carcass of affected animals putrefies rapidly because of high fever before death.

Leptospirosis

The **liver** is usually involved in acute, severe leptospirosis in **all domestic animals.** This is due to ischaemic injury to centrilobular areas as a result of intravascular haemolytic anaemia. Also, organisms are present in large numbers in the liver. Infection of **dogs** with *Leptospira grippotyphosa* is associated with chronic (chronic-active) hepatitis.

Other Bacterial Infections

These are those infections that cause systemic disease and because of bacteraemia, they also produce hepatocellular necrosis and hepatitis. Examples include *Yersinia tularensis, Yersinia pseudotuberculosis,* and *Pasteurella haemolytica* infection of **sheep; Salmonella** infection in many species (lesions in the liver are distinct accumulations cf mixed mononuclear inflammatory cells called **'paratyphoid nodules');** *Actinomyces pyogenes* infection of the **bovine foetus and neonate;** *Campylobacter foetus* subsp. *foetus* in **lambs;** *Actinobacillus equuli* infection of **foals,** and *Nocardia asteroides* infection of **dogs.** Lesions in these infections range from small foci of liver necrosis to many large abscesses. **Diagnosis** of the specific causative agent depends on bacterial isolation and characterization.

Parasitic Hepatitis

Nematodes

Migration of nematode larvae through the liver is common in domestic animals. As larvae travel through the liver, they produce tracts of hepatocellular necrosis which are accompanied by inflammation. With time, these tracts are filled with connective tissue which produces fibrous scars seen on the capsular surface. These scars appear as pale areas, and the term **'milk spotted liver'** has been used to describe such livers in **pigs** scarred by migrating larvae of *Ascaris suum.* Larvae sometimes become trapped within the liver or its capsule and are walled off within abscesses or granulomas. Examples of chronic hepatitis or hepatic scarring as a result of larval migration include that from migration of ascarids in several species of domestic animals, *Stephanurus dentatus* in **pigs,** and **Strongylus** sp. in **horses.** Infestation of liver with adult nematodes is less common than larval migration. *Capillaria hepatica* is sometimes found in the liver of **dogs** and **cats.**

Dogs with heartworm infection (*Dirofilaria immitis*) sometimes develop **'vena caval syndrome',** also known as **'postcaval syndrome'.** It is characterized by disseminated intravascular coagulation, intravascular haemolysis, and **acute hepatic failure.** The syndrome occurs particularly in **dogs** with large number of adult worms in the vena cava, as well as within the right atria and pulmonary artery. The liver is engorged with blood as a result of severe passive congestion from partial blockage of vena cava. Mechanical factors associated with the presence of large numbers of worms in the right atrium or vena cava are the cause of intravascular haemolysis that characterize vena caval syndrome.

Cestodes

A number of cestodes occur in the biliary system of domestic animals. The most important are the encysted forms of cestode parasites in the tissues of the intermediate hosts. Among these, the most important are larval cestodes of the genus **Taenia. Adults of Taenia live in the gastrointestinal tract of carnivores.** However, these are not harmful to their definitive hosts. The ova ingested by an intermediate host develop into embryos, which penetrate the wall of the intestine and are distributed through the blood to almost any site in the body. Parasitic cysts develop in the tissues of the intermediate host. The life cycle of the parasite is completed when cysts are ingested by the definitive host. Involvement of the liver in the intermediate host always occurs because portal blood, in which embryos migrate, first goes to the liver before flowing into the systemic circulation.

The cestode *Taenia hydatigena* occurs in **dogs**, but its intermediate stage, *Cysticercus tenuicollis*, occurs in the peritoneal cavity of a number of species, including **horses, ruminants**, and **pigs**. Immature cysticerci migrate in the liver and can cause extensive damage if infection is heavy. **Lesions** are similar to those caused by migration of immature **Fasciola hepatica**.

Hydatid liver disease is common in some countries. *Echinococcus granulosus* is a cestode that occurs in carnivores, and hydatid cysts can develop into many different animal species, including humans. The **dog-sheep cycle** is more important in some countries. **Cattle** in pastures are also commonly affected in some other countries. Embryos may develop into hydatid cysts in almost any organ in the intermediate host, **but liver and lungs are commonly affected.** These cysts are usually less than 10 cm in diameter, but can attain quite big size, particularly in humans. **Hydatid cysts, even when present in large numbers, rarely cause clinical signs of disease in domestic animals.**

Cestode worms that occur in the biliary system include *Stilesia hepatica* and *S. globipunctata*. Both can inhabit the bile duct of **ruminants**. Infections with these parasites may result in chronic inflammation of the biliary duct, but usually do not produce clinical signs of liver dysfunction.

Trematodes

Liver fluke disease of **sheep** and **cattle**, and sometimes other species, is usually due to *Fasciola hepatica*. **Hepatic fascioliasis** occurs in areas where climatic conditions (low swampy areas) are suitable for the snails that serve as intermediate hosts for the parasites. Adult *F. hepatica* lives in the biliary system. Their eggs pass through the bile to the intestinal tract and ultimately are passed in the faeces. Larvae then develop in the snail intermediate host (Genus **Lymnaea**). Cercariae which leave the snail encyst on grass, where they develop into **infectious metacercariae**. Metacercariae are ingested by the **ruminant host** and penetrate the wall of the duodenum to enter the peritoneal cavity, and afterwards, **enter the liver.** They migrate within the liver before settling in the bile ducts. Migration of immature flukes through the liver produces haemorrhagic tracts of necrotic liver parenchyma. These tracts in acute infestation are dark red, but with time become pale. Resolution is by fibrosis. A number of complications can occur following these migrations which include acute peritonitis, hepatic abscesses, death of the host as a result of acute, widespread liver necrosis associated with massive infiltration of immature flukes, and the proliferation of spores of *Clostridium haemolyticum* or *Clostridium novyi* in necrotic tissue and afterwards development of bacillary haemoglobinuria or **infectious necrotic hepatitis.**

Mature flukes live in the larger bile ducts and cause **cholangitis** and **cholangio-hepatitis.** Chronic cholangitis and bile duct obstruction lead to **ectasia** (dilation) and **stenosis** (narrowing) of the ducts. Obstruction of the ducts leads to extra-hepatic cholestasis. Animals with chronic liver fluke disease are in poor bodily condition.

In some areas, *Fasciola gigantica* and *Fascioloides magna* are important causes of liver fluke disease in **ruminants.** The adults of *F. gigantica* and *F. hepatica* live in the bile ducts. In contrast, *F. magna* migrate in the liver and cause widespread damage in **cattle** and **sheep.** In **cattle**, the immature *F. magna* flukes cause extensive tissue damage as they migrate through the liver, but the adults are enclosed by fibrous connective tissue in cysts. **In sheep,** the flukes continuously migrate through the liver and cause extensive damage.

Other trematodes that live in the bile ducts include *Dicrocoelium dendriticum* in **horses, ruminants, pigs, dogs,** and **cats;** *Eurytrema pancreaticum* in **ruminants;** and *Opisthorchis tenuicollis* in **pigs, dogs,** and **cats.** All can produce similar changes, but much milder than those associated with *Fasciola hepatica*. In addition, they sometimes cause obstruction of the biliary ducts.

Nutritional Diseases

Hepatosis Dietetica

Also known as **'nutritional hepatic necrosis'** hepatosis dietetica is a syndrome of **acute hepatic necrosis** that occurs in **young, rapidly growing pigs.** It is caused by a deficiency of either vitamin E or selenium. Pathogenesis of hepatosis dietetica is incompletely understood, but it is clear that vitamin E and selenium-containing enzymes destroy free radicals, and are therefore important for the maintenance of stability and integrity of cellular membranes.

Hepatosis dietetica is characterized by haemorrhagic centrilobular to massive hepatic necrosis. Areas of massive necrosis in the affected liver initially are distended and deep red and later form dense tracts of connective tissue (post-necrotic scarring) in animals that survive the acute disease.

Toxic Liver Disease

The liver is the most common site of toxic injury for two reasons:

1. Liver receives approximately 70% of blood from the portal vein, which drains blood from the gastrointestinal tract. Therefore, ingested toxic substances, including plant, fungal, and bacterial products, as well as metals, minerals, and

other chemicals that are absorbed into the portal blood, **are transported to the liver.**

2. Liver possesses enzymes capable of metabolizing a variety of endogenous and exogenous substances for elimination from the body. This process also activates some substances to a more toxic form, thereby causing liver injury.

Conversion of lipid-soluble substances into water-soluble substances for elimination from the body is known as **'biotransformation'.** Many exogenous chemicals **(xenobiotics)** are absorbed by digestive tract, lungs, or skin more readily because they are lipophilic (having an affinity for lipids) and cross membranes easily. In order to eliminate these compounds, they must be made water-soluble to facilitate their excretion into bile or urine. **There are two stages in the process of biotransformation: (1) During stage 1 metabolism,** functional groups are introduced or existing polar groups (i.e. having a positive charge at one end and a negative charge at the other) are exposed on the substrate (xenobiotic) by oxidation, hydrolysis, or reduction. **(2) In stage 2,** the product of stage 1 metabolism is conjugated with glucuronic acid, sulphate, or other groups, **and this water-soluble form is then excreted in bile or urine.** Stage 1 metabolism is performed by the mixed-function oxidase (MFO) system, also known as, the **cytochrome P-450 system.** This is the main enzyme system of the liver involved with drug metabolism and is located in the smooth endoplasmic reticulum. Activity of this enzyme system is greatest in liver cells in centrilobular regions. The MFOs are a collection of functionally similar enzymes (isoenzymes) with different substrate specificities, and therefore oxidize a variety of chemicals. Enzymes involved in stage 2 metabolism are found mainly in the cytoplasm.

Although hepatic biotransformation is a means of detoxifying and eliminating chemicals, **it can also generate toxic metabolites.** This process in which inert compounds are metabolized to toxic metabolites, **usually free radicals,** occurs during stage 1 metabolism and is called **'bioactivation'.** Free radicals can react with liver cell DNA, RNA, and proteins as well as produce **oxidative stress** within cells. **Antioxidants** particularly reduced glutathione and vitamin E, provide some protection against oxidative injury to cell membranes or organelles. **Animals deficient in antioxidants are especially prone to hepatocellular injury.**

An individual compound can be simultaneously metabolized by several different pathways. Some of these pathways produce **toxic metabolites,** whereas others produce **non-toxic compounds.** The proportion of a compound metabolized by a particular pathway influences the degree of injury caused by the compound. A number of factors influence the severity of injury induced by a toxin. These factors include age, sex, diet, endocrine function, and genetic constitution. **Therefore, responses of individual animals exposed to the same toxin can vary considerably.**

Toxic liver injury is better understood by the **acinus concept of the liver. The site of toxic injury in the acinus indicates the site of bioactivation of the chemical.**

For example, **carbon tetrachloride** (CCl_4) is metabolized by MFOs to CCl_3, a free radical. Lesions caused by carbon tetrachloride are most severe in the **periacinar (centrilobular)** areas, because this site is the area where the smooth endoplasmic reticulum is most abundant, and therefore, here the active form of the chemical is present in greatest concentration. On the other hand, **allyl alcohol** is activated by alcohol dehydrogenase, a cytosolic enzyme that is most abundant in **centroacinar** (periportal) areas. Therefore, hepatocellular injury caused by allyl alcohol is more severe periportally.

Toxic chemicals can be divided into **two groups**: (1) those that cause liver injury (**predictable hepatotoxins**), and (2) those that do not (**idiosyncratic toxin**). **Predictable toxins** are those that produce liver injury in almost all susceptible animals. **Most of the hepatotoxins in veterinary medicine fall into this category.** Examples include carbon tetrachloride and pyrrolizidine alkaloids. **Idiosyncratic toxins** are those chemicals that cause liver injury in only few of the exposed animals after prolonged or repeated exposure. The pathogenesis of idiosyncratic toxic injury is not well understood. An example is the inhalation anaesthetic halothane.

The **changes** of toxin-induced liver injury vary with the type, dose, and duration of exposure to toxin. The responses to acute toxic injury include cellular swelling and accumulation of lipid (**lipidosis** or **fatty change**) with or without cholestasis. This can progress to necrosis if the toxicosis is severe. Continuous or repeated toxic injury to the liver is characterized by three responses: (1) **fibrosis**, (2) **biliary hyperplasia**, and (3) **parenchymal regeneration**. Toxic liver injury can lead to **end-stage liver**, and with toxins such as **aflatoxins**, to **hepatic neoplasia**. Both acute and toxic injury to the liver can cause **liver failure**. Liver failure in acute toxic injury is due to the loss of functional liver mass from degeneration or necrosis of liver cells. In chronic toxic injury, liver failure is the result of fibrosis and disruption of liver architecture.

Toxic Plants

A variety of toxic plants cause liver injury in domestic animals. The **phytotoxins** (plant toxins) can be divided into **three groups**: (1) preformed hepatic phytotoxins, such as occur in blue-green algae, (2) pyrrolizidine alkaloids. These must be metabolized to an active form in the liver, and (3) toxins that are deconjugated by bacteria within the digestive tract to release a factor that is afterward bioactivated in the liver.

(i) **Blue-green algae:** Several genera of blue-green algae have been associated with lethal poisoning of **livestock**, and less commonly, small animals such as **dogs** and **cats**. Dead and dying algae contain **preformed toxins** such as microcystin LR which accumulate on the surface of water and are ingested by livestock. **Signs** develop rapidly and include diarrhoea, prostration (lying down), and death. **Gross lesions** include haemorrhagic gastroenteritis and massive liver necrosis. Other preformed toxins have also been identified in blue-green algae.

(ii) **Pyrrolizidine alkaloids:** These are found in many plant families that occur throughout the world. The most important genera in India are **Crotolaria** and **Senecio**. About 100 different alkaloids are known. Ingested alkaloids are converted to **pyrrolic esters** by the liver MFO system. These are alkylating agents and react with cytosolic and nuclear constituents. (**Alkylating agents** are those agents that bind to DNA and prevent complete separation of the two DNA chains during cell division). **Pigs** are particularly susceptible to pyrrolizidine alkaloid intoxication, **sheep** much less, and **cattle** and **horses**, are intermediate in susceptibility. The characteristic **lesion** of pyrrolizidine intoxication is the presence of megalocytes. **Megalocytes** are liver cells with enlarged nuclei and increased cytoplasmic volume. **Megalocytes can be many times the size of normal liver cells.** They form because of the **anti- mitotic effects** of pyrrolizidine alkaloids, which **prevent cell division** but not DNA synthesis during liver cell division to replace those that have undergone necrosis. This change, although it indicates pyrrolizidine alkaloid intoxication, is not pathognomonic, because it also occurs with other toxins such as aflatoxins and nitrosamines. **Chronic intoxication** is accompanied by liver fibrosis, biliary duct proliferation, and sometimes nodular regeneration of parenchyma. **Cattle** have regenerative nodules more often than **horses. Chronic hepatic damage can lead to hepatic failure.**

(iii) **Cycads:** These are primitive palm-like plants. They contain **cycasin**, a nontoxic glycoside that, following ingestion, is deconjugated by intestinal microflora to **release a toxic metabolite,** methylazoxymethanol. Metabolism of this compound produces **alkylating agents** which cause chronic hepatic lesions in **cattle** characterized by **hepatocellular megalocytosis** and nuclear hyperchromasia, and varying degree of hepatic fibrosis. **Acute intoxication** is more in **sheep** than in other species and produces acute gastrointestinal dysfunction and periacinar hepatic necrosis. **Chronic cycad poisoning** in **cattle** causes a nervous disease. **Dogs** can also be intoxicated by cycad.

Mycotoxins

Mycotoxins are secondary metabolites of fungi. That is, their production is not necessary for the survival of the fungus. Several **hepatotoxic mycotoxins** are important in veterinary medicine.

Aflatoxins are produced by the fungus *Aspergillus flavus* and *A. parasiticus*. There are **four major aflatoxins, B1, B2, G1 and G2. Aflatoxin B1 is the most common and is also the most potent toxin and carcinogen.** Aflatoxins are usually produced during storage of fungal-contaminated feed and may be present in many crops, such as maize, groundnuts, and cottonseed. Aflatoxins are converted to **toxic intermediates** by the smooth endoplasmic reticulum or liver cells. Carcinogenic, toxic, and teratogenic (causing developmental malformations) effects of aflatoxins are due to binding of the toxic intermediates to cell's DNA, RNA, or proteins.

Pigs, dogs, horses, cattle, and **poultry**, especially younger animals are sensitive to the toxic effects of aflatoxins, whereas **sheep** are more resistant. **Acute intoxication** is rare in domestic animals, except **dog**, because an animal will be required to consume excessively large amounts of contaminated feed at a time. **Lipidosis** and **biliary proliferation** also occur. **Chronic intoxication** is more common and results in increased susceptibility to infection, and sometimes, signs of hepatic failure. **Affected livers are firm** and **pale**, and **microscopically**, are characterized by lipidosis and necrosis of liver cells, biliary hyperplasia, fibrosis, and atypical liver cells.

Facial Eczema

Facial eczema is caused by mycotoxin **sporidesmin**, produced by fungus *Pithomyces chartarum*, a common plant in New Zealand and Australia. Ingestion of sufficient amounts of toxin produces necrosis of the epithelium of large bile ducts and **cholangio-hepatitis**. Cholestasis and failure to excrete **phylloerythrin** usually leads to **photosensitization** with lesions of the head, hence the common name **'facial eczema'**.

The disease is common in **sheep**, and less so in **cattle**. **Acute cases** are characterized by bile-stained liver with prominent bile ducts due to dilation and presence of bile in the lumen. **In chronic cases**, the bile ducts become thickened following epithelial necrosis and subsequent inflammation (chronic cholangitis and cholangio-hepatitis).

Hepatotoxic Therapeutic Drugs

Various therapeutic drugs can also cause liver injury in some animals. The mechanism by which these drugs can cause injury varies with species and with individual. **Cats are more susceptible than dogs to intoxication** by many chemicals because they are relatively deficient in the liver enzyme **glucuronyl-transferase** activity. This stage II enzyme forms conjugates between bioactivated (stage I) xenobiotics and glutathione. When stage II metabolism is disturbed, **injurious bioactivated products cause liver injury. Cats** are more sensitive to **acetaminophen** intoxication than **dogs** because of this relative enzyme deficiency. The tranquillizer **diazepam** can cause acute fatal liver injury in some **cats**. The mechanism of injury is not known.

Acute liver injury can occur in **dogs** following treatment with **trimethoprim-sulphonamide** antibiotic preparations. The anti-inflammatory drug carprofen can cause acute liver necrosis in **dogs. Chronic liver toxicity** occurs in **dogs** receiving anticonvulsants, such as primidone, phenytoin, and phenobarbital, for prolonged periods. The mechanism of hepatotoxicity is unknown.

Hepatotoxic Chemicals

Phosphorus occurs in **two forms: red** and **white**. Red is unimportant as a toxin, white phosphorus is sometimes used as a rodenticide. The mechanism of toxicity is not clear. Poisoning is indicated by the signs of gastroenteritis. **Microscopic lesions** include lipidosis of liver cells and centroacinar (periportal) necrosis. **Carbon tetrachloride** is a compound that must be bioactivated by MFO system to become toxic. Sometimes used as an anthelmintic, carbon tetrachloride produces centrilobular liver necrosis and lipidosis of surviving liver cells.

Metals

Metals also cause toxic liver injury. Copper toxicity may cause acute intravascular haemolytic anaemia in **ruminants,** or as chronic liver injury and end-stage hepatic disease in **dogs**. Two important syndromes of **iron poisoning** are **iron-dextran intoxication of piglets** and **ferrous fumarate intoxication of newborn foals.** These two toxicities are characterized by massive liver necrosis. Ferrous fumarate is used in foals as a component of a specific dietary supplement. Iron-dextran is usually administered intramuscularly to **suckling pigs** to prevent anaemia, but its administration has sometimes resulted in significant mortality and affected **pigs** die soon after infection. Excessive iron supplementation to **dogs** and **cats** may result in excessive storage of iron and subsequent liver disease due to iron overload, called **'haemochromatosis'.**

Diseases of Unknown Aetiology

Canine Chronic Hepatitis (Chronic-Active Hepatitis)

Chronic-active hepatitis is a chronic inflammatory and fibrosing disorder of humans, which may occur during chronic infections with the viruses of hepatitis B or hepatitis C. **In dogs,** hepatic disorders which have microscopic changes similar to those of the human disease have also been termed **chronic-active hepatitis.** The cause in most cases is unknown, although some cases have been associated with **leptospira** and **infectious canine hepatitis virus infection.** Chronic-active hepatitis is characterized by **progressive destruction of individual liver cells and infiltration of mononuclear inflammatory cells.** It is proposed that destruction of individual cells is mediated by an immune mechanism. The liver is usually small. Severely affected liver are characterized by architectural distortion which may be coarsely nodular texture to an end stage liver (cirrhosis). **Microscopically,** the disorder is characterized by necrosis of individual liver cells (piecemeal necrosis), periportal fibrosis, accumulation of inflammatory cells, especially lymphocytes in portal tracts and adjacent periportal areas of the lobules, and intrahepatic cholestasis.

Equine Serum Hepatitis

This disease occurs in horses. However, it is not always in those horses that have received an injection of a biological that contains equine serum; for example, equine antisera such as tetanus antitoxin or pregnant mare serum gonadotropin. Probably an **infectious agent** appears responsible, but none has been identified. The **clinical course** of the disease is very rapid and always fatal. Affected **horses** have liver failure that appears as hepatic encephalopathy and jaundice. The liver of affected animals is small with an increased lobular pattern.

Chronic Lymphocytic Cholangitis of Cats

Affected **cats** usually present jaundice as a result of intrahepatic cholestasis. **Microscopically,** liver is characterized by extensive aggregations of inflammatory cells, mainly lymphocytes and plasma cells that are present in portal areas, particularly around small bile ducts. Inflammation is accompanied by bile duct proliferation, liver or biliary fibrosis, and intra-hepatic cholestasis. The cause is unknown. The disease might have an immunological basis and has been compared with primary biliary cirrhosis of human beings.

Hepatic Injury as a Result of Systemic Disease

Many systemic diseases can cause liver injury and liver dysfunction. For example, acute haemorrhagic pancreatitis of **dogs** is sometimes accompanied by jaundice. The liver is particularly susceptible to the effects of **hypoxia**. Therefore, any disease that causes **anaemia** can produce centrilobular (paracentral) degeneration and necrosis.

Hepatocellular Nodular Hyperplasia

Hepatocellular nodular hyperplasia is common only in the **dog.** Incidence increases with age. The disease is not associated with significant dysfunction, **but hyperplastic nodules must be differentiated from regenerative nodules and liver neoplasms, with which they are usually confused.** Often many nodules are present. They can be seen on the capsular surface and are typically raised. On incision, they are well demarcated from normal parenchyma and usually compress adjacent parenchyma. Hyperplastic nodules are similar to normal liver, but the lobular pattern is distorted. The lobules contain an increased proportion of liver cells and decreased numbers of portal areas and central veins compared to normal liver. Liver cells usually contain lipid or glycogen-containing vacuoles.

Regenerative Nodules

Regenerative nodules are a different type of nodular lesion. They are not related to nodular hyperplasia, because regenerative nodules originate from the proliferation of liver cells in response to loss of hepatocytes. The cause is unknown. Regenerative nodules are easily differentiated from nodular hyperplasia by fibrosis and disruption of normal liver parenchymal architecture.

Cholangio-Cellular (Bile Duct) Hyperplasia

Hyperplasia of bile ductules commonly occurs as a non-specific response to a variety of liver injuries. Reactive proliferation of the ductular elements of the liver must be differentiated from neoplastic proliferation.

Neoplasms

Primary neoplasms of the hepatobiliary system can originate from liver cells and biliary epithelium of bile ducts, or the gallbladder and connective tissue and blood vessels. **The liver is common site of metastasis for many malignant tumours. In fact, most of the neoplasms within the liver are metastases from other organs.**

Hepatocellular Adenoma

These are benign neoplasms of liver cells. They are seen usually in **ruminants.** They are often single, un-encapsulated, red or brown masses. They are usually spherical but may be pedunculated. They are composed of well-differentiated liver cells which form uniform plates that may be two or three cells thick. Portal areas and central veins are few within the neoplasm. In **diagnosis,** hepatocellular adenomas must be differentiated from nodular hyperplasia and hepatocellular carcinomas.

Hepatocellular Carcinoma

These are malignant neoplasms of liver cells. They are uncommon in all domestic animals, but occur more commonly in **ruminants,** particularly **sheep.** They are usually single, often involve an entire lobe, and are well demarcated. They consist of grey-white or yellow-brown tissue which is divided into lobules by multiple fibrous bands (Fig. 19). Malignant liver cells characteristically form irregular plates (trabeculae) three or more cells thick. Vascular spaces are present between the trabeculae. Cells range from well-differentiated liver cells to atypical or

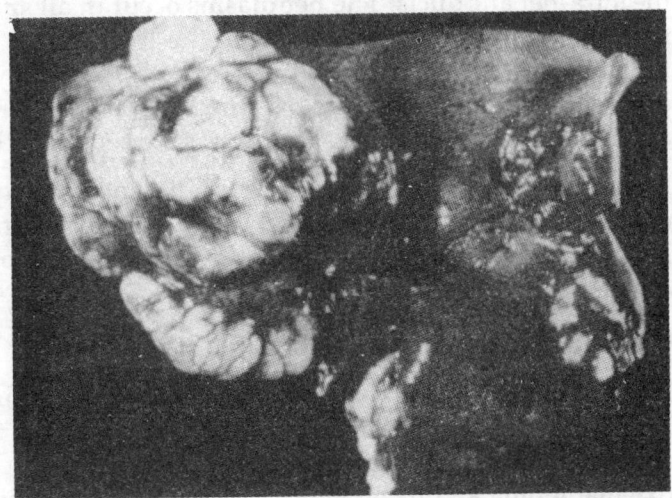

Fig. 19. Liver; cat. Hepatocellular carcinoma. Note that multilobular mass has replaced much of the normal liver.

177

bizarre forms. In the absence of metastasis, differentiation of well-differentiated carcinoma and adenoma is difficult. Metastasis to a number of sites occurs, particularly to lymph nodes, lungs, and seeding into the tissues lining the peritoneal cavity. Some hepatocellular carcinomas spread extensively within the liver (intra-hepatic metastasis).

Cholangio-Cellular (Bile Duct) Adenoma

Adenomas of the bile ducts are uncommon in most species. However, it is most common primary liver neoplasm in **cats.** They are usually distinct, firm, grey, or white masses composed of well-differentiated bile epithelium. **Cholangiomas** are gland-like structures formed by tubules lined with cuboidal epithelium and moderate amounts of stroma. The tubules may have narrow lumen or be distended by fluid, forming cystic structures. The stroma of the cyst wall consists of fibrovascular tissue with moderate amounts of collagen. Cysts are lined with benign biliary epithelium, which is simple cuboidal to flattened. Biliary epithelial cells may form papillary projections extending into the cystic spaces.

In cats, large cystic cavities lined by flattened biliary epithelium are considered as adenomas. However, some consider them as congenital malformations. Some of these lesions can involve extensive areas of liver. A similar, but congenital polycystic liver disease also occurs in **dogs**

Cholangio-Cellular (Bile Duct) Carcinoma

These are **malignant neoplasms** of biliary epithelium which usually originate from the intra-hepatic ducts. **The neoplasms occur in all species.** A large single mass or multiple nodules may be present in the liver. These neoplasms are firm, raised, umbilicated (having a central depression), pale-grey and un-capsulated. Well-differentiated carcinomas are organized into a tubular or acinar arrangement. The epithelial components of the neoplasms are separated by fibrous connective tissue.

Metastasis is common, particularly to adjacent lymph nodes of the abdomen, lungs, or by seeding into the abdominal cavity. Metastasis into the peritoneal cavity can produce nodules within the mesentery and on the serosal surface of the abdominal organs.

Miscellaneous Primary Neoplasms of the Liver

Primary neoplasms can originate from any of the cellular constituents of the liver. These include mesenchymal neoplasms derived from the liver's **connective tissue** (fibrosarcoma, osteosarcoma); **muscles** (leiomyosarcomas); **endothelium** (haemangioma and haemangiosarcoma), and carcinoids, which are neoplasms of neuroendocrine cells. Haemangiosarcoma primary to the liver occurs in **dogs**, although it is a relatively uncommon site compared to the skin and spleen

Metastatic Neoplasms

Liver and lungs are the two most common sites for metastatic spread of malignant neoplasms. Metastatic neoplasms must be differentiated from primary hyperplasia or neoplasia of the hepatocellular tissues. **Malignant lymphoma is the most common metastatic neoplasm found in the liver of most species.**

Some metastatic neoplasms have a typical appearance within the liver. For example, **melanomas** usually are black because of the presence of melanin, and **haemangiosarcomas** are usually dark red and brown. Haematopoietic neoplasms such as **lymphoma** and the **myeloproliferative disorders** can expand the liver and therefore produce hepatomegaly and an increased lobular pattern on the cut surface. This characteristic appearance is due to centrilobular degeneration because of **anaemia** in both malignant lymphoma and myeloproliferative disorders. In malignant lymphoma, neoplastic lymphocytes tend to infiltrate portal tracts and expand into the adjacent parenchyma in severe cases. Metastatic carcinomas often have an umbilicated appearance (characterized by depression) similar to that seen in cholangio-cellular carcinomas, **but umbilication is rarely a feature in sarcomas.**

Gallbladder

Biliary Obstruction, Cholelithiasis and Inflammatory Disorders

Biliary Obstruction

Obstruction of the bile ducts in domestic animals is usually caused by choleliths, foreign bodies such as parasites in the bile ducts, and stenosis (narrowing) of the ducts as a result of external compression by a neoplasm or periductular fibrosis. **Complete obstruction** of the common bile duct leads to extra-hepatic cholestasis and **jaundice**. **Obstruction of the individual intra-hepatic duct is usually asymptomatic.** Prolonged extra-hepatic cholestasis causes dilation of bile ducts, biliary hyperplasia in the portal areas, and hepatocellular injury due to retention of bile constituents. Rupture of calculi can lead to liver cell death and formation of pooled bile areas (bile lakes). The leakage of bile into portal areas causes **inflammation** and **fibrosis** that progress to extensive scarring of these areas, called **biliary fibrosis.**

Cholelithiasis

Choleliths or **gallstones** usually occur in all the domestic animals, but they are especially common in **ruminants**. Choleliths are concretions (calculi, stony masses) of normally soluble components of bile. They form when these components become supersaturated and precipitate. Choleliths in the gallbladder usually do not become clinically important unless they migrate and obstruct the biliary system

Cholecystitis

Cholecystitis is inflammation of the gallbladder. It can be **acute** or **chronic**. **Acute inflammation** of the gallbladder occurs in viral infections such as Rift Valley fever in **ruminants** and infectious canine hepatitis. Fibrinous cholecystitis occurs in **calves** with acute salmonellosis, particularly that caused by *Salmonella enteritidis*, serotype *dublin*. Other bacteria, either derived from the blood or coming from the intestine, can cause acute or chronic cholecystitis. **Chronic cholecystitis** is associated with prolonged bacterial infection of the biliary tree, or irritation from choleliths or parasites of the gallbladder. **Rupture of the gallbladder is rare**, but can occur as a result of acute or chronic infection. The release of bile can cause **fatal peritonitis** because of the irritating effect of bile on the serosal surfaces of the abdomen.

Hyperplastic and Neoplastic Lesions

Cystic Mucinous Hyperplasia

This has been reported in **dogs** and **sheep**. There are no external abnormalities, and cystic hyperplasia is seen only by opening the gallbladder. When the bile is removed, the affected **mucosa** is grey-white and has a thickened, sponge-like consistency. **Sessile** or **polypoid masses** are sometimes found. **At times large cysts also occur.** They appear as papillary projections into the lumen of the gallbladder. Most of the cysts contain a copious amount of mucus. The entire mucosa may be affected. However, **these lesions are usually of no importance to the host.** Cystic hyperplasia of the gallbladder usually goes undetected clinically. The **cause** is not known.

Adenoma

Adenomas of the gallbladder are rare neoplasms but are most common in **young cattle** and have been described in **dogs, cats,** and **sheep.** They are multi-nodular or papillary masses that protrude from the mucosal surface and consist of a loose connective tissue stack that is lined by well-differentiated biliary epithelium.

Carcinoma

Malignant neoplasms of the gallbladder epithelium are rare in domestic animals, but have been described in **dogs, cats,** and **cattle.** They are composed of mucin-secreting epithelial cells and usually have a papillary arrangement. Carcinoma of the gallbladder may involve the liver by direct extension and may metastasize to the hepatic lymph nodes and to more distant sites.

Exocrine Pancreas

Consequences of Dysfunction (abnormal function)

The exocrine pancreas has a lot of functional reserve. Therefore, only disorders that affect large portion of pancreas can cause abnormal digestion (maldigestion).

Maldigestion as a result of exocrine pancreatic insufficiency is most common in the **dog**, associated with either atrophy or chronic pancreatitis. However, the disorder also occurs sporadically in other species including **cattle**, especially **calves** with pancreatic hypoplasia, and in **cats**. Pancreatic insufficiency in small animals and calves is characterized by steatorrhoea (fat in the faeces), diarrhoea, and weight loss despite polyphagia (excessive eating).

Developmental Anomalies

Hypoplasia

Hypoplasia of the pancreas has been described in **calves** and is characterized by signs of pancreatic insufficiency. It has also been described in the **dog**, but it is usually considered as atrophy rather than true hypoplasia. In hypoplasia, pancreatic tissue is difficult to identify. The amount is small and the persisting parenchyma is neither distinct nor lobulated like the normal gland. The difference between atrophy and hypoplasia can be difficult to determine because both conditions lead to abnormally small organ with diminished function. Parenchymal cells of the hypoplastic pancreas do not usually contain **lipofuscin**, which is seen in atrophic cells.

Anomalies of the Duct System

The arrangement of the major pancreatic duct or ducts varies between and within species. For example, **sheep** have only one duct that drains into the common bile duct, whereas **cattle** and **horses** have two ducts. In **dogs**, several different arrangements of the pancreatic ducts have been described.

Specific anomalies include **congenital stenosis** of the pancreatic ducts and **cystic dilation** of the ducts. **Congenital cysts** within the pancreas sometimes occur in **lambs**.

Incidental Findings

Ectopic Pancreatic Tissue

Nodules of ectopic pancreatic tissue sometimes are present in the duodenum, stomach, gallbladder, and mesentery of the **dog** and **cat**. This type of anomaly in which normal tissue is present in an abnormal location, is called a **choristoma**.

Pacinian Corpuscles

These are **normally present in the interlobular connective tissue of the pancreas** and mesentery of the **cat**, and appear as distinct 1-3 mm **nodules. The corpuscles should not be mistaken for abnormal structures.**

Calculi

Formation of **concretions** or **stones** in the pancreatic duct is called **'pancreolithiasis'**, and is seen at times in **cattle**. It is usually an incidental finding at slaughter, and is more common in cattle more than 4 years of age.

Stromal Fat Cell Infiltration

Fat cell infiltration of the interstitial connective tissue of pancreas sometimes occurs in very fat **cats**. The pancreas itself is unaffected, therefore pancreatic function is normal.

Degeneration, Necrosis, Inflammation and Response to Injury

Degeneration

Degeneration of the acinar cells of the pancreas is a non-specific process. It can occur as a result of local and systemic diseases. Obstruction of the pancreatic ducts can also cause degeneration and atrophy of the pancreas. **Obstruction of the pancreatic duct(s)** can be caused by neoplasms, or chronic inflammation in which the accompanying fibrosis can compress the duct. Foreign bodies such as parasites or pancreoliths also occlude the duct. Atrophy may also be secondary to interstitial fibrosis of the pancreas, as occurs in **dogs** with chronic pancreatitis.

Juvenile Pancreatic Atrophy

This condition occurs in **dogs** and is characterized by atrophy of the exocrine pancreas. **Young animals are affected** (L. juvenile = young), usually between 6 and 12 months of age. Affected dogs show signs of maldigestion due to pancreatic insufficiency and rapidly lose weight despite a great appetite. The **pancreas** in affected dogs is **small**.

Necrosis

Pancreatic necrosis and **pancreatitis** have been described in a number of species. The cause is usually different in each species. **Causes** of necrosis of acinar cells **in calves** and **sheep** include zinc toxicosis and **in pigs** T-2 toxin (a trichothecene mycotoxin). However, spontaneous (idiopathic) necrosis and inflammation of the pancreas are most common in the **dog,** and to a lesser extent in the **cat**. Necrosis and pancreatitis may occur as either an acute or chronic disease. Although the pathogenesis is similar, the clinical signs and lesions of acute and chronic pancreatitis are different.

Inflammation

Inflammation of the pancreas is called **'pancreatitis'**. It may be **acute** or **chronic.**

Acute Pancreatitis

Acute pancreatitis is particularly common in the dog. Very fat sedentary bitches are especially predisposed. A similar situation also occurs, though less often, in cats. In **dogs**, pancreatitis occurs as a result of **release of activated pancreatic enzymes** into the pancreatic parenchyma and adjacent tissues. These activated enzymes particularly **phospholipase A** and **elastase,** digest pancreatic tissue, which results in release of inflammatory mediators. These further increase the process and attract inflammatory cells. The **mechanism** responsible for the release of pancreatic enzymes is incompletely understood. Acute pancreatitis usually occurs after **dogs** have eaten a meal high in fat.

Signs of acute pancreatitis include anorexia, vomiting, and abdominal pain. The **lesions** are due to proteolytic degradation of pancreatic parenchyma, vascular damage and haemorrhage, and necrosis or peri-pancreatic fat by lipolytic enzymes. Inflammation, which is characterized by accumulation of leukocytes around the affected tissue, occurs rapidly after the tissue necrosis. **Mild cases** of pancreatitis are characterized by oedema of the interstitial tissue of the pancreas. **Acute haemorrhagic pancreatitis is more severe.** The pancreas is oedematous and contains areas that are grey-white, the result of coagulative necrosis, and other dark-red or blue-black areas that are haemorrhagic. Areas of **fat necrosis** are seen as chalky-white foci as a result of saponification (conversion of fat into soap) of necrotic adipose tissue in the mesentery adjacent to pancreas. Portions of the normal parenchyma may be seen between the affected portions. The **peritoneal cavity** usually contains blood-tinged fluid, which may contain droplets of fat. **Peritonitis** is noticed by **fibrinous adhesions** between the affected portions of the pancreas and adjacent tissues.

The **microscopic appearance** of acute haemorrhagic pancreatitis is characterized by focally extensive areas of haemorrhage, accumulation of leukocytes and coagulative necrosis of the parenchyma, accumulation of fibrinous exudate in the interlobular septa, and necrosis and inflammation of fat in the mesentery near the affected portions of pancreas.

Acute, severe pancreatitis produces **systemic effects in affected dogs**. The release of inflammatory mediators and activated enzymes from the damaged pancreas may produce widespread vascular injury and subsequent widespread haemorrhage, shock and disseminated intravascular coagulation. **The liver is also affected.** This is indicated by increased concentration of serum hepatic enzymes such as alanine aminotransferase, and sometimes focal hepatic necrosis.

Pancreatitis is sometimes **caused by trauma**, usually in **dogs** and **cats** as a result of some crushing or impact trauma to the abdomen. Leakage of enzymes from the pancreas initiates necrosis. This is followed by trauma and inflammation of the pancreas and nearby tissues in the same manner as previously described for pancreatitis in the dog.

183

Acute pancreatitis that causes clinical disease is less common in species other than the **dog** and **cat**. Acute pancreatic necrosis and pancreatitis have been described in the **horse**, but the pathogenesis of pancreatitis in this species differs from that in the **dog** and **cat**. Necrosis and inflammation are the result of **migration of strongyle larvae** through the pancreas, which results in the release of pancreatic enzymes and enzymatic digestion of the pancreas and surrounding tissues.

Chronic Pancreatitis

Chronic pancreatitis is usually accompanied by **fibrosis** and **parenchymal atrophy.** It can occur in all species as a result of obstruction of the pancreatic ducts. **Chronic pancreatitis is most common and important in the dog,** but also occurs in **cat, horse,** and **cattle**, in which it is rarely of clinical importance. **In the dog,** pancreatic fibrosis and chronic pancreatitis are the result of progressive destruction of the pancreas by repeated mild occurrences of acute pancreatic necrosis and pancreatitis. **Pancreas has a poor regenerative capacity and responds to injury by replacement fibrosis and atrophy of parenchyma.** Thus, continuing destruction of pancreas causes loss of glandular tissue without replacement. If a fairly large portion of the pancreas is affected, **dogs** develop signs of exocrine pancreatic insufficiency **(diabetes mellitus). Grossly,** pancreas is a distorted, shrunken, and nodular mass with fibrous adhesions to adjacent tissues. **Fibrosis** of the pancreas also occurs in **cats**, and in **sheep** following necrosis of pancreatic cells from zinc toxicosis.

Chronic pancreatitis and **replacement fibrosis** occur sometimes in the **horse,** usually as a result of either parasitic migration or from ascending bacterial infection of the pancreatic ducts. Also, pancreatitis may occur in **horses** with chronic eosinophilic gastroenteritis. However, chronic pancreatitis usually is not clinically noticeable in the **horse**, because signs of pancreatic insufficiency rarely occur in this species.

Pancreatic cysts are fluid-filled fibrous sacs which may occur following pancreatitis is some **dogs** and **cats**.

Parasitic Infections

A number of parasites live in the pancreatic ducts of domestic animals. Parasitic infections of the pancreatic ducts are important if they occlude the ducts, either by physical obstruction or by causing inflammation within and around ducts. Examples include **flukes** such as *Opisthorchis tenuicollis, Clonorchis sinensis, Eurytrema pancreaticum,* and *Dicrocoelium dendriticum* that may inhabit the pancreatic ducts of a number of species. Nematodes, particularly **ascarids** and **cestodes** are common gastro-intestinal parasites of the domestic animals. Sometimes, they lodge in the pancreatic ducts.

Hyperplasia

Nodular hyperplasia of the pancreas occurs in **dogs, cats,** and **cattle**. It is particularly common in older dogs and cats. The lesion is clinically not important, but it must be differentiated from neoplasms of exocrine and endocrine pancreas.

The hyperplastic nodules are characteristically multiple, raised, smooth, and grey or white on cut surface. **Microscopically,** they consist of un-capsulated aggregates of acinar cells. The difference between hyperplasia and adenoma of the pancreas is poorly defined in domestic animals.

Neoplasms

Adenoma

Adenomas of the exocrine pancreas are rare, but have been described in the **cat**. Those of acinar cell origin share all the features of hyperplastic nodules, but are single and larger than normal pancreatic lobules, whereas hyperplastic nodules are not larger than normal lobules. However, this distinction is somewhat arbitrary.

Carcinoma

Carcinoma of the duct epithelium or acinar cells of the exocrine pancreas is **uncommon in all species.** However, it is usually reported in the **dog** and **cat**. The neoplasms are **single or multiple nodules** within the pancreas. Areas of haemorrhage or necrosis may be present in the neoplasm. The neoplasm is firmer than the adjacent pancreas because of proliferation of fibrous connective tissue. **Adhesions** of the affected pancreas to adjacent tissues occur. The neoplasm usually invades adjacent tissues and the peritoneal cavity. In the peritoneal cavity they are present as nodules over the mesentery, omentum, and serosa of the abdominal organs. **Metastasis** to the abdominal lymph nodes adjacent to the pancreas is also common. Some carcinomas metastasize widely.

Microscopically, carcinomas range from well-differentiated adenocarcinomas with tubular pattern to undifferentiated carcinomas with a solid pattern. The amount of fibrous stroma varies greatly and is usually greatest in poorly differentiated neoplasms. Zymogen granules seen in normal acinar cells are usually absent in the cytoplasm of the neoplastic cells.

Peritoneum

Abnormal Contents

Foreign bodies or substances may produce local or diffuse peritonitis and death. **Ingesta** may come from a ruptured stomach or intestine, **urine** or **bile** from rupture of the urinary bladder or gallbladder, respectively; **blood (haemoperitoneum)** from rupture of the liver, spleen, ovarian cysts, rupture of the gravid uterus, or of any large abdominal vessel. **Eggs** may be found in birds, and foetuses in other animals.

Hydroperitoneum (Ascites)

Accumulation of watery fluid in the peritoneal cavity is called 'hydroperitoneum'. As the fluid is non-inflammatory (**transudate**), hydroperitoneum is an oedematous condition and is called **'ascites'**. Ascites usually occurs in **dogs** and **cats**, and less commonly in **sheep** and **cattle**, and seldom in other animals. Sometimes, fluid in the peritoneal cavity may represent inflammatory oedema (**exudate**) such as in serous peritonitis, or may result from a severe acute urinary obstruction with or without rupture of the bladder, especially in **cattle** and **sheep**. Except the inflammatory form, **the amount of fluid that accumulates in the peritoneal cavity may be huge and causes distension of the abdomen** and all the symptoms associated with excessive abdominal pressure.

Ascites, or true oedema of the peritoneal cavity, may occur as part of a syndrome of generalized oedema and involve several causes of that condition. **The causes of ascites include:**

1. **Chronic passive congestion of the portal venous system.** The causes of this congestion are conditions which incompletely obstruct the flow of blood through the portal vein, most common being **hepatic cirrhosis.** Other causes of obstruction include pressure of neoplasms, abscesses, granulomas, and enlarged lymph nodes on the vein, as well as thrombus in the vein.

2. Local passive hyperaemia

3. Hypoproteinaemia

4. Increased permeability as in shock and oedema disease of **pigs,** and

5. Lymphatic obstruction when lymph nodes of the mesentery and viscera are invaded by tumours or infectious agents.

Like all oedema, fluid in ascites is a transudate with a specific gravity less than 1.017 and protein content below 3 percent. Accumulation of inflammatory exudate is characterized by the presence of signs of inflammation and elements of the exudate, mainly leukocytes and fibrin. The specific gravity and concentration of protein are higher in inflammatory exudate.

Peritoneal fluid of urinary tract origin, coming from a ruptured bladder as urine has the odour and other characteristics of urine. Evidence of urinary obstruction in the form of calculi, cystitis, hydronephrosis, or related lesions is usually present.

Grossly, the peritoneal cavity contains a clear or straw-coloured fluid. The maximum amount reported in **horses** is 170 litres, and in **dogs** 20 litres. In oedema disease of **pigs** as much as 500 ml has been found. Coagulation is absent or slight. The peritoneum is smooth, but later it becomes rough because long continued ascites acts as irritant to the serosa, and produces a mild inflammation.

The **clinical complications** of ascites are those of pressure which interferes with the abdominal organs and movement of the diaphragm during respiration. If the fluid is removed by abdominocentesis (surgical puncture of the abdomen), it again accumulates rapidly. The underlying disorders responsible for its accumulation, produce other characteristic clinical abnormalities, such as **uraemia** in the case of urinary obstruction.

Haemorrhages

Haemorrhages in the peritoneum usually occur in several septicaemic and toxaemic diseases, such as anthrax, pasteurellosis, and enterotoxaemia of lambs. Haemorrhages are usually present on the serosa of the diaphragm, stomach, and intestine.

Inflammation

Inflammation of the peritoneum (**peritonitis**) is **common in nearly all species of domestic animals.** According to the cause, it may be **acute** or **chronic**, and according to the character of the inflammatory process - **serous, fibrinous, suppurative, haemorrhagic, necrotic,** and **gangrenous**. Peritonitis is caused by bacteria. These include streptococci in **horses**, and *Actinomyces pyogenes* (previously *Corynebacterium pyogenes*), *Escherichia coli*, and members of the **Pasteurella** group in **cattle** and **pigs**. In visceral gout in **poultry**, urates are found in the peritoneum where they produce chronic inflammation. Necrosis occurs if a very irritating drug is administered intraperitoneally. Since bacteria are usually introduced with the drug, an abscess or an acute suppurative inflammation of subcutaneous connective tissue (**phlegmon**) usually develops in the area. If the drug is administered with a long needle and penetrates the colon, the wall of the colon gets perforated. This allows bacteria to escape from the intestine. If the body defences cannot contain the bacteria within the colon, they invade the peritoneum and cause a diffuse suppurative, or gangrenous peritonitis.

Neoplasms

Neoplasms of the mesentery and omentum are not common. They are usually secondary malignant ones which either metastasize from the intestine, or become transplanted from other organs such as the uterus, liver, or ovaries. There are tumours originating in the peritoneum called **mesotheliomas**, which **do occur but are rare.** They can be confused with inflammatory changes or tumour metastases. They appear as nodular or papillary growths of mesenchyme covered by proliferating mesothelial cells which may be difficult to differentiate from true epithelial cells. **Although considered malignant, mesothelioma rarely metastasizes.**

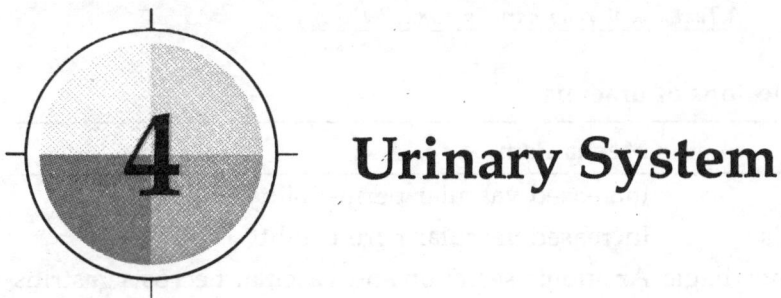

4 Urinary System

The kidney

Renal Failure

When renal functional capacity is damaged, kidneys fail to carry out their normal **metabolic** and **endocrine functions.** The glomerulus, tubules, collecting duct, and capillary blood supply are all closely inter-related in each nephron both anatomically and functionally. Therefore, alterations in tubular function or structure affect glomerular function and vice versa. **For example,** necrosis or atrophy of renal tubules results in loss of function of the affected nephrons and **secondary atrophy of the glomerulus.** Also, because most of the capillary blood supply to tubules is through post-glomerular capillaries, **reduction in glomerular blood flow reduces the blood supply to the tubules.**

Renal function can be diminished by pre-renal factors such as reduced renal blood flow, circulatory collapse, obstruction of vascular supply to the kidneys, shock, or severe hypovolaemia (decreased volume of circulating blood). Renal function can also be damaged by renal disease or by post-renal causes such as obstruction of urine outflow through the lower urinary tract. **Damaged renal function** results in the retention of those constituents of plasma that are normally removed by the kidneys. Estimation of plasma or serum concentrations of **urea, creatinine,** and **ammonia,** the nitrogenous waste products of protein catabolism, are routinely used as index of diminished renal function. The increase of these nitrogenous waste products in blood is called **azotaemia. Renal failure** can result in intravascular accumulation of other waste products such as guanidines, phenolic acids, and large molecular weight alcohols (e.g. myoinositol); reduced blood pH (**metabolic acidosis**); alterations in plasma ion concentrations, particularly potassium, calcium, and phosphate; and hypertension. The **result of tissue failure** is a toxicosis called **uraemia. Uraemia therefore is a syndrome associated with multi-systemic clinical signs and lesions due to renal failure.**

Animals that die from renal failure are because of cardiotoxicity from increased serum potassium, metabolic acidosis, and pulmonary oedema. Non-renal lesions of uraemia seen clinically and at postmortem are useful indicators of renal disease **(Table 6).**

Table 6. Non-renal lesions of uraemia

Lesion	Mechanism
Pulmonary oedema	Increased vascular permeability
Fibrinous pericarditis	Increased vascular permeability
Ulcerative and haemorrhagic	Ammonia secretion and vascular necrosis gastritis
Ulcerative and necrotic	Ammonia secretion in saliva and vascular necrosis stomatitis
Atrial and aortic thrombosis	Endothelial and sub-endothelial damage
Hypoplastic anaemia	Increased erythrocyte fragility and lack of erythropoietin production
Soft tissue mineralization	Altered calcium-phosphorus metabolism (stomach, lungs, pleura, kidneys)
Fibrous osteodystrophy	Altered calcium-phosphorus metabolism
Parathyroid hyperplasia	Altered calcium-phosphorus metabolism

The **severity of non-renal lesions of uraemia** depends on the length of time animal has survived in the uraemic state. **Therefore, in acute renal failure, non-renal lesions are few, whereas in chronic renal failure many lesions can be present.** Most of the lesions are due either to endothelial degeneration and necrosis resulting in thrombosis and infarction, or to the excretion of large concentrations of ammonia in the saliva and gastric juice. **Lesions of uraemia include** ulcerative and necrotic stomatitis characterized by a brown, foul-smelling, mucoid material adherent to the eroded and ulcerated lingual (of tongue) and oral mucosae. **Ulcers** are usually present on the underside of the tongue. Ulcerative and haemorrhagic lesions mostly occur in the **stomach** of **dogs** and **cats** and the **colon** of **horses** and **cattle**. Large areas of the gastric or colonic mucosa are usually oedematous and dark red because of haemorrhage. The gastrointestinal contents can be bloody and smell of ammonia. **Microscopically,** coagulative necrosis, haemorrhage, and neutrophilic infiltration occur in mucosa. Degeneration, necrosis, and mineralization (calcification) of the intima and media of arterioles are usually present in the gastric mucosa and sub-mucosa.

Increased vascular permeability in uraemic animals sometimes results in a fibrinous pericarditis, characterized by fine granular fibrin deposits on the epicardium (visceral pericardium), and diffuse pulmonary oedema. In pulmonary oedema, alveoli contain fibrin-rich fluid and usually mild infiltration of macrophages and neutrophils. This lesion is called **uraemic pneumonitis.**

In the uraemic animal, focal sub-endothelial degeneration can occur in the left atrial endocardium, and less commonly, the endothelial surface of the proximal aorta and pulmonary trunk. These arterial lesions are called **muco-arteritis,** and appear grossly as finely granular roughened plaque. Muco-arteritis along with loss of anticoagulant antithrombin III by glomerular leakage is favourable for the formation of large (in the wall) thrombi at these sites. Chronic renal failure usually causes **reduced production of erythropoietin** producing non-regenerative **anaemia.** Uraemia-associated increased erythrocytic fragility also contributes to the uraemia. Most animals in renal failure have **hyperphosphataemia** and normocalcaemia or **hypocalcaemia**. Alterations in calcium-phosphorusmetabolism in uraemic animal are characteristic of **chronic renal failure** and result from a set of complex events. When glomerular filtration rate is gradually reduced to less than 25% of normal, phosphorus is no longer properly secreted by the kidneys and **hyperphosphataemia** results.

Because of the interactions between serum calcium and phosphorus, ionized calcium concentration in serum is reduced as a result of precipitation of calcium and phosphorus. **Reduced ionized serum calcium stimulates parathyroid hormone secretion, causing calcium release from the stores in the bone and osteoclastic bone resorption.** These changes in the calcium-phosphorus metabolism are more severe because of the reduced ability of the diseased kidneys to hydroxylate 25-hydroxycholecalciferol to the more active 1, 25-dihydroxycholecalciferol **(calcitriol) resulting in decreased intestinal absorption of calcium.** Calcitriol production is further reduced by **hyperphosphataemia.** Also, calcitriol normally suppresses parathyroid hormone. Therefore, reduced calcitriol production further increases parathyroid hormone secretion. With time, these changes lead to **parathyroid chief cell hyperplasia (renal secondary hyperparathyroidism)**, fibrous osteodystrophy **(renal osteodystrophy)**, and **soft tissue calcification. Hyperparathyroidism** further increases disease by stimulating **nephrocalcinosis,** the process by which renal tubular epithelium is damaged by an increase in intracellular calcium. Calcium is precipitated in mitochondria and in tubular basement membranes.

Soft tissue calcification associated with uraemia occurs at many places and represents both dystrophic and metastatic calcification. The gastric wall can be gritty when cut because of calcification of the inner and middle layers of the mucosa, as well as sub-mucosal arterioles. Necrotic arterioles throughout the body are particularly susceptible to calcification during uraemia. A characteristic lesion, particularly in **dogs**, is calcification of the sub-pleural connective tissue of the cranial inter-costal spaces. These lesions are white-grey granular pleural thickenings with a horizontal 'ladder-like' arrangement. The inter-costal muscles are only superficially calcified. **Patchy or pulmonary calcification results in failure of the lungs to collapse,** areas of paleness, and mild to moderate firmness, sometimes in association with lesions of uraemic pneumonitis. **Microscopically**, the alveolar septa are calcified and can focally rupture, causing small emphysematous bullae. Although usually not seen at necropsy, **calcification occurs in the kidneys.** The kidneys can be gritty when cut because of the calcification of tubular basement membranes, Bowman's capsules, and necrotic tubular epithelium, especially in the medulla and inner cortex.

Developmental Abnormalities

Renal Aplasia (Agenesis)

This is **failure of development of one or both kidneys.** There is no recognizable renal tissue. The ureter may be present or absent. **Unilateral aplasia is compatible with life,** provided the other kidney is normal. **Unilateral aplasia** can go unnoticed during life and is seen only at necropsy. **Bilateral aplasia** is incompatible with life, and is rare.

Renal Hypoplasia

This is **incomplete development of the kidneys.** There are fewer nephrons, lobules, and calyces present at birth. **Hypoplasia** can be **unilateral** or **bilateral**. It occurs rarely and is difficult to diagnose. It has been reported in **pigs** and **foals**. Hypoplastic kidneys from **pigs** and **foals** have greatly reduced number of glomeruli. In **foals,** for example, 5 to 12 glomeruli are present per low-power field in affected kidneys compared to 30 to 35 glomeruli per low-power field for normal kidneys from adults. The shrunken kidneys in young animals, particularly **dogs**, are usually diagnosed as hypoplastic. However, in most of these cases the small kidneys are due to renal fibrosis resulting from renal disease developing at an early age, to progressive juvenile nephropathy, or to dysplasia (discussed next).

Renal Dysplasia

This is an **abnormality of altered structural organization.** It results from abnormal differentiation with the presence of structures not representative of normal nephrogenesis. Renal dysplasia is rare and like renal hypoplasia must be differentiated from renal fibrosis and progressive juvenile nephropathy. Dysplastic changes can be **unilateral** or **bilateral** and can involve much of an affected kidney or only as focal lesions. Dysplastic lesions can be small, misshapen, or both. The number of nephrons, lobules, and calyces are normal. Bilateral renal dysplasia has been described in **foals.** Cystic renal dysplasia has been described in **sheep.**

Progressive Juvenile Nephropathy (Familial Renal Disease)

This condition has been described in certain breeds of **dogs,** but could be an example of **renal dysplasia.**

Ectopic and Fused Kidneys

Ectopic kidneys are misplaced from their location due to their abnormal migration during foetal development. Ectopic kidneys mostly occur in **pigs** and **dogs** and usually involve only one kidney. Ectopic (away from normal) locations often include the pelvic cavity or inguinal region. Ectopic kidneys are usually structurally and functionally normal, but malposition of the ureter predisposes them to **obstruction and secondary hydronephrosis.**

Fused (horseshoe) kidneys result from fusion of the cranial and caudal poles of the kidneys during nephrogenesis. This fusion results in the appearance of **one large kidney with two ureters.** The histological structure and function of fused kidneys are usually normal.

Renal Cysts

Congenital renal cysts can occur in cases of renal dysplasia, or can occur as a primary entity. Kidneys can have **single or multiple cysts.** Some cysts cause no alteration in renal function, and are considered incidental findings. Such **incidental renal cysts** are common in **pigs** and **calves** and must be differentiated from hydronephrosis.

Cysts can originate anywhere in the nephron and be present either in cortex or medulla. Cysts vary from being just visible to several centimetres in diameter. They are usually spherical, thin walled, lined by flattened epithelium, and are filled with clear water fluid. The sources of fluid are glomerular filtrate, trans-epithelial secretions, or both.

Polycystic Kidneys

Polycystic kidneys have many cysts which involve numerous nephrons (Fig. 20). Cysts are of different sizes and are present both in the cortex and medulla. As cysts enlarge, they compress the adjacent parenchyma. When kidneys are polycystic, renal function is damaged. **Congenital polycystic kidneys** are rare in many species, but have been described in **pigs, lambs,**

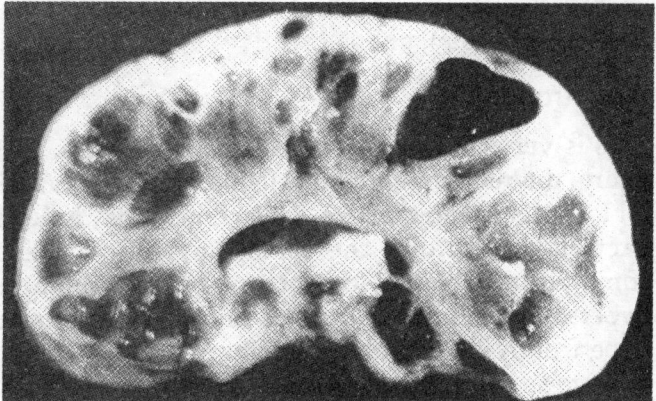

Fig. 20. Kidney; cat. Polycystic disease. Note numerous cysts of various sizes are present in the cortex and medulla.

and **dogs.** The pathogenesis of renal cysts is not entirely understood.

Acquired renal cysts can occur as a result of renal interstitial fibrosis (see 'chronic renal diseases'), or other renal diseases that cause intratubular obstruction. These cysts are usually small (1 to 2 mm) and occur mainly in the cortex. In all cases of renal cysts, the cysts must be differentiated from hydronephrosis (dilated renal pelvises), especially in **pigs** and **cows** with multilobular kidneys.

Inherited Abnormalities in Renal Tubular Function

Inherited abnormalities of tubular metabolism, in transport, or in reabsorption of glucose, amino acids, ions, and proteins have been described in **dogs**. **Cystinuria** is excretion of large quantities of cystine in the urine. It is a sex-linked inherited disease seen sometimes in **male dogs**. Cystinuria predisposes the affected dogs to **calculus formation** and **obstruction** of the lower urinary tract. Primary renal **glucosuria** is also an inherited disorder described in **dogs**. It occurs when the capacity of tubular epithelial cells to absorb glucose is reduced. Glucosuria predisposes the **dogs** to bacterial infection of the lower urinary tract and urinary bladder.

Growth Disturbances

Atrophy

Atrophy of the kidney is very common. Nephrons deprived of an adequate blood supply may show atrophic changes. Likewise, pelvic calculi, tumours, and parasites by the mechanical effect of pressure produce localized area of atrophy. Some of the larger pelvic calculi and the giant nematode *Dioctophyma renale* which localizes in the pelvis and also in the perirenal tissue and abdominal cavity interfere with the escape of urine into the ureter, and therefore produce atrophy through direct pressure and also through the secondary pressure of accumulated urine (**hydronephrosis**).

Hypertrophy

This is very common in all domestic animals. Following glomerular or tubular injury, the remaining renal cells become larger, and are thus able to compensate for loss of renal epithelium. When one kidney is destroyed, (ureteral obstruction or bacterial infection), the remaining kidney becomes greatly enlarged and compensates for the loss of renal tissue (**compensatory hypertrophy**). The hypertrophic kidney may be as much as twice its normal size. Histologically, the hypertrophy involves the epithelium of the nephron unit and the cells may be twice as large as the normal cells.

Hyperplasia

Hyperplasia of the glomerular and tubular structures of the kidney is **uncommon**.

Metaplasia

Metaplasia of the kidney involves the interstitial white fibrous connective tissue only. It is usually the result of bacterial infection. When metaplasia occurs, **masses or plates of bones may be found in the kidney.**

Metabolic Disturbances

Cellular Swelling

Previously known as 'cloudy swelling', **cellular swelling** is due to various inorganic, organic, and bacterial toxic substances. These toxic substances reach the kidney through the bloodstream. They first injure the glomeruli and convoluted tubules, and then the collecting tubules. The proximal convoluted tubules are usually the only tubules affected due to their high susceptibility to injury. The cells usually recover unless the injury is of a more severe type.

Macroscopically, the kidney is swollen, has a bulging out surface, and cooked appearance. **Microscopically**, the cells appear cloudy, their cytoplasm is granular, and they stain more intensely with eosin. Because the cells contain more fluid than normal, they are swollen and protrude into the lumen of the tubules. Postmortem autolysis should not be mistaken for cellular swelling. **In postmortem autolysis, cells do not swell.**

Hydropic Degeneration

This is characterized by the formation of **clear cytoplasmic vacuoles**, which do not contain glycogen, fat, or mucin, and are presumed to be tissue fluids. Causes include over-dosages of ether, chloroform, or carbon tetrachloride.

Fatty Change

The **disturbance of fat metabolism**, which causes fatty change in renal epithelium, occurs under the same conditions as it does in the heart, liver, adrenals, and skeletal muscles. It is the expression of **a severe injury to kidney cells. In most cases it is the result of a toxic injury.** The toxic substances reach the kidneys by means of the general circulation. Fatty change is a common alteration in many severe acute infectious diseases, particularly those that are septicaemic.

Macroscopically, the kidneys are enlarged, swollen, have a bulging cut surface, are friable and greasy in consistency, and white, yellow, or orange in colour. The colour depends on the species of the animal. **Cat kidneys are white**, while **horse kidneys are orange** in colour. The kidneys often have a mottled appearance due to variations in the amount of blood in various portions of the kidney. **Microscopically**, the tubular cells, particularly the convoluted cells, contain **distinct vacuoles of variable size**. Nuclei may be dark and pyknotic. Fatty change can be confirmed by staining sections with a fat stain.

Amyloidosis

Amyloid is an insoluble fibrillar protein with a beta-pleated sheet conformation. It is produced after incomplete proteolysis of several soluble amyloidogenic proteins. The cell responsible for degradation of amyloidogenic proteins is

macrophage. Amyloid deposits in human patients with plasma cell myelomas or other B-lymphocyte dyscrasias (**AL amyloidosis**) are composed of fragments of the light chains of immunoglobulins. **In domestic animals**, amyloidosis is usually an example of **reactive amyloidosis (AA amyloidosis)**. This form of the disease is usually associated with chronic inflammatory diseases. The amyloid deposits are composed of fragments of a serum acute-phase reactant protein called serum amylod associated (SAA) protein. Amyloid fibrils form either source are deposited in tissues along with a glycoprotein called **amyloid-P-component**.

Glomeruli are the common site for deposition of amyloid in most domestic animals. However, in **cats** medullary interstitium is the common site for deposition. **Renal amyloidosis** usually occurs in association with other diseases, particularly chronic inflammatory or neoplastic diseases. However, idiopathic renal amyloidosis is also described in **dogs** and **cats**. The underlying mechanisms of idiopathic amyloidosis are not known. However, **proteinuria** could be a factor. A hereditary predisposition for reactive **amyloidosis (AA)** has been found in **cats** and **dogs**. **In cattle**, renal amyloidosis is always due to chronic systemic infectious diseases. **Glomerular amyloidosis is a protein-losing nephropathy** resulting in marked **proteinuria** and **uraemia**. It can, like immune-complex glomerulonephritis, result in nephrotic syndrome. **Medullary amyloidosis** is usually asymptomatic unless it results in papillary necrosis (see 'circulatory disturbances').

Grossly, kidneys affected with glomerular amyloidosis are often enlarged, pale to yellow, and have a smooth to finely granular capsular surface. Glomeruli heavily loaded with amyloid can be seen as fine yellowish-brown dots on the capsular and cut surfaces. The cortex may have a finely granular appearance. **Treatment of kidneys with an iodine solution,** such as Lugol's iodine, stain glomeruli brown which become purple when exposed to dilute sulphuric acid (Fig. 21). This technique provides a rapid presumptive diagnosis of renal amyloidosis. Long-standing glomerular amyloidosis results in diminished blood flow from the glomeruli to the vasa recta. Such reduced renal vascular perfusion can lead to tubular atrophy, degeneration, and diffuse fibrosis. **Medullary amyloidosis** is usually not grossly visible.

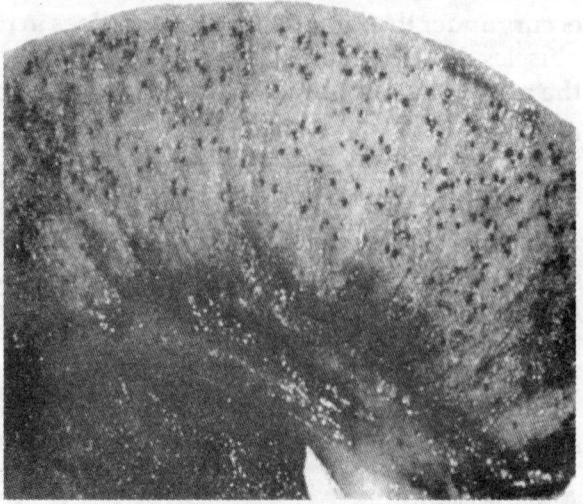

Fig. 21. Kidney; dog. Amyloidosis. The cut surface of a kidney is stained with Lugol's iodine and treated with sulphuric acid to demonstrate amyloid-infiltrated glomeruli.

Microscopically, glomerular amyloid is deposited in the mesangium and sub-endothelial locations. Amyloid is acellular and can accumulate in segments in glomerular tufts. **Therefore, a portion of the normal glomerular architecture is replaced by eosinophilic, homogeneous to slightly fibrillar material.** When amyloidosis involves the entire glomerular tuft, the glomerulus is enlarged, capillary lumina disappear, **and the tuft appears as a large eosinophilic hyaline sphere.** Amyloid can be present in renal tubular basement membranes, and these membranes are hyalinized and thickened. Affected renal tubules are markedly dilated and contain proteinaceous material. Amyloid is confirmed microscopically by staining with **Congo red stain.** When seen with polarized light, amyloid has green birefringence. Loss of Congo red staining after treatment of a section of affected kidney with potassium permanganate indicates that the amyloid present is AA-amyloid, that is, of acute-phase protein origin.

Circulatory Disturbances

Renal Blood Supply

The kidney has a rich blood supply. Knowledge of the normal renal blood supply is important in understanding the pathogenesis and distribution of various kidney lesions. Arterial blood comes from the **renal arteries.** After entering at the hilus, each renal artery branches into several **interlobar arteries** which then form **arcuate arteries.** Arcuate arteries send branches, the **interlobular arteries,** into the renal cortex. Finally, short vessels, the **afferent arteriole,** originate from interlobular arteries and give rise to **glomerular capillary tufts, efferent arterioles,** and the **peritubular capillary plexus.**

Hyperaemia and Congestion

Renal hyperaemia and congestion can be physiological, active, passive, or hypostatic. Hyperaemic kidneys are darker red than normal, swollen, and ooze blood from the cut surface. At postmortem, unilateral renal hypostatic congestion is present in animals that died in lateral recumbency (lying on one side) because of the force of gravity pulling unclotted blood downward

Haemorrhage

Renal cortical haemorrhages occur in many septicaemic diseases and result from vasculitis, vascular necrosis, thrombo-emboli, and dissociated intravascular coagulation. **Petechial haemorrhages** are usually seen on the surface and throughout the cortex of kidneys from **pigs** that die from septicaemia caused by diseases such as swine fever (hog cholera), African swine fever, erysipelas, streptococcal infections, salmonellosis, and other embolic diseases. Renal cortical ecchymotic haemorrhages associated with multifocal tubular and vascular necrosis are diagnostically important lesions of herpesvirus septicaemia in newly born **puppies.**

Large intra-renal or **sub-capsular haemorrhages** can result from direct trauma, renal biopsy, bleeding disorders such as haemophilia and disseminated intravascular coagulation.

Infarction

Red infarcts are areas of coagulative necrosis which result from local ischaemia of vascular occlusion and are usually due to thrombo-embolism, mural thrombosis, or aseptic emboli. **Grossly,** infarcts appear red or pale white depending on several factors including the interval after vascular occlusion and whether arteries or veins are occluded. Occlusion of arteries results in infarcts which are first **haemorrhagic** and slightly swollen, but become pale yellow-grey within 2 to 3 days because of lysis of erythrocytes and loss of haemoglobin. **Pale infarcts** have a central area of coagulative necrosis and are surrounded by a zone of congestion and haemorrhage as well as a pale margin because of surrounding zone of leukocytes.

Infracts are usually wedge-shaped (or cone-shaped) with the base against the cortical surface and the apex pointing toward the medulla. This conforms to the distribution of the obstructed vessel(s). **Infarcts can involve only the cortex, or cortex and medulla, depending on the size of the occluded vessel and the size of obstruction. For example,** thrombosis of an arcuate artery, which supplies both cortex and medulla, will result in an infarct involving the cortex and medulla. Thrombosis of a **cortical interlobular artery,** which supplies mainly the cortex, will result in an infarct of the cortex only.

Microscopically, in **acute renal infarction,** nephrons and interstitium in the central zone of the infarct become necrotic. At the margin of the infarct, only the proximal tubules become necrotic because of their high metabolic rate; **the glomeruli are spared.** Along the margin of the necrotic zone, infiltration in the beginning consists of neutrophils with a few macrophages and lymphocytes. Adjacent capillaries are markedly engorged with blood. **Healing of the infarct** occurs by lysis and phagocytosis of the necrotic tissue, leaving a **fibrotic scar. Scars** vary from linear to broad depending on the size of the acute infarct.

Endocardial thrombosis (vegetative valvular endocarditis, mural endocarditis) usually results in **thrombo-embolism of renal vessels** because of the great amount of cardiac output (20% to 25%) that goes to the kidneys. Therefore, infarcts occurring from thrombo-emboli are usually present in **cats** with left atrial thrombosis associated with cardiomyopathy, **or in any animal species with endocarditis involving the left heart.** In rare cases, emboli may be large enough to occlude the renal artery, causing infarction of the entire kidney. **Usually emboli obstruct many smaller vessels (e.g. inter-tubular arteries) and cause multiple small infarcts in the kidney.**

Renal infarcts in horses are rarely due to emboli originating from thrombosed mesenteric arteries associated with migrating larvae of *Strongylus vulgaris.* In such cases, **large mural thrombi** in the mesenteric artery protrude into thelumen of the aorta, and fragments, when loosened, cause thrombo-embolism of the kidneys. Thrombosis of pulmonary, coronary, splenic, or renal arteries and resultant infarction are common in **dogs** with renal amyloidosis because of loss through the urine of plasma anticoagulants such as antithrombin III. Endotoxin-mediated arterial or capillary thrombosis is a common cause of infarction in Gram-negative sepsis or endotoxic shock.

Septic emboli, particularly those from the bacterial **valvular endocarditis,** can also cause renal infarcts. Examples include *Actinomyces pyogenes* infection in **cattle,** *Erysipelothrix rhusiopathiae* in **pigs**, and *Staphylococcus aureus* in **small animals.** **Septic infarcts** are first haemorrhagic, but because of the presence of pyogenic bacteria, the necrotic tissue undergoes liquefactive necrosis and the infarcts can eventually develop into abscesses.

Necrosis

Renal Cortical Necrosis

Renal cortical necrosis occurs when **disseminated intravascular coagulation** causes widespread thrombosis in the glomerular capillaries, interlobular arteries, and afferent arterioles. Partial or complete renal necrosis is usually a bilateral lesion which occurs in all animal species, especially in association with Gram-negative septicaemias or endotoxaemias, and is related to endotoxin-induced endothelial damage, activation of the clotting mechanism and widespread capillary thrombosis.

The resulting **microthrombosis** of vessels causes widespread ischaemia and small and large areas of hypoxia-induced coagulative necrosis and haemorrhage throughout the renal cortex. The cortex is diffusely pale with a zone of hyperaemia separating the necrotic cortex from the viable medulla, or the cortex has large, irregular haemorrhagic areas resembling haemorrhagic infarcts interspersed with large yellow-grey areas resembling pale infarcts.

Papillary (Medullary Crest) Necrosis

Necrosis of the renal papillae, or their counterpart the medullary crest, **is a response of the inner medulla to ischaemia.** Papillary necrosis can be a **primary** lesion or be **secondary** to other renal lesions. **The inner medulla,** including the **papillae, is the zone least well supplied with blood than other zones of the kidneys.** This is because the inner medulla has very poor direct blood supply. On the other hand, most of the medullary blood supply is from the cortical blood through the vasa rectae. **Because of this limited blood flow,** any lesion or disease process that further reduces medullar blood flow can cause ischaemic necrosis (infarction) of the papillae.

Papillary necrosis occurs as a **primary disease** in animals treated with non-steroidal anti-inflammatory analgesic drugs and is similar to **analgesic nephropathy** in human beings. The primary disease has been described in **horses** treated with phenylbutazone for long periods. The condition is important in **dogs** and **cats** because of accidental ingestion of or treatment with ibuprofen, aspirin, or acetaminophen at excessive dosages. **Drugs causing papillary necrosis are called 'papillotoxins'.** Some of these drugs inhibit prostaglandin synthesis. Since prostaglandins are important for the maintenance of normal blood flow, these compounds can reduce blood flow and cause **ischaemic necrosis** of the cells in the **inner medulla.** In addition, they may cause direct oxidative damage to medullary tubular epithelium, further increasing necrosis of the **renal papillae.**

Papillary necrosis is usually an incidental finding at postmortem. Lesions include irregular, discoloured areas of necrotic inner medulla sharply demarcated from the surviving medullary tissue. The affected tissue, which is undergoing coagulative necrosis, is yellow-grey, green, or pink. With time, the necrotic tissue sloughs. Large pieces of sloughed tissue can obstruct the ureter and cause hydronephrosis, or form a focus for precipitation of minerals, resulting in the formation of pelvic or ureteral calculi.

Tubular Necrosis

Acute tubular degeneration and necrosis, usually referred to as **nephrosis,** occur from ischaemia or toxic damage to the renal tubular epithelial cells. Tubular epithelial cells respond to prolonged ischaemia or to nephrotoxins by undergoing degeneration. This is followed by necrosis and desquamation of the cells into the tubular lumen. **The proximal convoluted tubular epithelium is most susceptible to ischaemia or toxic injury because of its high metabolic rate.** Animals with severe tubular necrosis usually have signs of **uraemia.** Uraemia is associated with a decrease in urine production (**oliguria**) or absence of urine production (**anuria**). Acute tubular necrosis causes oliguria by several mechanisms. These include leakage of urine from damaged tubules through the disrupted basement membranes into the renal interstitium (interstitial tissue), or intratubular obstruction resulting from desquamated necrotic epithelium.

At postmortem, detection of acute tubular necrosis is usually difficult. However, at the beginning kidneys are swollen, and pale. The cut surface of the renal cortex bulges and is also pale. The medulla is pale or congested. The **microscopic appearance** of kidneys varies. Initially, proximal tubular epithelium is swollen, microvilli are absent, and the cytoplasm vacuolated or is granular and intensely eosinophilic. **The changes indicate coagulative necrosis.** In such tubules, nuclei exhibit pyknosis, karyorrhexis, or karyolysis. Necrotic tubular epithelium is desquamated into lumens, resulting in dilated tubules that contain necrotic cellular debris and hyalinized or granular casts.

If injury to the renal tubules is not lethal to the animal and the tubular basement membrane remains intact, tubular regeneration occurs from the surviving epithelium with restoration of renal function. Recent evidence indicates that epidermal growth factor secreted by distal convoluted tubules mediates the tubular repair process. The alternative to regeneration is loss of tubules subjected to nephrotoxins or ischaemia. This occurs if the toxin is not removed, the basement membrane does not remain intact, or the tubular epithelium does not survive the toxic dose to allow complete repair. **In such cases, tubules are replaced by fibrous connective tissue**. Affected tubules are non-functional, can be dilated, or be markedly atrophic, appearing shrunken.

Causes of Tubular Necrosis

Two general mechanisms are responsible for acute tubular necrosis: **ischaemia** and **nephrotoxicity**. Greatly reduced blood supply to kidney from any cause can result in **tubular necrosis.** Renal ischaemia can produce tubular cell injury and dysfunction, or cause cell death by necrosis or apoptosis. **Complete ischaemia for** more than two hours results in tubular necrosis, especially of the proximal convoluted tubules. Cell death is manifested by decreased adenosine triphosphate (ATP) production, increased membrane permeability, calcium ion influx, phospholipase activation, and generation of free radicals. **Disruption of mitochondrial respiration causes further cell membrane damage. The proximal convoluted tubules are most severely affected**. Prolonged ischaemia can produce necrosis of epithelium of the proximal and distal convoluted tubules, loops of Henle, and collecting ducts throughout the cortex, and to a lesser extent, the medulla. Glomeruli usually remain normal even when ischaemia is prolonged. **A characteristic lesion of ischaemic tubular necrosis is disruption of the tubular basement membranes,** called 'tubulorrhectic necrosis' (Fig. 22). Tubular repair in such kidneys is imperfect because regenerating

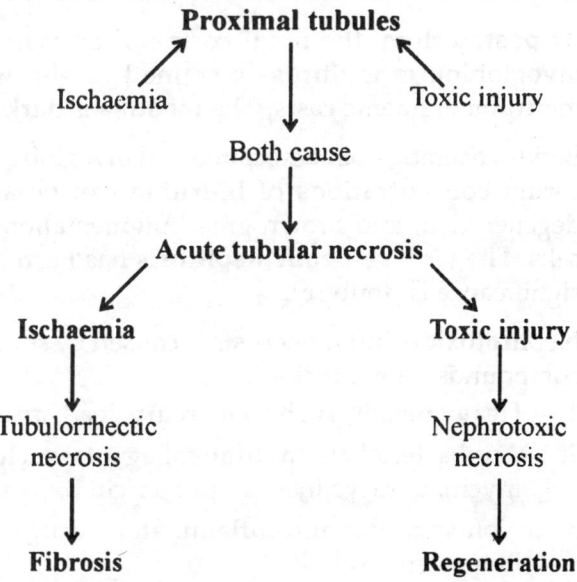

Fig. 22. Kidney, proximal tubules. Acute tubular necrosis occurs from ischaemia, or nephrotoxin. Both insults cause necrosis. **Ischaemia** results in **tubulorrhectic necrosis**, and disrupts the basement membrane. Since basement membrane is disrupted, **fibrosis** and tubular atrophy occur. In **nephrotoxic necrosis, the** basement membrane remains intact allowing **regeneration** to take place.

201

epithelial cells do not have their basement membranes. Failed regeneration leads to **tubular atrophy** and **interstitial fibrosis** (Fig. 22). **Gross** and **microscopic lesions** are similar to those described under tubular necrosis.

Haemoglobinuria occurs in cases of severe **intravascular haemolysis** and **haemoglobinaemia** as observed in **chronic copper toxicity in sheep; leptospirosis** or **babesiosis in cattle; red maple toxicity in horses,** and **babesiosis** or **autoimmune haemolytic anaemia** in **dogs. Myoglobinuria** accompanies acute **rhabdomyolysis** as occurs in **azoturia (Monday morning disease)** of **horses, captive myopathy** of **wild animals,** or severe trauma. In these cases, serum concentrations of haemoglobin or myoglobin are increased, and these products pass into the glomerular filtrate producing greatly increased concentrations in tubules causing **haemoglobinuric nephrosis** or **myoglobinuric nephrosis. Haemoglobin and myoglobin are not nephrotoxic in themselves.** However, large concentrations of haemoglobin or myoglobin in the glomerular filtrate can increase the tubular necrosis that occurs as a result of renal ischaemia. Haemoglobinuria and myoglobinuria can increase the harmful effect on tubular epithelium undergoing ischaemic necrosis.

At postmortem, the renal cortex of animals with severe haemoglobinuria or myoglobinuria is diffusely stained red-brown to blue-black and usually has intratubular **haeme casts.** The medulla is dark and has red streaks.

Besides haemoglobin-associated and myoglobin-associated renal changes, increased serum concentrations of bilirubin can be associated with cellular swelling, degeneration, and brown-green pigmentation of the proximal tubular epithelial cells. The term **cholemic nephrosis** has been applied to this lesion. However, its significance is doubtful.

Nephrotoxic tubular necrosis is caused by several naturally occurring or synthetic compounds. These include:

1. Heavy metals, such as mercury, lead, arsenic,
2. Antibacterial and antifungal agents, such as gentamicin, neomycin, strepto-mycin, tetracyclines, amphotericin B,
3. Non-steroidal anti-inflammatory drugs, such as aspirin, phenylbutazone, ibuprofen,
4. Plants, such as pigweed, oaks, yellow wood tree,
5. Oxalates,
6. Vitamin D and vitamin D supplements, and
7. Antineoplastic compounds, such as cisplatin

Gross and **microscopic lesions** resemble those described in acute tubular necrosis. **Nephrotoxins** can directly damage renal epithelial cells, **particularly the proximal convoluted tubules,** and can stimulate vasoconstriction and ischaemia. However, **nephrotoxins usually do not damage tubular basement membranes.**

Certain heavy metals, such as mercury, inorganic arsenic, lead, **are nephrotoxins.** Their common sources include herbicides (**arsenic**), old paint, batteries, and automobile components (**lead**), and environmental contaminants. Acute tubular necrosis is because of damage to membranes of proximal convoluted tubular epithelial cells or to mitochondrial damage produced by these toxins. Damage occurs from interaction of these metals with protein sulphydryl groups. **In mercury toxicosis,** mercuric ions enter the proximal tubular cells, become concentrated in the rough endoplasmic reticulum and cause tubular changes. The changes are followed by mitochondrial swelling and cellular death. **In lead toxicity,** the epithelial cells of the affected tubules have acid-fast intranuclear inclusions composed of lead-protein complexes.

Certain pharmaceutical agents are nephrotoxic and cause acute tubular necrosis when administered at excessive doses or too frequently. Antibacterials, such as gentamicin, neomycin, amikacin, and streptomycin **are nephrotoxic. Neomycin,** which is highly nephrotoxic, concentrates in the renal cortex; **streptomycin,** the least nephrotoxic, does not concentrate much in the renal cortex. Although **gentamicin** is intermediate in its nephrotoxicity between neomycin and streptomycin, tubular toxicity occurs because gentamicin is a commonly used drug in veterinary medicine.

Oxytetracycline is sometimes nephrotoxic in **cattle** and **dogs.** The mechanism of tubular damage has not been determined. **Amphoteric B**, an antifungal antibiotic, is also nephrotoxic. It causes disruption of cellular membranes. The membrane damage causes potassium ion loss, intracellular hydrogen ion accumulation, acute cellular swelling, and necrosis. **Sulphonamide-induced** tubular necrosis is now uncommon because the currently used sulphonamides have greater solubility. **Monensin** is an ionophore antibiotic used as a feed additive to control coccidiosis in **poultry** and **cattle. Horses are particularly susceptible to toxicosis.**

Non-steroidal anti-inflammatory drugs (NSAIDS), such as phenylbutazone, aspirin, and ibuprofen have been associated with acute renal failure in small animals, especially **dogs.** The mechanism of acute renal failure is that NSAID decrease synthesis of renal prostaglandins. Prostaglandins are responsible for maintaining normal renal blood flow. Among the **naturally occurring nephrotoxins** are ochratoxins and citrinins, mycotoxins produced by **Aspergilus** sp. and **Penicillium** sp. Ochratoxin A is nephrotoxic particularly for **pigs**, and has been associated with tubular degeneration and necrosis.

Acute tubular necrosis can result from the ingestion of **nephrotoxic plants.** This has been described in **pigs** and **cattle.** The toxic principle has not been identified and the mechanism of tubular damage is unknown. Acutely affected **cattle** usually have swollen, pale kidneys that sometimes have cortical petechial haemorrhages. The kidneys in chronic cases are fibrotic and pale.

Oxalate-induced tubular necrosis occurs in **sheep** and **cattle** after ingestion of toxic quantities of oxalates that accumulate in plants of various genera. After absorption of plant-derived oxalates from the intestine, calcium oxalates form and precipitate in vessel walls and in renal tubules, where they cause obstruction and epithelial cell necrosis.

Nephrosis occurs in **dogs** and **cats** given **excessive doses of vitamin D** (vitamin D intoxication, **vitamin D nephropathy**), or by accidental ingestion of calciferol-containing rodenticides. **In livestock,** chronic ingestion of plants such as **Solanum** which contain vitamin D-like biological activity can also cause nephrosis. Ingestion of excessive amounts of vitamin D can induce hypercalcaemia. Absorption of calcium by tubular epithelial cells causes mitochondrial calcification and cell death. Tubular and glomerular basement membranes are also calcified. **Microscopically,** tubular epithelium is necrotic and atrophic with calcific deposits in tubules scattered throughout the cortex.

Incidental Lesions of Renal Tubules

In dogs, granules of haemosiderin are usually seen in the epithelial cells of proximal convoluted tubules in kidneys that are otherwise normal. They result from degradation of haemoglobin reabsorbed from the glomerular filtrate by proximal tubular epithelium. Fine golden granules of **lipofuscin** ('**wear and tear pigment**') can accumulate in renal proximal and distal convoluted tubules of **old cattle** as well as striated muscle, resulting in **lipofuscinosis**. **Grossly,** the renal cortex shows streaks of brown discoloration, but renal function is not affected.

Klossiella equi is a sporozoan parasite of the **horse.** Various stages of its schizogony can be found in the proximal convoluted tubular epithelium, and to a lesser extent, in the glomerular epithelium. Sometimes, *K. equi* causes **mild tubular necrosis** and interstitial infiltrates of lymphocytes and plasma cells.

Glomerular Diseases

Damage to glomeruli can cause renal disease and various clinical signs. An important feature of glomerular disease is the leakage of small molecular size proteins into the glomerular filtrate and then into the urine. Renal lesions that result in **proteinuria** are called '**protein-losing nephropathies**'. A large quantity of plasma protein, **particularly albumin**, is filtered through the damaged glomeruli. This overloads the proximal convoluted tubules capacity for reabsorption to such an extent that protein-rich glomerular filtrate accumulates in the tubular lumens and afterwards appears in the urine. In such diseases, proximal tubular cells show microscopic eosinophilic intracytoplasmic bodies referred to as **hyaline droplets.** These are accumulations of intracytoplasmic protein absorbed from the filtrate. **Microscopically,** tubular lumens are usually dilated and filled with proteinaceous material. Prolonged, severe protein loss results in **hypoproteinaemia,** reduced colloid osmotic pressure, and loss of antithrombin III. Protein-losing nephropathy is an important cause of severe hypoproteinaemia in animals. Prolonged, severe protein-losing nephropathy, the **nephrotic syndrome**, is characterized by generalized oedema, ascites, and pleural effusion.

Glomerulitis

Inflammation of the glomerulus is called 'glomerulitis'.

1. Viral Glomerulitis

Glomerulitis occurs in acute systemic viral diseases, such as acute infectious canine hepatitis, septicaemic cytomegalovirus infection (inclusion body rhinitis) in **newborn pigs,** equine arteritis virus infection, swine fever (hog cholera), and Newcastle disease in birds. The **lesions** are mild, usually short lived, and result from viral replication in capillary endothelium. Proteinuria is transitory. Intranuclear inclusions are present in the glomerular capillary endothelium during viraemia in infectious canine hepatitis and cytomegalovirus infections. **Microscopically**, lesions in viral glomerulitis include endothelial hypertrophy, thickened and oedematous mesangium (thin membrane supporting the capillary loops in glomeruli), haemorrhages, and necrosis of endothelium. In addition to the lesions, infectious canine hepatitis virus can cause a transient immune-complex glomerulitis (see 'immune-mediated glomerulitis') and transient tubulo-interstitial nephritis (see 'interstitial nephritis').

2. Embolic Nephritis (Suppurative Nephritis)

Acute embolic nephritis, also called **suppurative glomerulitis,** occurs from bacteraemia. Bacteria randomly lodge in glomeruli and interstitial capillaries and cause the formation of multiple foci of inflammation throughout the renal cortex. **Microscopically,** glomerular capillaries have many bacterial colonies. Necrosis and extensive neutrophilic infiltration destroy the glomeruli. Glomerular or interstitial haemorrhage may also occur. If the affected animals survive, the neutrophilic infiltration will gradually have more numbers of lymphocytes, plasma cells, and macrophages.

Actinobacillosis of **foals,** caused by *Actinobacillus equuli,* is a specific example of **embolic nephritis.** Foals with actinobacillosis usually die within a few days after birth and have small abscesses in many organs, especially renal cortex, and a fibrino-purulent polysynovitis.

Embolic nephritis also occurs in **other animals** as a result of bacteraemia with any one of the several bacterial species. **In pigs, Erysipelothrix** sp., **Streptococcus** sp., and **Corynebacterium** sp. are usually isolated from the lesion.

3. Immune-Mediated Glomerulonephritis

Glomerulonephritis usually occurs from immune-mediated mechanisms. These mostly involve antibodies against glomerular basement membranes, or deposition of soluble immune complexes in the glomeruli. Immune-mediated glomerulonephritis is **diagnosed by** demonstrating immunoglobulin (Ig) and complement components, usually C3 in the glomeruli by immunofluorescent or immunohistochemical techniques.

Antibodies against basement membrane bind to glomerular basement membranes and damage the glomerulus through fixation of complement and result in leukocytic infiltration. The condition is known as **antibasement membrane disease**. To confirm the diagnosis of antibasement membrane disease, Ig and C3 must be demonstrated in the glomeruli, and antibodies must be eluted (separated out) from the kidneys and found to bind to normal glomerular basement membranes of the appropriate species.

4. Immune-Complex Glomerulonephritis

Immune-complex glomerulonephritis occurs in persistent infections or other diseases that have a prolonged antigenaemia which increase the formation of soluble immune complexes. **In domestic animals, immune-complex glomerulonephritis usually occurs in dogs and cats.** Dogs with protein-losing glomerular disease usually have glomerulonephritis of immune complex origin. Immune-complex glomerulonephritis is associated with **specific viral infections** such as feline leukaemia virus or feline infectious peritonitis virus in **cats,** infectious canine hepatitis virus in **dogs,** equine infectious anaemia in **horses**, bovine viral diarrhoea in **cattle**, swine fever (hog cholera) in **pigs; bacterial infections** such as pyometra or pyoderma; **chronic parasitism** such as dirofilariasis (**dogs**), trypanosomiasis (**cattle**); **autoimmune diseases** such as canine systemic lupus erythematosus; or **neoplasia (dogs** and **cats).** However, despite being well-documented disease, the specific cause of immune-complex glomerulonephritis is not known in **feline progressive membranous glomerulitis.**

Immune-complex glomerulitis begins with the formation of soluble immune complexes (**antigen-antibody complexes**) in the presence of antigen-antibody in equal amounts or slight antigen excess in the plasma. **These complexes are deposited in the glomerular capillaries** where they stimulate complement fixation with formation of C3a, C5a, and C567, which are chemotactic for neutrophils. In the early stages, **infiltrating neutrophils** damage the basement membrane through release of proteinases, arachidonic acid metabolites (such as thromboxane), and oxygen-derived free radicals and hydrogen peroxide. In the later stages, **monocytes** infiltrate into the glomeruli and cause continuing damage to the glomeruli by the release of biologically active molecules.

Many factors determine the extent of deposition of soluble immune complexes in the glomerular capillary walls. **Small and intermediate complexes are most damaging,** since large complexes are removed from circulation through phagocytosis by cells of the mononuclear-phagocytic system in the liver and spleen. An increase in local glomerular vascular permeability is necessary for immune complexes to leave capillaries and deposit in the glomerulus. This process is facilitated by **vasoactive amine** release from **platelets, basophils,** or **mast cells.** Mast cells or basophils release vasoactive amines by the interaction of immune complexes with antigen-specific IgE on the surface of these cells by **two ways:** by stimulation of the mast cells or basophils by cationic proteins released from neutrophils, or by the anaphylatoxin activity of C3a or C5a. **Platelet activation factor (PAF)** is released from immune complex-stimulated mast cells, basophils, or macrophages and causes platelets to release **vasoactive amines.** Localization of complexes in the basement membrane or in sub-epithelial locations depends on their molecular charge. Once small soluble immune complexes are deposited in the capillary, they can then become greatly enlarged as a result of interactions of immune complexes with free antibodies, free antigens, complement components, or other immune complexes.

After immune complex deposition, glomerular injury can also occur in the absence of leukocytic infiltration from the aggregation of platelets and activation of Hageman factor with the formation of fibrin thrombi that cause glomerular ischaemia. Also, damage to glomerular epithelial cell and extracellular matrix can directly result from the **terminal membrane attack complex** of the activated complement cascade (C5 to C9), which can cause epithelial detachment and proteinuria.

Finally, if exposure of the glomerulus to immune complexes is short lived, as in infectious canine hepatitis, **immune complexes will be phagocytosed by macrophages or mesangial cells** (cells present in the membrane supporting the capillary loops in glomeruli)**and removed,** and the glomerular lesions and clinical signs will disappear. On the other hand, intermittent exposure of glomeruli to soluble immune complexes, such as persistent viral infections (e.g. feline leukaemia virus infection and chronic heartworm disease) can **produce progressive glomerular injury** with severe lesions and clinical manifestations of glomerular disease.

Ultrastructurally (electron microscopically), immune complexes in the glomerular basement membrane appear as **electron-dense bodies.** Other changes include loss of visceral epithelial cell foot processes, and infiltration of neutrophils and monocytes.

Immune-complex glomerulonephritis can be diagnosed by demonstration of Ig and C3 in glomerular tufts. **In dogs,** IgG or IgM are the most common immunoglobulins. Both the immunoglobulins and C3 are usually seen in a granular ('**lumpy-bumpy'**) pattern using immunofluorescent or histochemical techniques. Sometimes the deposits have a linear distribution. The **diagnosis** of immune-complex glomeruonephritis can be confirmed only by ruling out antibasement membrane disease after demonstrating that the antibodies eluted from glomeruli do not bind to normal glomeruli.

Grossly, the kidneys are swollen, have a smooth capsular surface, are of normal colour or pale, and on the cut surface of the cortex show glomeruli as pinpoint red dots. **In horses**, this criterion cannot be used for diagnosis since their normal glomeruli are usually visible. If lesions do not resolve and become chronic, renal cortex is shrunken and the capsular surface has fine granularity. On the cut surface, the cortex is thin and granular, and glomeruli appear as pinpoint grey dots. With time, more severe scarring can develop throughout the cortex (see "renal fibrosis").

Microscopically, immune-complex glomerulonephritis appears in different histopathological forms. Glomerular lesions have been described as **proliferative, membranous**, or **membrano-proliferative**. Lesions may be distributed **diffusely** when most of the glomeruli are involved; **focally** when only a certain proportion of glomeruli are involved; **globally** when an entire glomerular tuft is involved; and **segmentally** when only a portion of glomerular tuft is affected. **Most of the lesions in immune-complex glomerulitis are diffuse.**

- **Proliferative glomerulonephritis:** This is characterized by increased cellularity of the glomerular tufts caused by proliferation of glomerular endothelial, epithelial, and mesangial cells and an accumulation of neutrophils and other leukocytes. Both capillary loops and the mesangium are involved.

- **Membranous glomerulonephritis:** This is characterized by diffuse glomerular capillary basement membrane thickening. **This is the most common form of immune-complex glomerulonephritis in cats.**

- **Membrano-proliferative glomerulonephritis:** This is characterized by both hypercellularity and capillary basement membrane thickening in affected glomeruli. **This is the most common form in immune-complex glomerulonephritis in the dog.**

Several other changes usually accompany the above lesions. These include adhesions between the epithelial cells of the glomerular tuft and Bowman's capsule (synechiae), hypertrophy and hyperplasia of the parietal epithelium lining Bowman's capsule, deposition of fibrinogen and fibrinous thrombi in glomerular capillaries, and tubular dilatation with homogeneous proteinaceous fluid. If the damage is mild and the cause is removed, glomeruli can heal without residual lesions. However, if the lesion is severe and prolonged, chronic granulomatous changes develop. Bowman's capsule can become thickened and hyalinized. In severe cases, proliferation of parietal epithelium, accumulation of monocytes, and deposition of fibrin can occur in Bowman's capsule. This results in the formation of a semicircular, hypercellular lesion in the glomerulus known as **'glomerular crescent'**. The glomerular crescent can also undergo fibrosis, and if Bowman's capsule ruptures, glomerular fibrosis can become continuous with interstitial fibrosis.

Glomerulosclerosis

In chronic glomerulonephritis, affected glomeruli shrink and become hyalinized due to an increase in fibrous connective tissue and mesangial matrix and a loss of glomerular capillaries. These glomeruli are hypocellular and non-functional. This process is called **'glomerulosclerosis'.** Glomerulosclerosis can be **diffuse,** involving all glomeruli, or **multifocal.** Also, it can involve a whole glomerular tuft (**global**), or only a portion of the tuft (**segmental**).

Because tubules receive their blood supply from the vasa recta, derived from glomerular capillaries and afferent arteriole, glomerulosclerosis reduces the blood flow through the vasa recta thus decreasing oxygen tension (pressure) in the tubules. **The resulting hypoxia causes tubular epithelial cell death through apoptosis which results in tubular atrophy.** Glomerulosclerosis is not the end stage of glomerulonephritis only, but can develop in any chronic disease in which severe damage to nephrons or loss of nephron function occurs.

Miscellaneous Glomerular Lesions

Glomerular Lipidosis

Glomerular lipidosis is characterized by small aggregates of foamy macrophages in glomerular tufts heavily loaded with lipid. It is an occasional incidental finding in **dogs. Microscopically,** glomeruli contain foamy macrophages, characteristic of glomerular lipidosis.

Tubulo-Interstitial Disease

Interstitial Nephritis

In various systemic infectious diseases of domestic animals, accumulations of inflammatory cells can be seen in the renal interstitium (interstitial tissue). In most of these diseases, inflammatory cell infiltrations, visible only microscopically, are not associated with renal failure and are of no importance (example 'equine infectious anaemia'). In other diseases, the renal interstitium may show moderate to severe interstitial inflammatory cell infiltrates that are grossly visible and associated with renal failure. When interstitial inflammation is the main lesion without embolic nephritis or pyelonephritis, this lesion is called **'interstitial nephritis'.** More recently, the term **'tubulo-interstitial nephritis'** has been used. This is because inflammatory and degenerative changes are usually present and are involved in the development of the main lesion. **Interstitial nephritis** can be **acute, subacute,** or **chronic,** and is associated with a lymphoplasmacytic infiltration. **Chronic interstitial nephritis** is associated with renal interstitial fibrosis (see 'renal fibrosis'). Besides interstitial nephritis, leukocytes are also found in the interstitium in pyelonephritis and embolic nephritis.

Interstitial nephritis occurs from bacterial and viral septicaemias. **The causes include:**

Cattle:	*Escherichia coli* septicaemia, (White spotted kidney)
	Malignant catarrhal fever
	Theilaria parva
Sheep:	Sheep-pox
Horses:	Equine viral arteritis
Pigs:	*Leptospira interrogans* serovar *pomona*
	Porcine reproductive and respiratory syndrome
Dogs:	*Leptospira interrogans* serovar *canicola, icterohaemorrhagiae,* and others
	Infectious canine hepatitis virus, recovery phase

These infectious agents first infect the kidney tubules and then produce an inflammatory response in the interstitium. **However, the pathogenesis of these infections is often not known.**

The pathogenesis of leptospirosis (both in dog and pigs) will be described as an example of an acute bacterial interstitial nephritis. Following infection, leptospiraemia occurs and organisms localize in renal interstitial capillaries, migrate through vascular endothelium, persist in the interstitial spaces, and migrate through the intercellular junctions of tubular epithelial cells to reach renal tubular lumen. In tubules, leptospira enter into epithelial microvilli and occur in the phagosomes of the epithelium of the proximal and distal convoluted tubules. **These tubular epithelial cells undergo degeneration and necrosis** as a result of either direct toxic effect of the leptospira or the associated interstitial inflammatory reaction. The main lesion is in the interstitium, which becomes infiltrated with monocytes, macrophages, lymphocytes, and plasma cells. **In affected dogs,** plasma cells secrete **Leptospira**-specific antibodies. However, the role of these antibodies in the pathogenesis or resolution of the lesion is not known. *Escherichia coli* septicaemia in **calves** can result in interstitial nephritis (called **'white spotted kidneys'**). The pathogenesis is not known but appears similar to that of leptospirosis.

Another well understood mechanism in the production of interstitial nephritis is the immune response against the virus of **infectious canine hepatitis** in **dogs.** During the viraemic phase of the disease, virus first localizes in the glomeruli (viral glomerulitis) and produces immune-complex glomerulonephritis. As the dog recovers from the acute phase of the disease and with the onset of systemic immune response, virus disappears from the glomeruli but reappears in tubular epithelial cells of the nephron. **Virus persists in tubular epithelium for weeks to months and causes tubular necrosis.** This is followed by lymphocytic and plasmacytic interstitial nephritis. Basophilic intranuclear inclusion bodies typical of canine hepatitis virus are present in infected renal tubular epithelial cells.

Deposition of immune-complexes in the tubular basement membranes, or interactions between antibasement membrane antibodies and tubular basement membranes, can initiate immune-mediated tubulo-interstitial disease in **human beings.** However, depositions of Ig and complement have been rarely identified in renal tubular basement membranes in **domestic animals.** The role of immune-mediated mechanisms is not clear as a cause of interstitial nephritis in **domestic animals.**

Infection with **equine arteritis virus** or **porcine reproductive** and **respiratory syndrome** virus usually results in multifocal **lymphohistiocytic interstitial nephritis** with interstitial oedema. **Lesions** are especially intense at the cortico-medullary junction and in the medulla. A severe vasculitis is characterized by fibrinoid necrosis and lymphohistiocytic infiltrates in the cortical and medullary interstitial arteries and veins. Virus can be found in endothelium and in interstitial and vascular macrophages.

Gross lesions of interstitial nephritis can be classified as **acute, subacute,** or **chronic.** Chronic interstitial nephritis is described later (see 'renal fibrosis'). The **distribution of lesions** can be **diffuse** as in canine leptospirosis, or **multifocal** as in 'white spotted kidneys' of **calves** due to *Escherichia coli* septicaemia (Fig. 23), infectious canine hepatitis, malignant catarrhal fever, or porcine leptospirosis. In diffuse

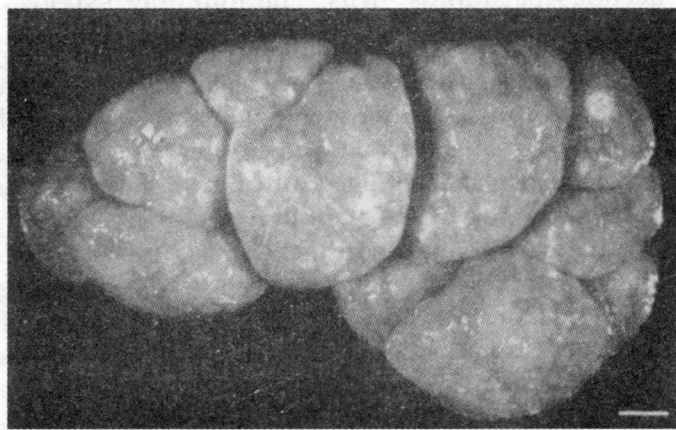

Fig. 23. **Kidney; calf. Multifocal interstitial nephritis (white spotted kidney).** Multiple white foci of inflammation are randomly scattered throughout the kidney. On cut surface, these foci extend well into the cortex.

interstitial nephritis, kidneys are swollen and pale with a grey mottling of the capsular surface. The cut surface bulges. Grey infiltrates of varying sizes blur the normal radially striated cortical architecture. These renal lesions appear as grey foci which are particularly intense in the cortex. Focal lesions are less severe and

211

composed of grey areas in the cortex and sometimes outer medulla.

Microscopically, collections of lymphocytes, plasma cells, and monocytes and a few neutrophils are randomly scattered, or localized throughout the oedematous interstitium. Tubular epithelial cells in the severely inflamed areas can be degenerate, necrotic, or both.

Granulomatous Nephritis

Granulomatous nephritis is a tubulo-interstitial disease. It usually occurs in chronic systemic diseases that are characterized by **granulomas** in various organs. **In domestic animals,** granulomatous nephritis is associated with a number of infectious agents including viruses, bacteria, fungi, and parasites. However, a common feature to each is the formation of grossly visible granulomas randomly scattered throughout the kidneys, but especially in the cortex.

Cats with **feline infectious peritonitis,** particularly the non-effusive (dry) form, usually have multifocal pyogranulomatous nephritis, characterized grossly by multiple, large, irregular, pale grey cortical foci that are firm and granular on cut surface. **Microscopically,** accumulations of macrophages are mixed with lymphocytes, plasma cells, and neutrophils (**pyogranulomas**). Its pathogenesis is thought to be related to a cell-mediated hypersensitivity (type IV) reaction to feline infectious peritonitis virus. The immune response causes a granulomatous necrotizing vasculitis and development of pyogranulomas.

Granulomatous nephritis is also caused by a variety of granuloma-inducing infectious agents, including fungi such as **Aspergillus** sp., Phycomycetes, or *Histoplasma capsulatum*, and higher bacteria such as **Mycobacterium** sp. *Mycobacterium tuberculosis* can cause granulomatous nephritis, particularly in **cattle.** Small, grey-white, **granulomatous foci** (2 to 5 mm) are scattered throughout the kidneys of animals with generalized miliary tuberculosis. A coarse nodular form of renal tuberculosis also occurs. In this form, **large granulomas** up to 10 cm in diameter are spread throughout the kidneys. These foci are white to yellowish-brown, dry, granular, and may have calcified, caseous centres. **Microscopically,** lesions are characterized by central foci of necrosis surrounded by epithelioid macrophages and giant cells that contain acid-fast bacteria.

Migratory *Toxocara canis* produce small, grey to white **granulomas** scattered throughout the renal cortex of dogs. These lesions appear to be due to cell-mediated immune responses to the migrating larvae and are composed of macrophages, lymphocytes, and eosinophils surrounded by fibroblasts in the fibrous connective tissue. In recent lesions, nematode larvae can usually be seen in the centre of these lesions. **After death, larvae become fragmented and the debris is phagocytized and eliminated.** Lesions heal by fibrosis, leaving a few finely contracted foci on the capsular surface.

Pyelonephritis

Pyelitis is inflammation of the renal pelvis. **Pyelonephritis** is inflammation of both renal pelvis and renal parenchyma. **It is an excellent example of suppurative tubulo-interstitial disease**. Both pyelitis and pyelonephritis occur from an extension of bacterial infection of the lower urinary tract that climbs through the ureters to the kidneys and then establishes infection in the pelvis and inner medulla. Rarely, pyelonephritis may occur from descending bacterial infections, in which bacterial infection of the kidney occurred through the haematogenous route, that is, embolic nephritis. **Ascending infection, however, is the most common cause of pyelonephritis.** Although **cattle** do not have a true renal pelvis, inflammation of the proximal ureter and renal pelvis in **cattle** is also called pyelonephritis.

The **pathogenesis of ascending pyelonephritis** depends on the abnormal reflux (backward flow) of bacteria-contaminated urine from the lower tract to the renal pelvis and collecting duct. This abnormal reflux is called **'vesico-ureteral reflux'**, that is, **backward flow of urine from bladder into the ureter.** Vesico-ureteral reflux occurs easily when pressure is increased within the urinary bladder as in urethral obstruction. In addition to physical causes that increase vesico-ureteral reflux, **bacterial infection of the lower urinary tract can increase vesico-ureteral reflux by several mechanisms.** When wall of the bladder is inflamed (**cystitis**), the normal working of the vesico-ureteral valve is interfered with. This allows urine to flow backward. **Cystitis** and **urethritis**, which occur with narrowing of the urethra or obstruction by urinary calculi or bladder neoplasms, can increase pressure in the bladder and increase reflux. Endotoxin liberated from Gram-negative bacteria infecting ureter and bladder can inhibit normal ureteral peristalsis, increasing reflux.

Bacteria which colonize the pelvis can easily infect inner medulla. **The medulla is highly susceptible to bacterial infection because of its poor blood supply** (see 'papillary necrosis'), its great interstitial osmolality **that inhibits neutrophil function,** and its **large ammonia concentration which inhibits complement activation.** Thus, bacteria can infect and ascend collecting ducts, cause tubular epithelial necrosis and haemorrhage, **and produce an inflammatory response.** Bacterial infection can gradually ascend in the tubules and the interstitium until the inflammatory lesions (**tubulo-interstitial inflammation**) extend from pelvis to capsule.

Since pyelonephritis is mostly an ascending infection and because females are more susceptible to lower urinary tract infections, **pyelonephritis occurs more frequently in females than males.** *E. coli*, especially uropathogenic strains which produce virulence factors such as alpha-haemolysis and adhesins, is one of the most common causes of lower urinary tract diseases and pyelonephritis. **Proteus** sp., **Klebsiella** sp., **Staphylococcus** sp., **Streptococcus** sp., *Pseudomonas aeruginosa* are also common causes of lower urinary tract infection and pyelonephritis in all species. *Corynebacterium renale* and *Eubacterium* (*Corynebacterium*) *suis* are especially pathogenic for the lower urinary tract of **cattle** and **pigs**, respectively, and are common causes of pyelonephritis.

Diagnosis of pyelonephritis is reached by finding out the presence of acute or chronic pyelitis and inflammation of the renal parenchyma. **Pyelonephritis can be unilateral, but is usually bilateral.** The pelvic and ureteral mucous membranes are acutely inflamed, red, roughened, or granular, and coated with a thin exudate. The pelvis and ureters are markedly dilated and have purulent exudate in the lumen. **The medullary crest (papilla) is usually ulcerated and necrotic.** Kidney involvement is seen by the presence of irregular, radial, red or grey streaks involving the medulla, extending toward the kidney surface. Usually patches of inflammation distributed on the kidney's capsule and cut surfaces are separated from each other by areas of normal renal parenchyma. Inflammation is usually most severe at the renal poles. Lesions of chronic pyelonephritis, in which an active bacterial infection exists, include acute inflammation as well as extensive necrosis with destruction of the medulla, and fibrosis with scarring in a patchy distribution in the outer medulla and cortex. **Sometimes, inflammation extends through the surface of the kidneys and produces extensive sub-capsular inflammation and localized peritonitis.**

Microscopically, the most severe lesions of pyelonephritis are in the **inner medulla.** The transitional epithelium is necrotic and desquamated. Necrotic debris, fibrin, neutrophils, and bacterial colonies may be attached to the denuded surface. Medullary tubules are markedly dilated and their lumens contain neutrophils and bacterial colonies. Tubular epithelium is focally necrotic. An intense neutrophilc infiltration, present in the renal interstitium, may be accompanied by marked interstitial haemorrhages and oedema. If obstruction of vasa recta occurs, coagulative necrosis of the inner medulla (**papillary necrosis**) can be severe. Lesions are similar in the tubules and interstitium, but they are less severe. When lesions become subacute, severity of the neutrophilic infiltrations decreases and lymphocytes, plasma cells, and monocytes infiltrate the interstitium. **Chronic lesions have severe fibrosis** (see 'renal fibrosis').

Hydronephrosis

Hydronephrosis is dilatation of the renal pelvis due to **obstruction of urine outflow** and is associated with increased pelvic pressure, dilatation of the pelvis, and atrophy of the renal parenchyma. **Hydronephrosis occurs in all domestic animals.** Obstruction causing hydronephrosis is sometimes caused by congenital malformation of the ureter, vesico-ureteral junction, or urethra, but the **common causes of hydronephrosis are ureteral or urethral blockage due to urinary tract calculi** (see 'lower urinary tract'), **chronic inflammation, or neoplasms of the ureter or bladder. Hydronephrosis can be unilateral or bilateral.** When hydronephrosis is **unilateral,** cystic enlargement of the kidney may become extensive before the lesion is seen. If the obstructive process causes partial or intermittent blockage,

bilateral hydronephrosis can become severe because of continued urine production and pooling of urine in the pelvis. **When obstruction is complete,** hydronephrosis is limited in development (discussed below). When increase in pelvic pressure is substantial, intra-tubular pressure is increased and glomerular filtration is greatly reduced. However, even with complete obstruction, glomerular filtrate does not stop completely because of continued reabsorption of the filtrate into the interstitium and lymphatic vessels. **When the obstructive lesion is bilateral and complete, death due to uraemia occurs before cystic enlargement becomes extensive.**

The **increased intra-tubular pressure** following ureteral obstruction results in **renal tubular dilatation.** Glomeruli remain functional, but much of the glomerular filtrate diffuses into the interstitium where it is removed by lymphatic vessels and veins. As pressure in the pelvis increases, the interstitial vessels collapse and renal blood flow is reduced, resulting in hypoxia, tubular atrophy, and if the increase in pressure is continued **interstitial fibrosis.** The glomeruli have a normal appearance for a long time, but ultimately become atrophic and sclerotic (hard).

Early changes of hydronephrosis include dilatation of the pelvis and calyces and blunting of the renal crest and papillae. When pelvic dilatation is increased, kidney is enlarged and rounder than normal, and the cortex and medulla are gradually thinned. Interstitial vascular obstruction results in cortical ischaemia, sometimes infarction, and necrosis. **In its most advanced form, hydronephrotic kidney is a thin-walled (2 to 3 mm thick), fluid-filled sac.** Continued pelvic dilation causes loss of tubules by degeneration and atrophy, **followed by fibrosis of the renal parenchyma.**

Sometimes, a severely hydronephrotic kidney becomes contaminated by bacteria and the thin-walled sac becomes filled with pus instead of urine. This lesion, called **pyonephrosis,** occurs from blood-borne bacteria lodging in a hydronephrotic kidney.

Chronic Renal Diseases

Renal Fibrosis (Scarring)

Renal fibrosis may occur as a primary event, but usually is a manifestation of the healing phase of a pre-existing renal lesion. Renal fibrosis occurs after many renal lesions including inflammation of glomeruli, tubules, or interstitial tissue, and degeneration or necrosis of renal tubules. The **mechanisms** by which fibrosis is caused are related to destruction and loss of nephron components by the inflammatory process and initiation of the healing process. Non-inflammatory mechanisms can also incite renal fibrosis.

Renal fibrosis and **chronic renal disease** are the most common pathological processes in **mature or aging domestic animals,** particularly **dogs** and **cats.** When renal fibrosis and loss of nephrons are severe, these lesions are manifested clinically

215

as **chronic renal failure** and **uraemia.** One of the most common signs is the inability of an animal to concentrate urine resulting in frequent urination (**polyuria**) of dilute urine (**isosthenuria**). Polyuria is accompanied by dehydration and excessive water drinking (**polydipsia**). **Hypoplastic anaemia** occurs as a result of the kidney's failure to synthesize and secrete **erythropoietin.** Fibrous osteodystrophy can develop due to abnormal calcium-phosphorus metabolism and renal secondary hyperparathyroidism.

In areas of renal fibrosis, **loss of renal parenchyma** includes tubules, glomeruli, and vessels and their replacement by fibrous connective tissue. **Therefore, fibrotic kidneys are pale to white, shrunken, and firm, with adhesions of the capsule to the underlying cortex.** Such kidneys should not be mistaken for chronic interstitial nephritis, end-stage kidney, or nephrosclerosis. Renal fibrosis usually follows a pattern characteristic of the preceding lesion. **Fibrosis** can be diffuse with fine granularity on the capsular surface. In contrast, fibrosis can be coarser as deep and irregularly shaped depressions of the capsular surface in either a diffuse, multifocal, or patchy distribution. **These fibrotic areas are pale when compared with more normal parenchyma.**

Diffuse fibrosis with a finely granular pattern can also occur following widespread necrosis of renal tubular epithelium (acute tubular necrosis). **Ischaemia** from obstruction of large arteries causes areas of coagulative necrosis. Healing results in large depressed scars which involve mainly cortex, but can extend into the medulla. Obstruction of smaller arteries results in smaller areas of coagulative necrosis which heal as small-diameter pits on the renal surface. A coarser pattern of diffuse renal fibrosis occurs in chronic interstitial nephritis of **dogs**. Both cortex and medulla can be fibrotic.

Microscopically, renal fibrosis is characterized by an increase in interstitial connective tissue and atrophy and disappearance of adjacent renal tubules. Foci of lymphocytes and plasma cells can be seen scattered throughout the endothelium. Multiple acquired cysts may be present throughout the cortex and medulla, and are lined by flattened epithelial cells. These cysts can be due to either dilated Bowman's capsules or atrophic glomerular tufts or to dilated or blocked tubular segments that have become isolated by connective tissue. Glomerulosclerosis is common in areas of severe interstitial fibrosis. **Calcification** of vessels, tubular basement membranes, Bowman's capsules, and degenerate tubular epithelium is common in fibrotic kidneys due to changes in calcium-phosphorus metabolism associated with chronic renal failure.

Progressive Juvenile Nephropathy

Progressive juvenile nephropathy, also known as **familial (hereditary) renal disease** is a **severe bilateral renal fibrosis** described in **young dogs**. A familial tendency has been demonstrated in **many dogs. Clinically,** the disease is characterized by polyuria, polydipsia (excessive thirst), and uraemia. The signs and gross lesions are similar to those of chronic renal disease and renal fibrosis in **mature or aging dogs.** Generally, kidneys are markedly shrunken, pale to white, and firm. **Microscopically,** the lesion is a membrano-proliferative glomerulonephritis.

Neoplasms

Primary renal neoplasms in domestic animals are less than 1% of the total neoplasms reported. They are usually **unilateral** and can be of **epithelial, mesenchymal,** or **embryonal** origin.

Epithelial Tumours

Renal Adenomas

These are rare. They are incidental finding at postmortem, and usually appear as small, white to yellow; solitary, well-circumscribed mass in the cortex. **Microscopically,** adenomas are composed of solid sheets, tubules, or papillary proliferations of cuboidal epithelial cells that are uniform in size and have granular eosinophilic cytoplasm and small, round to oval nuclei. **Mitotic figures, necrosis, and fibrosis are rare.**

Renal carcinomas

These are the most common primary renal neoplasms and occur usually in older dogs. The neoplasms are large (up to 20 cm in diameter), spherical to oval, and firm. They are usually pale yellow; contain dark areas of haemorrhage and necrosis, and foci of cystic degeneration. The masses usually occupy and obliterate one pole of the kidney and grow by expansion, compressing the adjacent normal renal tissue (Fig. 24). Metastasis to the lungs occurs frequently.

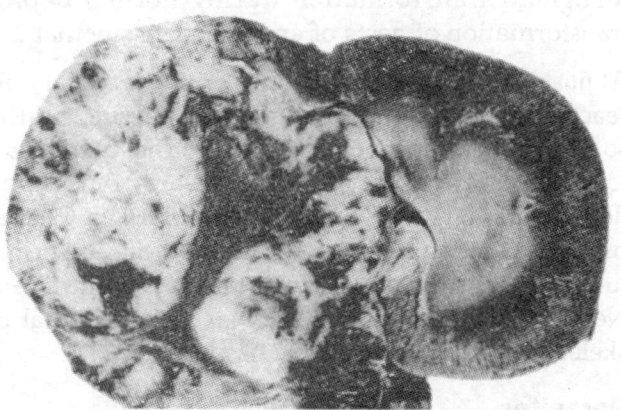

Fig. 24. Kidney; dog. Renal carcinoma. The neoplasm has infiltrated and replaced one half of the kidney.

As in adenomas, neoplastic cells form solid sheets, tubules or papillary growth patterns, but the cells in carcinomas are more atypical and neoplastic. Cells vary in

217

shape from cuboidal, columnar to polyhedral, also vary in size, and have clear or granular eosinophilic cytoplasm. Nuclei range from small, round, granular, and uniform to large, oval, vesicular, and pleomorphic. **Mitotic figures are numerous.** These neoplasms have a moderate fibrovascular stroma.

Mesenchymal and Metastatic Tumours

At times, **fibromas, fibrosarcomas,** or **haemangiosarcomas** originate in the kidneys. **Carcinomas** and **sarcomas (metastatic tumours)** originating in other organs can metastasize to the kidneys and are composed of scattered multiple nodules, usually involving both kidneys. **Renal lymphosarcoma** has been described in **cattle** and **cats,** particularly as a part of generalized or multicentric lymphosarcoma. They appear as single or multiple grey-white nodules or as diffuse lymphomatous infiltrates that cause uniform enlargement and pale discoloration of the kidney. Renal lymphosarcoma must be differentiated from the renal granulomas of feline infectious peritonitis by histopathological examination.

Tumours of Embryonal Origin

Nephroblastomas (Embryonal Nephroma, Wilms' Tumour)

These are common renal neoplasms of **pigs** and **chickens** in which they are usually seen at slaughter. They occur in **cattle** and **dogs** as well, but less commonly. These neoplasms are of embryonal origin, originate from metanephric blastema, and therefore occur in **young animals**. It is believed that neoplasms occur from malignant transformation during normal nephrogenesis, or from neoplastic transformation of nests of embryonic tissue that persist in the post-natal kidneys.

At postmortem, nephroblastomas may be solitary or multiple masses which usually reach a great size and in which renal tissue is difficult to detect. They are usually soft to rubbery and grey with foci of haemorrhage. On cut surface they are often lobulated. **Microscopic features** vary, but are morphologically similar to the developmental stages of embryonic kidneys. Characteristically, loose myxomatous tissue predominates. Scattered in this tissue are primitive tubules lined by elongated, deeply staining cells and structures that resemble primitive glomeruli. Nephroblastomas also have such mesenchymal components as cartilage, bone, skeletal muscle, and adipose tissue.

Parasites

Nematodes

Dioctophyma renale, the **giant kidney worm of dogs,** occurs worldwide. Because of a long and complex life cycle, this nematode is seen only **in dogs two years old or older.** The adult nematode lives in the renal pelvis, where it causes severe haemorrhage or purulent pyelitis and ureteral obstruction. The renal parenchyma is destroyed, resulting in kidney that becomes a cyst containing the nematode and purulent exudate.

The kidney worm *Stephanurus dentatus* of **pigs** is usually found in **adult pigs.** Adult worms often encyst in perirenal fat. However, some cysts with the nematode can be found in the kidneys.

Capillaria plica and *Capillaria feliscati,* occur in **dogs** and **cats** worldwide. These nematodes are attached to the renal pelvis, ureter, or bladder of animals of various ages. Microscopic inflammatory cell infiltrates and focal haemorrhages occur at the sites of attachment.

Lower urinary tract

The lower urinary tract consists of the **ureters, urinary bladder,** and **urethra**. At death, the urinary bladder can contract to such an extent that the normal bladder wall appears thick at postmortem. **Urine** should be clear **except in horses**, where because of the normal presence of mucus or fine crystals, it is **cloudy.**

Developmental Anomalies

Ureteral aplasia (agenesis) is rare. It can occur alone, or in animals with renal aplasia.

Ectopic ureters are usually found in **dogs**. Certain breeds are at greater risk. The involved ureter empties into the urethra, vagina, neck of the bladder, vas deferens, prostate, or other secondary sex organs. Ectopic ureters are more prone to obstruction or infection. Therefore, they predispose animals to pyelitis and pyelonephritis.

Patent Urachus

Urachus is a foetal canal that connects bladder with the umbilicus.

The most common malformation of the urinary bladder is **patent urachus (pervious urachus)**. This **lesion** develops when the foetal urachus fails to close, and therefore forms a direct channel between the bladder's apex and the umbilicus. Usually **foals** are affected and have dribbling of urine at the umbilicus. **Affected animals have increased susceptibility to bacterial infections of the urinary bladder.** Failure of the urachal remnant and the umbilical arteries and vein to involute (to regress) is usually observed in cases of 'neonatal' omphalitis and can result in a patent urachus. **Patent urachus** also occurs because of congenital urethral obstruction. Increased bladder pressure due to the obstruction forces urine out into the urachus.

At times, during urachal closure, the mucosa closes, but closure of the bladder musculature is incomplete. When this occurs, a **bladder diverticulum** (outpouching) of the apex of the bladder can develop. Urine stasis can occur in the diverticulum, predisposing the animal to·cystitis or urinary calculi.

Hydro-Ureter and Hydro-Urethra

Hydro-ureter and hydro-urethra are dilatation of the ureter and urethra, respectively. They are due to obstruction of urine outflow by blockage of the ureter(s) or urethra by calculi, chronic inflammation, or neoplasms. Depending on the location of the obstruction, hydronephrosis, hydro-ureter, and hydro-urethra can occur at the same time (see 'hydronephrosis').

Urolithiasis

Urinary calculi (uroliths) are concretions (calculi, inorganic masses) formed in the urinary tract. They are usually composed of salts of inorganic or organic acids, or other materials such as cystine or xanthine. **Struvite (magnesium ammonium phosphate hexahydrate), oxalate, apatite, carbonate, silica, urate, cystine, xanthine, or benzocoumarin ('clover stone') calculi have been seen in domestic animals.** Calculi can form in the renal pelvis, ureter, or in any portion of the lower urinary tract. Calculi vary in size and shape. Large renal pelvic calculi have a 'stag-horn' appearance because they take the shape of the renal calyces in animals which have true calyces. These calculi predispose the animals to **pyelitis** and **pyelonephritis**. **Urinary bladder calculi** can be single or multiple, variable in size, sand-like material that causes cloudy urine. Calculi may have smooth or rough surfaces. They are solid, soft, or friable. Calculi vary in **colour** depending on their composition. The calculi can be **white or grey** (e.g. struvite and oxalate), **yellow** (e.g. urate, cystine, benzocoumarin, and xanthine), or **brown** (e.g. silica, urate, and xanthine) depending on their composition. **Urinary calculi can cause urinary obstruction or traumatic injury to the urinary bladder mucosa.** Lesions of the urinary bladder appear as difficult or painful urination (**stranguria; dysuria**), with or without **haematuria**.

Both males and females are prone to urolithiasis but **calculi cause urinary obstruction usually in males** because of the narrow urethral diameter and longer urethra of males. When obstruction or dysuria occurs in females, calculi are usually large and located in the renal pelvis or urinary bladder (Fig. 25). **In males,** dysuria can result from large calculi, but urinary tract obstruction with uraemia usually occurs because of

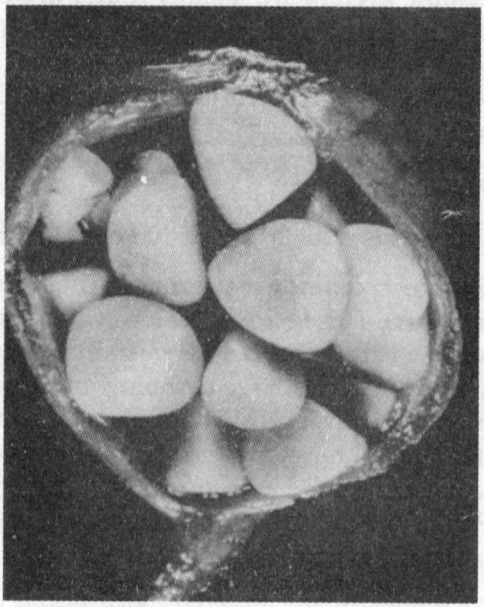

Fig. 25. Urinary bladder; dog. Urolithiasis. Multiple smooth calculi are present in the urinary bladder. The bladder wall is diffusely thickened.

obstruction of the urethra with small calculi. The sites of lodgment of urethral calculi vary with the animal species. **In male cattle,** calculi lodge in the urethra at the ischial arch and at the proximal end of the sigmoid flexture; **in rams and wethers** (castrated ram), the urethra process (vermiform appendage) is the most common site, and **in dogs,** calculi lodge proximal to the base of the os penis. **In cats,** fine struvite crystals (sand) in a rubber-like protein matrix can fill the entire urethra and such calculi are characteristic of the disease called **'feline urologic syndrome'.** **Urethral calculi are not commonly seen in horses and pigs.**

Calculi form because of the precipitation of salts in urine, usually along with an organic (protein) matrix. A number of factors can predispose the lower urinary tract to calculus formation.

1. **Urine pH** is important because some salts precipitate easily at acid pH (oxalates) and others easily at alkaline pH (struvite and carbonate).

2. **Bacterial infections** predispose to urolithiasis, for example, struvite calculi in **dogs.** Bacteria are involved in more than 60% of urolithiasis **in dogs.** Bacterial colonies, exfoliated epithelium, or leukocytes serve as the **nidus** (nucleus) for the precipitation of mineral constituents. **In cats,** a cell-associated herpesvirus is one of the several factors which predispose to struvite urolithiasis.

3. **Nutritional and dietary factors** have also been associated with the formation of urinary calculi. **In sheep,** diets containing sorghum or milo products, which have large concentrations of **phosphate,** predispose to struvite urolithiasis. **In cats,** consumption of dry commercial food rich in **magnesium** is an important predisposing factor for feline urologic syndrome. Ingestion of **oxalate-accumulating plants** predisposes to oxalate urolithiasis. **Vitamin A deficiency** can predispose to urolithiasis by causing squamous metaplasia of transitional epithelium. This results in desquamated squames (cornified epithelial cells) which serve as a nidus for calculi formation. **Dehydration,** as occurs when water intake is limited, can initiate or increase calculus formation by producing mineral constituents in a supersaturated state in concentrated urine. Super-saturation is unstable and predisposes to spontaneous precipitation. Ingestion of oestrogens, such as implantation or injection of oestrogens, can predispose sheep to so-called **clover stones (benzocoumarin)** or **carbonate calculi.**

4. **Hereditary defects** which result in urinary excretion of xanthine **(xanthinuria)** or cystine **(cystinuria)** can cause urinary calculi of the appropriate compound (see 'inherited abnormalities in renal tubular function'). Urate calculi form usually in **Dalmatian dogs** because of their large urinary excretion of uric acid.

At postmortem, animals which have died of urinary obstruction have greatly distended, swollen, or ruptured bladders and dilated ureters and renal pelvises. The bladder wall is thin and usually has haemorrhages. When urine is released from the bladder either because of rupture or incision at surgery or postmortem, the wall of the bladder is not stiff or firm, the mucosa is usually ulcerated, and the urine contains blood clots. Mucosal ulceration, localized haemorrhage in lamina propria, and mucosal necrosis are usually present in the ureter, bladder, or urethra adjacent to an obstructive calculus. If the bladder ruptures while animal is alive, blood clots and fibrin are at the site of rupture and in some cases an acute, localized chemical (urine-induced) peritonitis.

Microscopically, inflammation and haemorrhage are present in the lower urinary tract. Lesions are most severe in cases where obstruction is complete. The mucosa is usually ulcerated, and areas of transitional epithelial cell hyperplasia are scattered with goblet cells. Lamina propria is infiltrated with inflammatory cells. Neutrophils are present at foci of ulceration, and lymphocytes and plasma cells infiltrate perivascularly or uniformly throughout the lamina propria. Haemorrhage is most noticeable in the mucosa, but is also present in the wall and can cause separation of the smooth muscle bundles. Degeneration and necrosis of smooth muscle occurs in severe cases.

Inflammatory Diseases

Inflammation of the urinary bladder, called **cystitis,** is common in domestic animals. Since inflammation of the ureter (**ureteritis**) or urethra (**urethritis**) in the absence of cystitis are rare, this discussion focuses on cystitis. **Cystitis** can be **acute** or **chronic.**

Acute Cystitis

Cystitis can occur from several causes:

1. **Bacterial infections:** In all species, **bacterial infection** of the mucosa is the **most common cause of cystitis.** Bacterial cystitis is **more common in females** because their relatively short urethra provides a shorter barrier to ascending infections than the longer and narrow diameter of the male urethra. Bacteria commonly associated with cystitis are uropathogenic *Escherichia coli* (alpha-haemolysin-producing strains) **in all animal species;** *Corynebacterium renale* in **cattle;** *Eubacterium (Corynebacterium) suis* in **pigs;** and **Klebsiella** sp. in **horses.** In addition, **Proteus** sp., **Streptococcus** sp., **Staphylococcus** sp. have been isolated from cases of cystitis **in several animal species.**

2. **Chemical causes:** Active metabolites of **cyclophosphamide,** a drug used to treat neoplastic and immune-mediated diseases of **dogs** and **cats,** can cause a sterile haemorrhagic cystitis. **Cantharidin toxicosis** in **horses** occurs from ingestion of blister beetles in alfalfa hay, and haemorrhagic and necrotic cystitis develops as cantharidin is excreted through the urinary tract. Chronic ingestion of **bracken fern** by **cattle** can result in the syndrome **enzootic haematuria,** which can appear as acute urinary bladder haemorrhage, chronic cystitis, or urinary bladder neoplasia.

3. **Virus: In cats,** a cell-associated **herpesvirus** has been found in some cases of mild cystitis.

Pathogenesis

The lower urinary tract is normally free of bacteria, except distal urethra. Sterility (freedom from bacteria) of the urinary bladder is achieved by normal repeated emptying of urine and because of the antibacterial properties of urine. These antibacterial properties are due to the **acidic urine of carnivores, secretory IgA,** and **secreted mucin** which inhibit bacterial adhesion. It is also due to the large concentration of urea and organic acids, and to high urine osmolality.

Cystitis occurs when bacteria are able to overcome normal defence mechanisms and attach to or invade (colonize) the urinary bladder mucosa. Several factors can increase colonization and predispose animals to cystitis. **Colonization** is more common for strains of those bacteria which express molecules on their surfaces that increase adhesions. Example: the P and type 1 fimbriae of **certain strains of E. coli. Retention of urine** as a result of obstruction or neurogenic causes related to spinal cord diseases usually leads to cystitis.

Trauma of the urinary bladder mucosa due to calculi, faulty catheterization, and parturition causes erosion and haemorrhage and predisposes to bacterial invasion of the lamina propria. **Hydrolysis of urea** by urease-producing bacteria, such as *C. renale* and *E. suis*, releases excessive ammonia and can damage the mucosa. Bacterial growth is increased when **glucosuria** is present, as in diabetes mellitus. **Urinary bladder emphysema** can occur along with glucosuria-associated cystitis due to fermentation of glucose by certain bacteria. The **gas** is absorbed into lymph vessels in the lamina propria, tunica muscularis, and sub-mucosa and small bubbles are present throughout the bladder wall. Damage to the host immune system as occurs with infection by the **immunodeficiency virus** can increase susceptibility to bacterial cystitis. **Other bacterial virulence factors,** such as the *E. coli* haemolysin, increase pathogenicity and help bacteria overcome antibacterial factors of the urinary bladder and urine.

Once bacteria enter into the lamina propria, they cause vascular damage and inflammation. Acute cystitis can be **haemorrhagic, fibrinopurulent, necrotizing,** or **ulcerative.** However, in each case, the urinary bladder wall is usually thickened by oedema and inflammatory cell infiltration, and is diffusely or focally haemorrhagic. Haemorrhage is most common when obstruction is also present or after direct trauma due to catheterization. Urine in such cases is cloudy, flocculent, foul-smelling, ammoniacal, and red-tinged. The mucosa can have foci of erosion or ulceration, patches or sheets of adherent exudate and necrotic debris, or adherent blood clots.

Microscopically, acute cystitis is characterized by epithelial denudation with bacterial colonies present on the surface. The lamina propria is intensely oedematous and has a diffuse neutrophilic infiltrate. Superficial hyperaemia and haemorrhage are always present. A mild perivascular leukocytic infiltration can occur in the tunica muscularis.

Chronic Cystitis

Chronic cystitis occurs in several forms. Usually, the lesions include diffusely thickened, hyperplastic mucosa with increased number of goblet cells, and chronic lymphoplasmacytic infiltrate and fibrosis in the lamina propria. Hypertrophy of the tunica muscularis can be seen. This response is particularly common when cystitis is associated with chronic urolithiasis.

Several specific anatomical forms of chronic cystitis can occur. **Chronic polypoid cystitis** is a form found especially in **dogs**. The mucosa has a single or multiple, nodular mucosal masses composed of fibrous connective tissue and infiltrated with neutrophils and mononuclear leukocytes. The masses are ulcerated, or covered by hyperplastic epithelium with increased number of goblet cells. Chronic cystitis also takes the form of **disseminated nodular, sub-mucosal lymphoid proliferations.** The mucosa has a cobblestone appearance (**follicular cystitis**).

Mycotic Cystitis

Mycotic cystitis is sometimes seen when opportunistic fungi, such as *Candida albicans* or **Aspergillus** sp. colonize the urinary bladder mucosa. Such fungal infections usually occur secondary to chronic bacterial cystitis, especially when animals are immunosuppressed or **subjected to prolonged antibiotic therapy.** The urinary bladder is usually **ulcerated** with proliferation of underlying lamina propria. The generalized thickening of the urinary bladder wall is due to extensive inflammation consisting of neutrophils, lymphocytes, plasma cells, macrophages, oedema, and fibrosis.

Neoplasms

Neoplasms of the lower urinary tract occur mainly in the **urinary bladder.** They occur usually in **dogs,** sometimes in **cats,** and **rarely in other species.** Lower urinary tract neoplasms usually cause **mucosal ulceration** resulting in clinical signs of dysuria, haematuria, or obstruction. Urinary bladder neoplasms can block the ureters, causing obstruction of ureteral urine flow, increased ureteral pressure, and **hydronephrosis.** Urinary bladder neoplasms comprise less than 1% of total canine neoplasms. Most occur in **old dogs** without a sex predisposition.

Many chemicals including intermediate components of aniline dyes, aromatic hydrocarbons, and tryptophan metabolites have been found experimentally and epidemiologically to induce urinary bladder neoplasms. **Bracken fern** contains **quercetin, a carcinogen. Cattle** grazing **bracken fern** have developed sever different neoplasms of the urinary bladder (see 'enzootic haematuria, below).

Epithelial Tumours

Epithelial tumours are most common and are classified as transitional cell papillomas, transitional cell carcinomas, squamous-cell carcinomas, adenocarcinomas, and undifferentiated carcinomas.

Papillomas have a papilliferous (bearing papillae) or pedunculated appearance. **Microscopically,** they have a papillary growth pattern consisting of multiple papilliferous fibrosis stalks covered by transitional epithelium. **Carcinomas** are focal raised nodules or diffuse thickenings of the urinary bladder wall. **Transitional cell carcinomas** are composed of pleomorphic to anaplastic transitional epithelium. They usually occur in the trigone area (triangular region of the wall) of the bladder. Neoplastic transitional cells cover the mucosal surface as irregular layers, invade the lamina propria in the form of solid nests and acini and are found within lymphatic vessels of the sub-mucosal and muscle layers. **Squamous-cell carcinomas, adenocarcinomas,** and **unclassified carcinomas** probably arise from transitional epithelium. **In the bitch,** carcinomas are multicentric in origin, develop not only in the urinary bladder, but also in the urothelium (a layer of transitional epithelium external to the lamina propria) of the ureters, urethra, renal pelvis, and often extend to the vagina and vestibule. Metastasis of urinary bladder carcinoma is usually first to regional lymph nodes at the aortic bifurcation including the deep inguinal, medial, iliac, and sacral lymph nodes. Other potential sites of metastasis include lungs and kidneys with metastasis to other parenchymatous organs occurring later.

Mesenchymal Tumours

Mesenchymal tumours include **fibromas, fibrosarcomas, leiomyomas, leiomyosarcomas, rhabdomyosarcomas, lymphosarcomas, haemangiomas,** and **haemangiosarcomas.** They occur in the lower urinary tract.

Leiomyomas are the most common neoplasms and are solitary or multiple, circumscribed, firm, pale white **masses in the urinary bladder wall.** **Macroscopically,** their consistency and **microscopically** their appearance are similar to that of normal smooth muscle. **Fibromas** originate from connective tissue of lamina propria and project into the bladder lumen as solitary nodules. **Primary fibrosarcomas, leiomyosarcomas, haemangiomas, haemangiosarcomas are rare.** **Lymphosarcoma** sometimes infiltrates the wall, not only of the bladder, but also of the ureters and renal pelves in **cattle** with malignant lymphoma. **Rhabdomyosarcomas are rare,** but occur in bladder of **young dogs** (younger than 18 months old) suggesting an embryonal origin. These masses are described as **botryoid** (grape-like) because they are large, fungating masses (i.e. producing fungus-like growths) which protrude into the bladder lumen. They infiltrate the urinary bladder wall and can metastasize. **Microscopically,** neoplasms are composed of sheets of fusiform cells scattered with pleomorphis cells.

Enzootic Haematuria

Enzootic haematuria is a disease of cattle caused by chronic ingestion of **bracken fern.** The urinary bladder lesion is initially haemorrhagic cystitis causing marked persistent haematuria, hence the name **enzootic haematuria.** The mucosa is haemorrhagic with marked capillary congestion and ectasia (dilatation, distension). With time, epithelial (**papilloma** or **carcinoma**), mesenchymal (**fibromas, haemangiomas, and their malignant counterparts**), or mixed epithelial-mesenchymal neoplasms develop along with the lesions of chronic cystitis. **These neoplasms usually ulcerate the mucosa and bleed freely into the lumen.**

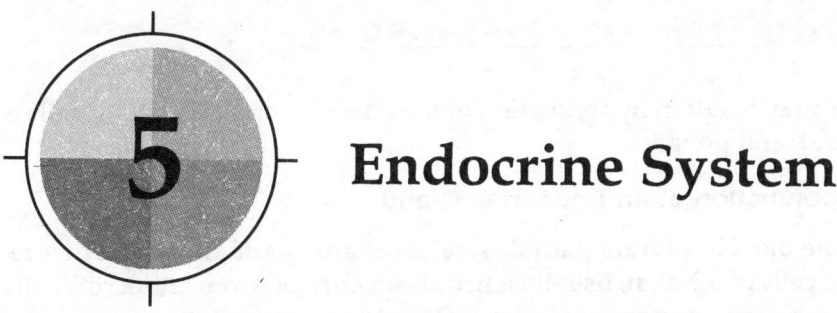

Endocrine System

Pathogenic Mechanisms of Endocrine Diseases

Many diseases of the endocrine glands are characterized by sudden and striking functional disturbances and characteristic clinico-pathological alterations which affect one or several body systems. For example, changes may primarily involve the skin (loss of hair caused by hypothyroidism), nervous system (seizures caused by hyperinsulinism), urinary system (polyuria caused by diabetes mellitus, diabetes insipidus, or hyper-adrenocorticism), or skeletal system (fractures induced by hyper-parathyroidism). **Briefly, the pathogenic mechanisms of endocrine diseases are as follows:**

1. Primary Hypofunction of an Endocrine Gland

In this mechanism, hormone secretion is subnormal (below normal) due to: (1) destruction of secretory cells by a disease process, (2) failure of an endocrine gland to develop properly, or (3) the result of a specific biochemical defect in the synthetic pathway of a hormone. In animals, **immune-mediated injury** causes hypofunction of several endocrine glands, such as parathyroid glands, adrenal cortex, thyroid gland, pancreatic islets, and hypothalamus. Thyroiditis caused by this mechanism is characterized by marked infiltration of lymphocytes and plasma cells and deposition of immune complexes with progressive destruction of secretory parenchyma.

Failure of development also results in a primary hypofunction of an endocrine gland. Classical example is the failure of oro-pharyngeal ectoderm to differentiate into trophic hormone-secreting cells of the adenohypophysis (anterior pituitary) in **dogs**. This results in pituitary dwarfism.

2. Secondary Hypofunction of an Endocrine Gland

In this mechanism, a destructive lesion in one organ such as the pituitary gland interferes with the secretion of a trophic hormone (i.e., hormone having nourishing and stimulating action). The reduced secretion of a hormone from that gland results in hypofunction of the target endocrine gland (i.e. the gland affected by that particular hormone). Thus, in this mechanism hypofunction of the target endocrine gland is secondary. For example, neoplasms of pituitary gland in **adult dogs, cats,** and **other animals** can interfere with the secretion of several pituitary trophic hormones. This may result in hypofunction of the adrenal cortex, follicular cells of the thyroid gland, and gonads.

3. Primary Hypofunction of an Endocrine Gland

This is one of the most important pathological mechanisms of endocrine disease in animals. The cells of a lesion, usually a neoplasm derived from endocrine cells, synthesize and secrete a hormone autonomously (independently) at a rate in excess of the body's ability to use and to degrade. **This results in a syndrome of hormone excess. Examples** are given **in Table 7.** These include hyperfunction of parathyroid chief cells, thyroid C (parafollicular) cells, beta cells of the pancreatic islets, secretory cells of the adrenal medulla, and follicular cells of the thyroid gland.

Table 7. Primary hyperfunction of an endocrine gland

Neoplasm	Hormone	Species	Lesion/Sign
Thyroid follicular cell adenoma	Thyroxine (T4) Triiodothyronine (T3)	Cat	Increased basal metabolic rate
Parathyroid gland chief cell adenoma	Parathyroid hormone	Dog	Fibrous osteodystrophy
Pancreatic Beta-cell adenoma/carcinoma	Insulin	Dog	Hypoglycaemia
Pheochromocytoma (adrenal medulla)	Norepinephrine	Dog	Hypertension
Acidophil adenoma (pituitary gland)	Growth hormone	Dog	Acromegaly
C cell adenoma/ carcinoma (thyroid gland)	Calcitonin	Bull	Osteosclerosis
Adrenal cortical adenoma/carcinoma	Oestrogen	Dog	Feminization

4. Secondary Hyperfunction of an Endocrine Gland

In this mechanism of endocrine disease, a lesion in one organ, for example, adenohypophysis (anterior glandular lobe of the pituitary gland), secretes an excess of a trophic hormone that leads to long-term stimulation and hypersecretion of a hormone by a target organ. **The classical example in animals** is the adrenocorticotrophic hormone (ACTH)-secreting neoplasm derived from pituitary corticotrophs in **dogs.** The functional disturbances and lesions occur from **increased blood cortisol concentrations** resulting from the ACTH-stimulated hypertrophy and hyperplasia of the zona fasciculata and reticularis of the adrenal cortex. In some **aging dogs** with marked adrenal cortical enlargement and functional disturbances of cortisol excess, no gross or histopathological evidence of a neoplasm is present in the pituitary gland.

5. Hypersecretion of Hormones or Hormone-like Factors by Non-endocrine Neoplasms:

Certain neoplasms of non-endocrine tissues **in both human beings and animals either secrete new humoral substances or hormones** which share chemical or biological characteristics or both with the original hormones secreted by an endocrine gland. Most of the humoral substances secreted by non-endocrine neoplasms are **peptides** rather than steroids, iodothyronines, or catecholamines. The non-peptide hormones require more complex biosynthetic pathways and are rarely produced by cancer cells. **Humoral hypercalcaemia of malignancy** ('pseudo-hyperparathyroidism') is a clinical syndrome produced by the autonomous hypersecretion of parathyroid hormone-related peptide (PTH-rP) **by cancer cells.** PTH-rP interacts with the parathyroid hormone receptor in target cells (e.g. bone and kidneys) and results in **persistent, usually life-threatening hypercalcaemia. A typical example** of this disease mechanism **in animals** is the adenocarcinoma of the apocrine glands of the anal sac **in dogs.** These neoplasms produce PTH-rP that mimic the action of PTH and results in an **increased mobilization of calcium from the bone** by osteoclasts causing **persistent hypercalcaemia.** Serum PTH concentrations are lower in dogs with apocrine carcinomas than in controls and PTH concentrations are undetectable in neoplastic tissue.

6. Endocrine Dysfunction (Abnormal Function) due to Failure of Target Cell Response

A failure of target cells to respond to a hormone can be due to either a lack of adenylate cyclase in the cell membrane or to an alteration in hormone receptors on the cell surface. **Hormone is secreted in normal or increased amounts by the cells of the endocrine gland.** For example, **insulin resistance associated with obesity in both animals and human beings** can occur from a decrease or down-regulation of receptors on the surface of target cells. The down-regulation of receptors develops in response to a chronic increase in insulin stimulated by the hyperglycaemia resulting from **excessive food intake.** Secretory cells in the corresponding endocrine gland (i.e. pancreatic islets) undergo compensatory hypertrophy and hyperplasia in an attempt to secrete additional hormone.

7. Endocrine Hyperactivity due to Diseases of Other Organs

A typical example is the **hyperthyroidism** that occurs **from chronic renal failure or nutritional imbalance. In the renal form,** retention of phosphorus occurs, resulting in a reciprocal decrease in serum calcium and parathyroid stimulation. Following this, progressive destruction of cells of the proximal convoluted tubules interferes with the metabolic activation of vitamin D by 1-alpha-hydroxylase in the kidneys causing decreased intestinal calcium absorption and continued parathyroid stimulation. The rate-limiting step in the metabolic activation of vitamin D is controlled by many factors. The intestinal absorption of calcium is disturbed and results in the development of progressive**hypocalcaemia**. The hypocalcaemia leads to parathyroid gland stimulation and to the development of generalized demineralization (decalcification) of the skeleton. **Nutritional hyperparathyroidism** develops in animals fed abnormal diets that are either too low in calcium, or too high in phosphorus or deficient in cholecalciferol.

Hyperfunction of an endocrine organ can also result from hormonal imbalances caused by **xenobiotic chemicals** (i.e. chemical compounds that are foreign to a living organism).

8. Failure of Foetal Endocrine Function

Subnormal function of the foetal endocrine system, seen usually in **ruminants,** can disrupt normal development and result in prolonged gestation. For example, in **cattle,** a genetically determined failure of development **(aplasia) of the adenohypophysis** has been described. However, the neurohypophysis develops normally. This aplasia results in a lack of foetal pituitary trophic hormone secretion during the last trimester and hypoplasia of target endocrine organs, namely, adrenal cortex, gonads, and follicular cells of the thyroid gland.

A very long duration of the gestation period occurs in **ewes** that ingest the plant *Veratrum californicum* early in gestation. **Toxins in the plant** cause extensive malformations of the central nervous system (CNS) and hypothalamus in **lambs.** Although the adenohypophysis is present, it is unable to secrete normal amounts of trophic hormone (ACTH) because it lacks the necessary fine control derived from the releasing hormones of the hypothalamus. Target endocrine organs in the foetus are hypoplastic and the adrenal cortex does not differentiate completely into the three distinctive zones that secrete corticosteroid hormones.

These observations suggest that: (1) foetal hormones are necessary for final growth and development of the foetus in certain animals, and (2) normal parturition at term in these species requires an intact foetal hypothalamic-adenohypophyseal-adrenocortical axis working in association with trophoblasts of the placenta.

9. Endocrine Dysfunction Resulting from Abnormal Degradation of Hormone

In this mechanism, the rate of secretion of a hormone by an endocrine is normal, but because of the decreased rate of degradation, blood concentrations are increased, thereby producing a syndrome of hypersecretion. A typical example of this mechanism is the syndrome of feminization due to hyper-oestrogenism and from decreased hepatic degradation of oestrogens in patients with cirrhosis. **Chronic renal disease** in **dogs** is sometimes associated with **hypercalcaemia**, due in part to a decrease in the ability of the diseased kidneys to degrade PTH, along with a decrease in urinary excretion of calcium.

10. Iatrogenic (Physician-Induced) Syndromes of Hormone Excess

Administration of an exogenous hormone can influence the activity of target cells either directly or indirectly and causes important functional disturbances. For example, chronic administration of potent preparations of **adrenal cortical steroids** at large daily doses, for symptomatic treatment of various diseases, can produce functional disturbances associated with an endogenous hypersecretion of cortisol. Increased concentrations of exogenous cortisol cause **marked atrophy of the adrenal cortex.** Similarly, administration of large doses of **insulin** can cause **hypoglycaemia,** and an excess of thyroxine (T4) or triiodothyronine (T3) can result in **hyperthyroidism,** particularly in certain species, for example **cats,** which have limited capacity to conjugate T4 with glucuronic acid, and therefore increase bile secretion.

Administration of progestogens to dogs indirectly **causes a syndrome of growth hormone excess.** For example, the injection of medroxyprogesterone acetate for the prevention of oestrus stimulates expression of the growth hormone gene in the mammary glands and causes increased circulating growth hormone concentrations producing many kinds of clinical manifestations of **acromegaly.**

Pituitary Gland (Hypophysis)

Pituitary gland is composed of **two functionally separate components**: (1) the **anterior pituitary** (or lobe), also known as **'adenohypophysis',** and (2) the **posterior pituitary** (or lobe), also known as **'neurohypophysis'. Adenohypophysis** is made up of a mixture of secretory cells, whereas the **neurohypophysis** represents an extension of the brain. **Histologically also, the adenohypophysis and neurohypophysis are totally different.** The adenohypophysis is composed of epithelial cells arranged in cords and nests, whereas the neurohypophysis is composed of tangled nerve fibres.

Adenohypophysis

Adenohypophysis consists of three portions: (1) pars distalis, (2) **pars tuberalis,** and (3) **pars intermedia.** The **pars distalis** is the largest and is composed of populations of different endocrine cells that secrete the pituitary trophic hormones. The secretory cells are surrounded by abundant capillaries. The **pars tuberalis** consists of dorsal projections of cells. Its primary function is to act as a scaffold for the capillary network. The **pars intermedia** is located between the pars distalis and pars nervosa of the neurohypophysis. It has two populations of cells in certain species. **In the dog,** one of these cell types (B cells) synthesizes and secretes adrenocorticotropic hormone (ACTH).

Secretory cells in the adenohypophysis are classified as **acidophils, basophils,** and **chromophobes** (see **Table 8**) based on the reaction of their secretory granules with pH-dependent histochemical stains. Based on specific immunocytochemical staining, **acidophils** are further classified functionally into **somatotrophs** that secrete growth hormone (GH; somatotropin) and **luteotrophs** that secrete luteotropic hormone (LTH; prolactin). **Basophils** include both **gonadotrophs** that secrete luteinizing hormone (LH) and follicle-stimulating hormone (FSH) and **thyrotrophs** that secrete thyrotropic hormone (thyroid-stimulating hormone; TSH). **Chromophobes** include the pituitary cells that synthesize ACTH and melanocyte-stimulating hormone (MSH).

Table 8: Cell types of the adenohypophysis and their function

Cell type	Hormone produced	Effect on
1. Acidophils		
i) Somatotrophs	Growth hormone (GH) (somatotropin)	Growth
ii) Luteotrophs	Luteotropic hormone (LTH) (prolactin)	Lactation
2. Basophils		
i) Gonadotrophs	Luteinizing hormone (LH)	Ovarian follicles Interstitial cell of testis
ii) Thyrotrophs	Thyroid-stimulating hormone (TSH)	Thyroid
3. Chromophobes	Adreno-corticotrophic hormone (ACTH)	Adrenal cortex
	Melanocyte-stimulating hormone (MSH)	Melaoncytes

Each type of endocrine cell in the adenohypophysis is under the control of a specific releasing hormone or factor from the **hypothalamus**. These releasing hormones are small peptides synthesized and secreted by neurons of the hypothalamus. Each hormone stimulates the rapid release of secretory granules containing a specific preformed trophic hormone.

Neurohypophysis

Neurohypophysis is divided into three parts. Pars nervosa (posterior lobe) is the distal component of neurohypophyseal system. It is composed of numerous capillaries that are supported by modified glial cells (pituicytes). The neurohypophyseal hormone (i.e. **oxytocin** and **antidiuretic hormone**, ADH or vasopressin) are synthesized in the cell body of hypothalamic neurons, packaged, into secretory granules, transported by long axonal processes, and released into the bloodstream in the **pars nervosa**.

Production and release of both anterior and posterior pituitary hormones are under the control of hypothalamus.

Developmental Disturbances of Adenohypophysis

Pituitary Dwarfism and Pituitary Cyst

Pituitary dwarfism in **dogs** is usually associated with a failure of the oropharyngeal ectoderm of Rathke's pouch (a diverticulum from the embryonic buccal cavity from which the adenohypophysis is developed) to differentiate into trophic hormone-secreting cells of the pars distalis. This results in **an enlarged, multiloculated cyst** in the sella turcica (a depression on the upper surface of the sphenoid bone, lodging the pituitary gland) and an absence of the **adenohypophysis.**

Juvenile panhypopituitarism (i.e. decreased secretion of all the pituitary hormones in young animals) occurs usually in **dogs.** The **dwarf pups** appear normal from birth to two months of age. Afterwards, slower growth and retention of puppy hair coat becomes noticeable. **Alopecia** (absence of hair from skin areas) develops gradually and progresses to **complete alopecia** for the head and tufts of hair on the legs. There is **hyperpigmentation of the skin** until the skin is uniformly brown-black over most of the body. **Adult dogs** vary in size from as small as two kg to nearly half normal size, depending on whether the failure of formation of the adenohypophysis is almost or only partially complete.

Neoplasms of Adenohypophysis

Adenoma of Pars Intermedia

Adenoma derived from cells of the pars intermedia is the **most common type of pituitary gland neoplasm in horses.** It is the **second most common** type **in dogs,** and **rare in other species.** Adenomas develop in **older horses,** usually in **females.**

In dogs, adenomas of the **pars intermedia** cause only moderate enlargement of the pituitary gland. The **pars distalis** is easily identified and clearly demarcated from the anterior margin of the neoplasm. The neoplasm can extend and cause **compression atrophy,** but it usually does not invade **pars distalis.**

Adenomas of the pars intermedia in dogs are either functionally inactive or associated with hypopituitarism and diabetes insipidus, or endocrinologically active and secrete excessive ACTH. This causes adrenal cortical hyperplasia and a syndrome of cortisol excess. These active (ACTH-secreting) adenomas of the pars intermedia have prominent groups of corticotrophs which have eosinophilic cytoplasm and scattered follicles.

In horses, adenomas of the pars intermedia are usually large neoplasms which extend out of the sella turcica (depression in bone lodging pituitary gland) and compress the overlying hypothalamus. The adenomas are yellow to white, multi-nodular, and enclose pars nervosa. When the neoplasm is cut, a sharp line of demarcation is present between the neoplasm and the compressed pars distalis. **The clinical syndrome in horses** with neoplasms of pars intermedia is characterized by polyuria, polydipsia (excessive thirst), huge appetite, muscle weakness, somnolence (sleepiness), intermittent hyperpyrexia, and generalized hyperhidrosis (excessive sweating). The affected horses usually develop hypertrichosis ('hirsutism') because of failure to seasonally shed hair. (Hypertrichosis and hirsutism mean an excessive abnormal growth of hair). The hair over the trunk and extremities is long (up to 10 to 12 cm), abnormally thick, wavy, and usually matted (i.e. thick and twisted).

The **neoplastic cells** are arranged in cords and nests along the capillaries and connective tissue septa. They are large, spindle-shaped, or polyhedral with an oval hyperchromatic nucleus. More cuboidal neoplastic cells sometimes form follicular structures that have eosinophilic colloid.

Horses with large neoplasms may have **hyperglycaemia** (insulin-resistant) and **glycosuria** (presence of glucose in urine). The disturbances in carbohydrate metabolism, huge appetite, hypertrichosis, and hyperhidrosis are due to deranged hypothalamic function caused by compression of overlying hypothalamus by the large pituitary neoplasms. The hypothalamus is the centre for regulation of body temperature, appetite, and shedding of hair.

ACTH-Secreting (Corticotroph) Adenoma

Functional neoplasms (i.e. endocrinologically active) of the pituitary gland are derived from corticotroph (ACTH-secreting cells) either in the pars distalis or the pars intermedia of **dogs**. These neoplasms cause symptoms of cortisol excess (**Cushing's disease**). They usually occur in **dogs**.

The pituitary gland is enlarged. Because the diaphragma sella is incomplete in the **dog**, the line of least resistance favours dorsal expansion of the enlarging pituitary gland mass.

Bilateral enlargement of the adrenal glands occurs in dogs with functional corticotroph adenomas. Pituitary corticotroph adenomas are composed of large or small, chromophobic cells supported by fine connective tissue septa. Their cytoplasm is devoid of secretory granules, but stains immuno-cytochemically for ACTH and MSH.

Endocrinologically Inactive Chromophobe Adenoma

Non-functional pituitary neoplasms occur in dogs and cats, but are uncommon in other species. Although chromophobe adenomas are endocrinologically inactive, they can cause important functional disturbances and clinical signs due to compression atrophy of adjacent portions of the pituitary gland and dorsal extension into the overlying brain. The **clinical disturbances** occur either from the lack of secretion of pituitary trophic hormones and decreased target organ function (e.g. adrenal cortex), or dysfunction of the CNS. Affected animals have incoordination and other disturbances of balance, are weak and sometimes collapse after exercise.

Chronically affected animals are blind. **Clinical signs** associated with non-functional pituitary adenomas and hypopituitarism are **not specific** and could be confused with other disturbances of the CNS, such as brain neoplasms and encephalitis, or with chronic renal disease.

Cranio-pharyngioma

Cranio-pharyngioma is a **benign neoplasm** derived from epithelial remnants of the oro-pharyngeal ectoderm of the cranio-pharyngeal duct (Rathke's pouch). It occurs in animals younger than those with other types of pituitary neoplasms. Cranio-pharyngioma is one cause of **panhypopituitarism** and **dwarfism** in **young dogs.**

Cranio-pharyngiomas are large and grow along the ventral aspect of the brain, where they can surround several cranial nerves. In addition, they extend dorsally into the hypothalamus and thalamus. **The resulting signs are usually due to:**

1. **Lack of secretion of pituitary trophic hormones.** This results in trophic atrophy and subnormal function of the adrenal cortex and thyroid gland, atrophy of the gonads, and failure to attain somatic maturation due to a lack of secretion of growth hormone.

2. **Disturbances of water metabolism** (polyuria, polydipsia, low urine specific gravity, and osmolality) from interference in the synthesis and release of antidiuretic hormone (ADH) by the large neoplasm.

3. Deficiency in cranial nerve function.

4. CNS dysfunction due to extension into the overlying brain.

Microscopically, cranio-pharyngiomas have alternating solid and cystic areas. The **solid areas** are composed of nests of epithelial cells (cuboidal, columnar, or squamous) with focal areas of mineralization (calcification). The **cystic spaces** are lined either by columnar or squamous cells and contain keratin debris and colloid.

Pituitary Gland Carcinoma

Pituitary gland carcinomas are uncommon neoplasms than adenomas, but have been described in **older dogs** and **cows.** They are usually endocrinologically inactive, but can cause important functional disturbances by destruction of the pars distalis and neurohypophyseal system. This causes panpituitarism and diabetes insipidus.

Carcinomas are large and invade into the overlying brain. Metastases occur rarely to regional lymph nodes or to distant sites such as the spleen or liver. Carcinomas are highly cellular and usually have large areas of haemorrhage and necrosis. Giant cells, nuclear pleomorphism, and mitotic figures are seen more frequently than in adenomas.

Disorders of Neurohypophysis

Diabetes Insipidus

Diabetes insipidus occurs when antidiuretic hormone (ADH) is produced in inadequate amounts or target cells in the kidneys lack the biochemical pathways necessary to respond to the secretion of normal or increased circulating concentrations of ADH. Diabetes insipidus results from compression and destruction of the pars nervosa, infundibular stalk, or supraoptic nucleus in the hypothalamus. This may result from a large pituitary neoplasm, an expanding cyst, or inflammatory granuloma, and by traumatic injury to the skull with haemorrhage. Compression or disruption of the posterior lobe, infundibular stalk, and hypothalamus by neoplastic cells interrupts the transport of ADH in non-myelinated axons from its site of production.

The **clinical manifestations of diabetes insipidus** are polyuria (excessive urination), polydipsia (excessive thirst) and low specific gravity of the urine (usually less than 1.010). Affected animals (usually **dogs**) excrete large amounts of hypotonic urine, which in turn makes them to drink equally large amounts of water to prevent dehydration and hyperosmolality of body fluids. Diabetes insipidus can also occur from renal disease. It is then called **nephrogenic**, as against the hypophyseal or pituitary form.

Adrenal Glands

Adrenal glands consist of **two distinct parts** that differ morphologically, functionally, and in embryological origin. Because of their close structural relationships, the **outer cortex** and **inner medulla** of the adrenal glands have been usually considered as parts of one organ.

Adrenal Cortex

The **adrenal cortex** microscopically and functionally is divided into **three layers or zones:** (1) zona glomerulosa, (2) zona fasciculata, and (3) zona reticularis. The **zona glomerulosa (outer zone)** is about 10% to 15% of the cortex and is responsible for the secretion of **mineralocorticoid hormones.** The secreting cells of the **zona fasciculata (middle zone)** are about 65% to 70% of the cortex and are responsible for the secretion of **glucocorticoid hormones.** The **zona reticularis (inner zone)** is the remaining 15% of the cortex. The secreting cells are responsible for the secretion of **sex steroids.**

Mineralocorticoids are adrenal steroids that affect ion transport by epithelial cells and cause excretion of potassium and conserve sodium. The most important mineralocorticoid is **aldosterone.** The electrolyte 'pumps' in epithelial cells of the renal tubule and sweat glands respond to mineralocorticoids by conserving sodium and chloride and by excreting potassium. In the distal convoluted tubule, a cation-exchange mechanism is responsible for the resorption of sodium from the glomerular filtrate and secretion of potassium into the lumen. **Mineralocorticoids accelerate these reactions.** A lack of secretion of mineralocorticoids, such as in the **Addison's-like disease of dogs,** can result in a lethal retention of potassium and loss of sodium.

Glucocorticoids: Cortisol and lesser amounts of **corticosterone** are the most important glucocorticoid hormones. **Glucocorticoids act on carbohydrate, protein, and lipid metabolism.** This results in sparing of glucose and a tendency to hyperglycaemia and increased glucose production. Also glucocorticoids decrease lipogenesis (formation of fat) and increase lipolysis (breakdown of fat) in adipose tissue, which results in release of glycerol and fatty acids. **Glucocoticoids also suppress both inflammatory and immunological responses,** and thus reduce associated necrosis and fibroplasia. However, under the influence of increased concentrations of glucocorticoids, an animal has **reduced resistance to bacterial, viral, and fungal diseases. Glucocorticoids can damage the immunological response.** Glucocorticoids also exert a **negative effect on wound healing.** They inhibit fibroblast proliferation and collagen synthesis, causing **decreased scar tissue formation. Dogs** with hypercortisolism can have wound dehiscence (splitting open of wound).

Sex hormones (progesterone, oestrogens, and **androgens**) are synthesized in small amounts by secretory cells of the **zona reticularis** of the adrenal cortex. Rarely, a neoplasm of the zona reticularis may cause an excessive secretion of adrenal sex steroids. This can result in clinical symptoms of virilism (development of male secondary sex characters in a female), precocious (premature) sexual development, or feminization. This depends on which steroid is secreted in excess, sex of the patient, and the age at onset.

Developmental Disturbances

Hypoplasia of the adrenal gland occurs from an abnormal development of the pituitary gland. This is associated with **anencephaly** (absence of brain), in some cases **cyclopia** (fusion of eyes, thus having one eye) and in hypophyseal aplasia. The adrenal cortex is small but medulla is normal.

Degenerative Lesions

Calcification

Extensive deposition of calcium salts usually occurs in the **adrenal glands of adult cats.** The cause is unknown. The calcium deposits are usually bilateral, but are not associated with clinical signs. Calcified adrenal glands are nodular, firm, and have many yellow-white, gritty foci throughout the cortex.

Amyloid

Amyloid deposition in the adrenal glands occurs in all species and usually involves only the **cortex.** The affected cortex is widened and the amyloid deposits are greatly visible as translucent areas. Amyloid deposition begins around the sinusoids in the inner portions of the zona fasciculta and is usually confined to this zone. Clinical signs of adrenal cortical insufficiency are usually not observed.

Inflammatory Lesion

Adrenalitis

Bacterial and parasitic agents usually localize in the adrenal glands and produce inflammation and necrosis. **Focal inflammations** are usually **suppurative,** originating during the course of bacterial septicaemias. Adrenal capsule provides an effective barrier against direct invasion by inflammatory reactions in adjacent tissue. **Granulomatous adrenalitis** due to *Histoplasma capsulatum, Coccidiodes immitis,* or *Histoplasma neoformans* sometimes occurs in **dogs** and **cats.** Granulomas with central areas of necrosis and calcification can destroy almost an entire adrenal cortex. *Toxoplasma gondii* produces necrosis with infiltration of histiocytes in the adrenal cortex in many animals. Large concentration of anti-inflammatory steroids in the adrenal cortex (e.g. cortisol and corticosterone) suppresses local cell-mediated immunity and allows the growth of certain fungi (**H. capsulatum, C. immitis**), protozoa (**Babesia** sp., or *Toxoplasma gondii*), and bacteria (e.g., *Mycobacterium tuberculosis*).

Hyperplasia of Adrenal Cortex

Accessory Adrenal Tissue

Accessory (additional) cortical nodules are common in the adrenal glands of **adult to aged animals.** They are found in the capsule, cortex, and medulla.

Hyperplasia

Nodular hyperplasia is common in the adrenal glands. They appear as spherical nodules in the cortex or attached to the capsule. Hyperplastic nodules are usually multiple, bilateral, and yellow and involve any of the three zones of the cortex. **Microscopically,** nodules near the capsule resemble zona glomerulosa. The lipid content in these hyperplastic nodules is not depleted. The h**yperplastic cortical nodules are most common in older horses, dogs, and cats.** Nodular hyperplasia of the zona reticularis is seen in animals with functional disturbances. This suggests an androgen excess (e.g. greater muscle mass, involution of mammary gland).

Diffuse cortical hyperplasia causes a uniform, bilateral enlargement of the adrenal cortex. Marked hypertrophy and hyperplasia of the cells of zona fasciculate and zona reticularis occur in response to hypersecretion of ACTH by a corticotroph adenoma of the pituitary gland. The cytoplasm of the hyperplastic cells is vacuolated because of lipid content.

Neoplasms of Adrenal Cortex

Adenomas

Adenomas of the adrenal cortex usually occur in **older dogs and sometimes in horses, cattle, and sheep. Castrated male goats** have a greater incidence of cortical adenomas than intact males. Usually seen as incidental findings at postmortem, sometimes adenomas are endocrinologically active. They are well demarcated and are usually present as a single nodule. Larger adenomas are yellow to red, distort the shape of the gland, and compress the adjacent cortical parenchyma. Adenomas usually develop in an adrenal gland with many nodules of hyperplasia. **Grossly,** it is difficult to differentiate adenomas from hyperplastic nodules. However, nodular hyperplasia consists of many small foci, and is usually associated with extra-capsular nodules of hyperplastic cortical tissue. Cortical adenomas are composed of well-differentiated cells which resemble secretory cells of the normal zona fasciculata or zona reticularis. The cytoplasm of neoplastic cells is eosinophilic, vacuolated, and filled with lipid droplets. Adenomas are surrounded by a fibrous connective tissue capsule and a rim of compressed cortical parenchyma.

Carcinomas

Adrenal cortical carcinomas are less common than adenomas and have been reported usually in **cattle and older dogs,** but sometimes occur in other species. Carcinomas develop in **adult to older dogs.** Adrenal carcinomas are larger than adenomas and are usually bilateral. **In dogs,** they are composed of yellow-red friable tissue and may invade into surrounding tissues and into the wall of the caudal vena cava resulting in thrombus formation. **In cattle,** they attain a very big size (up to 10 cm or more in diameter) and have many areas of calcification or ossification.

Carcinomas are composed of more highly pleomorphic secretory cells than adenomas and are divided by a fine fibrovascular stroma. The affected adrenal gland is completely destroyed by the carcinoma. The pattern of growth of nodular cells can be trabecular, lobular, and focal. **Neoplastic cells** are usually large and have prominent nucleoli and densely eosinophilic or vacuolated cytoplasm.

Carcinomas and adenomas of the adrenal cortex in dogs are sometimes functional and secrete excessive amounts of cortisol. Functional cortical adenomas and carcinomas cause severe atrophy of the cortex in the opposite adrenal gland because of negative feedback inhibition of the pituitary ACTH secretion by the increased blood cortisol concentrations. The medulla appears more prominent because of the lack of cortical tissue.

Hyper-Adrenocoticism

Hyper-Cortisolism (Cushing's Disease or Syndrome)

The clinical signs and lesions in the syndrome of hyper-adrenocorticism occur from **overproduction of cortisol** by hyperactive cells of adrenal cortex. **Affected dogs** develop a number of functional disturbances and lesions from the combined glyconeogenetic, lipolytic, protein catabolic, anti-inflammatory effects of glucocorticoid hormones on many organs. The disease is slowly progressive. **Cortisol excess is one of the most common endocrinopathies in adult and aged dogs,** occurs sometimes in **cats**, but is rare in other domestic animals.

There are several causes of increased circulating cortisol concentrations in **dogs.** The most common cause is a functional corticotroph (ACTH-secreting) adenoma of the pituitary gland that causes bilateral adrenal cortical hypertrophy and hyperplasia. The cortex of each adrenal gland is widened as a result of diffuse and nodular hyperplasia. Functional adrenal gland neoplasms are a rare cause of Cushing's syndrome of cortisol excess in the **dog.**

Functional Disturbances and Lesions of Cortisol Excess

The **appetite** and **intake of food** are usually increased as a result of either hypercortisolism or damage due to compression of hypothalamic appetite centres by a large dorsally expanding pituitary gland neoplasm. The **muscles** of the extremities and abdomen are weakened and atrophied, resulting in abdominal enlargement, muscle trembling and an abnormal posture to support the body's weight. Hepatomegaly caused by increased deposition of fat and glycogen contributes to the development of distended, pendulous abdomen. Muscular asthenia (weakness) and wasting result from increased catabolism of structural proteins and decreased protein synthesis under the influence of cortisol excess. **Cutaneous lesions** usually occur in **dogs** with hyperadrenocoticism. Cutaneous calcification is a characteristic lesion in **dogs** with hypercortisolism. These calcium deposits occur in **dogs** with normal blood calcium and phosphorus concentrations. Severe calcification also occurs in other tissues such as the lungs, skeletal muscles, and the wall of the stomach.

Hypoadrenocoticism (Addison's Disease)

Dogs with hypoadrenocorticism have **bilateral adrenocortical atrophy** involving all layers of the adrenal cortex. **Production of all three corticosteroids (mineralocorticoids, glucocorticoids, and adrenal sex steroids) is deficient.** The adrenal cortex is reduced to one tenth or less of its normal thickness and consists mainly of the adrenal capsule. Therefore, the medulla becomes more prominent, and along with the capsule, makes up the bulk of the remaining adrenal gland.

The **pathogenesis** of idiopathic adrenal cortical atrophy is unknown, but the lesion is probably immune mediated. Early in the disease many foci of lymphocytes and plasma cells are present between sinusoids and parenchymal cells. The entire three zones of the cortex are almost absent in dogs that die from untreated hypoadrenocorticism. The capsule is thickened due to collapse of adrenal cortex and fibroblastic proliferation.

Chronic adrenal gland insufficiency is recognized as a separate endocrinopathy of **dogs**. Adrenal cortical insufficiency occurs usually in **young adult dogs** and probably has an immune-mediated pathogenesis. The synthesis and secretion of **mineralocorticoids** are reduced, resulting in marked changes in potassium, sodium, and chlorine concentrations. Less potassium is excreted by the kidneys (**hypokaluria**), resulting in severe **hyperkalaemia** (excess of potassium in blood). Less sodium and chloride are reabsorbed from renal tubules leading to varying degrees of **hypernatremia** (excess of sodium in blood) and **hyperchloruria** (excretion of chlorides in urine) and a corresponding decrease in blood concentrations of these ions. Severe hyperkalaemia usually produces cardiovascular disturbances. Bradycardia (slowness of the heartbeat) that develops in some dogs (heart rate of 50 or less beats per minute), predisposes to weakness and circulatory collapse after minimal exertion.

Decreased production of glucocorticoids results in several functional disturbances of hypoadrenocorticism. Failure of gluconeogenesis and increased sensitivity to insulin leads to moderate hypoglycaemia. **Hyperpigmentation of the skin** occurs in some **dogs** with long-standing adrenocorticoid insufficiency and is a common finding in Addison's disease of human beings. This lesion occurs from a lack of negative feedback on the pituitary gland and increased release of ACTH (and pituitary MSH). The **plasma cortisol concentrations in dogs** with hypoadrenocoticism are low. Because of the severe atrophy of the adrenal cortex, no increase in blood cortisol concentration results after the administration of ACTH.

Adrenal Medulla

Adrenal medulla is derived from neuroectoderm of the neural crest and **produces catecholamine hormones (norepinephrine**, also called **noradrenaline**; and **epinephrine** also called **adrenaline**) from the amino acid **tyrosine. In mammals** medulla is completely surrounded by the adrenal cortex, and venous blood from the cortex flows to medullary cells. This blood has the greatest concentration of corticosteroids of any fluid in the body. This close anatomical association between the adrenal cortex and medulla is not by chance because the enzyme that converts norepinephrine to epinephrine is corticosteroid hormone dependent.

Proliferative Lesions

Medullary Hyperplasia

Diffuse or nodular medullary hyperplasia precedes the development of pheochromocytoma in **bulls** and **human beings** with C cell neoplasms of the thyroid gland. The proliferated chromaffin cells compress the surrounding adrenal cortex. The hyperplastic cells are round to oval and have a lightly basophilic cytoplasm. Some **bulls** with diffuse medullary hyperplasia have a few small nodules of proliferated medullary cells. Medullary hyperplasia is **diagnosed** on the basis of increased adrenal weight, decrease in cortico-medullary ratio due to an increase in the size and number of medullary cells, and numerous mitotic figures in the adrenal medulla.

Neoplasms

Neuroblastomas

Neuroblastomas usually occur in young animals. They originate from primitive neuro-ectodermal cells, and form a large mass in the abdomen. Neuroblastomas are composed of small neoplastic cells that have a hyperchromatic nucleus and a scant amount of cytoplasm and therefore **resemble lymphocytes**. They tend to aggregate around vessels to form pseudo-rosettes. Neurofibrils or unmyelinated nerve fibres can be demonstrated in neuroblastomas.

Ganglioneuromas

Ganglioneuromas are benign neoplasm composed of multipolar (having more than two processes) ganglion cells and neurofibrils and have a prominent fibrous connective tissue stroma. The surrounding adrenal tissue is usually severely compressed. Sometimes, neoplastic cells in adrenal medullary neoplasms differentiate into two cell lines. This results in pheochromocytoma and ganglioneuroma in the same adrenal gland.

Pheochromocytoma

Pheochromocytomas are the **most common neoplasms in the adrenal medulla of animals.** They occur mostly in **cattle** and **dogs,** and are uncommon in other species. Pheochromocytomas in **bulls** and **human beings** develop together with calcitonin-secreting C cell neoplasms of the thyroid gland. **Malignant pheochromocytomas** invade through the capsule of an adrenal gland and into adjacent structures (e.g. caudal vena cava) or metastasize to different sites (e.g. liver, regional lymph nodes, or lungs).

Pheochromocytomas are neoplasms of catecholamine-secreting ('chromaffin') cells. They are usually located in the medulla, and only rarely at extra-adrenal sites in the abdomen. **They are unilateral or bilateral.** Pheochromocytomas are usually large (10 cm or more in diameter) and replace most of the affected adrenal gland. Smaller neoplasms are surrounded by a thin rim of adrenal cortex. Large pheochromocytomas are multilocular (having many compartments) and light-brown to yellow-red, as a result of haemorrhage and necrosis.

Neoplastic cells vary from small, round to polyhedral to large pleomorphic cells with multiple hyperchromatic nuclei. The cytoplasm is lightly eosinophilic, finely granular, and usually indistinct. **Pheochromocytomas are composed of either epinephrine or norepinephrine-secreting cells, or both types of cell.**

Functional pheochromocytomas are rare in animals. Tachycardia (abnormally rapid heart rate), oedema, and cardiac hypertrophy reported in **dogs** and **horses** with pheochromocytomas are due to excessive catecholamine secretion. Arteriolar sclerosis and widespread medial hyperplasia of arterioles has been reported in **dogs** along with clinical signs of hypertension.

Norepinephrine is the main catecholamine extracted from pheochromocytomas in dogs. This is similar to the finding in **normal pups,** in which norepinephrine is the main catecholamine. In **adult dogs,** epinephrine predominates in adrenal medullary tissues. The catecholamine content of pheochromocytomas in bulls also having C cell neoplasms of the thyroid was greater than in the normal adrenal medulla.

Thyroid Gland

The **thyroid gland** in most animals occurs as **two lobes** on the lateral surfaces of the trachea. It is the largest endocrine gland in the body. **Histologically,** thyroid gland consists of **follicles** of varying size that contain **colloid** produced by the **follicular cells. Thyroid produces two biologically active hormones, namely, thyroxine (T4) and triiodothyronine (T3).** They are secreted into the bloodstream. T4 and T3 once released into the circulation, act on many different target cells in the body. The overall functions of T4 and T3 are similar. The mechanism of action of thyroid hormones resembles that of steroids in that free hormone enters target cells and binds first to cytosol-binding proteins, and afterwards, to high-affinity nuclear receptors. Binding of thyroid hormone to receptors on the inner mitochondrial membrane is responsible for the **early activation of energy metabolism and increased oxidative phosphorylation.**

Developmental Disturbances

Accessory Thyroid Tissue

Because of the complex embryogenesis of the thyroid, occurrence of accessory thyroid tissue is common. This accessory thyroid tissue is usually located in the mediastinum, but can be located anywhere from the base of the tongue to the diaphragm. **About 50% of the adult dogs have nodules of accessory thyroid tissue** embedded in the fat around the base of the heart and origin of the aorta. The follicular structure and function are the same as those of the main thyroid lobes. The accessory thyroid tissue may undergo neoplastic transformation.

Thyroglossal Duct Cysts

Thyroglossal duct cyst develops usually in **dogs** and **pigs** and sometimes in other animals. The word **'thyroglossal'** means related to the **thyroid gland** and **tongue**. These cysts are formed as a result of persistence of portions of the midline embryological primordial of the thyroid gland.

The cysts are present in the ventral aspect of the cervical region in **dogs** as moving masses. They rupture and form a tract to the exterior. Their lining epithelium consists of layers of follicular cells, sometimes with colloid-containing follicles. These cells can undergo neoplastic transformation and give rise to **papillary carcinomas.**

Degeneration and Inflammatory Lesions

Follicular Atrophy

In follicular atrophy, loss of follicular epithelium and disruption of follicles is progressive and, in time, the gland is replaced by adipose connective tissue with minimal inflammatory response. The gland is smaller and lighter in colour than normal. **In dogs,** the early lesion with mild clinical signs of hypothyroidism is confined to one part of the thyroid gland. A more advanced form of **follicular atrophy** occurs in **dogs** with clinical hypothyroidism and low blood concentrations of thyroid hormones. These thyroid glands are greatly reduced in size and are composed mainly of adipose connective tissue with only a few groups of small follicles containing vacuolated colloid.

Lymphocytic (Immune-Mediated) Thyroiditis

Lymphocytic thyroiditis in dogs and **very fat chickens** closely resemble Hashimoto's disease in humans. Although pathogenetic mechanism in the **dog** is not completely understood, a polygenic pattern of inheritance similar to that in humans is believed to occur. The **immunological basis** of chronic lymphocytic thyroiditis in both human beings and **dogs** is through the production of **autoantibodies.** These are usually directed against thyroglobulin or a microsomal antigen (thyroperoxidase) and sometimes against the TSA receptor protein, nuclear antigen, and a colloid antigen from thyroid follicular cells. **Thyroglobulin autoantibodies** have been found in 48% of **dogs** with hypothyroidism.

Microscopic changes consist of multifocal to diffuse infiltrations of lymphocytes, plasma cells, and macrophages, and sometimes, lymphoid nodules. Thyroid follicles are small and lined by columnar epithelial cells. Lymphocytes, macrophages, and degenerate follicular cells are usually present in vacuolated colloid. **Thyroid C cells** are present between follicles and are more prominent than those in normal **dogs**.

Goitre

Goitre is a clinical term. It is used to describe **a non-neoplastic and non-inflammatory enlargement of the thyroid gland.** It develops **in all domestic animals and birds** as a result of **hyperplasia of follicular cells.** Certain forms of thyroid hyperplasia, especially nodular, are difficult to differentiate from adenomas.

The important mechanisms for the development of thyroid hyperplasia include: iodine deficient diets, goitrogenic (producing goitre) compounds that interfere with the production of thyroxine, excess dietary iodine, genetic defects in the enzymes or thyroglobulin that are essential for the biosynthesis of thyroid hormones. **All these result in inadequate thyroxine synthesis and decreased blood concentrations of T4 and T3.** This decreased concentration of thyroid hormone is detected by the hypothalamus, which in turn stimulates the pituitary gland to increase the secretion of thyroid-stimulating hormone (TSH), which results in hypertrophy and hyperplasia of follicular cells.

Diffuse Hyperplastic and Colloid Goitre

Dietary iodine deficiency causes diffuse hyperplastic goitre. **Iodine-deficient goitre still occurs worldwide in domestic animals,** but cases are sporadic and few animals are affected. Marginally iodine-deficient diets which contain goitrogenic compounds can cause a severe thyroid follicular cell hyperplasia and goitre. **Goitrogenic substances** include thiouracil, sulphonamides, and a number of plants of the family **Brassicacceae**. Offspring of females fed iodine-deficient diets may develop severe follicular cell hyperplasia of thyroid and have clinical signs of hypothyroidism. **Both lobes of the thyroid gland are uniformly enlarged in young animals** as a result of diffuse hypertrophy and hyperplasia of follicular cells. The enlargements, when big, produce palpable or visible swellings in the cranial cervical area. The affected lobes are firm and dark red because of extensive capillary network.

Colloid goitre is the involutionary phase (i.e. regressive phase) of diffuse hyperplastic goitre in young adult and adult animals. The hyperplastic follicular cells continue to produce colloid, but endocytosis (uptake by cells) of colloid from the lumen is decreased. This is due to the decreased pituitary TSH concentrations produced in response to the return of blood T4 and T3 concentrations to normal. Both thyroid lobes are diffusely enlarged but are more translucent and lighter in colour than in hyperplastic goitre. These differences in gross appearance are because of **less vascularity** in colloid goitre and development of **macrofollicles** (large follicles).

Colloid goitre develops either after sufficient amounts of iodine have been added in the diet or after requirements for thyroid hormones have decreased in an older animal. **Blood T4 and T3 concentrations return to normal and the secretion of TSH by the pituitary gland is decreased. Follicles are distended with densely eosinophilic colloid due to decreased TSH-induced endocytosis.** The follicular cells lining the macrofollicles are flattened and atrophic. The interface (boundary) between the colloid and luminal surface of the follicular cells is smooth and the cells have no endocytotic vacuoles of actively secreting thyroid follicular cells.

The changes in diffuse hyperplastic and colloid goitre are similar throughout the diffusely enlarged thyroid lobes. Follicles are irregular in size and shape in hyperplastic goitre because they contain varying amounts of colloid which is lightly eosinophilic and vacuolated. Some follicles collapse because of the lack of colloid. The follicles are lined by single or multiple layers of hyperplastic follicular cells which, in some follicles, form **papillary projections into the lumen** (Fig. 26).

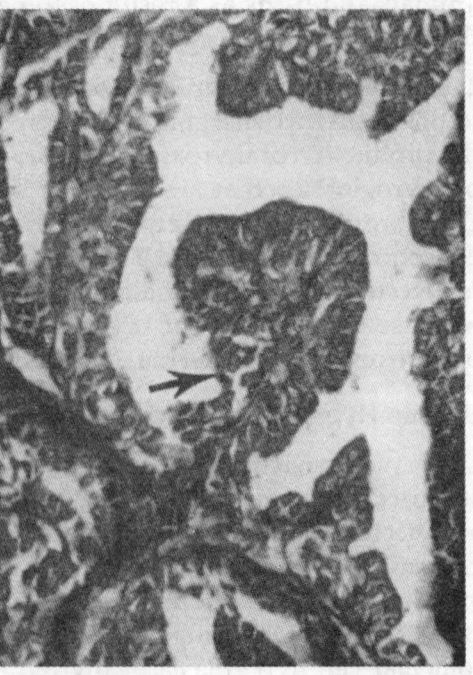

Fig. 26. Thyroid gland; dog. Hyperplastic goitre. Note papillary projection (arrow) extends into follicular lumen.

Although seemingly contradictory, **an excess of iodine in the diet can also result in thyroid hyperplasia in animals and human beings. Foals** of mares fed dry seaweed containing excessive iodine develop thyroid hyperplasia and clinically visible goitre. Thyroid glands of the young are prone to greater blood iodine concentrations than the dam because iodine is concentrated first in the placenta and then by the mammary gland. **Increased blood iodine interferes with thyroid hormone synthesis and secretion.** This causes decreased blood T4 and T3 concentrations with a compensatory increase in pituitary TSH secretion. Excess iodine appears to block the release of T3 and T4 by interfering with proteolysis of colloid by lysosomal enzymes in thyroid follicular cells.

Multifocal Nodular Hyperplasia (Goitre)

Multifocal nodular hyperplasia occurs in thyroid glands of **old horses, cats, and dogs.** It appears as multiple, white to yellowish-brown nodules of variable size, giving affected lobes moderately enlarged and irregular shape. **Multifocal nodular goitre in most animals except cats is endocrinologically inactive** and is an incidental lesion at postmortem. However, functional thyroid adenomas usually develop in a thyroid gland of **aged cats** with hyperthyroidism and multinodular hyperplasia of follicular cells. In contrast to thyroid adenomas, areas of nodular hyperplasia are not encapsulated and cause no compression of the adjacent parenchyma. **Thus, nodular goitre consists of multiple foci of hyperplastic follicular cells that are closely demarcated but not encapsulated from the adjacent thyroid tissue.**

Microscopic appearance of nodular hyperplasia varies. Some hyperplastic follicular cells form small follicles **with little or no colloid.** Other nodules are composed of larger follicles lined by one or more layers of columnar cells that form **papillary projections** into the lumen. Some of the follicles undergo colloid involution and are filled with densely eosinophilic colloid. These changes are due to alternating periods of hyperplasia and colloid involution inthe thyroid gland of **aged animal.**

Congenital Dys-hormonogenetic Goitre

Congenital dys-hormonogenetic goitre in **sheep, cattle,** and **goats** is inherited as an autosomal recessive trait. Most **lambs with congenital goitre** die soon after birth, or are very sensitive to the adverse environmental conditions, particularly cold.

Thyroid lobes are enlarged at birth because of intense diffuse hyperplasia of follicular cells. Thyroid follicles are lined by tall columnar cells, but are usually collapsed because of lack of colloid.

Neoplasms of the Thyroid Gland

Follicular Cell Adenoma

Adenomas are usually white to yellowish-brown, small, solid nodules which are well demarcated from the adjacent thyroid parenchyma. The affected thyroid lobe is only moderately enlarged and distorted. **Only a single adenoma is present in a thyroid lobe.** A distinct, white, fibrous connective tissue capsule separates adenoma from the compressed parenchyma. Some thyroid adenomas are composed of thin-walled cysts filled with yellow to red fluid. **Adenomas are classified into the follicular and papillary types. The follicular type is more common in the thyroid gland of animals.**

Follicular Cell Carcinoma

In dogs, thyroid **carcinomas are more common** than adenomas, **but in cats adenomas are more common.** About 60% of thyroid carcinomas in **dogs** are detected clinically by palpation as a firm mass in the neck and by signs of respiratory distress due to compression of the trachea. Carcinomas become fixed in position by extensive local invasion of adjacent structures, whereas adenomas (which do not invade) are freely movable under the skin. Neoplasms of thyroid origin also occur in accessory thyroid tissue which is located anywhere from the base of the tongue to the cranial mediastinum.

Thyroid carcinomas grow rapidly and invade adjacent structures, such as trachea, oesophagus, and larynx. The most common site of metastasis is **lungs** because thyroid carcinomas in the course of development invade branches of the thyroid vein. The retro-pharyngeal and caudal cervical lymph nodes are rare sites of metastases.

Hyperthyroidism

Proliferative lesions which secrete thyroid hormones (e.g. adenomas and multinodular hyperplasia) are common in the thyroid glands of **adult and aged cats.** Follicular cell adenomas, which develop in thyroid gland with multinodular hyperplasia, occur more commonly than thyroid carcinomas. **In aged cats,** a syndrome of hyperthyroidism associated with multinodular hyperplasia, adenomas, or carcinomas derived from follicular cells of the thyroid gland, is common.

Hyperthyroidism in cats also occurs in association with bilateral multinodular ('adenomatous') hyperplasia ('goitre'). These multiple areas of thyroid gland hyperplasia usually cause only slight enlargement of the affected lobe. In contrast to adenomas, areas of nodular hyperplasia are not encapsulated and the adjacent thyroid tissue is not compressed. **Microscopically,** hyperplastic nodules are composed of colloid-filled follicles lined by cuboidal follicular cells. These multiple nodules of follicular cell hyperplasia are considered a preneoplastic lesion as they can coalesce and form a thyroid follicular cell adenoma.

Hyperthyroidism is one of the two most common diseases in **adult to aged cats, diabetes mellitus** being the other. **Cats** with hyperthyroidism usually have greatly increased serum T4 and T3 concentrations. **Hyperthyroid cats** usually have disturbances of calcium homeostasis and diffuse chief cell hyperplasia in the parathyroid glands.

Thyroid neoplasms in the dog can secrete sufficient thyroid hormones to produce mild clinical signs of hyperthyroidism. These include weight loss polyphagia (excessive eating), weakness and fatigue, intolerance to heat, and nervousness.

Hypothyroidism

Hypothyroidism is a clinically important disease in dogs, but is seen only sometimes in other animals. **Certain breeds of dogs** are more commonly affected than others. **Hypothyroidism in dogs** usually occurs from primary lesions in the thyroid gland, **particularly lymphocytic thyroiditis** and idiopathic follicular collapse. Less common causes of hypothyroidism include bilateral non-functional thyroid cell neoplasms and severe iodine-deficient goitre. Hypothyroidism due to pituitary gland or hypothalamic lesions which prevent the release of either TSH or thyrotropin-releasing hormone (TRH) is seen sometimes in the **dog.** In these cases the thyroid is reduced in size and composed of colloid-distended follicles lined by flattened follicular cells.

Many functional disturbances are associated with hypothyroidism. These are due to decreased basal metabolic rate. A gain in body weight without any change in appetite occurs in some hypothyroid dogs. Thinning of the hair coat is usually associated with a bilaterally symmetrical alopecia (loss of hair). Affected areas include tail and cervical area.

Hyperkeratosis (thickening of the outer horny layer of the skin) is a constant finding in hypothyroidism. When severe, it occurs as circular scaling patches resembling **seborrhoea** (excessive secretion of sebum, oily secretion of sebaceous glands). **Microscopically,** hyperkeratosis involves the external root sheath. This causes follicular keratosis. **Hyperpigmentation** in areas of alopecia, such as dorsal aspect of the nose and distal portion of the tail, occurs in many **dogs** with hypothyroidism. **Myxoedema** occurs and is the result of accumulation of **mucins** (neutral and acid mucopolysaccharides combined with protein) in the dermis and subcutis. These substances bind large amounts of water, which results in marked thickening of the skin. **Microscopically,** mucins appear as granular or fibrillar material in H & E-stained sections.

Abnormalities in reproduction include lack of libido, reduction in sperm count, abnormal or absent oestrus cycles, and reduced conception rates.

Hypothyroidism in dogs is accompanied by decreased circulating **thyroid hormone concentrations** and decreased iodine uptake by the thyroid gland. The **serum cholesterol concentration** is usually increased greatly (300 to 900 mg/dl) in many hypothyroid dogs (normal serum cholesterol is 40 to 80 mg/dl). **Marked hypercholesterolaemia** in severe hypothyroidism causes a number of secondary lesions. These include atherosclerosis, hepatomegaly, and glomerular and corneal lipidosis. **Atherosclerosis** of coronary and cerebral vessels develops in **dogs** that have severe hypothyroidism and long-standing hyperlipidaemia.

Thyroid (Parafollicular) Cells

Thyroid gland also has a **second endocrine cell population** known as **'parafollicular cells'** or **'C cells'**. They secrete hormone **calcitonin** and are situated either in the follicular wall within the basement membrane between follicular cells, or as small groups of cells close to inter-follicular capillaries between follicles. **A characteristic feature** of C cells is the presence of numerous small, membrane-limited **secretory granules in their cytoplasm.** Immunocytochemical techniques have localized **calcitonin activity of C cells in these secretory granules.**

Calcitonin is a polypeptide hormone. The calcium ion concentration in plasma and extracellular fluids is the main stimulus for the secretion of calcitonin by C cells. The rate of secretion of calcitonin is greatly increased in response to increased blood calcium concentrations.

C cells store great amounts of **calcitonin** in their cytoplasm. In response to

hypercalcaemia the hormone is released rapidly from C cells into inter-follicular capillaries (Fig. 27). **Hyperplasia of C cells** occurs in response to long-term hypercalcaemia. When blood calcium concentration is reduced, the stimulus for calcitonin secretion is decreased, and numerous secretory granules accumulate in the cytoplasm of C cells (Fig. 27). Calcitonin exerts its function by interacting with target cells located in bone and kidneys. The actions of parathyroid hormone and calcitonin are antagonistic on bone resorption but synergistic in decreasing the renal tubular reabsorption of phosphorus.

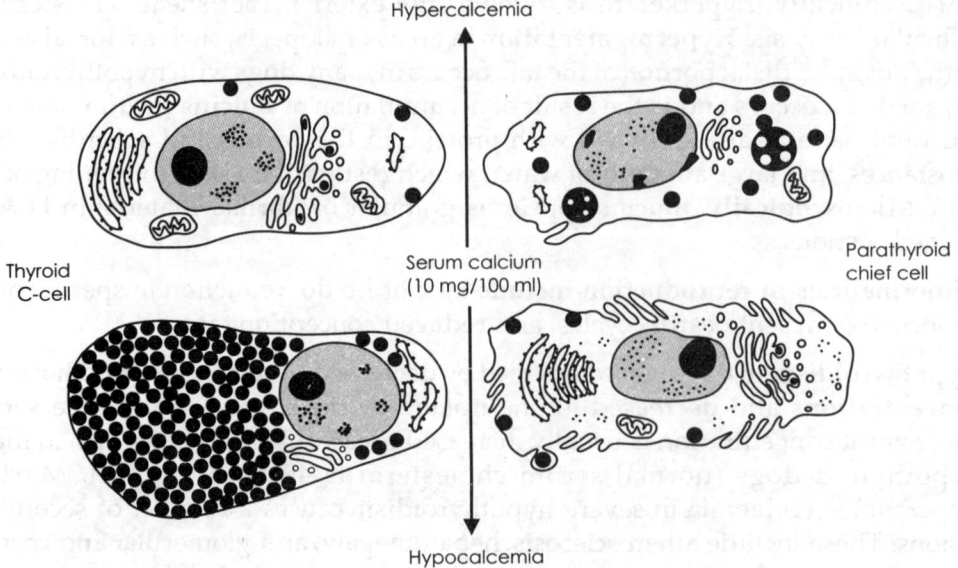

Fig. 27. Response of thyroid C cells and parathyroid chief cells to hypercalcaemia and hypocalcaemia. Thyroid C cells accumulate secretory granules in response to hypocalcaemia, but parathyroid chief cells are degranulated. However, they have an increased development of synthetic and secretory organelles. **In response to hypercalcaemia,** C cells are degranulated, and parathyroid chief cells are mainly in the inactive stage of the secretory cycle.

Thyroid C Cell Neoplasms

Neoplasms derived from C cells of the thyroid gland are usually seen in **adult to aged bulls,** but not in cows fed similar diets. Sometimes they are also seen in **horses** and **dogs,** but are rare in other species. A high percentage of **aged bulls** fed calcium-rich diets develop C cell neoplasms (30%) or hyperplasia of C cells (15% to 20%). **The incidence of C cell neoplasms increases with advancing age in bulls** and has been associated with the development of increased vertebral bone density.

Adenomas

C cell adenomas occur as **single or multiple** grey to yellowish-brown **nodules in one or both thyroid lobes. Adenomas are smaller** (1 to 3 cm in diameter) **than carcinomas** and are separated from the adjacent compressed thyroid gland parenchyma by a thin, fibrous connective tissue capsule. Larger C cell adenomas replace most of the thyroid lobe, but a rim of dark, brown-red thyroid gland is usually present on one side. **Microscopically,** thyroid C cell adenoma is an expanding mass of cells larger than a colloid-distorted follicle. The adenoma is well circumscribed or partially encapsulated, and adjacent follicles are compressed to varying degrees. The neoplastic cells are well differentiated and have palely eosinophilic cytoplasm.

Carcinomas

Thyroid C cell carcinomas cause extensive multinodular enlargement of one or both thyroid lobes and can replace the entire thyroid gland. Thyroid C cell neoplasms in **bulls, other animal species,** and **human beings** are **firm. Multiple metastases** occur to the cranial cervical lymph nodes. These are usually large and have areas of necrosis and haemorrhage. **Pulmonary metastases** appear as yellowish-brown nodules, but are rare. C cell carcinomas are composed of neoplastic cells that are more pleomorphic than cells of C cell adenomas. The carcinomatous cells are poorly differentiated; polyhedral to spindle shaped, and have palely eosinophilic, finely granular, indistinct cytoplasm. **Both adenomas and carcinomas have deposits of amyloid.**

The aetiology of C cell neoplasms is unknown. However, chronic stimulation of C cells by **large concentrations of calcium** absorbed from the digestive tract can be responsible for their high incidence. A significant decrease in the incidence of C cell neoplasms occurs when the excessive calcium intake of **bulls** is reduced. **Cows** fed similar rations rarely develop proliferative lesions of C cells because of the greater physiological requirements of pregnancy and lactation.

The source of the localized amyloid deposits in the thyroid C cell neoplasms is uncertain. However, the amyloid appears to be produced by the neoplastic cells, and amyloid deposits are not present in other organs. Amyloid deposition always occurs in medullary thyroid carcinoma in human beings, and amyloid has been reported also in certain other endocrine neoplasms. Amyloid in C cell neoplasm is present between neoplastic cells, around vessels, and in the interstitium. **Amyloid has been observed in bulls, horses, and dogs,** but in varying amounts from case to case. Chemical differences exist between amyloid fibrils of immunoglobulin origin and those produced by endocrine neoplasms.

Parathyroid Glands

Parathyroid glands consist of two pairs of glands situated in the cranial cervical region. The **dog** and **cat** have both the external and internal parathyroid glands located near the thyroid gland. Other animal species, such as the **pig**, have only a single pair of parathyroid glands. In **cattle** and **sheep**, the larger external parathyroid gland is located away from the thyroid gland. The smaller internal parathyroid glands are situated on the dorsal surface of the thyroid gland. In **horses**, the larger (lower) parathyroid gland is located away from the thyroid gland, while the smaller (upper) parathyroid gland is situated near the thyroid gland.

The parathyroid glands consist of secretory cell that produces one hormone. Parathyroid glands are mainly composed of chief cells in different stages of secretory activity, or in transition to oxyphilic cells in certain species. Chief cells secrete **parathyroid hormone (PTH)**. Parathyroid glands have a unique feedback control system based mainly on the concentration of calcium ion in the blood. Calcium ion concentration controls not only the rate of biosynthesis and secretion of PTH, but also other metabolic and intracellular degradative processes within chief cells. **PTH is the main hormone involved in the regulation of blood calcium concentration in mammals.** It does this by directly influencing the function of target cells in **bone** and **kidneys** and indirectly acting in the **intestine** to maintain sufficient plasma calcium concentration. The overall action of PTH on **bone** is to mobilize calcium into extracellular fluids.

PTH has a rapid and direct effect on renal tubular function. The ability of PTH to increase the renal absorption of calcium is important in the maintenance of calcium homeostasis. **Calcitonin** (hormone secreted by C cells of the thyroid gland) **and PTH** act together and provide a double negative feedback control mechanism to maintain within narrow limits the concentration of calcium in extracellular fluids. **The third major hormone involved in the regulation of calcium metabolism is cholecalciferol or vitamin D3.**

Developmental Disturbances

Parathyroid Cysts

Small cysts within the parenchyma of the parathyroid glands usually occur in **dogs**, but only rarely in other animal species. **Parathyroid gland cysts** are usually multiloculated and are filled with a densely eosinophilic proteinic material. These cysts develop from persistent and dilated remnants of the duct that connect the parathyroid and thymic primordia during embryonic development.

Degenerative Lesions of Parathyroid Chief Cells

Multinucleated Syncytial Cells

Multinucleated syncytial giant cells can develop in parathyroid glands of **dogs** and **cats**. These cells are usually more numerous near the periphery of the parathyroid glands. However, large numbers can be present in the more central portions of some glands. These cells are formed by the fusion of the cytoplasm of adjacent chief cells. The cytoplasm is densely eosinophilic and homogeneous. The nuclei are oval, smaller and more hyperchromatic than the adjacent chief cells. The **aetiology** and **functional significance** of syncytial chief cells is uncertain. **Usually they are incidental findings.**

Inflammatory Lesions and Hypoparathyroidism

Lymphocytic Parathyroiditis and Hypoparathyroidism

In hypoparathyroidism, the parathyroid glands either secrete subnormal amounts of PTH, or the hormone secreted is unable to interact with target cells. **Hypoparathyroidism has been described in dogs,** but occurs only rarely in other animal species. **In dogs,** hypoparathyroidism is usually caused by **diffuse lymphocytic parathyroiditis** and is characterized by **extensive degeneration of chief cells** and **replacement fibrosis.** With time, parathyroid gland is completely replaced by lymphocytes, fibroblasts, and neocapillaries with only a few viable chief cells.

Lymphocytic parathyroiditis develops by an immune-mediated mechanism. Other rare causes of hypoparathyroidism include invasion and destruction of parathyroid glands by primary or metastatic neoplasms and trophic atrophy of parathyroid glands occurring from hypercalcaemia.

The **functional disturbances and clinical signs of hypoparathyroidism** are the result of increased neuromuscular excitability and tetany. Because of the lack of PTH, bone resorption is decreased and blood calcium concentration decrease gradually to 4 to 6 mg/dl. **Affected animals** are restless, nervous, ataxic (have muscular coordination), weak and have intermittent tremors of muscle groups. Tremors can progress to generalized tetany and convulsive seizures. At the same time, blood phosphorus concentrations are increased because of increased renal tubular reabsorption.

Hyperplasia of Chief Cells

Hyperparathyroidism Secondary to Nutritional Imbalances

Nutritional hyperparathyroidism occurs usually in **cats, dogs,** and **horses.** The increased secretion of parathyroid hormone is a compensatory mechanism caused by nutritional imbalances. Such imbalances occur in diets low in calcium or diets with an increase of phosphorus and normal or low content of calcium. **The result is hypocalcaemia which stimulates parathyroid glands.** Blood phosphorus concentration, when increased, contributes indirectly to parathyroid stimulation by decreasing blood calcium.

In response to the diet-induced hypocalcaemia, chief cells undergo hypertrophy and hyperplasia. The organelles involved in protein synthesis (endoplasmic reticulum) and packaging of secretory products (Golgi apparatus) are well developed.

The most common nutritional imbalance causing **hyperparathyroidism in horses** is the ingestion of excessive amounts of phosphorus. **Hyperphosphataemia** stimulates parathyroid gland indirectly by lowering blood calcium. A diet deficient in calcium fails to supply the daily calcium requirement, and **hypocalcaemia** develops. Changes in concentrations of calcium and phosphorus in urine are useful in the **clinical diagnosis** of nutritional secondary **hyperparathyroidism in horse** than changes in blood concentrations of these minerals.

Hyperparathyroidism Due to Renal Disease

Hyperparathyroidism as a complication of chronic renal failure is accompanied by excessive production of parathyroid hormone in response to hypocalcaemia. When the renal disease is severe and reduces glomerular filtration rate, phosphorus is retained and **hyperphosphataemia** develops. The increased blood phosphorus concentration causes parathyroid stimulation by decreasing blood calcium. Chronic renal disease damages the production of vitamin D3 by the kidneys, and thereby, decreases intestinal calcium transport and increases mobilization of calcium from the skeleton. All parathyroid glands undergo marked chief cell hyperplasia, and bones develop varying degrees of generalized fibrous osteodystrophy.

Acute Parathyroid Stimulation:

Hypocalcaemia Associated with Parturition

Milk fever (parturient paresis) in dairy cattle is complex metabolic disease characterized by the development of severe **hypocalcaemia** and **hypophosphataemia** near the time of parturition and the initiation of lactation. The serum calcium concentration decreases to less than 50% of normal in spite of an increased secretion of PTH by cow's parathyroid gland.

The composition of the diet fed to dairy cows is an important factor in the pathogenesis of milk fever. Diets with **excessive calcium** increase incidence of the disease. On the other hand, **diets low in calcium** or diets supplemented with therapeutic doses of vitamin D reduce the incidence of parturient hypocalcaemia. Calcium homeostasis in pregnant cows fed an excessive calcium diet is maintained by intestinal calcium absorption (Fig. 28). This greater dependence on intestinal absorption rather than on PTH-stimulated bone resorption is an important factor in the development of severe **hypocalcaemia** near parturition in **cows** fed excessive calcium prepartal (before parturition) diets. Hypocalcaemia, in turn, stimulates release of **calcitonin hormone** into the circulation from thyroid C cells. The actions of PTH and calcitonin are antagonistic to each other in respect of bone resorption. An increased secretion of calcitonin prepartum prevents secretion of PTH to mobilize calcium from skeletal reserves and maintain blood calcium concentration

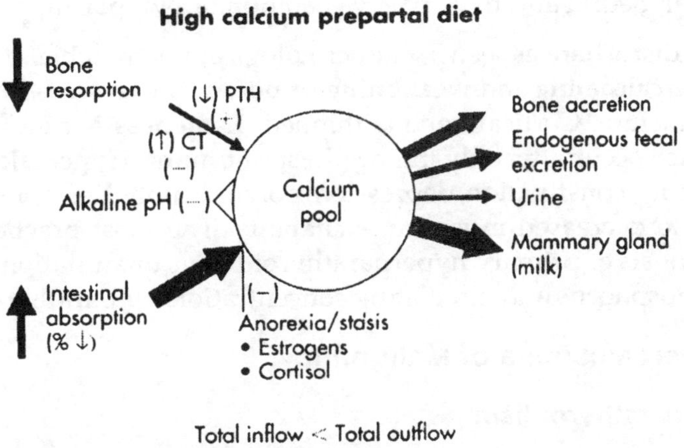

High calcium prepartal diet

Bone resorption

(↓) PTH (+)

(↑) CT (−)

Alkaline pH (−)

Intestinal absorption (% ↓)

Calcium pool

(−)

Anorexia/stasis
• Estrogens
• Cortisol

Bone accretion

Endogenous fecal excretion

Urine

Mammary gland (milk)

Total inflow < Total outflow

Fig. 28. Calcium homeostasis in cows fed a high-calcium prepartal diet. The homeostasis depends mainly on intestinal calcium absorption. The rate of bone resorption is low and parathyroid glands are inactive. Anorexia and gastrointestinal stasis, which usually occur near parturition, interrupt the major inflow into the extracellular fluid calcium pool. Outflow of calcium with the onset of lactation exceeds the rate of inflow into the calcium pool, **and the cows develop a progressive hypocalcaemia and paresis.**

during the critical period near parturition. **This leads to parturient hypocalcaemia (milk fever).** In milk fever, the thyroid content of calcitonin is reduced, many C cells are degranulated, and plasma concentrations of calcitonin are increased in **cows** before the development of profound hypocalcaemia.

Functional Neoplasms of Chief Cells:

Primary Hyperparathyroidism

Adenomas and carcinomas of parathyroid glands usually secrete excessive amounts of parathyroid hormone (PTH). This produces a syndrome of primary hyperparathyroidism. An increased secretion of PTH increases osteolytic and osteoclastic bone resorption. Mineral is removed from the skeleton at an increased rate, and bone is replaced by immature fibrous connective tissue. The **lesions of fibrous osteodystrophy** are generalized throughout the skeletal, but are more in certain areas such as maxilla, mandible, and sub-periosteal areas of long bones.

Adenomas of parathyroid glands occur in older animals, particularly dogs, but parathyroid carcinomas are uncommon. Chief cell adenomas usually cause enlargement of a single parathyroid gland which is grossly light brown to red. Parathyroid adenomas are encapsulated and sharply demarcated from the adjacent thyroid gland.

Parathyroid gland adenomas are composed of small groups of chief cells enclosed by vascular connective tissue septa which have many capillaries. The **chief cells**

are round to polyhedral and have palely eosinophilic cytoplasm.

The **functional disturbances** seen in endocrinologically active chief cells neoplasms are due to **hypercalcaemia** and **weakening of bones** by excessive PTH-stimulated resorption of calcium. Cortical bone is thinned. **Lameness** is due to fractures of long bones which occur after only minor physical trauma. **Hypercalcaemia causes** anorexia, vomiting, constipation, depression, polyuria, polydipsia, and generalized weakness due to decreased muscular excitability. The most practical laboratory test in the **diagnosis** of primary hyperparathyroidism is quantitation of total blood calcium and phosphorus and circulating concentrations of parathyroid hormone.

Humoral Hypercalcaemia of Malignancy:

Pseudo-hyperparathyroidism

Hypercalcaemia is a common disorder in animals. It has many causes. **The most common form is cancer-associated hypercalcaemia.** Neoplasms increase serum calcium by three mechanisms: (1) humoral hypercalcaemia of malignancy (HHM), (2) hypercalcaemia caused by metastases and solid neoplasms to bone, and (3) haematological malignancies. **Hypercalcaemia** occurs from an imbalance of calcium released from bones, calcium excreted by the kidneys, or calcium absorbed from the intestinal tract.

The clinical signs of hypercalcaemia are similar regardless of the underlying cause. They depend on the rapidity of onset of increased concentrations of serum ionized calcium. Metabolic acidosis increases the severity of clinical signs since it causes an increase in the ionized fraction of serum calcium. Increased serum ionized calcium induces clinical signs of gastrointestinal, neuromuscular, cardiovascular, and renal systems.

A **syndrome of HHM** in aged, mainly **female dogs** with adenocarcinomas of apocrine glands of the anal sac has been described. The dogs have persistent hypercalcaemia and hypophosphataemia, both of which return to normal following surgical excision of the neoplasm. **Clinical signs** include generalized muscular weakness, anorexia, vomiting, bradycardia depression, polyuria, and polydipsia. **These signs are due to severe hypercalcaemia.** Renal calcification has been detected microscopically in about 90% of dogs with HHM and anal sac apocrine gland adenocarcinomas.

Hypercalcaemia Associated with Lymphosarcoma

Lymphosarcoma is the most common neoplasm associated with **hypercalcaemia in dogs** and **cats.** The hypercalcaemia occurs from the production by neoplastic cells of humoral substances, or from physical disruption of trabecular bone by lymphosarcoma in bone marrow, or from both mechanisms.

Neoplasms Metastatic to Bone

Neoplasms that metastasize to bone and grow locally can produce **hypercalcaemia** by inducing local bone resorption. **This is not common in animals, but is an important cause of cancer-associated hypercalcaemia in human beings,** particularly patients with breast and lung carcinomas.

Pancreatic Islets

The **endocrine function of pancreas** is performed by small groups of cells ('islets of Langerhans'). These are completely surrounded by acinar (exocrine) cells which produce digestive enzymes.

The **pancreatic islets** contain many types of cells. **Beta cells,** the predominant secretory cells, biosynthesize insulin but co-secrete amyloid polypeptide. **F cells** or **PP cells** secrete pancreatic polypeptide. The glucagon-secreting **alpha cells** are less numerous.

The major stimulus for the release of insulin from beta cells is glucose. The main function of insulin is to stimulate anabolic reactions involving carbohydrates, fats, proteins, and nucleic acids. Hepatocytes, adipose cells, and muscles are three target sites for insulin. In general, **insulin increases the transfer of glucose** and certain other monosaccharides, some amino acids and fatty acids, and potassium and magnesium ions across the plasma membrane of target cells. It also increases glucose oxidation and glycogenesis, and stimulates lipogenesis and formation of ATP, DNA, and RNA. Insulin also decreases the rate of lipolysis, proteolysis, and gluconeogenesis.

Glucagon is a hormone which stimulates **energy release** from target cells and is secreted in response to a **reduction in blood glucose concentration.** It mobilizes stores of energy-yielding nutrients by increasing glycogenolysis, gluconeogenesis, and lipolysis. **Thus, it increases the blood concentration of glucose. Insulin and glucagon** act together to **maintain concentration of glucose** in extracellular fluids within narrow limits. **Glucagon** controls glucose influx into the extracellular space from the liver cells, and **insulin** controls the glucose efflux from the extracellular space into such insulin-sensitive tissues as adipose cells, muscle, and hepatocytes.

Hypofunction: Diabetes Mellitus

Diabetes is a metabolic disorder. It occurs from **decreased availability of insulin** for the normal function of many cells of the body. In some cases, **increased concentration of glucagon** contributes to the development of persistent hyperglycaemia. **Deficiency of insulin** could be due to degenerative changes in beta cells of the pancreatic islets, reduced effectiveness of the hormone due to the formation of anti-insulin antibodies or inactive complexes, damage to beta cells from immune-mediated islet toxicity, or inappropriate secretion of hormones by neoplasms in other endocrine organs.

Diabetes mellitus is a common disease in dogs. Most cases of spontaneous diabetes occur in **mature dogs** and they are **about twice more common in females than in males.** An increased incidence of diabetes has been observed in certain **small breeds of dogs,** but all breeds of dogs can be affected.

Pathogenesis

In the pathogenesis of diabetes mellitus, **several factors are responsible** for the decreased availability of insulin. The destruction of islets following severe pancreatitis or the selective degeneration of islet cells **are the most common causes in the animals. In dogs,** pancreatic islets are usually destroyed because of inflammation of the exocrine pancreas. **Chronic relapsing pancreatitis** with loss of both exocrine and endocrine cells and replacement by fibrous connective tissue is a common cause of diabetes mellitus. **In these dogs,** pancreas becomes firm, multinodular, and has areas of haemorrhage and necrosis. **In young dogs,** diabetes mellitus is the result of idiopathic atrophy (i.e. cause unknown) of the pancreas, acute pancreatitis with necrosis and haemorrhage, and aplasia of pancreatic islets. Hypoplasia of pancreatic islets has also caused diabetes mellitus in young dogs (2 to 3 months of age).

Cats with diabetes mellitus have **specific degenerative lesions** localized selectively in the islets of Langerhans, whereas the rest of the pancreas is normal. Selective deposition of amyloid in islets, causing degenerative changes in alpha and beta cells, is the most common pancreatic lesion in **cats** with diabetes. Scattered amyloid deposits in pancreatic islets which increase with age occur in the islets of many cats without clinical diabetes mellitus. **Another lesion** in the islets of cats with diabetes mellitus is **hydropic (vacuolar) degeneration of the beta and alpha cells.** The cytoplasm of beta cells is distended with massive accumulation of glycogen particles. **Vacuolar degeneration** with glycogen accumulation in **cats** develops in beta cells in response to long-term over stimulation ('exhaustion') because of peripheral insulin resistance.

Clinical Signs and Lesions

The onset of diabetes is insidious, and the clinical course is usually chronic. The **signs in dogs** include polydipsia, polyuria, increased feed consumption, loss of weight, bilateral cataracts, and weakness.

Diabetic animals have reduced resistance to bacterial and fungal infections, and usually develop chronic or recurrent infection such as suppurative cystitis, prostatitis, bronchopneumonia, and dermatitis. This increased susceptibility to infection is due in part to impaired chemotactic, phagocytic, and microbial functions and decreased adherence of polymorphonuclear leukocytes. Infections of the urinary bladder with glucose-fermenting organisms, such as **Proteus** sp., *Aerobacter aerogenes*, and *Escherichia coli,* cause gas formation in the wall and lumen. Emphysema also develops in the gallbladder wall in some **diabetic dogs.**

Hepatomegaly occurs as a result of **fatty change** and **cirrhosis**. Lipids accumulate in the liver as a result of increased fat mobilization. Individual liver cells are greatly enlarged by multiple droplets of **neutral fat**. If the accumulation of fat is extensive and long-standing, cirrhosis develops. The liver is enlarged, and its surface becomes coarsely nodular because of extensive remodeling of hepatic parenchyma. Individual liver cells degenerate and are replaced by regenerative and hyperplastic nodules and interlobular fibrosis (Fig. 29). **Jaundice** and **bilirubinuria** usually occur in severe cirrhosis.

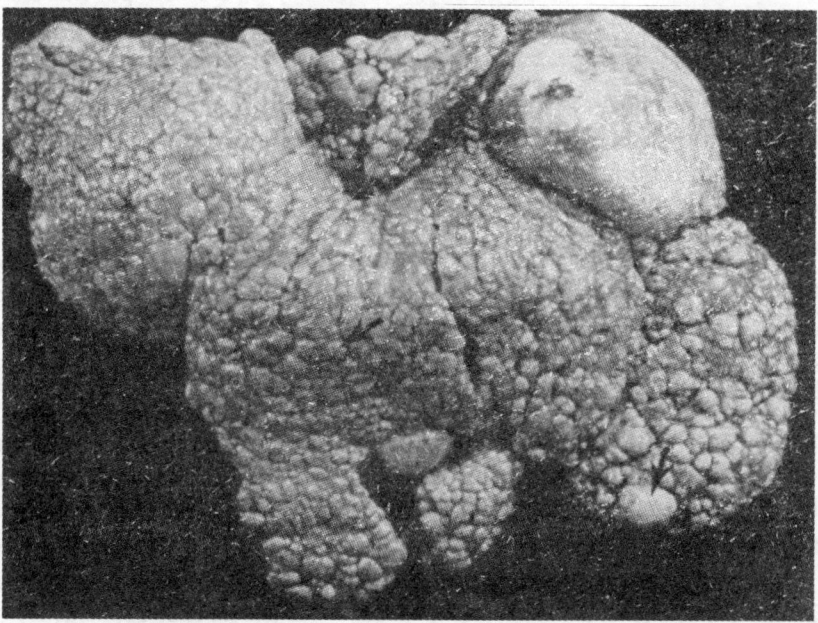

Fig. 29. Liver; dog. Cirrhosis. All lobes of the liver are considerably enlarged, firm, **and have a coarsely nodular surface.** The nodules (arrows) represent areas of regenerative hyperplasia of liver cells.

Cataracts usually develop in dogs with poorly controlled diabetes. Cataract formation is related to the **sorbitol pathway** by which glucose is metabolized. **Glucose** is first converted to sorbitol by the enzyme aldose reductase and afterwards to **fructose** by sorbitol dehydrogenase. These sugar alcohols accumulate in the lens and cause an intracellular accumulation of solute and hypertonicity. The change in the lens consists of swelling and hydropic degeneration of lenticular fibres. With time, disruption of lenticular fibres results in diffuse, often bilateral, opacity of the lens in animals with chronic diabetes mellitus.

Other lesions of diabetes mellitus include chronic renal disease, blindness, and gangrene. These are the result of microangiopathy characterized by thickening of the capillary basement membrane. **Dogs** develop nodular or diffuse glomerulosclerosis. Other renal lesions include accumulation of glycogen in cells of Henle's loop (intra-cytoplasmic) and distal convoluted tubule (intranuclear).

Hyperfunction of Pancreatic Islets

Beta-Cells (Insulin-Secreting) Neoplasms

Neoplasms originating from pancreatic islets are usually **adenomas** and **carcinomas** derived **from beta cells.** These are endocrinologically active and produce functional disturbances. **Beta cell neoplasms** are usually seen in **dogs** between 5 to 12 years of age (mean 9 years). These neoplasms also occur in **older cattle.**

Adenoma of the beta cells ('insulinomas') is usually a single yellow to dark red, spherical, small nodule. They occur as single or less often multiple nodules in one or multiple lobes of the pancreas. A thin layer of fibrous connective tissue separates the adenoma from the adjacent parenchyma.

Carcinomas of the pancreatic islets are more common in dogs than adenomas and are more common in the right (duodenal) lobe of the pancreas. Carcinomas can be differentiated from adenomas by their larger size, multilobular appearance, extensive invasion of adjacent parenchyma and lymph vessels, and metastasis in sites such as regional lymph nodes.

Adenomas are surrounded by a thin capsule of fibrous connective tissue. Numerous connective tissue septa containing small capillaries radiate from the capsule into the neoplasm and divide the neoplasm into small lobules. The **neoplastic cells** are well differentiated, are round to oval and have a palely eosinophilic and finely granular cytoplasm. **Carcinomas are larger than adenomas,** are multilobular, and invade into and through the fibrous capsule of the pancreas. The bands of dense fibrous connective tissue which go through the neoplasm divide the neoplasm into small lobules. The neoplastic cells are well differentiated, are closely packed, but are less uniform in size and shape than cells of adenomas. They are round to polyhedral and have a granular eosinophilic cytoplasm. Mitotic figures are not numerous. Microscopic evidence of clear local tissue invasion is the main feature for the diagnosis of islet cell carcinoma.

Clinical signs seen in functional beta cell neoplasms **are due to excessive insulin secretion and** the development of **severe hypocalcaemia.** The signs are not specific for hyperinsulinism produced by beta cell neoplasms. The clinical signs include weakness, fatigue, after vigorous exercise, generalized muscular, twitching, ataxia, mental confusion, and changes of temperament. The **dogs** are easily agitated have intermittent periods of excitability and restlessness. Periodic convulsive seizures occur later in the disease. The dominance of clinical signs relating to CNS indicates dependence of the brain on the metabolism of glucose for energy. Repeated episodes of severe hypoglycaemia result in the death of neurons and permanent neurological disability with terminal coma **and eventual death.**

Non-Beta (Gastrin-Secreting) Islet Cell Neoplasms

Gastrin-secreting, non-beta islet cell neoplasms of the pancreas have been reported in **human beings, dogs,** and **cats. Gastrin is a hormone** secreted by certain cells of the pyloric glands. It strongly stimulates secretion of gastric acid and pepsin. The hypersecretion of **gastrin** in human beings results in Zollinger-Ellison syndrome consisting of hypersecretion of gastric acid and recurrent peptic ulceration in the gastrointestinal tract. The non-beta islet cell neoplasms derived from ectopic APUD (amine precursor upake decarboxylase) cells in the pancreas produce an excess of gastrin, which is normally secreted by cells of the antral and duodenal mucosa. The incidence of gastrin-secreting pancreatic neoplasms in **dogs** and **cats** is uncertain, but is uncommon compared with insulin-secreting beta cells neoplasms. **Clinical signs in the dog and cat** include anorexia, vomiting of blood-tinged material, intermittent diarrhoea, progressive weight loss, and dehydration.

Animals with Zollinger-Ellison-like syndrome have single or multiple neoplasms in the pancreas. The neoplasms are firm, have increased amounts of fibrous connective tissue, and partial encapsulation, but the neoplasm usually extends into the surrounding pancreas. **Microscopically,** the basic pattern of pancreatic islet cell neoplasms in animals is similar irrespective of whether they are secreting insulin or gastrin.

Gastrin-secreting islet cell neoplasms in dogs invade locally into the adjacent pancreas and usually metastasize to regional lymph nodes and to the liver. These **dogs** have either single or multiple ulcerations in the gastric or duodenal mucosa, or both, and with blood in the lumen.

Other non-beta islet cell neoplasms reported in animals are the glucagon-secreting alpha cell neoplasms. **Glucagonomas** have been reported rarely in **dogs** and are associated with **superficial necrolytic dermatitis.**

Chemoreceptor Organs

Chemoreceptor tissue is present at several places in the body. These include carotid body, aortic bodies, nodose ganglion ofthe vagus nerve, and bodies on the internal jugular vein below the middle ear. The chemoreceptor organs are sensitive barometers of changes in the blood carbon dioxide content, pH, and oxygen tension. This way they help in the regulation of respiration and circulation.

Although chemoreceptor tissue is widely distributed in the body, **neoplasms develop mainly in the aortic and carotid bodies of animals. Aortic body chemodectomas** are seen more commonly in animals than those of the carotid body, but the reverse is true for human beings. These neoplasms develop mainly in **dogs** and rarely in **cats** and **cattle**.

Neoplasms

Neoplasms of Aortic Body

Aortic body neoplasms usually appear as a **single mass or as multiple nodules** near the **base of the heart**. In general, carcinomas are larger than adenomas. Aortic body carcinomas are less common than adenomas in **dogs. Carcinomas** infiltrate the wall of the pulmonary artery and form papillary projections into the lumen or invade through the wall into the lumen of the atria. Although neoplastic cells usually invade blood vessels, metastases to the lungs and liver are uncommon in **dogs** with aortic body carcinomas.

Neoplasms of the aortic bodies in animals are not functional. That is, they do not secrete excess hormone into circulation, but as a space-occupying lesion they can produce a number of functional disturbances. **Larger aortic body adenomas and carcinomas** put pressure on the atria, vena cava, or both and produce signs of cardiac decompensation. More aortic body neoplasms than carotid body neoplasms are benign. Aortic body carcinomas invade locally into the atria, pericardium, and adjacent vessels.

Neoplasms of the Carotid Body

Carotid body neoplasms originate near **bifurcation of the common carotid artery** in the cranial cervical area. They are usually unilateral, only rarely bilateral, and are slow growing. **Adenomas** are firm, white with scattered areas of haemorrhage, and are extremely vascular.

Carotid body carcinomas are larger, more multinodular than adenomas, invade the capsule, and penetrate into the walls and adjacent blood and lymph vessels. Metastasis of carotid body carcinomas can occur to the lungs, lymph nodes, liver, pancreas, and kidneys.

The **microscopic features of chemoreceptor neoplasms ('chemodectomas')** are basically similar whether they are derived from carotid or aortic body. The neoplasm is divided into lobules by branching trabeculae of connective tissue that originate from the fibrous capsule and are further subdivided into nests by fine septa of collagenous and reticulin fibres and small capillaries. Neoplastic cells are usually present along and around small capillaries and are round to polyhedral, closely packed, and have palely eosinophilic, finely granular, often vacuolated cytoplasm.

The **aetiology** of carotid and aortic body neoplasms is unknown. However, a **genetic predisposition** aggravated by chronic hypoxia has been observed in certain breeds of dogs. Carotid bodies of several animals, **including dogs**, have developed **hyperplastic foci** when animals are subjected to the **chronic hypoxia** of high altitudes. Human beings living at high altitudes have 10 times the frequency of chemodectomas as those residing at sea level.

Heart-Base Neoplasms Derived from Ectopic Thyroid Gland Tissue

Adenomas and **carcinomas** derived from **ectopic** thyroid gland account for about 5% to 15% of **'heart-base' neoplasms** in **dogs**. Ectopic thyroid gland neoplasms have a compact cellular (solid) pattern which is difficult to differentiate microscopically from aortic body neoplasms. Cells of ectopic thyroid gland neoplasms are smaller than those of aortic body neoplasms and have more hyperchromatic nuclei and an eosinophilic cytoplasm.

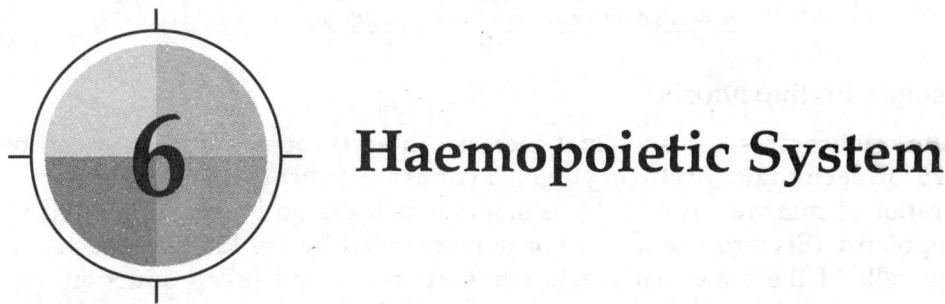

Haemopoietic System

Responses of the Haemopoietic System

Like other organs, bone marrow, lymph nodes, and spleen undergo atrophy, hyperplasia, hypertrophy, and neoplasm.

Atrophy of the bone marrow haemopoietic cells occurs after certain types of injury. Atrophy results in failure of erythropoiesis (**causes anaemia**), granulopoiesis (**causes neutropaenia**), and thrombopoiesis (**causes thrombocytopaenia**). Sometimes, injury to stem cells results in complete failure of haematopoiesis (**causes pancytopaenia,** that is, depression of all the cellular elements of the blood).

Hypertrophy of the bone marrow is extremely rare in animals because haemopoietic tissue is enclosed by bone. **Hyperplasia** of bone marrow haemopoietic tissue occurs after prolonged haemorrhage or haemolysis and bacterial infections. The haemopoietic tissue expands and replaces adipocytes (fat cells); yellow marrow becomes red. **Extra-medullary haemopoiesis** in organs such as liver and spleen usually accompanies hyperplasia of the bone marrow.

The **haemopoietic system** in some species, such as the **cat**, shows a significant incidence of **neoplasia**. **Sarcomas** of bone marrow can be derived from erythrocytic, granulocytic, and plasma cell populations. **Sarcomas of bone marrow have an important feature in that they release neoplastic cells into blood.** Identification of the sarcoma can be made by identifying the leukaemic cells in blood smears.

Erythrocyte Disorders

Erythrocytosis

Erythrocytosis is an increase in erythrocyte number, haemoglobin concentration, and packed cell volume. It may be **relative** or **absolute**.

(i) Relative Erythrocytosis

Relative erythrocytosis occurs from **dehydration** or **haemoconcentration**. Although the haematocrit and erythrocyte numbers are increased, the total erythrocyte mass is normal. Plasma proteins are affected by shifts in fluid volume in the same manner as erythrocytes. Estimation of the haematocrit or packed cell volume and plasma proteins gives some assessment of the degree of dehydration.

(ii) Absolute Erythrocytosis

Absolute erythrocytosis is an actual increase in erythrocyte number. It can be **primary** or **secondary erythrocytosis**. **Primary erythrocytosis** occurs from proliferation of marrow erythroid precursors which are no longer influenced by **erythropoietin**. (Erythropoietin is a hormone secreted by the kidney, which acts on stem cells of the bone marrow to stimulate red blood cell production, i.e., erythropoiesis). Although primary erythrocytosis is uncommon, it has been described in **dogs** and **cats**. Secondary erythrocytosis results from excessive production of erythropoietin. This occurs in response to hypoxaemia (deficient oxygenation in blood). **Secondary erythrocytosis** has been described in **older dogs**. The **clinical signs** of secondary erythrocytosis include cyanotic oral mucous membranes and depression. The increased viscosity of the blood causes impaired blood flow, cyanosis, and a tendency for thrombosis. Postmortem findings include generalized congestion, thrombosis of major vessels, and hyperplastic bone marrow.

Anaemia

Mechanisms of Anaemia

Anaemia is a reduction in the number of erythrocytes in an animal for that particular age, species, breed, and geographic location. Anaemia is an important indicator of underlying disease and should be investigated as a routine. Whether the **anaemia** is **regenerative** or **non-regenerative** depends on the presence or absence of compensatory erythropoiesis. **Regenerative anaemias** occur from haemorrhage or haemolysis, which is followed by stimulation of the bone marrow with release of immature erythrocytes. A blood film contains large **immature erythrocytes** that vary in size (**anisocytosis**). The immature erythrocytes stain blue (**polychromasia**). Polychromasia is a most useful indicator of compensatory erythropoiesis. Additional morphological indicators of rapid erythropoiesis include metarubricytes and rubricytes, and in **ruminants, basophilic stippling** (see Table 9). Incubation of blood with supravital stains, such as new methylene blue, causes aggregation of mitochondria, ribosomes, and remnants of the Golgi bodies in immature erythrocytes into the blue strands characteristic of reticulocytes. Reticulocytes appear in the blood within 2 to 3 days after haemorrhage or haemolysis. Evaluation of anaemia in **horses** is complicated because the **horse** does not release reticulocytes from the bone marrow.

1. Regenerative Anaemia

After finding out that anaemia is regenerative, that is, the result of erythrocyte loss, it is necessary to differentiate anaemia due to haemorrhage from that caused by haemolysis. However, such a differentiation is usually difficult. When haemorrhage has taken place within 36 to 48 hours, **hypoproteinaemia** occurs at the same time with the anaemia. This is because as the fluid enters the vascular

Table 9. Nomenclature of erythrocyte morphology

Term	Description
Acanthocyte	Erythrocyte with projections of variable length at different intervals around the cell
Basophilic stippling	Punctate (marked with dots) precipitate in cytoplasm
Codocytes (target cells)	Leptocytes with a dense, round, central concentration of haemoglobin
Discocyte	Normal biconcave disc. Degree of central pallor varies with species
Eccentrocyte	Haemoglobin displaced to one side of cell
Echinocyte	Spiculated erythrocyte with short, equally spaced projections over entire surface
Heinz bodies	Round, pale structures on the internal surface of themembrane, stain prominently with new methylene blue. They may project from the surface and when numerous may be free in the plasma
Keratocyte	Half-moon shape with spicules
Leptocyte	Thin erythrocyte with increased central pallor and dense peripheral haemoglobin
Macrocyte	Large erythrocyte
Microcyte	Small erythrocyte
Nuclear remnant	Small, single, black-staining, round inclusion in various locations within erythrocyte
Poikilocyte	Non-specific term for abnormally shaped erythrocyte
Polychromasia	Diffuse blue erythrocytes on Wright-Giemsa stains
Reticulocyte	Erythrocyte containing precipitated strands of RNA with supravital stains
Schizocytes	Small, irregular erythrocyte fragment that may have two or three pointed extremities
Spherocyte	Erythrocyte that assumes a spherical shape. Small, dense erythrocyte lacking central pallor (paleness), and therefore only seen in those species whose erythrocytes normally have central pallor, e.g., **dogs**
Spheroechinocyte	Spiculated spherocyte. Short, spiny projections around periphery

compartment to maintain blood pressure, the dilution that causes anaemia also causes hypoproteinaemia. **Detection of haemolysis may also be difficult.** Icteric mucous membranes, and bilirubin and haemoglobin in plasma and urine indicate haemolysis. Bilirubinuria is a more constant finding.

2. Haemorrhagic Anaemias

An important result of **chronic haemorrhage** is the depletion of iron stores which results in impaired erythropoiesis. This can occur in **parasitic diseases** such as **bovine pediculosis**, severe flea infestations of **puppies** and **kittens**, and **hookworms in puppies**. Chronic immune-mediated thrombocytopaenia in **dogs** and gastrointestinal neoplasms in **older animals** may also cause iron deficiency due to chronic extra-corporeal haemorrhage (i.e. occurring outside the body).

3. Haemolytic Anaemias

Most haemolytic aneamias in animals occur after injury to erythrocytes by infectious agents, antibodies, or strong oxidizing agents. Inherited haemolytic anaemias are less common and are due to an intracellular defect confined to a single protein. These anaemias in animals can result from abnormalities in haeme synthesis, membrane skeletal proteins, and glycolytic enzymes. Their severity varies depending on the abnormal protein and the location of the abnormality within the molecule.

(i) Intracellular Defects

In animals, inherited mutations in enzymes involved in haeme synthesis occur and produce accumulations of precursor molecules. **Congenital erythropoietic porphyria,** transmitted as an autosomal recessive trait, occurs in **cattle,** and is characterized by **red-brown discoloration of teeth, bones, and urine** due to accumulation of **porphyrins.** Because of the circulation of photodynamic porphyrins in blood, these animals have lesions of **photosensitization** in the non-pigmented skin and **haemolytic anaemia.** All affected tissues, including erythrocytes, show fluorescence with ultraviolet light. The premature **destruction of** developing and mature **erythrocytes** is caused by the accumulation of excess of **porphyrins. Bovine erythropoietic protoporphyria** is an inherited disorder of haeme synthetase, a terminal enzyme of the haeme synthetic pathway. This causes an accumulation of **protoporphyrins** in tissues and erythrocytes. **Photosensitivity** is the only clinical sign of the disease. There is no discoloration of the teeth and bone or anaemia. A congenital porphyria has been described in **cats,** and resembles congenital erythropoietic porphyria in **cattle.** These **cats** have brown teeth, photosensitization, and haemolytic anaemia.

Inherited disorders of the erythrocyte membrane skeleton are rare in animals, in contrast to human beings. A disorder similar to **hereditary spherocytosis** in human beings occurs in **cattle.**

Inherited glycolytic enzyme abnormalities in erythrocytes occur in animals. Pyruvate kinase deficiency in dogs and cats causes severe haemolytic anaemia with marked reticulocytosis. Affected dogs die at 3 to 5 years of age because of impaired erythropoiesis and liver disease resulting from haemochromatosis. Phosphofructokinase (PFK) deficiency has also been described in dogs. Affected dogs have mild to moderate haemolytic anaemia with increased numbers of reticulocytes. The disease is characterized by lethargy, fever, and pallor of mucous membranes. PFK-deficient erythrocytes are sensitive to changes in pH and are prone to haemolysis during periods of exercise, when panting results in alkalaemia (i.e. increased alkalinity of blood).

Most haemolytic anaemias in animals are caused by partial or complete phagocytosis of erythrocytes by monocytes of the mononuclear phagocyte system. This mechanism has been called extravascular haemolysis, in contrast to intravascular haemolysis in which erythrocyte lysis occurs within the blood vessels. Partial phagocytosis is important. In this, the erythrocyte loses a portion of its membrane and has a decreased surface area relative to its value. This change in shape from disk-to-sphere results in decreased deformability of the cells (i.e. decreased ability of erythrocyte to change shape when passing through narrow spaces, such as sinusoids and capillaries). Erythrocyte must be extremely flexible to travel through the splenic red pulp and sinusoidal walls. Spherocytes therefore get retained in the spleen along with macrophages with risk of further injury and eventual destruction.

Erythrocyte-macrophage interaction with spherocyte formation is important for the destruction of aged erythrocytes. This interaction is mediated by antibody fixation to erythrocyte membrane proteins, which become exposed as the cells age. Following erythrophagocytosis, the enzymes within phagolysosome dissolve the erythrocytes and haemoglobin is degraded. This releases bilirubin and iron from the porphyrin part of the molecule. The bilirubin is transported in the plasma combined with albumin to the liver. The iron is bound to plasma transferrin and transported to the marrow, where it is taken up by receptors in red cell precursors.

In intravascular erythrocyte lysis, haemoglobin released into the plasma is immediately bound to haptoglobin, its main transport protein. The haemoglobin-haptoglobin complex is then removed by hepatocytes and the haemoglobin is degraded. Haemoglobinuria an important indicator of intravascular haemolysis, is seen only when haptoglobin binding capacity is exceeded.

(ii) Infectious Causes

Infectious agents which cause haemolytic anaemia include viruses, bacteria, rickettsiae, and protozoa. Mechanisms of erythrocyte destruction by some of these agents involve antibody fixation on the erythrocyte membrane and then phagocytosis by macrophages.

Viral Infection

Equine Infectious Anaemia

Equine infectious anaemia is a disease of **horses, mules,** and **donkeys,** caused by an arthropod-borne **retrovirus. Horses may die of anaemia** during the viraemia or recover to undergo subsequent episodes of viraemia and anaemia. The **virus replicates in macrophages** and possibly other cells, which release large amounts of virus into the extracellular fluid.Each subsequent haemolytic crisis is caused by **a new antigenic variant of the virus.** Haemolysis is believed to be immune mediated. This is because C3 component is present on erythrocytes following adsorption of virus, antibody fixation and complement activation, which cause erythrophagocytosis.

During the viraemic phase, horses are depressed and have fever, jaundice, dependent pitting oedema, and pallor (paleness) of mucous membranes. Petechiae are usually present on the ventral surface of the tongue and conjunctivae. **Haemograms** show greatly reduced erythrocyte numbers and haematocrit as low as 0.10 L/L (10%). There is usually **bilirubinaemia.** The accompanying **leukopaenia** is caused by neutropaenia and a marginal lymphopaenia. Monocytes sometimes contain erythrocytes. **Thrombocytopaenia** (decrease in the number of platelets in blood) is seen within 1 or 2 days of infection, but its mechanism is unclear. At this stage **bone marrow** has marked erythroid hyperplasia, but magakaryocytes are not increased. This indicates that thrombocytopaenia, in part, is due to impaired thrombopoiesis. As the disease progresses, there is accumulation of haemosiderin-laden macrophages and plasma cells in the bone marrow and spleen. **Diagnosis** of equine infectious anaemia is made by **agar-gel immunodiffusion test,** in which a precipitin line develops in the presence of serum antibody to tissue culture-derived antigen.

Animals dying during haemolysis have jaundice, anaemia, and widespread haemorrhages. In more chronic cases, emaciated animals have serous atrophy of fat. The spleen and liver are enlarged, dark and swollen, and they and other organs have sub-capsular haemorrhages (Fig. 30). Petechiae are seen under the renal capsule and throughout cortex and medulla. The bone narrow is dark red due to replacement of fat by haemopoietic tissue. **Microscopic changes** are most significant in the **spleen, liver, and bone marrow.** Haemosiderin-laden macrophages in the spleen persist for months to years. Kupffer cell hyperplasia having haemosiderin and periportal infiltrations of lymphocytes are the most important changes in the liver. In most animals, the bone marrow is cellular because of the replacement of fat by intense erythropoiesis Granulocytes are less numerous and plasma cells are increased. As in the spleen, haemosiderin-laden macrophages are present in large numbers in chronic cases.

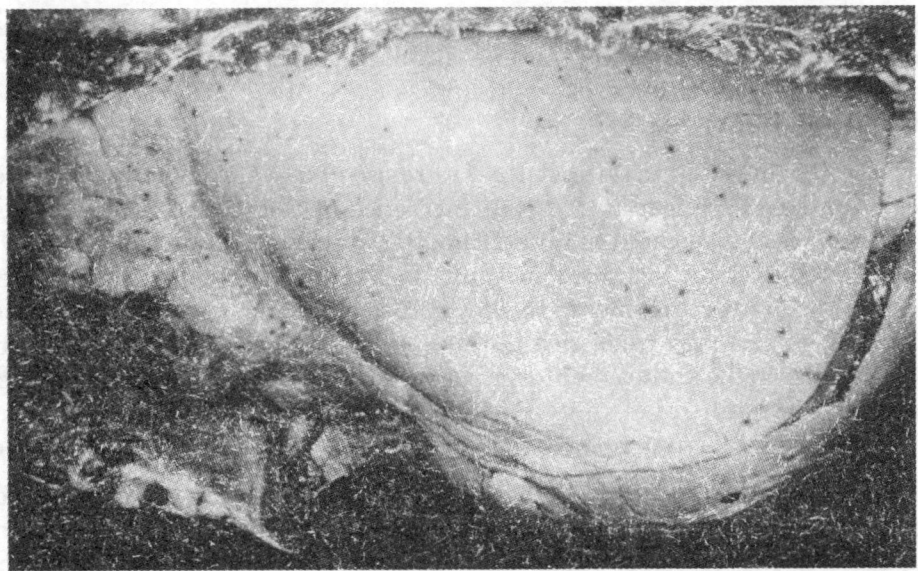

Fig. 30. Lung; horse. Equine infectious anaemia. Focal haemorrhages are visible beneath the visceral pleura.

Bacterial Infection

Leptospirosis

Leptospirosis is a **disease of domestic animals, rodents, and human beings** caused by serovars (serotypes) of *Leptospira interrogans*. Leptospira may survive for months in moist soil and stagnant water. Leptospira are best seen by dark-field microscopy of fluids, in which they appear as delicate motile spirilla.

Leptospira are not highly host specific. Therefore, several serovars may cause disease in several different species. In species that act as carriers, organisms persist in the **kidneys** or genital tract as a reservoir for contamination of the environment by urine and discharges following abortion. There is a lot of overlapping in clinical signs and laboratory and postmortem findings in the disease caused by different serovars in different animals.

Infection occurs through the skin and mucosal surfaces and is followed by **leptospiraemia.** Organisms then localize in the kidney, liver, and pregnant uterus. During the bacteraemic phase, animals may become jaundiced as a result of haemolysis and liver injury. **In calves, jaundice** is due to intravascular haemolysis. **Haemoglobinuria** may be transient or persist for several days. **In cows,** there is agalactia (failure of milk secretion) and blood-tinged milk. **Abortion** may occur in the acute phase or during convalescence. A subacute form of the disease in **cows** causes fever and decreased milk production. The udder is flabby and the milk resembles colostrum. **In pigs,** the most important form of leptospirosis is **abortion**

and birth of **weak piglets.** The dead piglets are heavily infected with leptospira. Leptospirosis in **pigs** and **cattle** causes a chronic intermittent nephritis usually seen at slaughter. A variety of serovars in **horses** cause **liver and kidney disease in foals** and **abortion in mares.**

Dogs are the maintenance host for *Leptospira canicola* serovar. However, vaccination has significantly reduced incidence of the disease. The *Leptospira icterohaemorrhagia* serovar, acquired from the environment contaminated by rats, causes acute hepatic injury, which results in hyperbilirubinaemia and increased concentration of liver enzymes in serum. This septicaemic phase of the disease can be very severe and may cause death in **pups.** Following septicaemia, all serovars in dogs localize in the kidney. Leptospira in the kidney cause focal diffuse interstitial nephritis. Although renal injury may be severe, death from renal failure is uncommon. **Animals that survive may excrete organisms in the urine for years.**

In the laboratory diagnosis, the old practice of demonstrating organisms by dark-field microscopy of fluids and tissue emulsions is now regarded as less sensitive compared to newer procedures such as **immunofluorescence of urine** or homogenates of foetal lung, kidney, or placenta.

In ruminants that die of acute leptospirosis, the most important findings are anaemia, jaundice, pulmonary oedema, and a pale, friable, bile-stained liver. The kidneys are swollen and dark from haemoglobin staining. Widespread ecchymotic haemorrhages may be present.

Dogs dying from the acute disease have widespread haemorrhage and focal hepatic necrosis. The kidneys are swollen, with sub-capsular and cortical ecchymotic haemorrhages. **Microscopic lesions** include tubular epithelial degeneration and necrosis, and interstitial oedema. This is followed by infiltration of lymphocytes and plasma cells. With time, kidneys become shrunken and have varying degrees of cortical fibrosis.

Protozoal Infections

Babesiosis (Piroplasmosis)

Babesiosis is a tick-borne disease caused by protozoa of the genus **Babesia.** They occur in all domestic animals, including wildlife ruminants. These protozoa cause **an acute disease** characterized by **haemolytic anaemia** and **injury to many organs.** They also cause a **chronic disease** associated with anaemia and weight loss, and a carrier state. **Calves** less than 3 months of age are resistant to Babesia infections. **In dogs** the acute disease occurs in **pups. In cattle** babesiosis is caused by *Babesia bigemina, B. bovis, B. divergens,* and *B. major;* **in sheep** by *B. motasi, B. ovis,* and *B. foliata;* **in horses** by *B. caballi* and *B. equi;* and **in dogs** by *B. canis* and *B. gibsoni.*

Babesia produce **acute disease** by **two mechanisms: haemolysis** and **circulatory disturbances.** Babesia invade erythrocytes and cause intravascular and macrophage-mediated haemolysis. The exact mechanisms of intravascular haemolysis are unclear, but they appear to be due to protozoa because there is a correlation between the severity of parasitaemia and the severity of anaemia, haemoglobinaemia, and haemoglobinuria. Phagocytosis of parasitized erythrocytes may be increased in the later stages of disease.

The **clinical signs of babesiosis** are due to variations in the pathogenicity of organisms and susceptibility of the animals. Organisms usually appear in erythrocytes within 8 to 16 days following vector-transmitted infection. Their appearance is accompanied by **fever**. Animals become listless, dehydrated, and weak with haemoglobinuria and jaundice. Subcutaneous oedema of the lower abdomen and thorax is seen **in horses**. *B. bovis* infections **in cattle** and *B. canis* infections **in dogs** cause nervous signs such as mania, recumbency with paddling of limbs, and coma. If animals recover, they may have relapses. Others suffer from chronic disease characterized by unthriftiness and weight loss.

Laboratory findings in acute babesiosis are those of anaemia with babesia visible in erythrocytes. Infected erythrocytes are large and most numerous in the edge of blood films. In vivo, infected erythrocytes accumulate in capillaries. Therefore, blood films prepared from capillary blood, for example from ear or tail incision, are useful for finding round to pyriform (pear-shaped) organisms.

At postmortem, animals dying from the acute disease have marked splenomegaly, jaundice, haemoglobinuria, swollen haemoglobin-stained kidneys, and sub-epicardial and sub-endocardial haemorrhages. The gallbladder is usually distended with thick bile. In *B. bovis* infection, grey matter throughout the brain shows congestion, which is easily seen against contrast of white matter. Parasitized erythrocytes are best seen in impression smears of kidneys, brain, and skeletal muscle. **Microscopic findings** in the liver and kidney are typical of haemolytic anaemia and include degeneration and loss of periacinar hepatocytes and cholestasis, and haemoglobinuric nephrosis with degeneration of tubular epithelium. Erythroid hyperplasia is present in the bone marrow. In animals that survive the acute disease, there is haemosiderin accumulation in the liver, kidney, spleen, and bone marrow.

Trypanosomiasis

Trypanosomiasis is caused by **flagellated protozoa** which occur in the blood and sometimes in tissues of animals and human beings. They have a widespread distribution, but cause disease mainly in warmer climatic areas such as Asia, Africa, and South America. Many species of trypanosomes infect animals without any host specificity. Thus, a particular trypanosome may infect several animal species, **and more than one species of trypanosomes may be found in the same animal.**

Some important trypanosomes of animals are *Trypanosoma congolense* (nagana disease), *T. vivax, T. brucei,* and *T. evansi* (surra disease) which infect **cattle**; *T. suis* infects **pigs,** and *T. equiperdum* (dourine disease) infect **horses**. *T. melophagium* in **sheep** and *T. theileri* in **cattle** are widespread, but non-pathogenic. Trypanosomes normally survive in wildlife reservoir hosts, and are non-pathogenic to them. They are transmitted by arthropod vectors, such as the tsetse fly, in which the organism survives in the salivary glands for the life of the fly. Other biting insects transmit trypanosomes mechanically.

The mechanisms by which trypanosomes cause disease are complex and incompletely studied. The considerable variation in the severity of the disease is due to factors such as strain of organism and immunocompetence of the host. **Some trypanosomal species cause rapidly fatal disease, others cause chronic debilitating disease, and some allow complete recovery with significant immunity.** Trypanosomes escape from the host's immune response following development of new ce¹¹ membrane proteins, which results in waves of parasitaemia and chronic disease. **Cattle** with acute trypanosomiasis have anaemia, which is initially regenerative with increased MCV, reticulocytosis, and bone marrow erythroid hyperplasia. With time, anaemia becomes less regenerative. Leukopaenia is caused by neutropaenia and lymphopaenia. Plasma proteins are low due to hypoalbuminaemia. In case of *T. vivax,* organisms are present in large numbers in blood. In contrast, *T. congolense* localize within the vasculature of the brain and skeletal muscle. **Cattle** with *T. congolense* develop chronic debilitating disease. Animals have rough hair coats, appear 'pot-bellied', and have fever, intermittent diarrhoea, and exercise intolerance. Mortality is greater with *T. vivax* due to intercurrent acute infectious diseases, such as salmonellosis. The development of a **severe haemolytic anaemia** in **Zebu cattle** infected with *T. vivax* is associated with a reduction in erythrocyte **sialic acid** concentration by **sialidase** with increased susceptibility of desialated erythrocytes to phagocytosis by MPS.

Postmortem findings in cattle include cachexia, generalized oedema with increased fluid in body cavities, and generalized lymph node enlargement. Bronchopneumonia, a flabby heart, and serous atrophy of pericardial fat may be present. Liver and kidneys are enlarged. The lymph nodes are enlarged up to 4 times their normal size because of lymphoid hyperplasia, and most of the fatty bone marrow is replaced by red haemopoietic tissue. The spleen is enlarged because of lymphoid hyperplasia and is firm when incised.

Theileriasis

Theileriasis is caused by a small protozoal parasite of the genus **Theileria,** which infects lymphocytes and erythrocytes of **ruminants**, especially **cattle, sheep,** and **goats**. The infection is spread by blood-sucking ticks. Several species are involved, but *T. parva* is the most important. It is the cause of East Coast fever of **cattle** in East and Central Africa. The mortality rate is almost 100% in susceptible **cattle**.

The organisms in erythrocytes are pleomorphic, and appear as rod-shaped, comma-shaped, oval, round, or anaplasma-like. *T. parva* is numerous in blood during the initial stage of infection, but not thereafter. *T. mutans* and *T. annulata* remain in blood in small numbers for a long period, as do *T. hirci* and *T. ovis* in **sheep** and **goat** blood. **Macroschizonts** and **microschizonts (Koch's bodies)** are found in the cytoplasm of lymphocytes in the peripheral blood and lymph nodes. These **schizonts** usually have blue cytoplasm which contains numerous reddish-purple, dot-like granules. Infected lymphocytes often undergo blast transformation.

The **incubation period** of *T. parva* following tick transmission in susceptible animals is 8 to 25 days. **Clinical signs** vary with the severity of disease. The disease is characterized by fever, swelling of the superficial lymph nodes, anorexia, lachrymation and nasal discharge, depression, and diarrhoea with blood in faeces. Anaemia is significant with *T. parva* but **leukopaenia** is marked with slight bilirubinaemia. Anaemia is inversely proportional to the degree of parasitaemia, and is regenerative. Red cell destruction in theileriasis may involve **erythrophagocytosis** from immune-mediated mechanisms. Serological tests, indirect fluorescent antibody test, and ELISA (enzyme-linked immunosorbent assay) are useful in detection of carrier animals. Control of the disease involves immunization, limiting transport of **cattle**, and vector control.

Cytauxzoonosis

Cytauxzoonosis caused by *Cytauxzoon felis,* a protozoal organism, is an acute, fatal disease of domestic **cats** in the southern United States. The mechanism of natural transmission is unknown, although arthropods are thought to be the vectors.

C. felis undergoes schizogony in monocytes and macrophages. The monocytes enlarge and accumulate within the walls of veins, eventually causing occlusion of the vessels. Merozoites are released and enter erythrocytes. **Cats become acutely ill** with fever, pallor, and jaundice and usually die within 2 to 3 days. Haematological findings include moderate to severe **haemolytic anaemia** and **neutropaenia**. In Wright-Giemsa-stained smears, the cytoplasm of the organism stains light blue, whereas the nucleus is purple. Erythrophagocytosis is an important finding in bone marrow aspirates and impression smears of the spleen.

Rickettsial Infections

Anaplasmosis

Anaplasmosis is a disease of **cattle** and **sheep** caused by organisms of the genus **Anaplasma**. In cattle, *A. marginale* causes severe **haemolytic anaemia,** whereas *A. centrale* is less pathogenic. *A. ovis* causes disease in **sheep** and **goats**. The organisms are transmitted by ticks and mechanically by biting flies and hypodermic needles.

Mechanism of disease caused by **Anaplasma** organisms involves penetration of the erythrocytes. Following penetration, the membrane of the red cell invaginates and engulfs the organism within the vesicle. The parasite then divides by binary fission into new infective units. Later, pores form in the erythrocyte membrane through which organisms escape to infect other cells. It is suspected that the organism exerts its effects on the red cell by release of **hydrolytic enzymes.** The presence of **Anaplasma** proteins on the erythrocyte results in the formation of antibodies that get attached on the erythrocytes and interact with macrophage receptors. The observation that non-infected erythrocytes are also destroyed indicates that antibodies produced interact with normal erythrocyte membrane proteins.

Young animals are susceptible to infection but do not develop disease. The immunity which develops following infection is that of a carrier state which results in a reservoir of domestic and wild ruminants that can infect other animals.

The **incubation period** of anaplasmosis is 1 to 3 months, followed by **haemolytic anaemia.** Affected animals have pale, jaundiced mucosae, are depressed and weak, and have reduced exercise tolerance. **In contrast to babesiosis, there is no haemoglobinuria.**

Laboratory findings are anaemia of varying severity. In case the disease is severe, as many as 50% to 60% of the erythrocytes contain organisms. There may be one or more dark blue to black organisms, of 0.3 to 1 μm in diameter, per erythrocyte. They must be differentiated from nuclear remnants. There may be moderate neutrophilia. During severe haemolysis, there is hyperbilirubinaemia. Recovery from acute anaplasmosis results in persistent infection in which animals serve as reservoirs for transmission within herds. Animals which die from acute anaplasmosis have blood of low viscosity, pale to jaundiced tissues, an enlarged spleen, and jaundiced liver with distended gallbladder.

Eperythrozoonoses

Eperythrozoonoses are diseases caused by erythrocytic rickettsial parasites of the genus **Eperythrozoon,** family Bartonellaceae. A carrier state exists in **cattle, sheep,** and **pigs,** in which they sometimes cause **haemolytic anaemia.** Transmission of the organism has not been extensively studied as in babesiosis and anaplasmosis, but incidence of disease in **sheep** and **pigs** accompanies heavy ectoparasite infestations. The mechanism of disease appears similar to those of other red cell parasites, in which immune-mediated haemolysis within macrophages follows attachment of the organisms to erythrocytes.

In both **sheep** and **pigs,** sudden death of one or two animals is followed by anaemia in other animals within the herd. *Eperythrozoon wenyoni* in **cattle** is less pathogenic than *E. ovis* in **sheep** and *E. suis* in **pigs.** It is important that blood smears are taken from anaemic **sheep** or **pigs,** because detection of the organism after death is difficult. In acute disease, the anaemia may be severe and many organisms are found on erythrocytes as well as free between erythrocytes. In less severe infections, anaemia may be mild, and it is necessary to search to find the few parasitized cells. The organisms closely resemble *Haemobartonella felis*. They are in ring forms with pale centres except on the edge of the cell, where they appear bacillary.

In animals dying of eperythrozoonosis, the findings are those of macrophage-mediated haemolysis with anaemia, jaundice, splenomegaly, and distended gallbladder. **Microscopic lesions** in the spleen include congestion, erythrophagia, macrophage hyperplasia, and haemopoiesis. Plasma cell numbers are increased in the spleen. Bone marrow has varying degrees of erythroid hyperplasia. Its severity indicates the duration of haemolysis.

Haemobartonellosis

Haemobartonellosis is caused by rickettsial organisms of the genus **Haemobartonella** (family Bartonellaceae) which resemble **Eperythrozoon** species. The disease occurs in **cattle, goats,** and **dogs** but is most important in **cats** as a cause of **feline infectious anaemia.** Transmission is by blood-sucking arthropods.

Haemobatonellosis in the cat may cause an acute haemolytic, regenerative, anaemia with marked parasitaemia. *Haemobartonella felis*-erythrocyte membrane interactions cause immune-mediated erythrophagocytosis in the spleen, liver, and bone marrow. **Cats** with acute form of the disease are weak and depressed and have pale, jaundiced, mucous membranes. Haematological findings in these **cats** are a regenerative anaemia with haematocrits as low as 0.10 L/L (10%). Detection of *H. felis* in erythrocytes requires a properly stained blood film of good quality and an experienced examiner. Differentiation of the organism from artefact may be difficult, especially when the organisms are rod forms on the edge of the erythrocyte. Finding ring forms away from the cell periphery is very helpful in differentiating organisms from artefacts.

Cats dying from haemolytic anaemia due to *H. felis* have pale mucous membranes with or without jaundice. There is usually splenomegaly, and bone marrow is particularly replaced by red haemopoietic tissue as a result of erythroid hyperplasia.

Haemolytic Anaemia from Non-Infectious Agents

Chemicals

Haemolytic anaemias can be caused by **chemicals** which inhibit erythrocyte metabolism or which cause denaturation and precipitation of haemoglobin and protein in the membrane skeleton of the erythrocytes. The erythrocyte survives by constantly generating ATP from glucose metabolism through the Embden-Meyerhof pathway. This **energy** is needed to maintain erythrocyte cation content, iron of haemoglobin in the divalent form, sulphydryl groups of haemoglobin and enzymes in the reduced form, and membrane integrity. The erythrocyte membrane consists of a lipid bilayer in which certain proteins are attached to an underlying cytoskeleton. The cytoskeleton provides the membrane both its strength and flexibility, allowing it to withstand deforming stress in capillaries and while traveling the walls of sinusoids. **Any disruption of the membrane cytoskeleton may lead to haemolysis.**

An important aspect of erythrocyte metabolism, in relation to injury by oxidative toxins, **is the capacity to maintain a reducing environment by efficient antioxidant mechanisms.** These mechanisms involve enzymes **methaemoglobin reductase** and **glutathione peroxidase,** as well as reduced pyridine nucleotides nicotinamide-adenine dinucleotide (NADH) and NADH phosphate (NADPH). **Oxidant injury** to erythrocytes in animals usually occurs when reducing capacity of the erythrocyte is overloaded after ingestion of the harmful chemicals. **Methaemoglobin formation** appears to be necessary requirement in the development and precipitation of denatured haemoglobin to form **Heinz bodies.** Heinz bodies are inclusions within erythrocytes. They are formed from the precipitated denatured haemoglobin following oxidative damage to erythrocytes. It is believed that the precipitated, denatured haemoglobin causes further oxidation of membrane proteins and inhibition of several erythrocyte enzymes. **The end result is erythrocyte injury leading to cation leak, loss of deformability, and fixation of immunoglobulin to altered membrane proteins. Both macrophage-mediated erythrocyte destruction and intravascular lysis occur.**

Onions

Onions contain an agent that can cause **oxidative haemolytic anaemia.** Poisoning sometimes occurs in **cattle,** and in **dogs** that ingest onions in cooked food or chew raw onions. **Clinical findings** include **acute haemolytic anaemia** with paleness, jaundice, and weakness. **Haemoglobinuria** has occurred in **cattle** that have ingested large quantities of onions.

Propylene Glycol

Cats are prone to erythrocyte oxidative injury because their globin chains contain more sulphydryl-containing amino acids than those of other mammals. For this reason, **Heinz bodies** are usually present in feline erythrocytes. Until recently, **propylene glycol** was a common additive to commercial pet foods and induced **Heinz body** formation **in cat erythrocytes.** Drugs such as **aspirin** and related products contain strong **oxidants** that can cause **haemolytic anaemia in cats.**

Miscellaneous Substances

Oxidative injury to erythrocytes has occurred **in horses** following ingestion of leaves and bark of **red maple trees** in United Stares. **Heinz body haemolytic**

anaemias may' occur in **dogs** as a result of **zinc toxicity**, following ingestion of zinc nuts, bolts, and coins.

Laboratory findings in animals **with oxidative erythrocyte disorders** include **anaemia** and **compensatory erythropoiesis.** An important diagnostic feature of these anaemias is the presence of **Heinz bodies in erythrocytes.** In Wright's-Giemsa-stained blood films, there are distinct protrusions from the cell membrane or tiny pale spherule under the cell membrane. These inclusions are easily seen on new methylene blue-stained smears. **Eccentrocytes,** that is, erythrocytes with haemoglobin concentrated in one portion of the cell, occur following erythrocyte oxidative injury in **dogs.** Animals which die from **Heinz body haeomlytic anaemia** have **generalized paleness** and **jaundice.** There is usually pulmonary oedema with frothy fluid in the trachea. The spleen is enlarged and swollen. The liver is usually enlarged and jaundiced. Gallbladder is distended with bile.

Copper

Copper poisoning and haemolysis occur when copper is present in the plasma at concentrations greater than the binding capacity of its transport protein, albumin, and ceruloplasmin. This occurs in **sheep, cattle,** and **pigs following release of copper from the liver. At lower concentrations,** copper inhibits erythrocyte enzymes of the Embden-Meyerhof pathway, which results in ATP depletion and erythrocyte lysis. **At higher concentrations,** copper inhibits enzymes within the hexose-monophosphate shunt, leading to **impaired glutathione metabolism,** and as a result, Heinz body formation. Anaemia in all species occurs from a combination of these mechanisms, which lead to haemolysis followed by **haemoglobinaemia** and **haemoglobinuria.** Examination of blood films confirms severe anaemia and may reveal Heinz bodies.

Hypophosphataemic Haemolytic Anaemia

This haemolytic anaemia occurs as post-parturient haemoglobinuria in the dairy cow 3 to 8 weeks after parturition. It also occurs in **beef cattle** and **non-postpartum cattle** consuming **phosphorus-deficient diets. Cattle** dying from haemolytic anaemia have generalized paleness, jaundice, watery blood, and fluid in serous cavities. The liver is enlarged, swollen, and pale. Gallbladder is distended with bile. Spleen is enlarged and congested.

Erythrocytes require inorganic phosphorus for incorporation into phosphorylated intermediate molecules within Embden-Meyerhof pathway and for synthesis of ATP. **In phosphate depletion,** the erythrocytic glycolytic rate is slowed, and ATP synthesis decreases. The structure and function of erythrocytes are damaged, and when plasma phosphorus concentrations reach critical level, **haemolysis occurs.** Intravascular haemolysis, indicated by **haemoglobinuria,** is a common finding, but phagocytosis of abnormal erythrocytes (extravascular haemolysis) probably also occurs.

Laboratory findings include haemoglobinaemia and **haemoglobinuria**. The **anaemia** may be **severe** with **haematocrits as low as** 0.10 L/L (10%).

Immune-Mediated Haemolytic Anaemias

Immune-mediated haemolytic anaemias (IMHA) are those anaemias in which erythrocyte destruction occurs following attachment of an antibody to the erythrocyte membrane.

Idiopathic immune-mediated haemolytic anaemia is the most common type of haemolytic anaemia in dogs, but also occurs in other species. The **aetiology** in most cases is unknown. Probably the damaging antibody develops because infectious agents (such as **viruses**) or foreign substances (such as **drugs**) alter proteins of the erythrocyte membrane. Circulating immune complexes involving the antigens may be adsorbed on erythrocyte membranes. It was found that there was a higher incidence of IMHA in **dogs** recently vaccinated against canine distemper, adenovirus type 2, leptospirosis, parainfluenza, and parvovirus.

The decreased survival of antibody-coated erythrocytes is because **macrophages,** mainly in the spleen, but also in the liver (Kupffer cells) and bone marrow, **have receptors for the Fc region of IgG. Partial phagocytosis** which occurs from removal of those portions of the erythrocyte membrane that have the highest concentration of antibody results in **transformation of erythrocytes from biconcave disks to spheres. Spherocytosis** is the characteristic feature of this disease. **Spherocytes** are easily seen in smears of canine blood as small erythrocytes lacking central paleness. There is a direct correlation between the number of spherocytes and the rate of haemolysis. **Spherocytic erythrocytes are at risk for phagocytosis because they are no longer pliable (flexible) or deformable and are retained in the spleen, in close proximity to macrophages.** As these cells accumulate in the spleen, lactic acid from erythrocyte glycolysis causes a drop in the pH of the red pulp, and the function of erythrocyte glycolytic enzymes is damaged.

The IgG class of antibody is the most important cause of canine immunohaemolytic anaemia. As in human beings, it is likely that there is a direct correlation between the quantity of IgG bound to erythrocytes and haemolysis. The antibody may also fix complement-increasing phagocytosis. Sometimes, **dogs** in a haemolytic crisis have haemoglobinaemia and haemoglobinuria consistent with complement-mediated injury to the erythrocyte membrane followed by leakage of haemoglobin into the plasma. IgM antibodies are particularly efficient at binding complement and may also be present on erythrocytes of these animals.

Dogs with immune-mediated haemolytic anaemia are very sick and recumbent, but the disease may occur in a **sub-clinical** form. Acutely ill dogs may have pale mucosae with or without jaundice, and some may vomit and may have fever. A drop of blood should be placed on a slide for agglutination. If haemagglutination occurs, **haemoglobinuria** is a very serious sign. These animals are emergency cases and require rapid diagnosis and treatment.

Laboratory examination is essential for an accurate diagnosis. The degree of **anaemia** varies but may be severe with haematocrits of 0.05 to 0.15 L/L (5% to 15%). In most dogs, the aneamia is regenerative, however, in very acute cases, there will be **spherocytosis** without polychromasia in blood smears. Sometimes **dogs** with immune-mediated haemolytic anaemia remain reticulocytopaenic or compensatory erythropoiesis is delayed. In such **dogs**, bone marrow should be examined. Usually there is phagocytosis of erythrocytes, and metarubricytes and rubricytes are present, indicating that inadequate compensatory erythropoiesis is due to phagocytosis of erythrocytes precursors.

The prognosis is guarded in these reticulocytopaenic dogs. The blood in the tube and the stained blood film must be carefully examined for agglutination of erythrocytes. Agglutinated erythrocytes are easily detected in the thicker areas of the blood smear where they occur as irregular clumps, which should not be confused with the linear formation of erythrocytes in rouleaux. The presence of polychromatophilic erythrocytes in the clumps indicates agglutination because these cells do not participate in rouleaux. An important feature of the erythrocytes, seen at low magnification, is **marked anisocytosis.** This extreme variation in erythrocyte diameter is due to the presence of macrocytic, immature erythrocytes plus small spherocytes.

Polychromasia is pronounced, and metarubricytes and rubricytes may be present. **Platelets may be reduced** because of concurrent immune-mediated thrombocytopaenia. **Neutrophilia** is also common and appears to accompany the reticulocyte response. **Monocytosis** indicates traffic from the bone marrow to the spleen where monocytes become macrophages capable of erythrophagocytosis.

The direct antiglobulin test (DAT; direct Coombs' test) is a haemagglutination assay for antibody or complement bound to erythrocytes (Fig. 31). This test demonstrates the presence of anti-erythrocyte antibody, or activated complement components **on the surface of the patient's red cells. The indirect Coombs' test, demonstrates** the presence of anti-erythrocyte **antibody in the serum.** The **principle** involved in the **direct test** is that red blood cells of patients are coated with antibody *in vivo*, and for **indirect test** that patient's serum contains anti-erythrocyte antibody. Based on this principle, a washed saline suspension of the patient's erythrocytes (in direct test), or of normal homologous washed red cells exposed to the patient's serum (in indirect test) is incubated at 37° C and 4° C with species-specific antiglobulin (antisera containing goat- or rabbit-derived antibody for canine IgG, IgM, or complement C3 to induce visible agglutination of the red cells (Fig. 31). Erythrocytes coated with only anti-erythrocyte IgG do not agglutinate, **but they undergo agglutination after interaction with a species-specific anti-IgG.** Erythrocytes, coated with anti-erythrocyte IgM (**cold agglutinins**) undergo spontaneous agglutination in contrast to cells coated with anti-erythrocyte IgG.

281

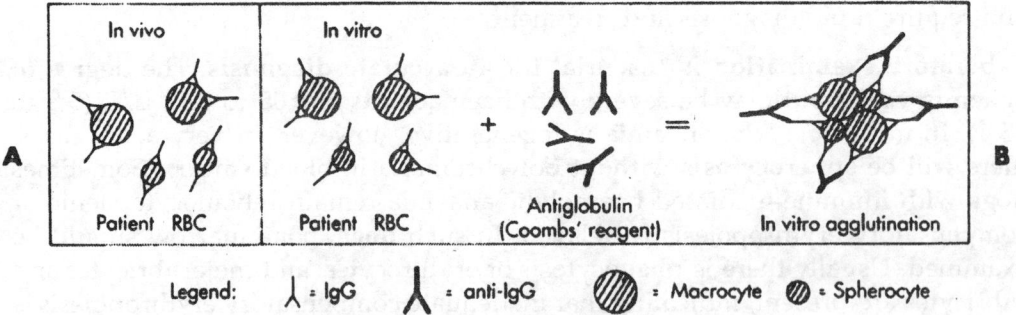

Fig. 31. Direct antiglobulin test (DAT). A. Red blood cells (RBCs) of patient are coated with antibody *in vivo*. **B.** *In vitro* detection of antibody is obtained by adding heterologous antiglobulin reagent, which results in cross-linking of RBCs and microscopic or macroscopic agglutination.

Although direct antiglobulin test is very useful in diagnosing immune-mediated haemolytic anaemias, the results must be carefully interpreted in the context of other laboratory clinical findings. For example, **dogs** previously treated with glucocorticoid drugs usually have a negative test result. The test results may also be negative when antibody molecules are of low avidity (binding strength) and are lost during erythrocyte washings, or when the numbers of antibody molecules are too low to be detected. **Therefore, a negative direct antiglobulin test (DAT)** in the presence of haematological and clinical findings consistent with immune-mediated haemolytic anaemia **should not prevent the diagnosis. Flow cytometry may replace the DAT in future because it detects lower numbers of antibody molecules on erythrocytes.** In the early stages of the disease, bone marrow aspirates show erythroid hyperplasia and erythrophagocytosis.

Postmortem findings in dogs with immune-mediated haemolytic anaemia include pale tissues, mild to moderate jaundice, pulmonary oedema, and frothy tracheal fluid. The heart may be rounded and dilated. Liver is usually enlarged and pale, and gallbladder is distended. The spleen is enlarged and is firm when incised. Lymph nodes are enlarged. In **dogs** with **thrombocytopaenia** (decrease in the number of platelets), haemorrhages are present on the serosal surfaces of visceral organs. **Microscopically**, macrophages in the liver, spleen, and bone marrow contain haemosiderin. There is a direct relationship between the numbers of haemosiderin-containing macrophages and duration of the disease.

Neonatal Alloimmune Haemolytic Anaemia

Neonatal alloimmune haemolytic anaemia (neonatal isoerythrolysis) occurs in **foals** that obtain anti-erythrocyte antibody in colostrum from **mares** which have been sensitized to erythrocyte antigens released from the foetus. The foetus inherited these erythrocyte antigens from the sire. Foal erythrocytes enter the maternal circulation at sites of focal placental haemorrhage, or the mare may have been sensitized to foal red cells during previous parturition. The incidence of the disease is 1% to 2%. Some blood groups are more antigenic than others.

Severely affected foals become lethargic and weak as early as 8 to 10 hours after birth, or anytime over the next 4 to 5 days. They have pale, jaundiced mucous membranes, and if haemolysis is severe, **haemoglobinuria. Haematocrits** may be as low as 12 to 15 L/L (12% to 15%). Within a few days erythroid hyperplasia occurs in the bone marrow. Serum bilirubin concentrations are usually increased. **Foals that die** during a haemolytic crisis are **markedly jaundiced** and have **splenomegaly.**

Kittens of blood group A born to females of blood group B are at risk for **neonatal haemolysis. Cats** with blood group B have naturally occurring antibodiesto the A antigen. However, blood group B is rare in most cats.

Non-Regenerative Anaemias

Whether the anaemia is regenerative or non-regenerative is based on the presence or absence of compensatory erythropoeisis (see 'mechanisms of anaemia').

Non-regenerative anaemias are due to impaired erythropoiesis, and are the most common anaemias in animals and humans. Therefore, haemogram is an essential part of thorough clinical examination **because non-regenerative anaemia is an indicator of occult (hidden disease).** For example, **dogs** with liver disease are usually anaemic. Therefore, additional laboratory testsare required to find out the underlying disorder. Bone marrow examination is indicated in animals with significant non-regenerative anaemia when an underlying disease is not clear.

The non-regenerative anaemias are:

1. Anaemia of Chronic Disease

The **anaemia of chronic disease (ACD) is an anaemia that occurs along with chronic inflammatory or neoplastic disorders.** The anaemia is mainly due to **impaired erythropoiesis,** which results in **low reticulocyte production.** The mechanisms by which chronic inflammation and neoplasia damage erythropoiesis are not known. However, **studies by cytokines** produced in inflammatory disorders, such as rheumatoid arthritis in humans, have thrown light on the mechanisms by which erythropoiesis is inhibited by anaemia of chronic disease (ACD). **Some concentrations of interleukin-1 (IL-1),** a polypeptide with a wide variety of activities in infection and immunity, **are increased in ACD.** IL-1 inhibits erythropoiesis indirectly by stimulating T-lymphocytes to produce **gamma-interferon,** which has been shown to directly inhibit erythroid precursor cells in culture.

Tumour necrosis factor, another cytokine with a significant role in inflammation and the immune response **causes a non-regenerative anaemia** when administered to animals and inhibition of the growth of erythrocyte precursor cells in culture. It is possible that **other cytokines** that help in regulating inflammatory and immune responses also damage erythropoiesis. **Erythropoietin concentrations** are increased, but they are low in comparison with the concentrations in equally anaemic individuals with ACD. **Interleukin-1** and **tumour necrosis factor** inhibit erythropoietin production, thus they increase development of ACD. The anaemia of ACD is usually accompanied by **low serum iron** despite the presence of adequate amounts of iron in the monocyte-macrophage system. The delayed release of iron from macrophages is due to the **cytokine-mediated inhibition of erythropoiesis.** Animals in renal failure are usually anaemic mainly because of inadequate production of erythropoietin by the kidney. The mechanisms of anaemia in chronic liver disease are unknown.

Animals with ACD usually have a mild to moderate anaemia. Despite the decreased availability of iron, the erythrocyte indices are usually normal. Changes in the shape of erythrocytes occur in **cats** and **dogs** with chronic liver disease. These include elongated erythrocytes with short irregular projections and acanthocytes. **In chronic inflammatory disorders,** concentrations of plasma proteins are usually increased and the albumin/globulin ratio decreased because of increased gamma globulin. Granulocyte hyperplasia may be present in animals with chronic suppurative inflammation somewhere in the body. **Microscopically,** haemosiderin deposits in bone marrow aspirates may be increased.

2. Nutritional Deficiency Anaemia

Nutritional deficiency anaemias are unknown in domestic animals. Because **piglets** have low iron contents at birth and a rapid rate of growth, they become iron deficient and suffer from **iron deficiency anaemia.** They become anaemic, and severely debilitated if they do not receive a supplement of iron soon after birth. Parenteral administration of iron is now common in **pigs,** and therefore, iron deficiency anaemias occur only sporadically. **Iron deficient piglets** have retarded growth, dyspnoea, and lethargy at about 3 weeks of age. The skin and mucosae are pale, and head and forelimbs show oedema. **Haematological findings include** erythrocyte numbers as low as 3 or 4×10^9/L (3 or 4×10^6/mm^3), haemoglobin concentrations of 20 to 40 g/L (2 to 4 g/dl), and haematocrits as low as 0.08 L/L (8%). Blood films may show microcytic, hypochromic erythrocytes and poikilocytes. There is usually marked thrombocytosis. Serum iron concentrations are decreased and may be as low as 5 μmol/L (28 μg/dl). Bone marrow aspirates show an accumulation of **rubricytes** and **metarubricytes** because of inadequate transport of iron for haemoglobin synthesis.

Nutritional iron deficiencies are rare in other species. A more common condition is iron deficiency secondary to chronic haemorrhage. **Chronic haemorrhage** may be caused by blood-sucking parasites such as hookworms (*Ancylostoma caninum*) and fleas (*Echidnophaga gallinacean*) in **dogs** and **haemonchosis** in **cattle** and **sheep**. Bleeding from mucosal surfaces, mainly in **dogs**, can exhaust iron contents. **Laboratory findings** of hypochromic, microcytic anaemia indicates hidden bleeding from lesions such as intestinal neoplasms, or the result of chronic immune-mediated thrombocytopaenia.

3. Aplastic Pancytopaenia

Aplastic pancytopaenia are a group of disorders characterized by pancytopaenia (abnormal depression of **all** the cellular elements of the blood) and **hypocellular bone marrow** (i.e. decrease in the number of cells in the bone marrow). They occur in **cats** with leukaemia virus infections and sporadically as an idiopathic disorder in **dogs**. Pure **erythrocytic aplasia** is failure of erythropoiesis while granulopoiesis and thrombopoiesis are normal.

Dogs are particularly prone to oestrogen toxicity. These dogs have neutrophilia and thrombocytosis, followed by thrombocytopaenia and **anaemia**. Dogs may recover if oestrogen concentrations in the body return to normal. The disease, however, may become irreversible in some **dogs**, and then they become **pancytopaenic.**

Ehrlichiosis

Ehrlichiosis is a tick-transmitted **rickettsial** disease. It affects several species of animals and human beings. **In dogs,** the disease is caused by *Ehrlichia canis* and several other species and in **horses** by *E. equi* and a few other species.

Following an incubation period of 8 to 20 days, *E. canis* causes acute disease in which organisms infect monocytes and then spread throughout the mononuclear phagocyte system. This is followed by invasion of the endothelial cells, which results in vasculitis. The disease then enters into a sub-clinical phase, from which **dogs** may either recover or develop pancytopaenic bone marrow failure.

Clinical findings during the **acute phase** are non-specific and include fever, ocular and nasal discharges, anorexia, and lymph node enlargement. The **sub-clinical phase** lasts for 40 to 120 days and is characterized by signs of multi-systemic disease.

Laboratory findings in the acute phase include **thrombocytopaenia** with large platelets and non-regenerative anaemia. *Babesia canis* infection may be present concurrently and can result in regenerative anaemia. Pancytopaenia develops in the chronic phases of the disease. Bone marrow examination reveals depletion of erythrocytic, granulocytic, and megakaryocytic cells. Serological diagnosis is based on indirect fluorescent antibody test.

Postmortem findings vary with the stage of the disease. **In acute disease** there are widespread petechiae and ecchymoses, with splenomegaly and lymphadenomegaly. Chronically infected dogs are emaciated. The bone marrow is hyperplastic and red in acute disease but becomes hypoplastic and pale in chronic disease. **Microscopic findings** include generalized perivascular plasma cell infiltration, which is most pronounced in the chronic disease. **Ehrlichia organisms are difficult to detect microscopically.** Examination of Wright-Giemsa-stained impression smears of lungs, liver, lymph nodes, and spleen is a more effective method for detecting **Ehrlichia** in macrophages.

E. equi **infection produces a disease in horses similar to the canine disease,** but mortality is low. **Equine ehrlichiosis is characterized by** fever, anorexia, depression, oedema of the lungs, and ataxia. **Laboratory findings** indicate mild anaemia, leukopaenia, and thrombocytopaenia. **Postmortem findings** include petechiae and ecchymoses, and jaundice of the subcutaneous tissues and fascia.

Bracken Fern Poisoning

Bracken fern poisoning is a **pancytopaenic disease** of **cattle** and **horses**. It occurs following several weeks of ingestion of the green plant or hay containing the fern. **In both species,** it causes haemopoietic stem cell injury. **In cattle,** haemorrhage is the main sign of disease. There is low morbidity and high mortality. **Laboratory findings** include leukopaenia and thrombocytopaenia. **Postmortem findings** include numerous haemorrhages in all tissues.

Leukocyte Disorders

Total and differential leukocyte counts should always be a part of clinical evaluations. This is because correlation of these data with clinical findings can confirm or exclude diseases characterized by inflammation, necrosis, or both. Knowledge of neutrophil kinetics (turnover, or rate of change) in health and disease helps in finding out the duration and severity of inflammatory processes. Animals which are ill and under stress, or receiving glucocorticoid drugs, have characteristic changes in the leukocyte profile. These include neutrophilia, eosinophilia, and lymphopaenia. In the **dog,** there is also monocytosis. Reversal of these changes means recovery from the stressful state and a favourable prognosis. Examination of blood monocytes provides information about the activity of the mononuclear phagocyte system. These cells play a very important role in chronic inflammation and haemolytic anaemia.

Neutrophils

Neutrophils are important in defence against infections. Therefore, evaluation of numbers and age of neutrophils is particularly useful in disease assessment. To interpret these changes, one must be familiar with species variations in **neutrophil kinetic in health and disease.**

Neutrophils (granulocytes) are produced in the bone marrow. It is useful to consider granulopoiesis (formation of neutrophils/granulocytes) as occurring in compartments or pools: **mitotic** and **post-mitotic maturation,** and **storage pools** (Fig. 32). In the circulating blood (compartment), neutrophils may marginate along the vascular endothelium or be free in the blood. **In the dog, horse,** and **calf** these **two pools (marginal** and **circulating**) are of equal size. **In cats,** the marginal pool is larger than the circulating pool. The size of the circulating pool (i.e. total neutrophil numbers) indicates the rate at which cells enter the blood from the bone marrow and leave the blood to enter the tissues. **Blood therefore serves as a vehicle to transport neutrophils,** with a transit time of about 10 hours. **Following migration into tissues, neutrophils do not re-enter capillaries.** There is continual removal of neutrophils from the blood as they migrate across mucous membranes, particularly the alimentary tract and into other tissues.

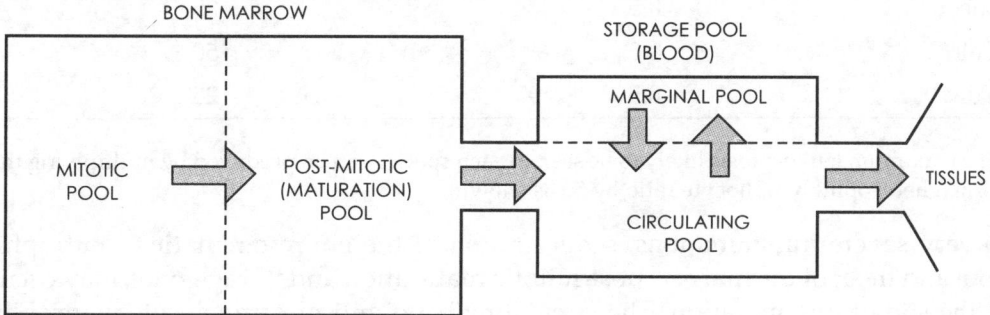

Fig. 32. Neutrophil kinetics.

The ability of animals to respond to increased tissue demand for neutrophil varies according to the species. It can be predicted from the numbers of circulating neutrophils or the neutrophil/lymphocyte ratio **(Table 10). Animals with greater numbers of circulating neutrophils in health are able to produce and deliver maximum neutrophils to tissues.** Animals respond to a greater tissue demand for neutrophils by releasing mature cells from the bone marrow post-mitotic maturation and storage pool (Fig. 32), followed if necessary, by the premature release of immature cells to the circulating pool (Fig. 32). At the same time, **humoral mediators** including granulocyte macrophage-colony stimulating factor (GM-CSF) and interleukin-3 stimulate differentiation of pluripotent stem cells into the committed neutrophil mitotic pool (Fig 32). **Therefore, the degree of neutrophilia or neutropaenia,** as well as the number of band and metamyelocyte neutrophils in a given species, **provides insight into the duration and severity of an inflammatory process. Table 10** makes it clear that the greatest neutrophilia, without release of band neutrophils in response to inflammation, would occur in the **dog;** whereas a lesser neutrophilia, with increased need for band neutrophils, would occur in the **cow.**

Table 10. Leukocyte responses in benign diseases

Species	Normal neutrophil/ lymphocyte ratio	Maximum expected* leukocytosis x 10^9/L
Dog	2.4	120
Cat	1.5	75
Foal	1.4	70
Horse	1.2	60
Pig	0.7	35
Goat	0.6	30
Sheep	0.5	25
Calf	1.0	50
Cow	0.5	25

*The maximum leukocytosis likely to be seen in each species can be predicted by multiplying the normal neutrophil:lymphocyte ratio by 50 as shown.

In very severe inflammations, sequestration of the entire circulating neutrophil pool and most of the marrow post-mitotic maturation and storage pool, may occur at the site of inflammation. The circulating band and metamyelocyte neutrophil numbers may be similar to or greater than mature neutrophils. **This is more common in cow and horse than in the dog and cat.**

The rate of restoration of the marrow neutrophil post-mitotic maturation and storage pool and the blood **neutrophil pool depends on the severity of the inflammatory process and how rapidly it is controlled. If the infection is controlled rapidly,** neutrophil numbers return to normal and band neutrophils disappear. **However, if the infection is not controlled,** stem cells are committed to continue production of neutrophils. Bone marrow hypertrophy occurs until more neutrophils are released than are required, resulting in **neutrophilia.** These inflammatory processes are moderately severe and of long duration.

Neutropaenia occurs from depletion of the circulating and marrow post-mitotic maturation and storage pools in animals with severe infections. Although rare, immune-mediated neutropaenias occur and should be considered in chronically neutropaenic animals.

Neutrophil dysfunction occurs in human beings in diabetes mellitus and uraemia. As in humans, impaired movement and phagocytic defects of neutrophils also occur in animals with these disorders. **Congenital leukocyte function disorders** have been described in **humans, dogs,** and **cattle.** These are characterized by recurrent bacterial and fungal infections and persistent neutrophilia in the young. The neutrophils have **defect in the integrin CD11/CD18** which is responsible for adhesion of neutrophils to surfaces and also serves as a receptor for complement C3b. Neutrophils with this defective integrin are unable to migrate across capillary walls into tissues. **Recurrent bacterial and fungal infections** have been described **in dogs** in which neutrophils had normal phagocytic function but impaired bacterial ability.

Eosinophils

Infiltration of tissues by eosinophils is somewhat independent of other leukocytes. Three cytokines, IL-3, IL-5, and GM-CSF, are particularly important in regulating the production of eosinophils. Eosinophils are attracted to tissues as a part of a T-lymphocyte-mediated immune response to certain antigens, **mainly allergens and those of helminthes.** T-helper lymphocytes are involved in the production of IL-5, which stimulates the release of eosinophils from the marrow. Once eosinophils arrive at a site of inflammation, they may undergo apoptosis and are rapidly phagocytosed by macrophages, but if they are stimulated by IL-3, IL-5, and GM-CSF, they survive for prolonged periods.

Eosinophils are mainly tissue cells, especially in those tissues with an epithelium exposed to the external environment, such as the respiratory and gastrointestinal tract. Eosinophil granules have constituents similar to other granulocyte, but their specific effector molecules are most important. **Major basic protein,** the most abundant cationic eosinophil protein, **is toxic to helminths, tumour cells, and host cells. Eosinophil peroxidase** is toxic to the helminthes, protozoa, bacteria, tumour cells, and host cells, whereas **eosinophilic cationic protein** has bactericidal and helminthotoxic activities.

It is now clear that eosinophils protect against parasites. The binding of eosinophils to helminths is mediated by anti-parasite IgG, IgE antibodies, or by C3b that have been deposited on the surfaces of parasites. **Another function of eosinophils** on body surfaces is the regulation of inflammatory reactions involving mast cells, basophils, and IgE antibodies. At sites of hypersensitivity inflammation, **eosinophils neutralize histamine** and are capable of inhibiting mast cells degranulation.

A number of syndromes occur in animals with marked tissue eosinophilia with or without blood eosinophilia. These include pulmonary eosinophilia and eosinophilic enteritis in **dogs** and **cats**, eosinophilic granulomatous inflammation of the alimentary tract and skin in **horses**, and a variety of neoplastic diseases.

Eosinopaenia is common in animals, usually in response to stress or the administration of glucocorticoid drugs, due to inhibition of T-lymphocyte subgroups that regulate eosinophil movement and functions.

Basophils and Mast Cells

Like eosinophils, **basophils and mast cells are specialized effector cells of the immune system.** They share the membrane glycoprotein CD45 with other cells in the bone marrow. This indicates that **mast cells are derived from haemopoietic stem cells.** Mast cells leave bone marrow to assume their special structure and function after settling in tissue sites such as under the epithelial surfaces.

Basophils and mast cells and their mediators are primary effectors of allergic inflammation. Both have **IgE binding sites,** and following formation of IgE-antigen **complexes,** activation of the cells results in secretion of their **histamine, neutral proteases,** and **cytokines** which are responsible for most of the early events that characterize **allergic reactions of the respiratory tract, intestine, and skin.** It is now clear that basophils and mast cells play both **pro-inflammatory and immune-modulatory roles in allergic disorders.**

Basophilia is rare in animals, but is at times seen along with eosinophilia. This is because basophils and eosinophils share many immuno-phenotypic properties. Sometimes basophils and mast cells are seen with eosinophils in tracheal washes of **dogs** and **horses** in intermittent chronic bronchitis, probably hypersensitivity disorders. The same is seen in tracheal washes from **dogs** containing *Oslerus osleri* larvae.

Monocytes and Macrophages

Monocytes are produced in bone marrow and then are transported in the blood to tissues and body cavities. Here, they rapidly differentiate into macrophages. Monocytes remain in the bone marrow for about 24 hours before entering the peripheral blood.

Macrophages are derived from monocytes. Monocytes undergo biochemical and immuno-phenotypic changes required for the purposes of liver, spleen, bone marrow, lymph nodes, lungs, central nervous system, and other tissues containing components of the mononuclear phagocyte system. This diversity covers the highly phagocytic activity of Kupffer cells in the liver, in contrast to macrophages with purely secretory activity in support of the immune response or hemopoiesis. **Tissue macrophage populations are continuously being renewed.** The turnover time for Kupffer cells is about 5 to 6 days.

Macrophages play an important role in the immune response. They show foreign antigens on their surface in a form that can be recognized by antigen-specific T-lymphocytes. T-lymphocytes, in turn, secrete cytokines that activate macrophages, which are more efficient at phagocytosis and cytocidal functions. Macrophages and lymphocytes, therefore, are mutually interactive.

Bone marrow macrophages not only secrete growth factors necessary for haemopoiesis, but also exert local control over stem cells within the haemopoietic microenvironment. Macrophages are the important cells in erythroblastic islands, where through cyto-adhesive protein fibronectin, **they nourish the development of erythroid precursor cells.** The **erythroid cells** migrate along macrophage membrane extensions until they reach a marrow sinusoid.

Monocytosis (increase in the number of monocytes in blood) in haemograms of animals indicates an increased demand for macrophages in the tissues. This is particularly seen in haemolytic anaemias. For example, blood smears from **cats** with severe *Haemobartonella felis* infections or **dogs** with immune-mediated haemolytic anaemia usually have numerous monocytes en route to the spleen. **Monocytosis** is also **present in suppurative inflammatory states,** such as **pyometra in dogs** and **traumatic pericarditis in cattle.** Monocytosis occurs in **dogs** following administration of glucocorticoid drugs.

Myeloproliferative Disorders

The myeloproliferative disorders refer to neoplastic transformation of one or more of the descendants of the myeloid stem cells. Myeloproliferative disorders may result in **release of abnormal cells into the peripheral blood (leukaemia),** or they may cause **pancytopaenia** because of the interference with haemopoiesis and leukaemia. Neoplasia of one myeloid cell line will cause impaired differentiation and maturation of other cell lines. Lymphosarcomas and lymphocytic leukaemias are considered in the discussion of lymph nodes. The **leukaemias** have been classified as **acute** or **chronic** based on clinical course and degree of differentiation of the neoplastic cells.

Acute Leukaemias

Acute Myelogenous Leukaemia

Acute myelogenous leukaemia (M1 and M2) is identified by stains that react with cytoplasmic enzymes. **In the FAB classification,** they are sub-classified into acute myeloblastic leukaemias without maturation (M1) and with maturation (M2). **Affected dogs and cats** are usually in good condition, but may show anorexia, depression, or weight loss. Some may have bleeding such as epistaxis. **Haematological findings** include non-regenerative anaemia, thrombocytopaenia, and neutropaenia. Bone marrow aspirates are dominated by one population of cells which is usually less differentiated than those in the blood. **The cells are mostly blast cells,** which have staining characteristics similar to granulocyte precursor cells.

At postmortem, paleness of tissue and petechiae are seen if the animals are thrombocytopaenic. The spleen may be enlarged. The fat in the medullary cavities of long bones is replaced by yellowish white to red, firm tissue. **Microscopically,** the spleen and bone marrow are filled by large, round cells, which require cytological examination and cytochemical staining to identify them and differentiate them from lymphoblasts.

Promyelocytic Leukaemia

This is a rare neoplasm of **dogs** and **cats.**

Myelomonocytic Leukaemia

Myelomonocytic leukaemia (M4) is a concurrent leukaemia of neutrophil and monocyte precursors. These are rare neoplasms of **dogs, cats,** and **horses.**

Monocytic Leukaemia

Monocytic leukaemia (M5) occurs sometimes in **dogs, cats, horses,** and **cattle. Affected animals** show weight loss, anorexia, and depression. **Haematological findings** include non-regenerative anaemia with variable neutropaenia, neutrophilia, and thrombocytopaenia. Postmortem findings are similar to other leukaemias. However, there may be more extensive involvement of other organs including spleen, liver, lungs, lymph nodes and kidneys. **Microscopically**, the masses consist of numerous large, round cells with large nuclei similar to those in the blood and bone marrow.

Malignant Histiocytosis

Malignant histiocytosis **is a disease of dogs and cats. It is characterized by neoplastic proliferation of macrophages** in many organs including the skin. **Affected dogs** show anorexia, weight loss, lethargy, and anaemia. Generalized lymph node enlargement is common. **At postmortem,** there may be widespread haemorrhage in thrombopaenic **dogs.** Lymph nodes are enlarged and firm, and there is usually splenomegaly and hepatomegaly. Numerous round to spindle-shaped cells and abundant erythrophagia (ingestion of erythrocytes by macrophages) are found on **microscopic examination** of the lymph nodes, liver, and splenic red pulp.

Erythrocytic Sarcoma

Erythrocytic sarcoma (M6) (erythraemic myelosis) **in cats** is characterized by lethargy, paleness, and a variety of haematological abnormalities including a severe, non-regenerative anaemia with haematocrits as low as 0.06 L/L (6%). Blood films usually contain erythrocyte precursors in various stages of differentiation.

In addition to watery blood **at postmortem,** there are prominent abnormalities in bone marrow cavities. In a sagittally cut femur, the medullary cavity is partially to completely filled by firm, red tissue. Splenomegaly and hepatomegaly may be present, usually in **cats** with many circulating neoplastic cells.

Megakaryoblastic Leukaemia

Megakaryoblastic leukaemia is **a rare disease of dogs and cats.** There is usually a rapid clinical course with variable degrees of pancytopaenia. In most cases, animals have low to normal numbers of platelets. This indicates that platelet synthesis by **neoplastic megakaryocytes** is impaired.

At postmortem, there is tissue paleness, lymph node enlargement, and splemomegaly. Impression smears for cytology and histological sections of lymph nodes, spleen, and liver have infiltrates of cells similar to those observed in the bone marrow.

Plasma Cell Sarcoma

Plasma cell sarcoma is not common, but does occur in dogs and cats. There are **two basic disease mechanisms:** (1) One is caused by neoplastic cell proliferation, and (2) the other is the result of protein released from the neoplastic plasma cells. Most of the plasma cell neoplasms occur in the **bone marrow** where they interfere with haemopoiesis and erode endosteal bone by focal osteolysis. Plasma cell neoplasms at times also occur in other tissues. Although lymph nodes and lamina propria of the intestine are the richest sources of normal plasma cells, they are not the sites where plasma cell sarcomas occur. **Cytokines** produced by the neoplastic plasma cells and others produced by bone marrow stromal cells favour preferential proliferation of neoplastic clone.

Most plasma cell sarcomas secrete protein. As the neoplastic cells originate from transformation of one cell, **the protein molecules are similar** and are partial to complete immunoglobulin molecules of one class (**monoclonal gammopathies**), in contrast to immunoglobulins in animals with chronic infections (**polyclonal gammopathies**). Sometimes **dogs** with chronic infections such as ehrlichiosis and blastomycosis have monoclonal gammopathies. Hyperviscosity of the plasma indicates the quality and structural properties of the protein and is therefore more severe if cells are producing IgM molecules rather than IgG or IgA molecules. **In dogs,** plasma hyperviscosity causes retinal haemorrhages, glomerular disease, and depression.

Epistaxis and **melena** (blood in faeces) have been observed **in dogs** with plasma cell sarcoma. Bleeding is caused by effects of the abnormal protein on platelets and coagulation proteins. When **hyperviscosity** is severe, bleeding can occur from distension and rupture of small vessels.

In dogs, renal disease is caused by the effects of **hyperproteinaemia** on glomeruli and deposition of protein in tubules. Neoplastic plasma cells usually fail to assemble normal combinations of light and heavy chain molecules. This results in release into the circulation of light chains or low-molecular weight proteins that appear in the urine and can be quantitated by heat precipitation.

Animals with plasma cell sarcomas have mild to moderate **non-regenerative anaemia,** or **pancytopaenia** if the marrow is severely involved. Marrow and splenic aspirates may have increased numbers of plasma cells in varying stages of differentiation. If the cells have abnormal (for example, binucleate cells), and there is interference with haemopoiesis, or focal osteolysis, a diagnosis of neoplasm should be made.

At postmortem, plasma cell sarcomas appear as soft, gelatinous, pink to red masses in bone marrow spaces including those of the vertebrae. Neoplasms may have eroded the bone and extended into the surrounding soft tissue. **Microscopically,** the tumours are composed of **sheets of atypical to well-differentiated plasma cells.**

Chronic Leukaemias

Chronic leukaemias are characterized by a **long clinical course** with large numbers of **circulating cells** which are **more differentiated than those in the acute leukaemias.**

Chronic Granulocytic Leukaemia

This is rare in animals, but occurs in **cats** infected with feline leukaemia virus. It also occurs in **dogs** and **horses. Dogs** are debilitated and spleen is so enlarged that it is detectable by palpation. There is non-regenerative anaemia, marked leukocytosis, and thrombocytopaenia. **Neutrophilic leukaemias are most common.** However, eosinophilic leukaemias have been reported in cats with feline leukaemia virus. Basophilic leukaemias are rare. Myelocytes, promyelocytes, and myeloblasts are usually identified by thorough smear examination.

At postmortem, these animals are usually emaciated. **Dogs** have marked splenomegaly and lymph nodes are usually enlarged. The bone marrow cavities are completely filled with red tissue. **Microscopically,** granulocytes infiltrate into the spleen, liver, and lymph nodes. The differentiation of neutrophilic leukaemia from a chronic inflammatory response (**leukaemoid reaction**) may be difficult.

Chronic Megakaryocytic Sarcoma

This is also **rare** but may occur in **cats** infected with the feline leukaemia virus. Platelet counts are high with marked variation in platelet size. **Marked thrombocytosis may cause thrombosis.** A macrocytic non-regenerative anaemia may be present. In bone marrow aspirates, there are numerous megakaryocytes in all stages of development. **At postmortem,** these **cats** have paleness of tissue, splenomegaly, hepatomegaly, and bone marrow cavities occupied by solid red tissue. **Microscopically,** marked accumulations of megakaryocytes occur in the splenic red pulp, hepatic sinusoids, and lymph nodes.

Mast Cell Leukaemia

Mast cell leukaemia is **a rare disease of dogs,** but has a somewhat higher incidence in **cats. Clinical signs** which occur from excessive production of histamine include vomiting and diarrhoea. Splenomegaly occurs in most **cats.** Variable numbers of mast cells are found in blood smears. Gastric and duodenal ulceration are usually seen at postmortem. The spleen is consistently enlarged and firm, and there is usually hepatomegaly. Large numbers of mast cells infiltrate the splenic red pulp, and occupy hepatic sinusoids and parenchyma, bone marrow, and kidneys.

Platelet Disorders

Thrombocytosis

Thrombocytosis is **an increase in the number of blood platelets.** Platelet numbers fluctuate in the blood of animals and increase greatly in response to most haemopoietic stimuli. Neutrophilia and anaemia with reticulocytosis are usually accompanied by thrombocytosis.

Thrombocytopaenia

Thrombocytopaenia is **a decrease in the number of blood platelets.** It is an important disorder in animals. Thrombocytopaenia, like neutropaeniaor anaemia, is due to premature cellular destruction or defective production. **Platelet life span** may be decreased because of consumption of platelets following their adhesion to injured vascular endothelium, e.g., in diseases such as infectious canine hepatitis and swine fever (hog cholera). Platelet adhesion followed by platelet activation may initiate intravascular coagulation and more platelet consumption. Thrombocytopaenia due to phagocytosis of antibody-coated platelets may occur alone, or it may accompany other immune-mediated diseases such as haemolytic anaemia and systemic lupus erythematosus. An **isoimmune thrombocytopaenia** occurs **in neonatal pigs** at 1 to 3 days **following ingestion of colostrum.** The syndrome is characterized by severe haemorrhage and high mortality.

A **cyclic thrombocytopaenia** occurs in **dogs** as a result of infection of platelets by rickettsial organism *Ehrlichia platys.* **Thrombocytopaenia** as a result of failure of platelet production can occur in any bone marrow disorder. **Oestrogen toxicity in dogs** is usually detected clinically by haemorrhages which are typical of thrombocytopaenia. The same is true of **bracken fern poisoning in cattle. Clinical signs** of thrombocytopaenia are petechiation observed on mucosae and ocular sclerae. The skin of **dogs** has petechial to diffuse haemorrhages. Mucosal bleeding at the gingival margin and into the intestine is significant in canine thrombocytopaenia. **Epistaxis** is also common in thrombocytopaenic animals, and haemorrhage can be severe following surgery or trauma. Unlike the erythrocyte direct antiglobulin test, tests for antiplatelet antibody have been difficult to develop.

Platelet Function Disorders

These disorders are characterized by spontaneous occurrence of petechiae and mucosal bleeding, and life-threatening haemorrhages following surgery, despite normal platelet counts. **These functional defects** may be **congenital** or **acquired.** They occur from defective platelet secretion, adhesion, or aggregation. The ability of the platelets to adhere to sub-endothelial collagen in spite of rapid blood flow in arterioles is mediated by **von Willebrand cytoadhesive protein.** Congenital absence or decrease in this protein results in **von Willebrand's disease** (discussed later).

Platelet secretion, adhesion, aggregation and prostaglandin metabolism are damaged in **uraemia,** and are responsible for the mucosal haemorrhage that occurs in animals with renal failure. Platelet aggregation is damaged following administration of aspirin and related compounds because of inhibited thromboxane synthesis from arachidonic acid. Bovine platelets synthesize little thromboxane, and platelet function is unaffected by the administration of aspirin. **Inherited bleeding disorders** with defects *in vitro* platelet aggregation occur in human beings and animals.

Platelet aggregates are mostly unstable and disintegrate before stabilization of the platelet plug by fibrinogen. A disorder of bleeding in **calf** is characterized by an inadequate content of adenosine diphosphate (ADP) in platelets. ADP released following platelet activation is an important activating agent for nearby platelets, thus facilitating platelet aggregation.

Coagulation Disorders

As discussed, **platelet disorders** result in bleeding from mucosal surfaces because of inadequate plugging at sites of endothelial damage. **Disorders of coagulation,** also known as **coagulopathies,** result from failure of fibrin synthesis within platelet aggregates. This causes inadequate stabilization of the platelet plug. Prolonged bleeding then occurs after temporary occlusion of the injured vessel wall by the unstable platelet plug.

Coagulation System

The **coagulation cascade** has undergone significant changes over the past decade. It is now clear that platelet and endothelial cell surfaces provide a framework for assembly and interaction of coagulation proteins. The **intrinsic** and **extrinsic** **pathways** of the **coagulation system** are now known to be **highly interdependent.** However, the general principle that coagulation events are all directed toward the **conversion of fibrinogen to fibrin remains unchanged. Fibrinogen,** an acute phase reactant, is synthesized by liver cells, circulates in plasma, and **is located in alpha granules of platelets and megakaryocytes.**

Briefly, the coagulation sequence is a series of enzymatic changes, converting inactive proenzymes into activated enzymes and ending in the formation of

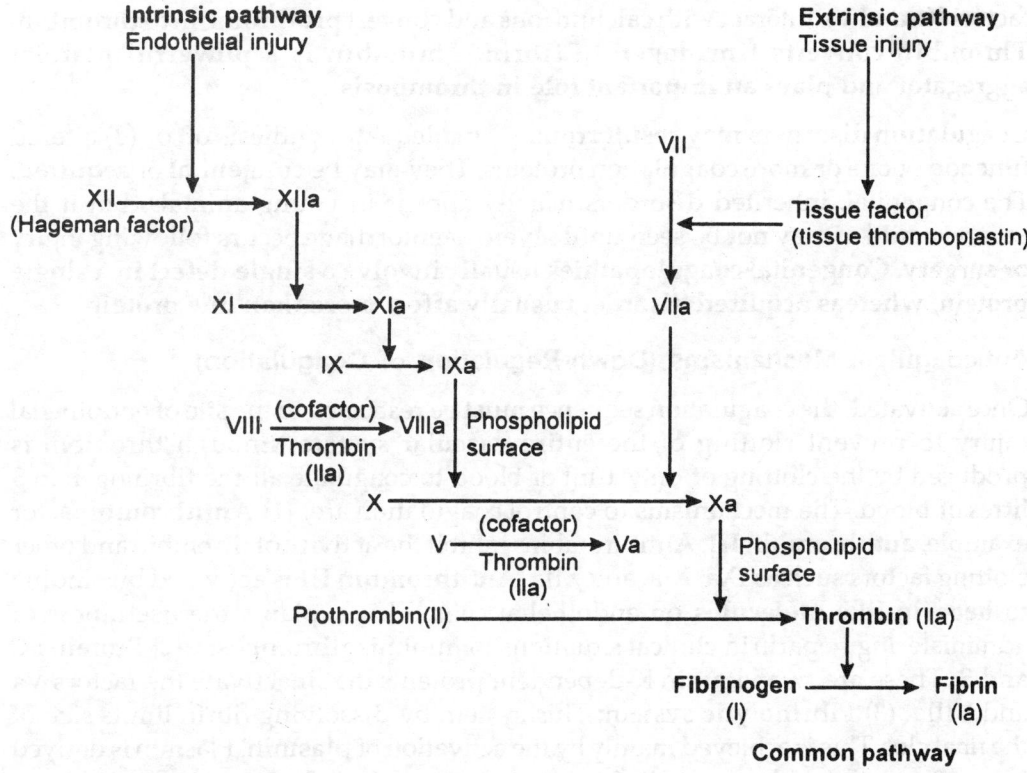

Fig. 33. The coagulation system. Note the common link between the intrinsic and extrinsic pathways at **factor X**. An activated factor is indicated by adding suffix 'a'.

thrombin. Thrombin then converts the **soluble** plasma protein **fibrinogen** into the **insoluble** fibrous protein **fibrin.** The blood coagulation system is divided, as mentioned above, into **an intrinsic and extrinsic pathway.** Both converge at the point where factor X is activated (Fig. 33).

The **intrinsic pathway** is activated following endothelial injury (Fig. 33). **First, factor XII (Hageman factor) is activated** by its surface contact with collagen, or other negatively charged substances, and in the reactions that follow, factors XI and IX are activated. Then factor X is activated to factor Xa, as follows. On the phospholipid surface of platelets, factor IXa (the enzyme), factor X (the substrate), and factor VIIIa (the reaction accelerator) are assembled (Fig. 33). Calcium ions hold the assembled components together and in the reaction that occurs, factor X is converted to factor Xa.

The **extrinsic pathway** is activated by **tissue factor (tissue thromboplastin)** released at sites of injury. Tissue factor activates factor VII, which in turn activates factor X. Then, in the **common pathway,** on the platelet surface (phospholipid complex), factors Xa and Va interact with calcium ions and convert **prothrombin to thrombin. Thrombin converts fibrinogen to fibrin. Thrombin is a powerful platelet aggregator and plays an important role in thrombosis.**

Coagulation disorders may result from: (1) inadequate synthesis of, or (2) altered function of one or more coagulation proteins. They may be **congenital** or **acquired**. The congenital, inherited disorders usually appear in young animals, but if the defect is mild, it may not be seen until severe haemorrhage occurs following injury or surgery. **Congenital coagulopathies usually involve a single defect in a single protein, whereas acquired disorders usually affect more than one protein.**

Anticoagulant Mechanisms (Down-Regulation of Coagulation)

Once activated, the coagulation sequence must be restricted to the site of endothelial injury to prevent clotting of the entire vascular system. Enough thrombin is produced by the clotting of only 1 ml of blood to coagulate all the fibrinogen in 3 litres of blood. The mechanisms to control coagulation are: **(1) Antithrombins,** for example, **antithrombin III.** Antithrombins inhibit the activity of thrombin and other clotting factors such as IXa, XIa, and XIIa. **Antithrombin III** is activated by binding to **heparin-like molecules** on endothelial cells. This explains the usefulness of administering heparin in clinical situations to minimize thrombosis. **(2) Proteins C and S:** These are two vitamin K-dependent proteins that inactivate the factors Va and VIIIa. **(3) Fibrinolytic system:** This system by dissolving fibrin limits size of the final clot. This is achieved mainly by the activation of **plasmin.** Plasmin is derived from enzymatic breakdown of its inactive precursor **plasminogen,** present in blood, either by a factor XII-dependent pathway or by **plasminogen activators (PAs).** The most important among plasminogen activators is the **tissue-type PA (t-PA). Tissue-type plasminogen activator** is synthesized mainly by endothelial cells and is most active when attached to fibrin. The affinity for fibrin makes t-PA a useful therapeutic agent. **Plasmin breaks down fibrin.** The resulting **fibrin split products (FSPs),** also called **fibrin degradation products** can also act as weak anticoagulants.

Congenital Coagulation Disorders

The **congenital coagulation disorders** occur **from molecular lesions in coagulation proteins.** In other words, there may be inadequate synthesis of a normal molecule, or synthesis of an abnormal molecule in which the abnormality in a critical location interferes with function. The latter situation may result from a **purine or pyrimidine base change in DNA.** Most coagulation factors undergo post-ribosomal modification, such as cleavage of a portion of the molecule before it becomes functional, **and this process also may be abnormal.**

Factor XII Deficiency

Factor XII deficiency occurs in cats and occasionally has been reported in **dogs.** It occurs as an autosomal recessive trait. Homozygotes have prolonged activated partial thromboplastin times (APTTs), **but no clinical evidence of bleeding.**

Factor XI Deficiency

Factor XI deficiency occurs in cattle and dogs. It is transmitted as an autosomal recessive gene in **cattle.** Spontaneous haemorrhage is of little importance in affected animals but can be severe following surgery. Homozygous factor XI-deficient animals have prolonged whole blood clotting times, APTTs, **and lack of factor XI activity.**

Factor IX Deficiency (Haemophilia B)

Factor IX deficiency occurs in dogs and cats. The inheritance is sex linked, because the gene is present on the X chromosome. Affected males have low factor IX activity, and carrier females have 40% to 60% of normal activity.

It is now clear that factor IX and other factor deficiencies in animals may result from **a wide range of molecular lesions** that have yet to be clarified. Bleeding in **male pups** is due to complete deletion of the factor IX gene. **Canine haemophilia B** closely resembles the human disease.

Haemorrhage in factor IX deficiency is **mild** in **cats** and **small dogs** and **more severe** in **large dogs,** probably because of the greater degree of trauma in large weight-bearing animals.

Factor VIII Deficiency (Haemophilia A)

Factor VIII deficiency is an important disease in dogs. It also occurs in **horses, cattle, sheep,** and **cats,** and in **all species.** It is an X chromosome-linked recessive trait. **Bleeding may be severe in large dogs and horses. Haemarthrosis** (bleeding in a joint), subcutaneous haematomas, and bleeding into the central nervous system and body cavities may occur in varying degrees in factor VIII deficiency. Laboratory evaluation reveals long APTTs. Factor VIII activity is low, and von Willebrand factor levels are normal. Carrier female animals have about 50% factor VIII activity and normal levels of von Willebrand factor.

von Willebrand's Disease

von Willebrand's disease is an inherited abnormality of von Willebrand glycoprotein synthesis. It is the **most important haemostatic disorder in human beings and many breeds of dogs.** It also occurs in **cats** and **horses.**

The **von Willebrand protein or factor (vWF) is synthesized in endothelial cells and megakaryocytes.** The mature canine subunit of 2813 amino acids is glycosylated and joined to another subunit by disulphide bonds to form multimers. (A multimer is a protein molecule made up of more than one polypeptide chain). **Multimers are very large molecules with high molecular weights.** The glycoprotein is found in plasma, megakaryocytes, platelets, sub-endothelium, and endothelial cells. In the plasma, von Willebrand protein forms a complex with factor VIII. This increases the concentration of factor VIII at sites of vascular injury and protects it from proteolytic degradation. **Platelet von Willebrand glycoprotein is mainly located in alpha granules and is secreted on the surface following platelet activation.**

Mature vWF facilitates adhesion of platelets to exposed vascular sub-endothelium following injury. This is especially important in small vessels with rapid blood flow (high shear rate). vWF acts as a bridge between platelet surface receptor, **glycoprotein Ib (GPIb),** and exposed collagen (Fig. 34). Although platelets can adhere directly to collagen, **vWF-glycoprotein Ib association** is the only interaction sufficiently strong to overcome the high shear rate of flowing blood. Genetic deficiencies of vWF **(von Willebrand's disease),** or its receptors, result in **serious bleeding disorders,** highlighting the importance of these

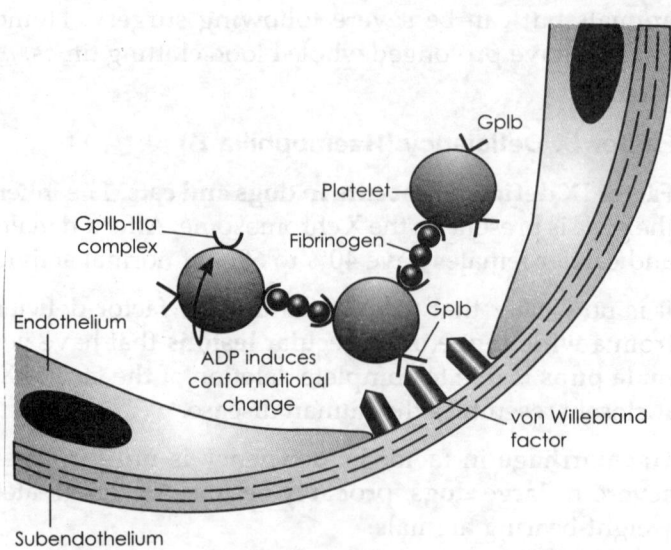

Fig. 34. Platelet adhesion and aggregation. Von Willebrand factor functions as an adhesion bridge between sub-endothelial collagen and the glycoprotein Ib (GpIb) platelet receptor. Aggregation is achieved by fibrinogen's binding to platelet GpIIb-IIIa receptors and bridging many platelets together. ADP = adenosine diphosphate.

interactions. Studies in human beings have revealed that **the largest vWF molecules have the most GPIb binding sites, and bleeding times are prolonged in humans and dogs which are unable to assemble large molecules.**

Intensive study of **humans** with von Willebrand's disease has established that there is molecular heterogeneity (molecular variations). **A similar heterogeneity occurs among breeds of dogs.** The disease in **dogs** is of three types: **(1) Type I, the most common** is characterized by **decreased levels** of a normal multimetric glycoprotein pattern, that is, decreased levels of large vWF molecules. **(2) In type II, dogs lack the large multimers (i.e. large vWF molecules),** and **(3) Type III dogs** have very low or no detectable von Willebrand glycoprotein.

Clinically, animals with von Willebrand's disease have a **bleeding disorder** due to defective platelet adhesion. **Epistaxis, oozing of blood from mucous membranes, petechiation, and serious post-operative haemorrhage** are the most common findings. **Despite being a congenital defect,** variation in the expression of von Willebrand's disease may present a different clinical picture. For example, it may result in bleeding in some mature dogs, whereas dogs with mild form of the disease may only bleed because of another disease such as urinary or intestinal tract carcinomas or inflammation of a mucosal surface.

Laboratory diagnosis of animals suspected of having von Willebrand's disease is achieved by quantitative and multimeric analysis. **Plasma vWF concentrations** are measured by an **ELISA** using polyclonal antibodies specific for canine vWF. The protein measured in this assay is referred to as **von Willebrand antigen (vWF:Ag).**

Acquired Coagulation Disorders

Toxicities causing haemorrhage usually follow ingestion of one from a group of related substances known as **coumarins. Coumarins** are synthesized by moulds in sweet clover and **are used in rodenticides** (agents to kill or control rodents). **Sweet clover poisoning** is most common in **cattle,** but can also occur in **sheep** and **horses. Dogs** and **cats** that accidentally ingest rodenticides develop life-threatening haemorrhages. Repeated ingestion of coumarins is necessary to exhaust vitamin K stores.

Coumarins and Related Compounds

Coumarins and related compounds interfere with the vitamin K-dependent coagulation factors II, VII, XI, and X. The **clinical signs** vary depending on the degree and location of **haemorrhage. Spontaneous bleeding** causes large **haematomas** and haemarthroses (bleeding in the joints). **Cattle** with sweet clover poisoning bleed severely following minor surgery. **Calves** born to dams ingesting mouldy sweet clover may die of internal haemorrhage at birth, although the dam is unaffected.

Rodenticide toxicity in dogs causes a variety of clinical signs which occur from hypovolaemia (decreased volume of circulating blood) from haemorrhage, organ dysfunction, or bleeding into body cavities. Haemorrhage into the brain may produce neurological dysfunction and sometime sudden death. Haemarthrosis causes sudden lameness. Haematomas occur following venipuncture and trauma.

Liver Disease

Liver disease, in which there is inadequate synthesis of coagulation factors, can cause severe bleeding. Significant depletion of these factors occurs either late in progressive liver diseases when most of the organ is destroyed, or in cases of acute, severe liver cell necrosis. Accurate laboratory assessment of coagulation factor function in animals with liver disease is difficult because this may be complicated by subnormal platelet function and simultaneous disseminated intravascular coagulation.

Disseminated Intravascular Coagulation

Disseminated intravascular coagulation (DIC) and fibrinolysis are important coagulation disorders. They occur from a variety of mechanisms in neoplastic diseases, severe haemolysis, and other disorders. **These disorders cause unregulated and excessive production of thrombin,** which is the most important factor in the pathogenesis of DIC. The **overproduction of thrombin** results in the consumption of coagulation factors which are its substrates, such as fibrinogen, factor V, and factor VIII. **Thrombin** binds to its receptors on platelets and endothelial cells and is a potent agonist (stimulator) causing platelet activation and aggregation. **Thrombin** also causes endothelial cells to release tissue plasminogen activator. Newly formed fibrin stimulates the production of **plasmin** from plasminogen and results in aggressive **fibrinolysis**.

Therefore, the **clinical and laboratory manifestations** of DIC occur **from the overproduction of thrombin and plasmin.** The overproduction of thrombin with relatively reduced expression of plasmin may result in either large-vessel thrombosis or microvascular fibrin deposition leading to organ dysfunction and ischaemic necrosis. Excessive thrombin production with severe secondary fibrinolysis may cause increased consumption of haemostatic factors and bleeding.

Thymus and Lymph Nodes

Thymus is essential for the development and function of the immune system. The epithelial portions are derived from branchial pouches, whereas **lymphocytes originate in bone marrow** and travel to the thymus through blood. Thymus provides a microenvironment for the development of **mature T-lymphocytes,** which **normally constitute 70% to 80% of peripheral blood lymphocytes.** The gland consists of sub-capsular, cortical, and medullary zones.

Following release from the thymus into the blood, T-cells travel to the splenic periarteriolar lymphatic sheaths and the cortical areas around germinal centres in lymph nodes. The critical balance of production and distribution of T-lymphocytes is extremely important in immune homeostasis. **Immunodeficiency** or **autoimmunity** may occur from inadequate or too much activity of a particular group, for example, CD4 (helper) or CD8 (cytotoxic) T-cells.

Thymus is large before birth and involutes following sexual maturity. The lymphoid and epithelial components are gradually replaced by loose connective tissue and fat.

Thymic Disorders

Developmental Disorders of the Thymus

Congenital disorders discussed here are those which result in inadequate T-lymphocyte function, and also those which result in B-lymphocyte and plasma cell dysfunction. Many have been described in humans and have been very helpful in learning more about mechanisms of immunity and immune regulation. The animal counterparts of immunodeficiency serve as valuable models in comparative immunology research. **Combined immunodeficiencies (CIDs) are diseases affecting both B and T-lymphocytes.**

Combined Immunodeficiency (CID)

Equine Combined Immunodeficiency

Equine CID is a genetic disorder of foals. It is inherited as an autosomal recessive trait. That is, both sire and dam are carriers of the defective gene. **There is a failure of functional B and T-lymphocyte production.** Therefore, **foals are extremely susceptible to a variety of microbial agents and usually die before 5 months of age. Adenoviruses** which are resisted by normal foals are the major causes of death in foals with CID. The viral infection is usually complicated by various bacterial or protozoal infections that result in **pneumonia.** The underlying biochemical defect for failure of B and T-lymphocyte differentiation must occur at an early stage of lymphocyte development. **In children,** this is the result of adenosine deaminase deficiency, which may cause defective DNA synthesis in lymphocytes. **This enzyme is not deficient in affected foals.** The exact mechanism of their lymphocyte stem cell failure remains unknown.

Affected foals usually have profuse nasal discharge, unthrifty hair coat, loss of condition, pneumonia, and sometimes diarrhoea. Varying degrees of neutrophilia and left shift and a mild anaemia occur due to chronic inflammation. **Lymphopaenia** is marked and persistent. Serum IgM, which is normally present in **newborn foals,** is absent. Maternally derived IgG decreases to very low concentrations by about 3 months of age. Thus, **diagnosis** of CID in such a foal requires fulfilment of these conditions: (1) persistent lymphopaenia, (2) absence of serum immunoglobulin, or (3) hypoplastic lymphoid tissue.

Postmortem findings are severe bronchopneumonia and small spleen and lymph nodes. The thymus may be difficult to identify or may consist of a few isolated lobules within the mediastinal fat. The spleen has markedly reduced white pulp due to the absence of germinal centres and periarteriolar lymphatic sheaths. Lymph nodes are similarly depleted of lymphocytes.

Inflammatory and Degenerative Disorders of the Thymus

Injury to the thymus which may result in immunodeficiency may be caused by infectious agents (usually viruses), toxins, neoplasms, malnutrition, and aging. The feline leukaemia virus (FELV) and feline immunodeficiency virus (FIV), are examples of infectious agents that infect **T-lymphocytes,** resulting in chronic respiratory and digestive system infections. Viruses with similar capabilities are those of canine distemper, bovine virus diarrhoea, equine rhinopneumonitis (equine herpesvirus-1), and feline parvovirus.

One of the T-lymphocyte surface glycoproteins (CD4) is the receptor for attachment of the human acquired immunodeficiency (AIDS) virus. **In FIV-infected cats,** there is depletion of CD4 lymphocytes, and this results in **reversal of the CD4/CD8 T-lymphocyte ratio.** In FIV-infected **cats,** thymic cortex has a high viral load and lymphoid follicles become hyperplastic. Later there is lymphoid depletion and follicular involution. Therefore, thymic and lymph node atrophy are seen at postmortem in animals with these viral infections.

Thymic function is damaged in severe dietary protein deficiencies of young animals. This leads to reduced immunoglobulin synthesis. Environmental toxins such as lead and mercury have a suppressive effect on the immune system.

A syndrome called **'idiopathic thymic haemorrhage'** has been reported in **dogs,** which involves thymus, thymic mediastinum and thymic remnants in **young dogs. Affected dogs** die unexpectedly from massive mediastinal haemorrhage and hypovolaemic shock.

Neoplasms of the Thymus

Since thymus has both lymphoid and epithelial tissue, it is possible that either or both can be neoplastically transformed.

Thymic lymphosarcoma is **a T-lymphocyte neoplasm of young animals,** particularly **cats** and **cattle,** with a much lower incidence in **dogs. Clinical findings** include the presence of a large mass in the thoracic cavity. Thoracic aspirates (material obtained by aspirates) show many medium to large lymphocytes, which usually have vacuolated cytoplasm. This feature is characteristic of lymphocytes in fluid. If present, mitoses indicate neoplasm.

Bovine thymic lymphosarcoma usually occurs in **beef cattle** 6 to 24 months of age, and is characterized by massive thymic enlargement. The aetiology is unknown. The thymus is an important site of lymphosarcoma in **cats.** The tumours are large, white or grey mediastinal masses which displace adjacent structures and result in fluid accumulation (Fig. 35). In **cats,** thoracic fluid is

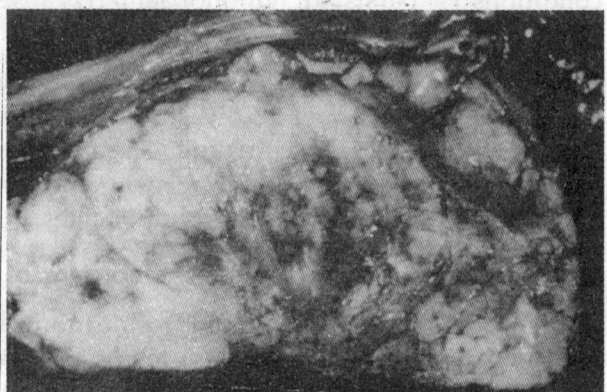

Fig. 35. Thymus; cat. Lymphosarcoma. The large tumour has been cut transversely. Note white tumourous masses.

usually chylous (milky) because of lipid accumulations. **Microscopically,** these tumours are diffuse lymphosarcomas containing large lymphocytes which are uniform in size, shape, nuclear morphology, and nuclear/cytoplasmic ratio.

Thymomas are primary **neoplasms of thymic epithelial cells** and are accompanied by varying proportions of non-neoplastic lymphocytes (**thymocytes**). They grow slowly and **are uncommon** but occur in **dogs, cats, cattle,** and **sheep.** They are usually encapsulated, nodular, firm masses with soft and cystic areas, located in the cranial mediastinum. They are cytologically dissimilar with small lymphocytes and are round to spindle-shaped epithelial cells present singly or in clumps. Variable number of mast cells, plasma cells, eosinophils, neutrophils, and macrophages may be present. **Microscopically,** connective tissue trabeculae of variable thickness subdivide the mass into lobules composed of solid sheets and cords of round to spindle-shaped epithelial cells. Variable numbers of mainly small lymphocytes are present accompanied by a smaller number of medium and large lymphocytes. The cystic structures are lined by epithelial cells, which may be ciliated.

Lymph Nodes

If a lymph node(s) is enlarged, it is called **lymphadenomegaly.** If a node(s) is small or absent it is called **lymph node hypoplasia, lymph node aplasia,** or **lymph node atrophy** depending on the case. **Lymphadenomegaly** may be **localized** involving a single node or **generalized** involving many nodes.

Lymph Node Disorders

Degenerative Disorders

Atrophy of lymph nodes and bronchial and gut-associated lymphoid tissues may occur from viral infections, toxins, and malnutrition. Examples of these are discussed with degenerative disorders of the thymus. Degenerative processes associated with aging also result in defective function and decreased numbers of lymphocytes causing deficient immunological responses.

Hyperplasia of Lymph Nodes

Arrival of **a large number of antigens** in a lymph node results in increased blood supply, increased numbers of macrophages, and recruitment of many lymphocytes. **Superficial lymph nodes** become palpably enlarged. Lymphocytes transform into large cells, which undergo cell division. Depending on the nature of the antigen, the transformed cells mature into T-lymphocytes or plasma cells. Aspirates of **hyperplastic lymph nodes** show a greater variation in lymphocyte morphology in comparison to normal lymph nodes, because of increased numbers of large lymphocytes among predominantly small lymphocyte population. There are also increased numbers of macrophages, which may be antigen-presenting cells, and a few neutrophils. **Mitotic figures are not common.** The nuclear chromatin pattern of lymphocytes varies in hyperplastic lymph nodes. **Plasma cells** are usually seen and indicate recent stimulation of the node by antigens that stimulate antibody synthesis. In contrast to hyperplastic nodes, aspirates of **lymphosarcomatous nodes** may have many disintegrated cells.

The **histological findings in hyperplastic lymph nodes** indicate the duration of stimulation. The venules with high endothelium are prominent. They indicate increased lymphocyte adhesion and migration soon after the arrival of antigen. **Germinal centres** with numerous macrophages become prominent in secondary follicles. The T-cell population is increased. As a result, the paracortex is expanded. Within a few days, increased numbers of plasma cells may be detected in the medullary cords. Chronically stimulated nodes have increased numbers of follicles. Differentiation of benign hyperplasia from a neoplasm may be difficult.

Inflammatory Disorders of Lymph Nodes

Inflammation of one or more lymph nodes is called **lymphadenitis.**

Caseous Lymphadenitis

Caseous lymphadenitis is a specific lymphadenitis of **sheep** and **goats** caused by *Corynebacterium pseudotuberculosis,* which is also the cause of **ulcerative lymphangitis** in **cattle** and **horses** and pectoral abscesses in **horses**. It is believed that the organism lives in the intestine and enters the skin through wounds contaminated with soil containing faecal material or purulent discharges. **Most sheep do not become ill.** Debilitation occurs only in a small percentage of sheep in which infection involves internal lymph nodes and other organs.

The **encapsulated abscesses** of cutaneous lymphadenitis in **sheep** are characteristically **green** and **caseous**, with **concentric rings** resembling those of an onion (Fig. 36). Similar abscesses may be found in the lungs, especially in **older sheep**. The abscesses in **goats** are usually more numerous and usually involve lymph nodes of the head and neck.

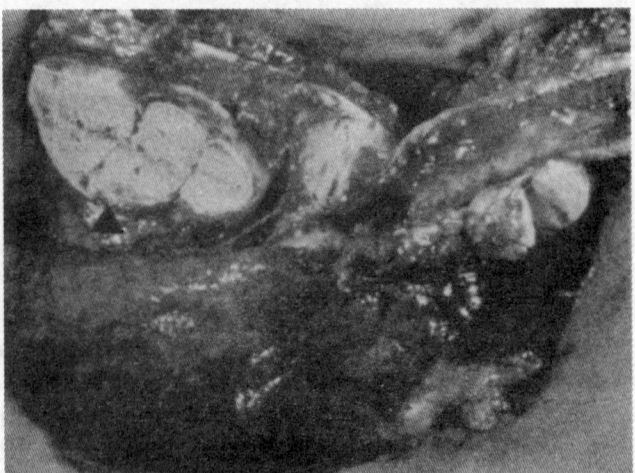

Fig. 36. Lung; sheep. Caseous lymphadenitis. Note that the incised mediastinal lymph nodes are completely filled with caseous material (arrowhead).

Histoplasmosis

Histoplasmosis is a diffuse disease of the monocyte-macrophage system caused by fungus *Histoplasma capsulatum*. The fungus grows as a mould in soil and as yeast in animal tissues. In most animals, the organism is inhaled and causes a mild, self-limiting infection with hypertrophy of tracheo-bronchial lymph nodes in **dogs** and **cats**. Since the fungus is confined to monocytes and macrophages, spread beyond the respiratory tract occurs by haematogenous and lymphatic spread of infected cells. **Disseminated histoplasmosis in dogs and cats** causes gastrointestinal or liver disease of a long duration. There are also reports of eye involvement in feline disseminated histoplasmosis.

Disseminated histoplasmosis is characterized by neutrophilia and monocytosis in some animals. Non-regenerative anaemia is common because of the chronic inflammation. **Cytology** is useful in the **diagnosis of histoplasmosis.** The procedures include examination of cells of buffy coat, body fluids, and tracheal wash preparations, and aspirates of bone marrow and lymph nodes. The organisms are visible in monocytes, neutrophils, and macrophages.

Dogs dying of this disease are emaciated. The large intestine is thickened with mucosal corrugations caused by infiltration of the sub-mucosa and the lamina propria with macrophages, lymphocytes, and plasma cells. Lymph nodes are enlarged, and in contrast to lymphosarcoma are firm when incised. The spleen and liver are enlarged and firm, and the liver is diffusely grey.

Epizootic Lymphangitis

Epizootic lymphangitis or **equine histoplasmosis** is a chronic **suppurative lymphadenitis** of **horses, mules,** and **donkeys** caused by *Histoplasma farciminosus*. The fungus exists in the soil and enters the body through contaminated wounds. Fungal spores are also inhaled and cause lesions of the upper and lower respiratory tracts.

Lesions, in most locations, **are nodules** which eventually discharge a mucopurulent exudate. The organism is seen in smears of the exudate as round to oval yeasts 2 to 3 μm in diameter. Spontaneous recovery may occur. **At postmortem,** suppurative and granulomatous **lesions** are most numerous **in the skin,** with occasional spread to the **lungs, liver,** and **spleen.**

Leishmaniasis

Leishmaniasis, like histoplasmosis, is a diffuse disease of the monocyte-macrophage system caused by protozoa of the genus **Leishmania.** It occurs in **humans, dogs,** and **other animals.** The protozoa proliferate by binary fission in the intestine of the sand fly and become flagellated organisms. They then develop a non-flagellated form in macrophages.

The **cutaneous lesions in dogs are ulcers** at the site of insect bites. These ulcers are due to proliferation of the organism in macrophages, accumulation of neutrophils, lymphocytes, and plasma cells, and focal disruption of the dermis and epidermis. In **visceral form of the disease, dogs** are emaciated and show generalized enlargement of lymph nodes. Lymph node aspirates contain macrophages with organisms. **Dogs** have a non-regenerative anaemia and a polyclonal hypergammaglobulinaemia.

At postmortem, dogs with visceral leishmaniasis are emaciated and have enlarged liver, spleen, and lymph nodes. The bone marrow is usually hyperplastic. In the **impression smears** of these organs, macrophages show numerous round organisms about 2 μm in diameter. A vesicular nucleus and a small kinetoplast help in differentiating them from *Histoplasma capsulatum.*

Neoplastic Lymphocyte Disorders

Neoplastic lymphocyte disorders occur as **leukaemia** and **lymphosarcoma.** **Leukaemia** is characterized by neoplastic cells in the blood and bone marrow, and **lymphosarcoma** by tumours in soft tissue. In **animals with leukaemia,** tumour in the bone marrow may cause interference with haemopoiesis, characterized by anaemia, neutropaenia, or thrombocytopaenia. **Animals with lymphosarcoma** usually have a normal haemogram except mild, non-regenerative anaemia in some animals because of chronic disease. However, **animals with lymphosarcoma** usually have more neoplastic lymphocytes in the circulation, and an absolute lymphocytosis occurs in about 20% of cases.

Lymphocytic Leukaemia

In **animals,** lymphocytic leukaemias caused by large, poorly differentiated lymphocytes have a **shorter clinical course** than those of chronic leukaemias caused by small lymphocytes.

Acute Lymphocytic Leukaemia

Acute lymphocytic leukaemias occur in all species, and the cells may be **of B or T-cell origin.** Except **calves,** most affected animals have mild lymph node enlargement. **Cats and dogs** show non-specific signs of illness such as anorexia and lethargy. Animals with leukaemia are sick because of sequestration (isolation) of cells with rapid metabolic rates in capillary beds, thus depriving normal cells access to glucose and other substrates. **When the tumor has replaced haemopoietic tissue in the bone marrow,** the haemogram findings include anaemia, neutropaenia, and thrombocytopaenia. **Blood smears** show mainly **large lymphocytes.** Although the number of leukocytes may be within normal range, they usually exceed 50 x 10^9/L (50 x 10^3/mm^3). The cells are uniformly large with nuclei and prominent nucleoli. Disintegrated neoplastic cells are common, because of their fragility. **Bone marrow aspirates** usually show marrow particles in which lymphocytes similar to those present in the blood, predominate. They are differentiated from granulocytes by cytochemical staining.

At postmortem, animals with acute lymphocytic leukaemia show varying degrees of paleness. **Calves** show generalized lymph node enlargement, hepatomegaly, and splenomegaly, **in contrast to other species** where lymph nodes, liver, and spleen are mildly enlarged. The spleen is firm. In **calves**, the marrow cavities are usually fully occupied by tumour. In these areas necrosis may be present. In **dogs** and **cats**, marrow may be partially or completely replaced by yellow-white tissue whose consistency is firmer than that of fat. **Microscopically**, bone marrow is dominated by a homogeneous population of large cells with large spaces within the nucleochromatin and one or more large nucleoli.

Cytological examination of marrow imprints (impressions) allows a much better identification of the cells and is helpful in differentiating neoplastic erythroid precursors from lymphocytes in **cats**. Therefore, at postmortem, tissues for both fixation and cytology should be taken. **In the liver,** sinusoids usually contain large lymphocytes in larger numbers than expected. Colonies of these cells may be present in portal areas. There is usually a diffuse population of large lymphocytes in the red pulp and the spleen.

Chronic Lymphocytic Leukaemia

Chronic lymphocytic leukaemia is less common than acute lymphocytic leukaemia. It is characterized by **a persistent increase in circulating small lymphocytes,** and vague, non-specific, clinical findings. It occurs in **older cats, dogs, and cattle. Haemograms** show a mild non-regenerative anaemia. The degree of neutropaenia and thrombocytopaenia indicates the extent to which the bone marrow has been occupied by lymphocytes. Lymphocyte counts vary and range from $10 \times 10^9/L$ to $100 \times 10^9/L$ ($10 \times 10^3/mm^3$ to $100 \times 10^3/mm^3$). **The cells are small to medium-sized lymphocytes.** These cells sometimes produce immunoglobulin, and the laboratory findings are similar to those seen in secretory plasma cell sarcomas, in which there is marked hyperproteinaemia. Sometimes, **in dogs and cats,** the cell type consists of lymphocytes with cytoplasmic granules. Bone marrow aspirates are usually very cellular and dominated by lymphocytes morphologically similar to those seen in the blood.

At postmortem, animals with chronic lymphatic leukaemia usually have paleness of tissues. There may be mild enlargement of lymph nodes and liver. Spleen may be markedly enlarged and fleshy when incised. **White tumour nodules** may be present on the liver and kidney. **Microscopically,** tumour nodules are densely packed with small lymphocytes with scant cytoplasm. These cells are crowded in portal areas in the liver and form dense foci in the kidney and other organs. Lymph node lesions are characterized by dense populations of small lymphocytes occupying significant portions of the node. These destroy the normal architecture in the cortex, resulting in an extension of monocytes without follicles.

Leukaemia in Other Species

Leukaemia is rare in other species. Sporadic cases have been reported in **sheep, goats, pigs,** and **buffaloes**. Lymphoma **in sheep** occurs mostly in adult animals, without sex and breed predilection. The tissues most commonly involved are lymph nodes, spleen, liver, kidney, small intestine, and heart. **Ovine lymphoma** is caused by a C-type oncovirus and the bovine leukaemia virus is oncogenic for sheep. Lymphoma **in goats** is rare, and presents as lymphadenopathy at postmortem. **In pigs**, lymphoma occurs mainly as a sporadic disease in young animals, without sex or breed predilection. **Clinical signs** include ataxia or paralysis, enlarged superficial lymph nodes, loss of body weight, dyspnoea, and sudden death. The **diagnosis** is difficult from the blood examination because the WBC count is usually normal and abnormal lymphocytes may not be present.

Lymphosarcoma

Lymphosarcoma is an important disease in domestic animals. However, there are species variations in aetiology, tumour distribution, and clinical and postmortem findings. **Animals with lymphosarcoma may or may not be leukaemic.** That is, may or may not have neoplastic cells in bone marrow and blood.

The classification system for human lymphosarcomas has been applied to animal lymphosarcomas. The **general rules** are that lymphosarcomas of **small cells** with low mitotic rate have a low rate of progression and thus respond poorly to therapy, whereas lymphosarcomas of **larger cells** with high proliferative rates are potentially curable diseases. The system requires the identification and correlation of tumour cell types and tumour growth patterns. The **neoplasms** are therefore graded as **low-grade** (slow clinical course), **intermediate-grade,** and **high-grade** (aggressive clinical course) lymphosarcomas.

Staining of lymphosarcoma cells with monoclonal antibodies has a prognostic significance. Dogs with B-cell lymphosarcomas have a better prognosis than those with T-cell neoplasms. **Proliferating cell nuclear antigen (PCNA),** a protein associated with DNA polymerase which is expressed only in the nuclei of cells actively synthesizing DNA, is one of the several proliferating markers which may be useful in the identification of neoplastic lymphocytes. The appearance and location of tumours at necropsy, cytological and histological appearance, and immunophenotyping are all used in the study of lymphosarcoma.

Canine Lymphosarcoma

In dogs, lymphosarcoma occurs mainly in the middle-aged animals. It occurs in **multicentric** (having many centres), **alimentary, cutaneous,** and **mediastinal forms, multicentric form being the most common.** In all forms of the disease, **dogs** are anorexic and lethargic, eventually becoming cachectic (having general physical wasting). The **multicentric form** causes generalized enlargement of lymph nodes, with or without hepatic and splenic enlargement and infiltration of bone marrow. **Dogs** with **mediastinal disease** are dyspnoeic (having difficult breathing) and have reduced exercise tolerance. In the **alimentary form,** vomiting, diarrhoea, and blood in the stool are seen. Nodules, plaques, and ulcers are present in the skin of dogs with **cutaneous form** of lymphosarcoma.

Mild to moderate non-regenerative anaemia is observed, and anaemia may be microcytic and hypochromic with mild reticulocytosis, because bleeding tumours of the intestine deplete dog's iron. Aspirates from enlarged lymph nodes, liver, spleen, and the bone marrow should be obtained, if suspect cells are seen in the blood film. Lymph node aspirates show **numerous large lymphocytes** of uniform morphology. These cells are usually fragile. Therefore, aspirates may contain numerous naked nuclei and free cytoplasmic fragments. The **nuclei** in intact cells are large with very small amount of coarse cytoplasm. **Cells in mitoses are more numerous than in hyperplastic nodules.** In lymphosarcoma of liver numerous large lymphocytes are present. The **diagnosis** is more difficult in splenic aspirates, which may also have normal lymphocytes, plasma cells, and numerous erythrocytes.

Postmortem findings in canine lymphosarcoma **vary with the form of the disease.** When lymph nodes are enlarged, they are white-grey and bulge when excised. Similar tissue is usually present in the spleen and liver. Long bones should be cut sagittally. to check the extent to which fat and haemopoetic tissues have been replaced by tumour. Histological differentiation of lymph node hyperplasia may be difficult. **In neoplastic areas,** a significant portion of the node with normal architecture is completely destroyed by cells with large open nuclei and prominent nucleoli. **Usually there are many lymphocytes in mitoses.** Infiltration of lymphocytes into the sub-capsular sinus and through the capsule into the adjacent fat indicates lymphoma.

Cutaneous lymphosarcoma occurs in two forms: (1) **epitheliotropic,** and (2) **non-epitheliotropic. Epitheliotropic cutaneous lymphoma** is characterized by infiltration of neoplastic T-lymphocytes into the epidermis and adnexal epithelium. The lymphocytes have clear cytoplasm with large pale nuclei which are usually pleomorphic. The **non-epitheliotropic tumours** are characterized by B-cell or T-cell infiltration into the dermis and sub-cutis. **Microscopically,** majority of the non-epitheliotropic lymphosarcomas consist of large lymphocytes, but immunoblastic and histiocytic types also occur.

Feline Lymphosarcoma

Lymphosarcoma is one manifestation of several haemopoietic diseases caused by the **feline leukaemia virus (FLV). Cats** become infected when the virus first colonizes the pharyngeal epithelium and pharyngeal lymphoid tissue. The virus stimulates an immune response in most cats, which results in neutralization of the virus at this stage. The virus replicates in the spleen, lymph nodes, and gut-associated lymphoid tissue which are unable to mount an effective immune response, and then replicates in the bone marrow cells and intestinal crypt epithelial cells. **Viraemia and excretion of virus in saliva and urine** follows infection of neutrophils and platelets and widespread epithelial infection. The **lymphosarcomas** have been **classified as multicentric, thymic, alimentary,** and **miscellaneous.** The miscellaneous includes ocular, renal, and neural forms. Lymphocytes with abnormal morphology may be found in blood or bone marrow from **cats** with any form of lymphosarcoma.

Clinical manifestation of lymphosarcoma varies with the form of the disease, that is, the location of the tumour or tumours. Non-specific signs include paleness of mucous membranes, lethargy, and wasting. **Cats** with thymic lymphosarcoma have dyspnoea. **Cats** with internal lymph node enlargement, hepatomegaly, or intestinal lymphosarcoma may have palpable abdominal masses. **Cats** with renal lymphosarcoma may have renal failure.

Laboratory findings in feline lymphosarcoma include non-regenerative anaemia, regardless of the form of the disease. If the bone marrow is involved, there may be neutropaenia, thrombopaenia, and anaemia as the tumour replaces haemopoietic tissue. Sometimes, *Haemobartonella felis* organisms are seen in erythrocytes as a result of the immunosuppressive effects of the virus. Agglutination of erythrocytes is also usually seen as a result of circulating FLV-antibody complexes. **Lymphocytes from cats with lymphosarcoma and leukaemia** are usually larger than normal large lymphocytes. They have large nuclei compared to cytoplasm, and nuclear shapes may be irregular. The bone marrow aspirates may have variable numbers of immature lymphocytes, and in some cases, complete replacement of haemopoietic cells by the tumour. **Cats** with abdominal masses are usually emaciated. If the masses are lymph nodes, aspirates contain mainly large lymphocytes, some of which are in mitosis. With liver and kidney lymphosarcomas, aspirates contain numerous lymphocytes along with hepatocytes and renal tubular epithelial cells, respectively.

At postmortem, cats with lymphosarcoma may have diffuse or nodular enlargement of organs such as the liver, kidneys, thymus, and lymph nodes. If enlarged lymph nodes are cut, the surface is soft, white, and bulges. With thymic lymphosarcomas, a large, grey, soft mass is present in the thoracic cavity. Marrow cavities of large bones are occupied by yellow-white tissue in animals with lymphosarcoma involving bone marrow. **Impression smears** should be made from these tissues as a supplement to histological examination.

Bovine Lymphosarcoma

Enzootic bovine lymphosarcoma is a disease of adult cattle caused by the bovine leukaemia virus (BLV), an RNA retrovirus similar to other oncogenic viruses. Its behaviour differs from the feline virus, in that its expression is minimal in spite of its persistence within lymphocytes for the life of the animal. Its spread is mostly through the transmission of infected lymphocytes as opposed to transmission of free virus in secretions. Following establishment of infection, circulating antibody appears and is present throughout life. Blood-sucking arthropods or other mechanical means of transferring small numbers of infected lymphocytes are the chief means of spread. **The disease has a much higher incidence in dairy cattle compared to beef cattle.** This is probably because dairy cattle husbandry favours viral transmission. Herd surveys have revealed high rates of infection but low incidence of the disease.

Clinically, enzootic bovine sarcoma has a peak incidence in cattle of 6 to 8 years. **Enlargement of one or more superficial lymph nodes is common.** On rectal palpation, enlarged abdominal and pelvic lymph nodes may be found. Unilateral or bilateral **exophthalmos** occurs following involvement of retrobulbar lymphoid tissue. Involvement of the digestive tract may cause **persistent diarrhoea**, and involvement of the right heart may cause congestive heart failure. Nervous system lymphosarcoma is usually manifested by **posterior paresis** (partial paralysis) **or paralysis** because of pressure by the external mass on the cauda equina or on the lumbar spinal cord or its nerve roots. In addition, most cattle have lesions of lymphosarcoma in the liver and spleen. Involvement of the bone marrow and leukaemia may occur in the terminal stages of the disease. **Persistent lymphocytosis** develops in about 30% of infected animals and may last for many years prior to clinical expression of the disease. **Serological detection** of BLV antibody helps in differentiating BLV-induced lymphocytosis from the lymphocytosis caused by chronic bacterial infections.

The **aetiology** of 'sporadic lymphosarcoma' is unknown. The **thymic form** is characterized by large cranial thoracic masses, respiratory distress, and weight loss in cattle less than 2 years of age. The **juvenile form** is a disseminated lymphosarcoma and has been reported in **foetuses** and in **calves** up to 6 months of age. **Lesions** are generalized lymph node enlargement, depression, weight loss, and usually leukaemia with greatly increased numbers of lymphocytes accompanied by anaemia and neutropaenia. The **cutaneous form** is rare, occurs in **young cattle**, and consists of distinct cutaneous plaques or large scabby lesions.

Postmortem findings in all forms reveal characteristic tumours whose location depends on the form of the disease. Enlarged lymph nodes bulge when incised and reveal soft, grey-white tissue which may exude a milky fluid. Large masses, as in thymic lymphosarcoma, may contain areas of necrosis. Besides tumours in lymph nodes, liver, and spleen, cardiac involvement is most common in the right atrium.

Equine Lymphosarcoma

The incidence of lymphosarcoma in horses is lower than that of cattle, dogs, and cats. The distribution of lymphosarcoma varies in the horse. Reports of concurrent leukaemia may vary from rare to more than 50%. With the exception of the

cutaneous disease, most forms cause debility with anaemia, hypoproteinaemia, and dependent oedema. The **multicentric form** is characterized by involvement of peripheral lymph nodes with tumour masses in the mediastinum and abdomen. **Cutaneous** and **subcutaneous lymphosarcoma** in horses like other species, are chronic diseases without leukaemia or internal organ involvement. The subcutaneous tumours are multiple, well-circumscribed, yellow to white, firm nodules in various locations over body, usually involving tendons at joint surfaces.

The **alimentary form** is a wasting syndrome, due to involvement of the small intestine, resulting in malabsorption. The large intestine and numerous lymph nodes, including thoracic, may be involved. The neoplastic lymphocytes from the intestine and enlarged adjacent lymph nodes are usually plasmacytoid. **Mitotic figures are rare. Splenic lymphosarcoma** in the horse is characterized by massive organ enlargement. Some cases are leukaemic with lymphocyte counts greater than $100 \times 10^9/L$ ($100 \times 10^3/mm^3$). In contrast to the alimentary form, most tumours in the other forms are composed of large lymphocytes. Immunophenotyping has identified both B and T-lymphocytes in these tumours, with an increased number of neoplastic B-lymphocytes. Sometimes, horses with lymphosarcoma have regenerative anaemia characterized by an increased MCV, and marrow erythroid hyperplasia, in the absence of haemorrhage.

Hodgkin's disease

Hodgkin's disease is a complex form of lymphoma which occurs in **humans**. It is a **chronic disease,** characterized by slowly enlarging lymph nodes that get replaced by nodular tumours which ultimately affect other organs such as the liver, spleen, and bone marrow. More diffuse replacement of lymph nodes can be seen, and the pattern of the tumours can vary from almost pure population of lymphocytes to nodules containing large numbers of plasma cells, histiocytes, eosinophils, and fibroblasts. Diffuse fibrosis of the lesions occurs in one form of the disease. The histological picture may be difficult to differentiate from that of lymphoma or from that of inflammatory granuloma depending on the predominant cell types. The characteristic feature present in all forms of Hodgkin's disease is the typical cell called the **Reed-Sternberg cell**. It is a large cell containing two large nuclei with prominent nucleoli which resemble inclusion bodies. **It has been described as a cell with mirror images.**

Cases in animals (dogs, cats) are reported from time to time with the diagnosis of Hodgkin's disease, but it is not clear whether they represent the same disease. **Typical Hodgkin's disease has not been found in animals.**

Plasma Cell Neoplasm

Multiple myeloma (close resemblance to plasma cell sarcoma) **is a malignant neoplasm of plasma cells originating in the bone marrow** and usually metastasizing in the liver, spleen, lymph nodes, and other organs. The cell type usually contains a significant number of **mature plasma cells,** often with Russell bodies (i.e. inclusions representing aggregates of immunoglobulin), and also less mature cells which may be totally undifferentiated or resemble lymphoblasts. The cells may form distinct masses or may diffusely replace pre-existing structures. **In humans,** there is extensive destruction of the skeleton. The cells produce **monoclonal immunoglobulins** which may be **complete** or **incomplete.** This has been termed **monoclonal gammopathy,** which leads to hyperviscosity of the blood. Due to their high molecular weight, these proteins are restricted to the plasma, but if incomplete immunoglobulins are produced mainly of L chains (light chains), they appear in the **urine (Bence Jones proteins).** Multiple myeloma is also associated with nephrosis, characterized by protein casts in the distal convoluted and collecting tubules associated with tubular atrophy and a cellular infiltrate of plasma cells, lymphocytes, histiocytes, and multinucleated giant cells. **Amyloidosisis** is usually associated with multiple myeloma. **Multiple myeloma is rarely seen in animals.**

Spleen

Splenic Disorders

Atrophy

Atrophy occurs from mechanisms such as haemosiderosis, old age, wasting disease, and induration (hardening) following prolonged splenic congestion. **Viral diseases** such as bovine virus diarrhoea and drugs such as corticosteroids destroy lymphocytes, causing splenic atrophy. The **atrophic spleen** is small and firm, with a shrivelled capsule. Accumulation of iron and calcium as sclerotic nodules below the capsule is a common finding in the spleen of **old dogs.** Haemosiderin is usually present in splenic macrophages, especially following prolonged congestion.

Rupture

Rupture of the spleen usually occurs in **dogs.** The spleen may exist in two or more portions with various irregular fibrotic fissures indicating trauma at some time in the animal's life.

Enlargement of the Spleen (Splenomegaly)

An enlarged, uniform spleen (splenomegaly) is a common postmortem finding in animals. It occurs following congestion, hyperplasia, or neoplasia. Congested spleens are swollen and ooze blood when cut. This is more noticeable if autolysis is rapid as in anthrax. Splenomegaly due to proliferation of cells results in a fleshy (muscular) spleen with little oozing of blood when cut.

Torsion of the spleen results in marked congestion and **splenomegaly** due to occlusion of the splenic vein. **Splenomegaly due to cellular proliferation** results in a **firm spleen.** This occurs in chronic haemolytic anaemias in which gradual accumulation of macrophages results in a less congested and **more cellular red pulp.**

Diffuse infiltration of neoplastic cells into the spleen results in a uniformly firm spleen and occurs in lymphocytic, granulocytic and mast cell leukaemias, and in plasma cell sarcomas. **Microscopically,** red pulp is completely occupied by tumour cells, and there is usually disappearance of lymphoid follicles in the white pulp.

Nodular Disorders of the Spleen

Presence of nodules below the capsule, or those which protrude from the cut surface of the spleen indicates **benign nodular lymphoid hyperplasia. It is most common in the dog,** but is seen in all species. The nodules may be up to 2 cm in diameter, and they vary from grey to red pink. The largest nodules may have yellow centres because of necrosis.

Splenic haematomas are common in dogs, but the cause is usually not known at postmortem. Small haematomas must be differentiated from nodular hyperplasia and large ones from haemangiomas and haemangiosarcomas.

Neoplastic Disorders of the Spleen

The endothelial cell neoplasms, **haemangiomas** and **haemangiosarcomas,** occur in the spleen. They occur usually in **older dogs** of large breeds and are prone to rupture and cause intraperitoneal haemorrhage. The presence of anaemia with reticulocytosis in many of these dogs indicates bleeding from these tumours over a period of time.

Splenic involvement in bovine lymphosarcoma is variable. However, a high incidence of splenic involvement occurs in canine, feline, and equine lymphosarcoma. In most cases, the organ is uniformly enlarged. Distinct masses of lymphosarcoma can occur in the spleen and are white to yellow when cut.

Granulocytic leukaemia in dogs usually results in marked splenomegaly, caused by infiltration and proliferation of neoplastic granulocytes. **Plasma cell sarcomas in dogs** and **mast cell** and **erythrocytic sarcomas in cats** usually cause splenomegaly.

The splenic parenchyma is not fertile ground for the establishment of metastatic carcinomas. They are only occasionally found late in the course of disseminated neoplastic disease. Although uncommon, implantation of mesotheliomas and carcinomas to the splenic capsule can occur.

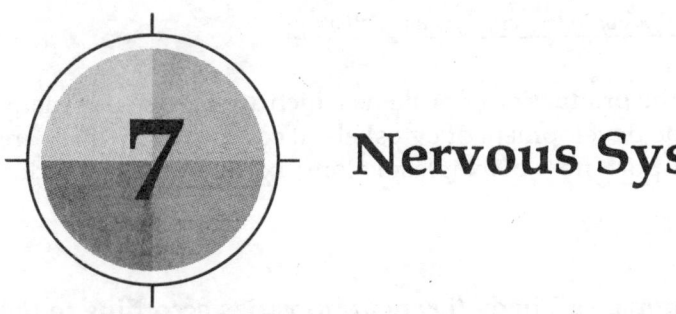

Nervous System

The **central nervous system (CNS)** consists of a **parenchyma** that contains **neurons, neuroglia, blood vessels, ependymal cells,** and **choroids plexus.** The exterior of the CNS is covered by meninges. Except meninges, these components form two parts of the CNS, the **grey** and **white matter.** The **grey matter** contains numerous neuronal cell bodies plus a network of axons and dendrites, their synaptic junctions, and processes of oligodendroglia, astrocytes, and microglia. **This network of processes in the grey matter is called neuropil.** The **white matter** is characterized by myelinated axons that extend from neuronal cell bodies of the grey matter, plus the presence of oligodendroglia, astrocytes, and microglia. **Neuroglia** includes astrocytes, oligodendroglia, microglia, and ependymal cells.

The cellular elements of the CNS vary in their susceptibility to injury. Neurons are the most sensitive. The more resistant glial cells usually react to injury by an increase in size, number, or both. Response of the neuron to injury is usually **necrosis** followed by its **disappearance.**

Neurons

Neuronal cell bodies vary considerably in size and shape. Their nuclei are vesicular to spherical in shape and usually centrally located. In large neurons, they contain a prominent central nucleolus. Their characteristic features include large granular basophilic bodies in the cytoplasm called **Nissl substance** or **body** (Fig. 37). They are composed of rough endoplasmic reticulum and polysomes (polyribosomes). Nissl

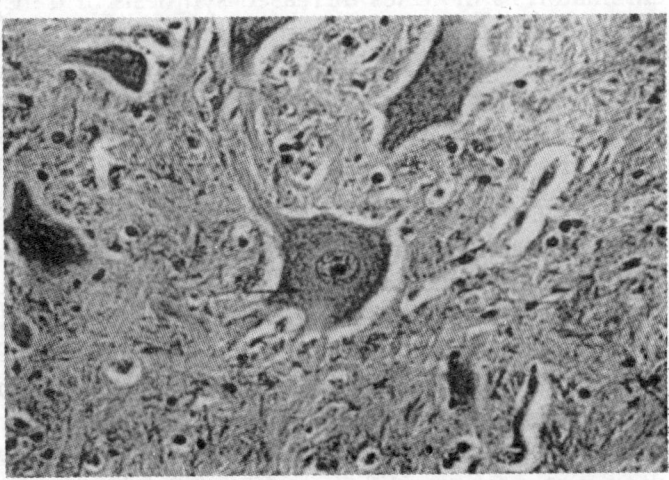

Fig. 37. Spinal cord, ventral horn; dog. Normal animal. This normal motor neuron (centre) has a centrally placed nucleus and contains **cytoplasmic Nissl substance** (arrow). H & E stain.

317

substance is responsible for the production of proteins which are involved in many vital processes. These include development of cytoskeletal components which are involved in axoplasmic transport (flow of axoplasm along axon) and regeneration of peripheral nerves.

Reaction to Injury

The appearance of the neuronal cell body (i.e. neuron) varies according to the injury. The characteristic changes include: with **axon injury**, there is central chromatolysis (loss of Nissl substance); **with ischaemia** (ischaemic cell change); **with lysosomal enzyme deficiencies** (enlargement of the cell body resulting from alteration of lysosomes); **with aging** (accumulation of lipofuscin pigment); and **with certain neuronal degenerative diseases** (excess accumulation of neurofilaments). Also certain special features occur in some viral infections. Examples include intranuclear and intracytoplasmic inclusion body formation or both (e.g. intracytoplasmic Negri body formation in rabies), and prominent cytoplasmic vacuolation (e.g. typical of spongiform encephalopathies such as scrapie and mad cow disease).

Response of Neurons Following Injury to Their Axons That Extend to the Periphery

An example of this type of injury is **motor neurons** whose cell bodies are in the brain and spinal cord and axons extend in peripheral nerves to innervate skeletal muscle. **After axonal injury,** (e.g., crush or transaction, i.e., cut), the change that occurs in the cell body is called **'central chromatolysis'**, or **'axonal reaction'**. Central chromatolysis indicates increased synthesis of transport and structural proteins required for regeneration of the axon and re-establishment of axonal transport system. The extent to which chromatolysis occurs depends on the degree and location of axonal injury. It is more pronounced, and can even be followed by neuronal death, if the axonal injury is severe and closer to the cell body. The time required for recovery of cell bodies can be several months (3 to 6 months), depending on the severity of the axonal injury and the length of axon regenerated.

Microscopically, central chromatolysis is characterized by swelling of the neuronal cell body, dispersion of central Nissl substance, and peripheral displacement of the nucleus (Fig. 38). The onset occurs within 24 to 48 hours and reaches its maximum in about 18 days following axonal injury. The change in the axon away from the point of injury is called **'Wallerian degeneration'**, and first appears within 24 hours of injury. It is characterized by fragmentation of the axon and myelin along its length. This axonal alteration is followed by disintegration, and usually there is no evidence of the axon remaining by the second week after the injury.

Changes in the myelin sheath surrounding myelinated axons are seen by 28 to 96 hours after injury when axonal disintegration is well advanced. Changes include lamellar splitting, fracturing, and fragmentation. The fragmented components of the sheath form droplets termed **'ellipsoids'**, which surround and enclose isolated fragments and debris of the former axon. Both axonal and myelin debris are then **removed by macrophages through phagocytosis.** Degeneration of myelin is usually completed by the end of the second week.

If the neuronal cell body survives the injury to its axon, regeneration from the proximal stump can occur.

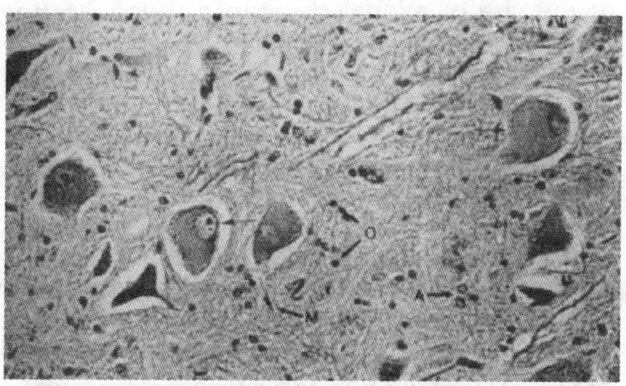

Fig. 38. Neurons, facial nucleus; dog. Central chromatolysis. Compare with Fig. 37. Two cells have eccentric nuclei (situated away from the centre; arrows). Neurons in the centre and to the right have pale central cytoplasm. The cell body of the neuron to the right is also swollen. Note the normal astrocytic **(A)**, oligodendroglial **(O)**, and microglial **(M)** nuclei. H & E stain.

The degree of axonal regeneration depends on the status of the endoneurial tube away from the original point of injury. The **normal endoneurial tube and its contents** from outside inward **consist of:** (1) a connective tissue layer called **endoneurium,** (2) the **basement membrane** that surrounds the Schwann cell plus the Schwann cell cytoplasm, (3) the **myelin sheath** of myelinated axons, and (4) the **axon**. About 24 to 72 hours after axonal injury, the endoneurial tube, formed from the persisting basement membrane, contains degenerating remnants of the previously existing axon along with Schwann cells. **Schwann cells begin to proliferate and eventually form a longitudinal column of cells called 'bands of Büngner'.**

If the endoneurial tube remains intact, as can occur following compression injury to a peripheral nerve, neural regeneration occurs through the formation of axonal sprouts. A regenerating sprout from the proximal axonal stump can enter the column of Schwann cells and regenerate along its original pathway to the periphery. This re-establishes innervation with an end organ, for example, skeletal muscle. Such axons can also become re-myelinated and **regain their physiological function of impulse transmission. A regenerating neuron lengthens at a rate of about 1 to 4 mm per day,** because of axoplasmic flow. However, the time required for axonal regeneration can vary depending on the length of axon to be regenerated. **If, however, the integrity of the endoneurial tube is destroyed,** which may occur after complete severance (separation) of a peripheral nerve, **regeneration may not occur.** In such a case, the proximal axonal stump may not reach the distal endoneurial tube because of fibrous connective tissue proliferation (**scar formation**) at the site of axonal severance. Regenerating axons may also enter wrong endoneurial tubes resulting in improper impulse transmission. For example, a sensory neuron axonal sprout may enter an endoneurial tube meant for a nerve innervating a muscle.

Response of Neurons Following Injury to Their Axons that Remain Within the CNS

The response of the cell body after injury of axons which remain within the CNS, for example, **upper motor neurons, can vary.** Upper motor neurons make up the motor system. This system remains confined within the CNS and is responsible for voluntary movement, maintenance of tone for the support of the body against gravity, and regulation of posture. **After injury,** some cell body may show **central chromatolysis,** others have central chromatolysis followed by **atrophy and death** (e.g., by apoptosis), and other undergo **atrophy.**

Wallerian degeneration within the CNS is similar to that described for the peripheral nervous system (PNS), except that in the CNS degenerated axons and myelin sheaths can remain for months before complete removal. **Affected axons and their sheaths** undergo a series of changes as they degenerate. In the beginning, axons form linear and round swellings at, and also some distance away from, the site of injury. These axonal enlargements can be seen within a few hours at the site of injury and remain prominent for the first week or so. The surrounding myelin sheath is usually distended to create a space between the sheath and the axonal swelling. With time, such affected axons and

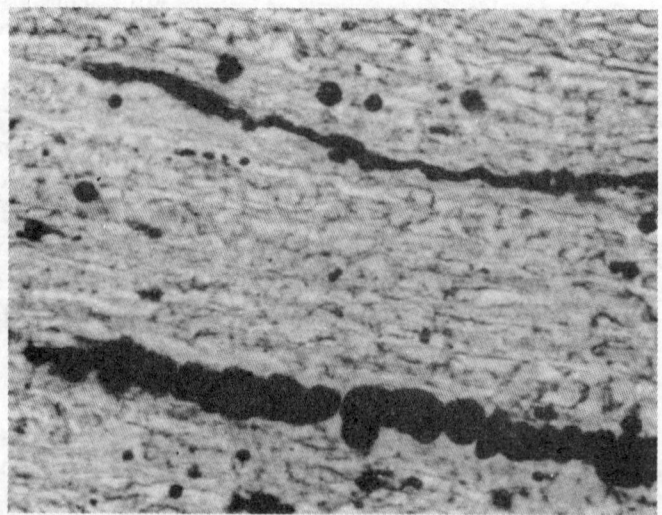

Fig. 39. Spinal cord, white matter; cow. Wallerian degeneration. Two myelinated axons are degenerated. The upper is minimally enlarged while the lower axon is markedly swollen and undergoing fragmentation. Also, note the scattered myelin debris. Marchi method for degenerating myelin.

myelin sheaths fragment along their length form **ellipsoids** (Fig. 39), described earlier in the case of PNS. These ellipsoids are eventually removed through degeneration and phagocytosis, leaving an empty space, or one containing myelin debris or macrophages, or both. With time, most of the lesion consists of enlarged empty spaces. The absence of axons in such dilated spaces does not necessary mean that the entire axon has degenerated and been removed. This requires several months. Instead, it may be the site of separation of an enlarged axon from the adjacent axon at the level of the section being examined.

Ischaemic Neural Injury

Neurons depend on a continuous supply of oxygen to remain viable. If the supply is interrupted for several minutes, the most susceptible neurons degenerate. Ischaemic neuron injury (ischaemic cell change) occurs following ischaemia which can result from obstruction of blood flow to the CNS or reduction in the available oxygen in the blood. This type of neuronal lesion can also occur from **metabolic disturbances** other than ischaemia, such as in nutritional deficiencies and toxicities that ultimately interfere with oxygen utilization. In H & E stained sections, the neuronal cell body is shrunken and deeply eosinophilic. The nucleus is reduced in size and is pyknotic (stains dark blue). The nucleus may not be detectable. Perineuronal and perivascular spaces are prominent because of swelling of astrocytic processes.

In contrast to neurons, cells such as **astrocytes swell** following ischaemia because of the increased uptake of sodium and chloride ions and water. Such **swelling** depends on the cell being viable and having a semi-permeable plasma membrane, even though its function is abnormal. If the degree and duration of the ischaemia is severe enough to cause cell death, the plasma membrane becomes fully permeable and the cell does not swell, but becomes shrivelled or shrunken and **undergoes disintegration,** as described for the ischaemic cell change of neurons. **It is emphasized that cells of the CNS are not equally sensitive to ischaemia, and the degree of ischaemia which causes swelling or death for one cell (e.g., astrocyte) is not the same for another cell (e.g. neuron).**

Astrocytes

Astrocytes are of **two types**: (1) **protoplasmic,** located mainly in grey matter, and (2) **fibrous,** which occur mainly in white matter. **Microscopically,** astrocytes have large vesicular nuclei, indistinct nucleoli, and no visible cytoplasm with routine H & E staining (see Fig. 37). With suitable special stains, or immuno-histochemical staining for **glial fibrillary acidic protein (GFAP),** the major intermediate filament reveals prominent cytoplasmic processes. Processes vary from short, bush-like to long branching processes in protoplasmic and fibrous astrocytes, respectively.

Astrocytes are the most numerous type of cells in the CNS. In the CNS, they **facilitate the reparative processes after injury** such as inflammation and necrosis and **are similar to fibroblasts** which bring about reparative processes in other organs. Astrocytes act as the main stromal cell population used for repair, but do not synthesize collagen fibres. Instead, repair is facilitated by the abundant proliferating astrocytic cell processes containing intermediate filaments composed of GFAP.

Structurally, astrocytic processes provide support for other cellular elements and insulate synapses. Processes of astrocytes (**foot processes**) also terminate on blood vessels throughout CNS. Astrocytes also have other diverse functions which include brain development, homeostasis of the microenvironment, and regulation of and participation in immune reactions. Interactions between astrocytes, microglia, and neurons carry out immune reactions in the brain. Astrocytes can express major histocompatibility (MHC) class I and II antigens, a variety of cytokines and chemokines, and adhesion molecules **which regulate inflammatory events in the CNS.**

Reaction to Injury: Common reactions of astrocytes in CNS injury are **swelling** and **hypertrophy (astrogliosis).** Swelling is an acute response, and may be the only change present or may progress to hypertrophy. Swollen astrocytes have clear or vacuolated cytoplasm. **If injury is severe,** astrocytic processes break into fragments and disappear. This is followed by lysis of the cell body. Hypertrophied astrocytes, also called **'reactive astrocytes'** indicate a response towards a more prolonged injury to the CNS. Because of increase in intermediate filaments, mainly GFAP, the cytoplasm becomes clearly visible along with branching of the processes with H & E staining. **In prolonged degenerative conditions,** astrocytes called **'gemistocytes'** can be observed. These cells have eccentric nuclei and abundant pink homogeneous cytoplasm with routine H & E staining. **Astrocytic proliferation (astrocytosis)** can occur in CNS injury. When it occurs, the most important examples of astrocytosis are attempts to 'ward-off' abscesses and neoplasms, or to fill in cavities (**porencephaly**) that occur following necrosis of large foci of neural tissue.

Oligodendroglia

Oligodendroglia are located in both white and grey matter of the CNS. In the white matter, they are called inter-fascicular oligodendroglia, while in grey matter as perineuronal satellite oligodendroglia. **Inter-fascicular oligodendroglia** in the white matter are **responsible for the formation and maintenance of the myelin sheaths.** Oligodendroglia also influence maturation and maintenance of axons. **Perineuronal satellite oligodendroglia** surround neuronal cells bodies in the grey matter, where they regulate the perineuronal microenvironment, and are also around blood vessels. When the perineuronal microenvironment is altered, or neuron cell bodies are injured in the grey matter, perineuronal satellite oligodendroglia hypertrophy and proliferate in a process called **'satellitosis'** in an attempt to regulate the environmental disturbance.

The **mature, small oligodendrocyte** has a spherical, hyperchromatic nucleus similar to that of a lymphocyte. Like astrocytes, the cell body and processes of this cell do not stain with H & E staining methods (see Fig. 37), and can only be demonstrated with special procedures which include silver impregnation.

Reaction to Injury: Reaction to injury includes degeneration and proliferation. Both perineuronal and inter-fascicular oligodendroglia degenerate, but only perineuronal oligodendroglia can proliferate.

Microglia

The current belief is that microglia originate from **circulating monocytes** which enter and populate the CNS during development and early postnatal life, like monocyte-macrophage system in other organs. After entry into the CNS, the cells become **'amoeboid microglia'**, phagocytosing old and worn-out cells and cellular debris during remodelling and maturation of the CNS. Amoeboid cells then enter into an inactive stage and transform into **'ramified microglia'**. Ramified microglia constitute up to 20% of the cells and are present throughout the mature CNS and serve as sentinels (soldiers on watch) of brain injury. Ramified microglia, also called as **'resting cells'**, are most numerous in perineuronal and perivascular areas. **The main function of microglia is participation in immunoregulation and in degenerative and inflammatory diseases of the CNS.** The CNS also contains macrophages, different from microglia. These macrophages are involved in immunological and phagocytic responses to disease processes and infectious organisms.

Ramified microglia have small, hyperchromatic ovoid, nuclei and no appreciable cytoplasm with routine H & E staining. The small hyperchromatic nuclei and nuclear shape differentiate microglia from astrocytes and oligodendrocytes (see Fig. 37).

Reaction to Injury: Microglia are the first cells to react in CNS injury. The magnitude of the response is in relation to the severity of damage. **After injury,** ramified microglia undergo activation and become fully immunocompetent reactive cells. These reactive cells, called **'rod cells'**, readily proliferate either focally forming **glial nodules** or more diffusely, depending on the nature of the injury. Resident microglia and blood-derived macrophages express major histocompatibility complex (MHC) class I and II antigens, serve as antigen-processing cells, and possess a number of adhesion molecules, cytokines, and chemokines. Once activated, these cells can also produce nitric oxide, reactive oxygen intermediates, and other chemical mediators of inflammation. When tissue necrosis occurs, foamy lipid-laden macrophages, sometimes called **'gitter cells'** accumulate in the damaged CNS. **Macrophages** acquire this **'foamy' appearance** because they phagocytize necrotic cellular debris.

Ependyma, Choroid Plexus, and Blood-Brain Barrier

The **ependyma** is a single-layered, cuboidal to columnar, ciliated epithelium that lines the ventricles and mesencephalic aqueduct of the brain, and central canal of the spinal cord. This layer of cells is thus situated between the cerebrospinal fluid

(CSF) and nervous tissue. Ependymal cells have cilia which project into the CSF and beat in the direction of the CSF flow. The choroid plexus is covered by highly specialized ependymal cells. The ependymal cells of the choroid plexus are less noticeably ciliated and have specialized tight junctions which are functional part of the **'blood-CSF barrier'** (discussed later). The ependymal cell layer regulates several processes which involve interaction between the CSF and brain parenchyma.

The **choroids plexus** is infoldings of blood vessels of the pia mater covered by a thin coat of ependymal cells which form tufted projections into the third, fourth, and lateral ventricles of the brain. **The important function of the choroids plexus is production of cerebrospinal fluid.**

The apposing surfaces of the epithelial cells that cover the choroid plexus form tight junctions. These barriers, along with the tight junctions that form between the cells of the arachnoid membrane, make up the blood-CSF barrier. Tight junctions between endothelial cells of cerebral blood vessels form the **'blood-brain barrier'** (BBB). This barrier system separates the blood from the parenchyma of the central nervous system.

Reaction to Injury: Responses of ependymal cells to injury include atrophy, degeneration, and necrosis. Atrophy usually occurs in response to enlargement of the ventricles which occurs in hydrocephalus. Ependymal cells are more like neurons than other neuroglia in that they do not regenerate and therefore do not repair denuded areas. After 1 to 2 weeks, **astrogliosis** occurs.

Inflammation of the ependyma (ependymitis) can also occur. The infection is the most common cause. Organisms usually enter into the ependyma through the circulation (haematogenous), and by direct contamination (e.g., rupture of a cerebral abscess into the ventricular system). **In the case of bacterial infection,** suppurative exudate which forms in the CSF can cause **obstructive hydrocephalus.**

Meninges

The **meninges**, which enclose the CNS, consist of three layers: **dura mater, arachnoid,** and **pia mater.** The arachnoid and pia together are called the **leptomeninges.** They form a single functional compartment called the **subarachnoid space** which contains the CSF and blood vessels. The meninges form a protective covering for the CNS and provide scaffolding which supports nerves and blood vessels that enter and leave the brain and spinal cord.

The **dura mater** is a strong and dense collagenous membrane. The **arachnoid mater** is a thin, but multilayered membrane composed of cells that overlap one another. The **pia mater** is closely adhered to the surface of the brain and spinal cord and is penetrated by a large number of blood vessels that supply the underlying nervous tissue.

Reaction to Injury: Pathological processes that invade the meninges, usually the leptomeninges, can secondarily invade into the CNS because of the close relationship between the two tissues. Similarly, processes that affect the CNS can secondarily affect the meninges, usually the leptomeninges.

Meningitis

Meningitis is inflammation of the meninges. Usually it refers to inflammation of the **leptomeninges** (pia mater, subarachnoid space, and arachnoid mater) in contrast to inflammation of the dura mater, which is called **pachymeningitis.**

Leptomeningitis can be acute, subacute, or chronic and, depending on the cause suppurative, non-suppurative, or granulomatous (see 'inflammation of the central nervous system'). **Infectious agents** spread to the meninges by the same routes (e.g., haematogenous, direct extension) which result in infection of the brain, excluding retrograde (backward) axonal transport which occurs in some viral infections (e.g., rabies virus). Inflammation of the specific parts of the dura mater of the cranial cavity can occur in the **external dura** (periosteal dura) following osteomyelitis, formation of extra-dural abscesses, and skull fracture, and involve the **inner dura** along with leptomeningitis.

Anomalies and Malformations

Anencephaly

Anencephaly means absence of brain, but in many cases only the rostral part of the brain (cerebral hemispheres) is absent, or very rudimentary; and to varying degrees the brainstem is preserved. Therefore, this abnormality should be called **'prosencephalic hypoplasia'** (i.e., hypoplasia of forebrain). Although the cause of these anomalies is unknown, **anencephaly** has been reported to be associated with anomalies in other body systems in **calves.**

Hydrocephalus

Hydrocephalus is an increased accumulation of cerebrospinal fluid (CSF) in the ventricular system. It can result from obstruction within the ventricular system (**non-communicating form**), or when there is communication of CSF with the subarachnoid space where the CSF can be in excess (**communicating form**).

Obstruction within the ventricular system at the lateral apertures of the fourth ventricle results in **non-communicating hydrocephalus.** An area particularly prone for obstruction is the mesencephalic aqueduct. When **congenital,** this type of hydrocephalus can be associated with enlargement (doming) before the sutures have fused, and the enlarged head can cause dystocia. Hydrocephalus of this type has a **predisposition for certain breeds of dogs. Acquired non-communicating hydrocephalus** has been associated with obstruction of lateral apertures of the fourth ventricle, aqueduct, or the inter-ventricular foramen. **Causes** of obstruction include infection or inflammation, neoplasms, and rarely, cholesteatomas in the choroids plexus of the **horse. (A cholesteatoma** is a cyst-like mass or benign tumour filled with desquamating debris, usually having cholesterol).

Communicating hydrocephalus, in which CSF of the ventricular system communicates with the subarachnoid space, **is the least common of the two forms.** Several causes have been proposed, including arteritis, subarachnoid haemorrhage, and meningitis.

In a **third type of hydrocephalus,** called **'hydrocephalus ex vacuo'** (or compensating hydrocephalus) the increase in size of the lateral ventricles with increase in the volume of CSF, is secondary to either absence or loss of cerebral tissue. This type of hydrocephalus can occur whenever there is lack of development or destruction and loss of cerebral tissue surrounding lateral ventricles.Examples include certain anomalies (hydranencephaly) and some storage diseases (e.g., ceroid-lipofuscinosis), and aging of the CNS, both of which are associated with cerebral atrophy. Interference in flow, or increased pressure, of the CSF would not occur in this type of hydrocephalus.

Lesions in either of the first two forms of hydrocephalus, particularly the **non-communicating form,** include enlargement of the ventricular system proximal to the point of obstruction. White matter near the dilated lateral ventricles is reduced in thickness. However, the grey matter retains its normal appearance. The ependyma may be atrophied and focally discontinuous.

Hydranencephaly

Hydranencephaly is characterized by the formation of a cavity in the area normally occupied by the white matter of the cerebral hemispheres. It occurs from lack of proper development of this part of the cerebrum. The cavity formation (cavitation) results from destruction of immature progenitor (ancestor) cells whose loss prevents normal development. Hydranencephaly is usually quite severe with little tissue present between the expanded ventricular lining and the outer meninges. **Such a lesion grossly appears as a thin-walled sac.** Because of the lack of resistance, ventricles expand into this space (**hydrocephalus ex vacuo**). The ependymal lining remains preserved or may be variably defective.

Causes include foetal viral infection (e.g., Akabane and bovine virus diarrhoea infection in **calves;** and bluetongue, border disease, and Rift Valley fever infections in **lambs**), and nutritional copper deficiency (affects ovine foetus in uterus).

Porencephaly

Porencephaly refers to **a cleft or cyst** in the wall of the cerebral hemisphere which communicates with the brain surface (e.g., subarachnoid space), **but can also** communicate with the lateral ventricle of the brain.

Syringomyelia

Syringomyelia is formation of a tubular cavity (syrinx means tube) in the spinal cord not lined by ependyma. It is separate from the central canal. It can extend over several spinal cord segments. **The lesion has been described in the dog.** The syrinx (tube) can communicate with the central canal, but should not be confused with **hydromyelia,** which means dilatation of the central canal with an abnormal accumulation of fluid. Proposed causes include trauma, infection, and neoplasms which cause parenchymal degeneration and cavity formation.

Dysraphic Anomalies

Dysraphia

Dysraphia literally means an abnormal seam (a line where two pieces of fabric are sewn together). It usually refers to **a defective closure of the neural tube during development.** This defect, which can occur anywhere along the tube, is seen in anencephaly, prosencephalic hypoplasia, cranium bifidum, and spina bifida.

Cranium Bifidum

Cranium bifidum is characterized by a dorsal midline cranial defect through which meningeal and brain tissue can protrude. The protruded material, which forms a sac is covered by skin and can be lined by meninges (**meningocele**), or meninges accompanied by a part of the brain (**meningo-encephalocele**). **Causes** include inheritance in **pigs** and **cats** and treatment of **cats** with griseofulvin.

Spina Bifida

Spina bifida is the spinal counterpart of cranium bifidum. This lesion, which usually affects the caudal spine, is characterized by a dorsal defect in one to several vertebrae of the dorsal spinal column. **The lesion results from a defective closure of the neural tube.**

There may be no herniation of the meninges or spinal cord through the defect (**spina bifida occulta**), or herniation of either meninges (**meningocele**) or meninges and spinal cord (**meningomyelocele**) can occur, forming a sac covered with skin. The lesion has been described in several species, including **horses, calves, sheep, dogs,** and **cats.** Another lesion, **myeloschisis,** is similar to spina bifida except that in its severe form results from failure of the entire spinal neural tube to close. This lesion is therefore characterized by lack of development of the entire dorsal vertebral column.

Lesions Resulting from Viral Infection of the Foetus

Viruses can affect the foetus directly or indirectly. That is, only the dam or the placenta is infected, and foetal lesions occur secondarily. **Direct infection** can cause malformation by affecting organogenesis (origin and development of organs) in the embryo, immature cells of the foetus, or differentiated cells of the foetus.

1. Viral Effect on Organogenesis

Two examples of this type of viral teratology (malformations) include:

- **Microencephaly** (abnormally small brain and **myeloschisis** (see 'spina bifida') caused by influenza viral infection, and

- **Myeloschisis** caused by Newcastle disease viral infection, both in young chicken embryos.

2. Viral Effect on Immature Cells

Lesions due to parvoviral infection and feline infectious enteritis virus (feline panleukopaenia virus) have been detected in the **cat. Grossly**, the size of the cerebellum is reduced (**cerebellar hypoplasia**).

Congenital defects in **neonatal calves** can occur from foetal infection with bovine virus diarrhoea virus (a pestivirus). The primary lesion is a **cerebellar hypoplasia-atrophy**, but other lesions of the CNS can also occur, including porencephaly, hydranencephaly, and dysmyelination.

Swine fever (hog cholera) virus, also a pestivirus, can be teratogenic to the **pig foetus**. The neural defects resulting from foetal infection are **hypomyelinogenesis (hypomyelination)** and **cerebellar hypoplasia**.

Border disease viral infection (also a pestiviral infection) can cause maldevelopment in the CNS and non-neural tissues (e.g., skeleton) of **lambs** and **goats** after natural infection of the dam during pregnancy. One important characteristic lesion is hypomyelinogenesis.

Akabane viral infection (caused by a bunyavirus) occurs in **cattle, sheep,** and **goats**. Characteristic lesions of the CNS include porencephaly-hydranencephaly and degeneration (with loss of neurons) of the ventral horns of the spinal cord.

Bluetongue viral infection (orbiviral infection) of **sheep** also causes porencephaly-hydranencephaly, cerebellar hypoplasia, and hypoplasia of the spinal cord following foetal infection during pregnancy.

3. Viral Effects on Differentiated Cells

Infection of the **neonatal dogs** with **parainfluenza virus** can cause hydrocephalus. The basic lesion is an aqueductal stenosis (incomplete closure) which results in the development of non-communicating hydrocephalus. The virus grows in and causes destruction of ependymal cells lining the ventricular system.

Inborn Errors of Metabolism

Disturbance of Amino Acid Metabolism

Aminoacidopathy

Two diseases characterized by **errors of amino acid metabolism** have been described in the **neonatal calf:** (1) **Maple syrup urine disease** occurs in **young calves** (see 'disorders of myelin formation and maintenance'), and (2) **Bovine citrullinaemia,** originally described in Australia, occurs in **neonatal calves**.

Bovine citrullinaemia is a rare inborn error of metabolism of the urea cycle which results in pronounced accumulation of citrulline (an alpha-amino acid) in the body fluids. **Grossly,** the livers of affected animals are pale yellow. **Microscopically,** brain shows mild to moderate diffuse astroglial swelling in the cerebro-cortical grey matter. Liver lesions are mild to severe hepatocellular hydropic change. The neurological signs, which occur during the first week of life, are due to increasing concentrations of **plasma ammonia.**

Lysosomal Storage Disease

Lysosomal storage is a cellular alteration in which an increased amount of material, which normally is degraded, **accumulates within lysosomes,** often causing **cell death. Lysosomal storage diseases** were originally thought to develop because of mutations that result in a reduction in lysosomal enzyme synthesis. However, more recently it has become clear that **other defects** are also involved. **These include:** (1) synthesis of enzymatically inactive proteins which resemble active normal enzymes, (2) defects in post-translational processing of enzyme protein destined for the lysosome, (3) lack of enzyme activator or protector protein, and (4) other defects include lack of substrate activator or protector protein, and lack of transport protein which is required for elimination of the digested material from lysosomes. **Characterization of lysosomal disorders has therefore been broadened to include any protein which is essential for normal lysosomal function.**

The best known diseases are characterized by accumulation of the substrate or substrate precursors and sometimes even by the absence of a critical metabolic product for normal lysosomal function. **As a general principle, cell swelling** and **cytoplasmic vacuolation** occur because of the accumulation of unprocessed substrate. Therefore, differences in the size and appearance of cells depend on the availability of the substrate in the organ system. Many lipids and glycolipids are unique to the nervous system and therefore only neural cells accumulate the substrate.

An example of lysosomal storage disease which affects **humans** and **animals** is **gangliosidoses** (one form is called as **Tay-Sachs disease** in humans). These diseases are mostly transmitted in an autosomal recessive pattern. They are often gene-dose dependent, and as such, recessive homozygotes manifest the disease, whereas heterozygotes are phenotypically normal, but the specific enzyme activity is reduced (about 50% of normal). The age and onset of **clinical signs** and severity of the disease process vary among different diseases, because deficiency of the involved enzyme is not always the same. If the gene defect is such that the **mutant enzyme is not synthesized at all**, there is an early onset of a disease. On the other hand, if there is some residual synthesis of the deficient enzyme, there is delayed onset of a milder form of the disease since partial catabolism of the accumulated substrate allows a longer period before the loss of cell function.

Accumulation of materials in lysosomes can also be acquired. Such lysosomal storage can occur following acquired toxicities (e.g., plant poisoning), accumulation of **iron** (e.g., haemosiderin after erythrocyte lysis), and excess absorption and accumulation of ingested **copper**. One unusual lysosomal storage disease, which has several forms, is **ceroid-lipofuscinosis**. Its lysosomal dysfunction is not completely understood. The disease resembles other lysosomal storage diseases in that it can have a recessive mode of inheritance, but differs in that it has no gene-dose effect or noticeable lysosomal enzyme defect.

Most of the lysosomal diseases of humans and animals, but not all, **affect the CNS and cause neurological disturbances.** The lesions of the different diseases vary. However, neurons and sometimes other cell types (e.g., neuroglia) are usually affected. **Gross lesions** also vary among different diseases. **Brain atrophy** occurs with **globoid leukodystrophy** and **ceroid-lipofuscinosis** in later stages of the diseases. With ceroid-lipofuscinosis, the atrophy, which usually involves the cerebral hemispheres (especially the cortex) but also sometimes the cerebellum, can result in a 50% reduction in brain weight. The cerebral hemispheres are increased in firmness and usually have yellowish-brown colour, whereas gyri are thinned and the sulci widened (**cerebral cortical atrophy**).

Brain atrophy is not prominent in other lysosomal storage diseases. However, brains of animals with gangliosidosis can have a firm, rubbery consistency. **Microscopically,** affected neurons usually have a foamy (finely vacuolated) or granular cytoplasm. This indicates the degree to which the stored material is removed during processing. The specific features of the stored material can be understood only by electron-microscopic examination.

One disease, **globoid cell leukodystrophy,** differs from the others in that **the primary lysosomal defect appears to involve oligodendrocytes rather than neurons.** Degeneration of oliogodendroglia results in the **disturbance of myelin formation and maintenance** and the accumulation of unprocessed myelin breakdown products (particularly degraded myelin membranes, galactosylceramide, and galactocerebroside) in macrophages called **globoid cells.** **Globoid cells are macrophages** which phagocytize the unprocessed myelin breakdown products that result from oligodendroglial destruction. **Psychosine** (galactosylsphingosine) which accumulates during the disease is directly toxic to oligodendrocytes (see 'diseases of myelin formation and maintenance').

Characteristic features of some of the important lysosomal storage diseases of animals are presented in Table 11.

Table 11. Classification of important lysosomal storage diseases that involve the CNS of animals

Disease	Storage Product	Deficiency Enzyme	Species Affected
GM1 gangliosidosis	GM1 ganglioside	Beta-galactosidase	Cattle, dog, cat, sheep
GM2 gangliosidosis	GM2 ganglioside	Beta-hexosaminidase	Dog, cat, pig
Globoid-cell leukodsytrophy (Krabbe's-like disease)	Galactosylceramide (galactocerebroside) and galactosylsphin-gosine (psychosine)	Galactosylceramidase (galactocerebroside beta-galactosidase)	Dog, cat, sheep
Alpha-mannosidosis	Mannose-containing oligosaccharide	Alpha-mannosidase	Cattle, cat
Beta-mannosidosis	Mannose-containing oligosaccharide	Beta-mannosidase	Goat, cattle
Mucopolysaccharidosis	Different glycosa-minoglycans	Several different enzyme deficiencies	**Dog** (type I, Hurler's disease; type VI, Maroteaux-Lamy disease; type VII, Sly disease) **Cat** (type I, Hurler's disease; type VI, Maroteaux-Lamy dsease; type VII, Sly disease) **Goat** (type III, Sanfilippo's disease)
Ceroid-lipofuscinosis	Subunit c of mito-chondrial ATPase	Prelysosomal defect?	Dog, sheep, cattle
	Sphingolipid Activating proteins A and D	Palmitoyl protein thioesterase	Dog Sheep
	Unknown	Unknown	Dog, sheep, cattle, cat
Niemann-Pick type c disease	Primarily ganglioside in neurons	Unknown	Cat, dog

Factors Influencing Susceptibility of the CNS to Trauma

In general, trauma of the central nervous system in animals is less common than in humans. Animals are not exposed so commonly to trauma-causing situations as are humans, and there are anatomical differences that help protect the brain of animals.

Among animals, trauma of the brain is usually seen in **dogs** as a result of automobile-induced injury. Trauma in small animals can result from falls from significant heights (e.g., balconies, roofs). **Cats** often have only minor injury to the CNS, even after falling from great heights. Other examples include fracture of the spinal column or cranium in jumping horses. Predisposition to cerebral trauma is also influenced by anatomical differences. Functional factors also play an important role in brain injury. **The brain of a freely movable herd is much more susceptible to injury than a stationary, supported one.**

Cerebral Trauma

Concussion

Concussion occurs after head injury. It is a clinical condition characterized by a temporary loss of consciousness followed by recovery. This type of injury is only part of the entire range which has been called **'diffuse brain injury'**. The severity of diffuse brain injury, depending on the degree of trauma, can vary from a mild, reversible concussion without loss of consciousness to severe injury which results in a permanent neurological damage or even death. Diffuse brain injury involves widespread disruption of neurological function.

Concussive injuries of the diffuse type also occur in animals, but there are some differences between animals and humans. For example, it is difficult to produce severe concussion in animals because the margin between stunning blow and fatal injury is very small. **The smaller the brain, the less prone it is to rotational forces and the larger are the forces necessary to cause concussion.** However, concussion can occur more frequently than realized in animals. As in human, a movable head is much more prone to trauma than a fixed, supported one.

Diffuse brain injury is usually not associated with gross lesions. Microscopically, lesions include axonal degeneration and neuronal loss as well as regenerative processes (central chromatolysis). The more severe forms of diffuse brain injury are also associated with generalized acute brain swelling that can be followed after some time by cerebral oedema.

Contusion

In contrast to the diffuse form of cerebral injury, contusion is characterized by **focal brain injury.** It is grossly seen, usually as haemorrhage, and like concussion, can result in unconsciousness and even death. Lesions can be superficial (e.g., cerebral gyri) or more central (e.g., brain stem), and there may even be skull fracture. Although **haemorrhage** is the most common lesion, contusion of the brain results in **tearing of CNS tissue.** Tearing results in **necrosis** and **neuronal loss.**

Haemorrhage

Trauma to the head is the **most common cause of haemorrhage,** although it can be caused by wide variety of injuries. **Following trauma to the head,** haemorrhages can develop in the epidural, subdural, and leptomeningeal (subarachnoid and pia mater) areas and in the brain parenchyma. Epidural haemorrhage has been reported in the **horse,** especially jumpers, resulting from falls while working. Subdural haemorrhage, which is an accumulation of blood between the dura mater and arachnoid membrane, occurs in **dogs** and **cats.** But leptomeningeal and parenchymal haemorrhages are most common in these species following head injury.

Spinal Cord Trauma

Assessment of spinal cord trauma should include examination not only of the spinal cord, but also of the vertebral column and spinal nerve roots. **Injuries** to the spinal cord can be **concussion, contusion, haemorrhage, laceration, transection** (division by cutting transversely), and **compression.**

Concussion

Spinal concussion is immediate and temporary loss of function. This may occur from severe direct blows to the spinal column. As with cerebral concussion, there is usually only a temporary functional disability of the cord after injury, but permanent neurological damage can occur, depending on the degree of trauma.

Contusion

This is characterized by **haemorrhage, necrosis,** and **tears** which are usually focal and grossly visible. Contusion can occur without fracture of the vertebral column, with fracture, and fracture plus dislocation of the spinal column.

Haemorrhage

The same types of haemorrhage that affect the brain (epidural, subdural, leptomeningeal, and parenchymal) also occur in spinal cord and meninges. **Causes** are similar to those affecting the brain and include stretching as a result of abnormal movement and severance of blood vessels associated with vertebral fracture.

Laceration and Transection

Both laceration and transection can occur following vertebral fracture, laceration by penetration of bony fragments and severance (transection) of the spinal cord by sharp fragments of bone associated with dislocation of the vertebrae.

Compression

Compression of the spinal cord can be **due to intramedullary** (within the spinal cord) **or extramedullary** (outside the spinal cord) **pressure.** Causes of intramedullary pressure include intra-parenchymal haemorrhages and neoplasms (e.g., nephroblastoma of the **young dog**). Extramedullary pressure can be caused by inter-vertebral disk herniation in the **dog**, cervical stenotic myelopathy (**wobbler syndrome**) in the **horse** and **dog**, vertebral fracture and dislocation, and neoplasms of the meninges, nerve rootlets or both.

Inter-vertebral disk disease occurs in **dogs**. Inter-vertebral disks are present between all vertebral bodies. Inter-vertebral disks in a significant percentage of **dogs** begin to degenerate after about one year of age, predisposing them to sudden herniation earlier.

An uncommon lesion in the **dog** called **'progressive haemorrhagic myelomalacia'** can follow spinal cord injury, particularly associated with severe type I disk herniation, but can also occur following other forms of spinal trauma. This lesion, which is characterized by softening to semi-liquefaction (**myelomalacia**) and haemorrhage of the tissue, can develop after injury.

Cervical stenotic myelopathy or **wobbler syndrome** is characterized by **stenosis** (narrowing) of the cervical vertebral canal which causes compressive trauma to the cervical spinal cord. It affects **horses** and **dogs**. The **disease in the horse** is known by several names: **wobbler syndrome**, wobbles, equine incoordination, and **cervical stenotic myelopathy**. Lesions of the CNS are similar to the lesions in inter-vertebral disk herniation.

Circulatory Disturbances

Effect of the Rate of Oxygen Deprivation on Lesion Development

The rate at which ischaemia occurs in the CNS determines the degree of injury that follows. The more rapid the onset of ischaemia, the more severe is the lesion. If the blood flow in an artery is gradually reduced (e.g., due to arteriosclerosis), there is often enough time for anastomotic vessels to dilate and compensate. However, if the obstruction is sudden (e.g., caused by an embolus), much of the tissue can die before an adequate anastomotic circulation can be established. This same principle applies to compressive injury to the CNS that produces a reduction in blood flow.

Susceptibility of Cells and Specific Anatomical Areas to Ischaemia

Susceptibility of cells and tissues of the CNS to ischaemia, in the decreasing order, are neurons, oligodendroglia, astrocytes, microglia, and blood vessels. Neurons are not equally susceptibility to ischaemia, and differences occur in relation to their location in the CNS. Susceptible neurons include those of the cerebral cortex, hippocampus, certain areas of the basal ganglia, and Purkinje cells of the cerebellar cortex. Neurons of the grey matter of the spinal cord and greater part of the brain stem are more resistant to ischaemia than cerebral cortex.

The time required for the death of neurons following ischaemia need not always be the same. This difference has been associated with the severity of the ischaemic insult; the more the ischaemia, the less time required for neuronal death (ischaemic cell change). On the other hand, the less severe the ischaemic insult, the longer the time required for neuronal death. This mechanism of injury has been referred to as **'delayed neuronal death'**.

Oedema of the CNS

Cerebral oedema is of **two distinct types**: (1) **vasogenic**, and (2) **cytotoxic**. **Vasogenic type** is characterized by an **increased extracellular fluid** resulting from increased vascular permeability and the **cytotoxic type** is characterized by an **increased intracellular fluid** with normal vascular permeability. Other types of cerebral oedema include **hydrostatic (or interstitial) oedema** which is associated with **increased hydrostatic pressure** (e.g., resulting from hydrocephalus), and **osmotic oedema**, which depends on the development of abnormal osmotic forces between the blood and nervous tissue.

1. Vasogenic Oedema

The underlying mechanism of vasogenic oedema is **breakdown of the blood-brain barrier** which results in movement of plasma constituents such as water, sodium, and plasma proteins into the **extracellular space**, particularly that of the white matter. In addition to extracellular accumulation of fluid, vasogenic oedema can also be accompanied by some cellular swelling (e.g., involving astrocytes). **Vasogenic oedema is the most common type and occurs following vascular injury.** It is usually adjacent to haematomas, contusions, infarcts, inflammatory foci, and neoplasms and occurs in certain toxicities.

2. Cytotoxic Oedema

Cytotoxic oedema is characterized by the **accumulation of fluid intracellularly** (e.g., in neurons, astrocytes, oligodendroglia, and endothelial cells) as a result of altered cellular metabolism, usually due to ischaemia. **Affected cells swell within seconds of injury**. It is due to energy deficiency which interferes with normal function of the ATP-dependent sodium-potassium pump. Thus, the cell cannot maintain homeostasis and secrete intracellular sodium. **An increased concentration of intracellular sodium is followed by an increased entry of water.** Both grey and white matters of the brain are affected. The fluid taken up by the swollen cells is mainly derived from the extracellular space, which becomes reduced in size and has increased concentration of extracellular solutes (dissolved substances).

To be described as cerebral oedema, there must be additional fluid movement into the brain and not merely a change of existing intra-parenchymal fluid from extracellular to intracellular compartment. The additional fluid originates from the circulation and from the CSF, which has extensive communication with the extracellular fluid of the brain. **The blood-brain barrier remains intact during the development of this type of odema,** so that fluid does not enter into the brain due to a disturbance in vascular permeability. **Specific causes** of cytotoxic oedema include hypoxia-ischaemia, intoxication with metabolic inhibitor such as 2, 4, dinitrophenol and ouabain, and severe hypothermia.

3. Hydrostatic (Interstitial) Oedema

Hydrostatic oedema is characterized by the **accumulation of a protease-free fluid** in the extracellular space of the brain because of increased ventricular pressure which accompanies **hydrocephalus.** Fluid moves across the ependyma of the ventricular wall and accumulates extracellularly in the peri-ventricular tissue, mainly white matter. Unlike the other forms of cerebral oedema that cause swelling of the affected CNS tissue, hydrostatic oedema causes degeneration and loss of the peri-ventricular white matter. The blood-brain barrier remains intact.

4. Osmotic Cerebral Oedema

Cerebral oedema also occurs in **'water intoxication',** which can result from an increased body hydration (accumulation of water) caused by: (1) excessive, faulty intravenous hydration, (2) compulsive drinking caused by abnormal mental function, or (3) altered anti-diuretic hormone secretion. The increased body hydration produces hypotonic plasma, with subsequent development of an osmotic gradient between the hypotonic plasma and the hypertonic state of the normal cerebral tissue. **Fluid moves from plasma into the brain.** In this type of oedema, the blood-brain barrier remains intact. Fluid accumulation occurs mainly intracellularly, but can also be present extracellularly.

Sequelae of Cerebral Oedema

The **gross lesions** which occur in cerebral oedema are due to enlargement of the **brain enclosed in a limited space.** The degree of swelling decides the type and extent of lesions which develop.

Because of compression against the cranium, the affected brain has flattened gyri and shallow sulci, and it can shift in position. If the oedema is confined to one side, the displacement is unilateral. **On cut surface,** the white matter is most commonly affected, usually in **vasogenic type of oedema which is the most common.** It is smaller and soft, has a moist appearance, and is light yellow in the fresh, unfixed state.

Microscopically, the extracellular fluid associated with vasogenic oedema is usually not detectable, except in cases of marked vascular injury. Only its effects, (separation of the parenchyma causing reduced staining intensity), can be seen. In addition, after prolonged vasogenic oedema, the lesions include hypertrophy and hyperplasia of astrocytes, activation of microglia, and demyelination. **Cytotoxic oedema is characterized by cellular swelling, including swelling of astrocytes.**

Infarction

Infarction means necrosis of a tissue following obstruction of its arterial blood supply. Anastomoses of the arteries which penetrate from the ventral and cortical surfaces of the brain are insufficient to prevent infarction following sudden occlusion of one or more of these arteries.

Cerebral necrosis, which is similar to infarction following vascular obstruction, can also result from other causes. These include stopping of cerebral circulation, sudden hypotension, and reduced or absent oxygen in inspired air. Additional causes include altered function of haemoglobin (e.g., as a result of carbon monoxide poisoning), inhibition of tissue respiration (e.g., cytochrome oxidase system following cyanide poisoning), toxic substances and poisons, and nutritional deficiencies. **Although resulting from different mechanisms, the necrosis which occurs has basically the same gross and microscopic characteristics as that which is associated with classical infarction.** The degree of injury will depend on the severity and duration of the inciting cause.

Areas of cerebral infarction differ somewhat in gross appearance from infarcts in other tissues. The large quantity of lipids and enzymes, plus the relative lack of fibrous connective tissue stroma in the brain and spinal cord, make affected areas eventually **soft (malacia) because of liquefactive necrosis.** Lesions affecting the **grey matter** tend to be haemorrhagic (**haemorrhagic infarction**), whereas infarction of the **white matter** is usually pale (**pale infarction**). This difference is due in part to the less dense capillary network in the white matter, in part to the fact that the vessels supplying the white matter have fewer anastomoses than those of the grey matter. **Infarcted tissue goes through a characteristic sequence of changes that can help to decide a relatively accurate assessment of the age of the infarct.**

Recent advances have improved our understanding of the **mechanisms involved in ischaemic injury of the CNS.** The CNS depends on blood for a continuous supply of the **oxygen and glucose, and interruption of this blood flow for only a few minutes results in death of vulnerable neurons.** If the stoppage of flow occurs for a longer period, all types of cells (neurons, oligodendroglia, astrocytes, and microglia) in the affected area die.

When an artery supplying the CNS is suddenly occluded, blood supply to cells at the centre of the affected area (the core) is rapidly stopped, and if maintained for a sufficient period, **all cells will die.** Neurons at the border of this area continue to receive some blood from non-obstructed vessels. It is believed that axonal terminals of degenerated ischaemic neurons in the centre of the infarct release excessive amounts of the neurotransmitter glutamate, causing injury to neurons still alive at the border. **This increases the extent of injury that can occur with infarction.** This process begins after binding of the neurotransmitter glutamate to receptors on live neurons at the border. This leads to an abnormal movement of calcium ions into the living cells **followed by an increase in intracellular calcium ion concentration.**

This gradual increase in calcium ions contributes to a series of events which lead to **neuronal death**. When infarction is also associated with haemorrhage, the mechanical injury from the pressure, plus tissue displacement by the haemorrhage, can cause additional damage.

Vascular Disease

The incidence of cerebro-vascular diseases similar to those in humans is low in animals, and neurological signs with these are unknown. **Arteriosclerosis** ('hardening' of arteries) can be classified as lipid (**atherosclerosis**) or non-lipid arteriosclerosis. The latter includes **arterial fibrosis, mineralization,** and **amyloid deposition**. Also, vascular diseases of the CNS can result from inflammation/ infection, either from a systemic disease or from extension of inflammatory meningeal or parenchymal disease. Some of the diseases are covered later in this chapter. Thrombosis of cerebral blood vessels or venous sinuses occurs rarely. Thrombosis can occur with or without evidence of a demonstrable local or systemic disease process.

Atherosclerosis

Atherosclerosis has been reported in a number of animals including **pigs, dogs,** and **several avian species. Older pigs** are most commonly and severely affected. Vessels involved include aorta and its major branches, extra-mural coronary arteries, and meningeal arteries. Affected arteries are rigid, irregularly thickened, and white to yellow-white. Arterial lumens are narrowed or almost obliterated, but there is usually no appreciable ulceration, thrombosis, or haemorrhage. Intimal thickenings in intracranial arteries contain fewer lipids and have a greater tendency for fibrosclerosis than other vessels. In arteries within the brain parenchyma, there is collagenous adventitial or transmural thickening. The arterial lesions can be associated with haemorrhage or infarcts involving basal nuclei, fornix, internal and external capsules, hippocampus, and thalamus. Atherosclerosis occurs rarely in the **dog** along with disturbed lipid metabolism of hypothyroidism. **Lesions** involve meningeal arteries as well as vessels elsewhere in the body and are most severe in the intima and media. **Haemorrhage, ischaemia, and infarction are uncommon, but can occur.**

Non-Lipid Arteriosclerosis

Arterial fibrosis usually occurs in older animals and has been described in **dogs** and **horses.** In the **dog,** fibrosis of the intima, media, or adventitia occurs in cerebrospinal vessels of all types and caliber. Collagenous thickening of the adventitia of small meningeal and parenchymal arteries can be accompanied by extension into other layers of the vessel wall. A common site is the choroid plexus. **In old horses,** a similar pattern of fibrosis occurs in vessels, but the intima is more prone. **Amyloid deposits** in meningeal and cerebral vessels are reported in **older**

dogs and **other animals. Mineralization** (deposition of calcium or iron salts) of cerebral blood vessels occurs in the brains of several species, but is especially common in **adult horses.** Meningeal vessels in **old cats, old horses,** and **cattle** are the other sites of vascular mineralization.

Specific Diseases Associated With Circulatory Dysfunction

Vascular-mediated injury can be associated with or complicate a number of diseases affecting the central nervous system. **Examples of such diseases include:**

1. Feline Ischaemic Encephalopathy

Feline ischaemic encephalopathy has a peracute to acute onset and affects **cats** of any age. **Clinical signs** usually indicate unilateral cerebral involvement and include depression, mild ataxia, seizures, behavioural changes, and blindness.

The **lesion** is unilateral, or rarely, bilateral necrosis of the cerebral hemisphere, usually in the area supplied by the middle cerebral artery. The necrosis can be multifocal or involve up to two thirds of one hemisphere. Haemorrhage can occur in the parenchyma or leptomeninges. In chronic cases, cerebral atrophy can occur. **Microscopically,** the lesions follow the sequence of changes which occur in infection.

The cause of the disease has not been established. Although specific vascular lesions (thrombosis or vasculitis) have been found in only a few cases, **an ischaemic mechanism is suspected** and is consistent with the character of the brain damage.

2. Ischaemic Myelopathy-Encephalopathy

Ischaemic (or necrotizing) myelopathy (pathological condition of spinal cord) has been described in the **dog, cat, horse, pig,** and **lambs. Clinically,** there are functional deficiencies of spinal cord, sometimes with cerebral involvement in certain species. **In dogs,** the **lesion** is an acute focal infarct involving cervical or lumbar spinal cord. **Microscopically,** emboli occlude meningeal or parenchymal arteries or veins or both, in affected areas.

3. *Clostridium perfringens* Type D Encephalopathy (Pulpy Kidney Disease, Overeating Disease)

Clostridium perfringens type D enterotoxaemia, associated with epsilon toxin production, is **a disease of sheep, goats,** and **cattle,** but only sheep show neurological signs of the disease. Sheep of all ages, except newborns, are susceptible. Incidence is at its peak between 3 and 10 weeks of age. Resistance of the newborn is due to the lack in the intestine of pancreatic proteolytic enzymes necessary for activation of the epsilon toxin, and also to trypsin inhibitors in colostrum. **Lambs in quite good condition are found dead.**

Gross lesions are usually absent in peracute cases, but when present, occur in the internal capsule, basal nuclei, thalamus, hippocampus, midbrain, cerebellar

339

peduncles, pons, and corona radiata of frontal cortex. **Lesions** are focal, bilaterally symmetrical and vary from yellowish-grey to red with malacia in advanced stages. Lesions in other tissues consist of pulmonary congestion and oedema, serous pericardial effusion, petechiation, and **soft (pulpy) kidneys.**

Microscopically, lesions in acute cases include perivascular and interstitial oedema. The fluid in perivascular spaces is usually protein rich and eosinophilic. Walls of arterioles may be hyalinized, and endothelial cell nuclei are swollen and vesicular. **Vasogenic** (interstitial) **oedema** gives a light or pink-staining, spongy appearance to the neuropil. Both grey and white matters are affected, but changes are more severe in the white matter. Peri-capillary haemorrhage and necrosis of neurons and microglia occur.

Brain damage is due to vascular injury and breakdown of the blood-brain barrier. Binding of **epsilon toxin** to endothelial cell surface receptors results in opening of tight junctions, disturbed transport processes, increased vascular permeability, oedema, swelling of astrocytic foot processes, and ultimately necrosis due to **hypoxic-ischaemic mechanisms.** Some of the effects of epsilon toxin can be mediated by an adenylcyclase- cyclic adenosine monophosphate (cAMP) system.

4. Oedema Disease (Enterotoxaemic Collibacillosis) of Pigs

Oedema disease is a disorder of rapidly growing, **healthy feeder pigs** being fed a high energy ration. Pigs are usually 4 to 8 weeks of age, but younger and older pigs can be affected. **Most affected pigs die within 24 hours.** Animals which develop CNS lesions survive for several days.

The basic lesion is an angiopathy which leads to oedematous and hypoxic-ischaemic injury in a number of tissues including the **brain. Grossly,** oedema is present in the subcutis, gastric sub-mucosa, gallbladder, colonic mesentery, mesenteric lymph nodes, larynx, and lungs. Serous effusions occur in the thoracic cavity and pericardial sac. Congestion and sometimes haemorrhage also occur. **The characteristic gross lesions in the brain** are bilaterally symmetrical foci of necrosis in the terminal brain stem. Lesions are yellow-grey, soft, and slightly depressed.

The main microscopic lesion is a degenerative angiopathy/vasculitis usually seen in the terminal brain stem and in cerebral and cerebellar meninges. Cerebral, cerebellar, and spinal blood vessels are also affected. In the beginning, perivascular oedema occurs from early vascular injury. Oedema is followed by necrosis of medial smooth muscle cells, deposition of fibrinoid material, and accumulation of macrophages and lymphocytes in the adventitia. Thrombosis is not a feature of this disease.

The disease is associated with strains of *Escherichia coli*, which produce a Shigella-like toxin (similar to toxins produced by *Shigella dysenteriae*) called **'Shiga-like**

toxin type IIe (SLT-IIe'). Glycolipid cell surface receptors on endothelial cells are binding sites for the toxin and their presence makes the animal susceptible to the disease. Binding of the toxin to these receptors can initiate a chain of inflammatory and immunological reactions that lead to vascular damage.

Metabolic /Toxic Brain Injury

Osmotic Encephalopathies

Sodium Chloride (Salt) Poisoning

Sodium chloride toxicity, also known as **'water deprivation syndrome'**, occurs in **pigs, poultry,** and sometimes in **ruminants**. The disease is due to **hypernatraemia** (an excess of sodium in the blood) caused by excessive intake of sodium salts, or severe dehydration followed by rehydration. During the hypernatraemic phase, the brain 'shrinks' because of the osmotic loss of water. Entry of sodium, potassium, and chloride ions into the brain, within minutes, is an acute adaptive response to equalize the sodium imbalance. **Maintenance of a normal ionic balance in the brain is critical for normal function,** and although a new ionic equilibrium is established, this response alone cannot compensate for severe or prolonged hypernatraemia.

A second, more delayed adaptive response of the brain is an entry or endogenous production of organic osmolytes such as certain amino acids and methylamines to equalize the osmotic imbalance created by hypernatraemia. This response requires hours or days to establish a new osmotic equilibrium. **When animals are given free access to fresh water, hypernatraemic to hyponatraemic shift occurs.** Within minutes, the brain attempts to compensate for this osmotic imbalance by eliminating sodium, potassium, and chloride ions. However, this early response cannot compensate for the osmotic stress created by the increased organic osmolytes in the brain. **As a result of the osmotic gradient, water enters the brain with subsequent brain swelling.**

Grossly, lesions include cerebral and leptomeningeal congestion and oedema. **Microscopically,** cerebrocortical neuronal necrosis is accompanied by astrocytic swelling. **In pigs,** leptomeninges and perivascular spaces have an infiltrate of eosinophils. With longer survival, an entry of macrophages takes place depending on the extent of necrosis. Paleness of subcortical white matter indicates oedema.

Metabolic Encephalopathy Due to Other Organ Dysfunction

Hepatic Encephalopathy

Acute and chronic liver failure and hepatic atrophy associated with congenital or acquired vascular shunts (passages or anastomoses between two natural channels, especially between blood vessels), **usually results in neurological disease.** This disorder is due to accumulation of toxic substances normally removed by the healthy liver and to disruption of normal metabolic functions in a number of organs and tissues. The **cause** of neurological dysfunction is build-up of ammonia and abnormal neurotransmission.

Nutritional Deficiencies

1. Thiamine Deficiency

Thiamine (vitamin B_1) deficiency is associated with neurological disease in **carnivores (dogs, cats, fox)** and **ruminants.** In carnivores there is an absolute dietary requirement for the vitamin. Dietary factors (i.e., ingestion of fish containing thiaminase), dietary deficiency, or diets in which the vitamin is destroyed by other means such as heating, **can all lead to thiamine deficiency.** Thiamine is a critical co-factor in carbohydrate metabolism, and brain damage is related to energy failure (depletion of high -energy phosphates). **Gross and microscopic lesions** are bilaterally symmetrical and usually involve brain stem, but cerebral cortex and cerebellum are also affected. Lesions consist of status spongiosus, neuronal necrosis, and myelin degradation.

The **disease in cattle, sheep,** and **goats** has been called **'polioencephalomalacia'** or **'cerebrocortical necrosis'.** This disease is usually seen in **cattle** of 6 to 18 months of age fed concentrate rations. **Polioencephalomalacia** usually occurs in **cattle** fed rations rich in carbohydrates with little roughage and is also associated with clinical or sub-clinical **acidosis. In sheep,** most cases occur in younger age groups (e.g., 2 to 7 months).

Gross lesions, if present, are limited to the cerebral cortex. Surface of the brain may be swollen as noticed by flattening of cerebrocortical gyri, and narrow sulci. In advanced cases with prolonged survival, areas of marked atrophy of cerebral gyri with thin or absent grey matter zone, remain covered by meninges. **Microscopically,** the earliest changes are astrocytic swelling and neuronal necrosis (ischaemic cell change) with oedema. Neurons in middle to deep lamina are preferentially affected. In mild cases, lesions are limited to the depths of cerebrocortical sulci, but usually there is involvement of entire gyri. After 4 to 5 days, neuronal necrosis and oedema are more severe. After 8 to 10 days, necrosis and oedema result in laminar separation (at the grey-white matter interface) in which there are prominent macrophages. Animals which survive may develop cerebral atrophy and hydrocephalus ex vacuo 1 to 2 years later.

2..Vitamin E Deficiency

Vitamin E (tocopherol) deficiency is associated with a variety of lesions in various tissues. **Vitamin E functions as an antioxidant, and protects cells from free radical-mediated injury.** Diseases in which vitamin A may be involved are **neuraxonal** dystrophy and **equine degenerative myeloencephalopathy** in **horses**. Low vitamin E concentrations have been found in some of these diseases. **Lesions** are **microscopic** and consist of **neuraxonal dystrophy** or **axonal spheroids** with or without other evidence of degeneration of axons and fibre tracts.

3. Copper Deficiency

Central nervous system disease produced by copper deficiency in animals is mainly a disorder of **sheep** and **goats**. It may be present at birth (**'swayback'** in **lambs** and rarely in **kids**), or onset may be delayed up to 6 months (**'enzootic ataxia'** in **lambs** and **kids**). **Copper is a component of several enzyme systems** which include cytochrome and lysyl oxidases, tyrosinase, and superoxide dismutase, as well as the protein **ceruloplasmin**. A deficiency of copper can affect several tissues such as skin (wool and hair growth and pigmentation), musculoskeletal development, and integrity of connective tissues. **Copper deficiency** can be **primary** (due to copper-deficient soils and inadequate intake from feed), or **secondary** (defective absorption due to interactions between copper, molybdenum, zinc, cadmium, or inorganic phosphates).

About 50% of congenitally **affected lambs** and rarely **kids** have gross bilateral and cerebrocortical lesions. **Microscopically**, astrogliosis is associated with the degeneration of white matter. **Lesions in the brain stem and spinal cords** in both congenital swayback and delayed-onset enzootic ataxia are microscopic, similar in **lambs** and **kids**, and affect both grey and white matter. Large multipolar neurons of the brain stem and ventral, lateral, and dorsal horns

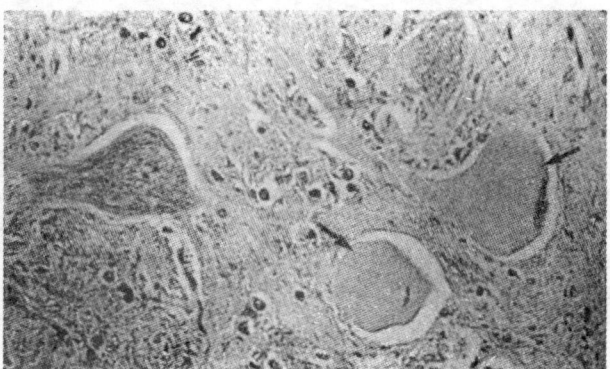

Fig. 40. Spinal cord, cervical level; kid. Swayback-enzootic ataxia. Central chromatolysis is seen in two motor neurons (arrows) of the ventral horn. The other neuron (left side) is normal. H & E stain.

of the spinal cord are affected. Neuronal cell bodies lack stainable Nissl's substance **(chromatolysis)**, the cytoplasm is dense, pink, and homogeneous and nuclei are often displaced to an eccentric position against the cell membrane (Fig. 40). Lesions in the white matter of the spinal cord consist of bilateral areas of paleness in the dorso-lateral aspect of the lateral funiculi. The paleness of the white matter is due to degeneration of myelinated axons. The **pathogenesis** of lesions which occur in swayback and enzootic ataxia is poorly understood.

Chemical Intoxications

1. Lead

Lead poisoning has been described in **cattle**. In **cattle** and other species, it is through the oral route, less commonly, through the respiratory system or skin (inorganic lead). Depending on the quantity absorbed, **poisoning** can be **peracute, acute, subacute**, or **chronic**. Lead poisoning can affect many tissues and organs including CNS, peripheral nervous system, liver, kidneys, gastrointestinal tract, bone marrow, blood vessels, and organs of the reproductive and endocrine systems. **Gross lesions in the CNS are usually absent. Microscopically,** lesions in peracute cases are absent. In acute cases, lesions consist of congestion, astrocytic swelling, and status spongiosus. Lesions in **dogs** resemble those in **cattle**, but vascular damage is more noticeable and consistent. Vascular lesions can progress to mural hyalinization.

Lead can damage the brain through several mechanisms. Direct toxic effects on neurons, astrocytes, and cerebral endothelial cells occur by disrupting metabolic pathways. Calcium homeostasis and its role in various biochemical reactions of the CNS can be the primary target. Direct injury to endothelial cells and astrocytes can lead to disruption of the blood-brain barrier, oedema, and subsequent CNS injury. **It is likely that multiple mechanisms contribute to the brain damage.**

2. Selenium

An acute paralytic syndrome called **'bilateral poliomyelomalacia'** has been observed in **pigs**. This is due to the incorporation, of toxic amounts of selenium in pig rations, by mistake. Cutaneous manifestations of the toxicity occur and include rough coats, partial alopecia, and separation and sloughing of the hoofs.

Grossly, bilateral areas of softening and yellow discoloration occur in the ventral spinal grey matter of the cervical and lumbar intumescences (swellings). **Microscopically**, acute lesions consist of status spongiosus and neuronal chromatolysis.

The **pathogenesis of the lesions** is not known, but may involve an induced nicotinamide or niacin deficiency.

3. Arsenic

Toxicity due to ingestion or cutaneous absorption can occur with **inorganic as** well as **organic arsenicals** and can affect many organs including the nervous system. Inorganic compounds are mainly herbicides or pesticides while organic arsenicals have been used as feed additives in the **pig** and **poultry** industries as growth promoters and to control intestinal diseases.

Poisoning with inorganic arsenicals is an acute enteric disease with hepatic and renal manifestations but neurological signs can occur. **In pigs, clinical signs include**

blindness resulting from damage to optic nerves and tracts, and incoordination, paresis, and paralysis related to spinal cord and peripheral nerve lesions. **Gross lesions are not present. Microscopically,** lesions in cranial and peripheral nerves consist of status spongiosus and fragmentation of myelin sheaths followed by axonal degeneration.

4. Organophosphates

Organophosphates are divided into **two groups** according to their use, mode of action, and type of toxicity. **In the first group,** which include organophosphate esters used as pesticides, fungicides, herbicides, or rodenticides, acute toxicity is produced by **inhibition of cholinesterase** either directly or indirectly. This allows acetylcholine to accumulate at synaptic or nerve-tissue junctions resulting in persistent depolarization. **Clinical signs** are variable and include hyperactivity or depression, respiratory difficulty, muscle tremors, and salivation. Seizures have been observed in **dogs** and **cats,** but are uncommon in **cattle. Death is due to respiratory failure. Gross** and **microscopic lesions** in the nervous system are absent.

The **second group of organophosphates** is the cresyl and related compounds. These compounds cause **delayed neurotoxicity** unrelated to cholinesterase inhibition. **Signs of toxicity** occur 1 to 2 weeks after exposure. Young animals tend to be less seriously affected, whereas recovery is slow and incomplete in adults. Susceptible animals include **cats, ruminants, chickens,** and **ducks. Dogs** are less sensitive. **Clinical signs** are those of sensory and motor neuropathy and spinal cord damage.

No specific gross lesions are present. Microscopically, there is degeneration in the spinal cord in the distal part of axons, especially those with a larger diameter. The degeneration has been called as **'dying-back neuropathy',** which is axonal injury extending from the periphery back toward the nerve cell body.

Organophosphorus compounds causing delayed neurotoxicity inhibit the activity of a target enzyme called **neurotoxic esterase.** The function of the enzyme in the peripheral and central nervous system is not fully understood.

Plant Poisoning

Astragalus, Oxytropis, and Swainsona Poisoning

These three genera of plants with various species are **toxic to livestock. Cattle, sheep,** and **horses** are generally affected. Toxicity is usually very slow and clinical signs are not observed until after the plants have been grazed for 14 to 60 days. There are no specific gross lesions. **Microscopically,** lesions involve neuron cell bodies throughout the neuraxis and visceral ganglia and are similar to the inherited lysosomal storage diseases.

345

Mycotoxins

Leuko-Encephalomalacia of Horses

Ingestion of mouldy feed, mainly **maize** or maize by-products, contaminated with the **fungus** *Fusarium moniliforme* causes an acute fatal neurological disease in **horses**. **Clinical signs** include depression, somnolence (sleepiness), head pressing, aimless wandering, or seizures. Rapid progression of these clinical signs followed by death is typical.

Gross lesions mostly involve the white matter of the cerebral hemispheres (frontal and parietal lobes). As a result of the white matter damage, including oedema, brain swelling is marked with flattening of cerebrocortical gyri. The lesions are usually bilateral but unequal in severity and are extensive. The **characteristic gross lesion** is **yellow gelatinous malacia and liquefaction** of the affected white matter (mainly breakdown of lipids) accompanied by haemorrhage.

Microscopically, affected white matter is coagulated or liquefied and the neuropil is disrupted by accumulation of pink-staining proteinaceous fluid with scattered neutrophils and macrophages. Blood vessels are degenerate or necrotic and some are infiltrated with neutrophils, plasma cells, and eosinophils. Less characteristic changes include oedema and perivascular cuffing in the leptomeninges and neuronal necrosis in deeper layers or the entire width of the overlying grey matter. **Similar lesions have been reported in the spinal cord where grey matter is especially affected.**

This equine mycotoxicosis can be associated with **hepatotoxicity,** or hepatotoxicity may be the only manifestation. Other animals including **pigs** and **various avian species (ducks, chickens)** are also susceptible, but clinical disease and lesions usually indicate pulmonary, hepatic, or renal injury.

The **toxin isolated** from *F. moniliforme* is called 'fumonisin B$_1$', although other fumonisins have been extracted. **Vascular damage** is the main injury caused. Fumonisins inhibit the enzyme **ceramide synthase,** which interferes with the synthesis of sphingolipids. Fumonisins disrupt cellular membranes, are associated with lipid peroxidation of cell and cellular membranes, inhibit synthesis of macromolecules and DNA, and may increase production of tumour necrosis factor-alpha by macrophages.

Disorders of Myelin Formation and Maintenance

Terminology

Disorders of myelin formation include **hypomyelinogenesis (hypomyelination)** and **dysmyelination. Hypomyelinogenesis (hypomyelination)** is a process in which there is under-development of myelin. **Dysmyelination** is abnormal formation of myelin which can be chemically defective. **Demyelination**, which means degeneration and loss of myelin **already formed,** can be of primary and secondary types. **Primary demyelination,** refers to a disease process in which the myelin sheath is selectively affected with the axon remaining intact. Unless indicated otherwise this is the type meant in the discussion that follows. **Secondary demyelination** refers to degeneration of myelin along with injury to the axon, as in Wallerian degeneration, **and is not a selective injury of the myelin sheath.**

Hereditary Diseases

Hypomyelinogenesis and Dysmyelination

Hypomyelinogenesis and dysmyelination usually occur in the early post-natal period and have similar clinical and pathological features. However, there are some differences in the lesions and the mechanisms by which they develop. The diseases have been described in **dogs, cattle, pigs,** and **sheep,** but are rare.

Globoid Cell Leukodystrophy

Globoid cell leukodystrophy is a lysosomal disease, its one main lesion being demyelination. Brain, spinal cord, and peripheral nerves can be affected. The disease, which is inherited as an autosomal recessive, is generally seen in younger animals. Oligodendroglia are deficient in the lysosomal enzyme galactosyl-ceramidase (galacto-cerebrosidase) which is normally responsible for the degradation of galactosylceramide (galacto-cerebroside) which is normally responsible the degradation of galactosylceramide (galacto-cerebroside), galactosyl-sphigosine (psychosine), monogalactosyl diglyceride, and lactosylceramide. **Galactosyl-sphingosine (psychosine) is highly toxic and causes death of oligodendroglia. Galactosyl-ceramide,** which is non-toxic and accumulates within oligodendroglia, is released into the extracellular space during degradation of these cells and **stimulates accumulation of macrophages** (called 'globoid cells'), which contain this storage material. Globoid cells, which are believed to originate outside the CNS, appear in the early stage of the demyelination, increase as degeneration of the white matter progresses, and tend to disappear in the terminal stage.

Gross lesions of the CNS are characterized by a grey discoloration of the affected white matter (central hemispheres and spinal cord). The lesion in the spinal cord involves the peripheral white matter. **Microscopically,** such areas have pronounced loss of myelin. Peripheral nerves are also affected and lesions include demyelination and axonal degeneration.

Spongy Degeneration

Under this heading of **spongy degeneration is a group of diseases of young animals** characterized by a **spongy lesion** called **'status spongiosus'** which occurs mainly in the white matter of the CNS, but also extend into grey matter. **Status**

spongiosus can develop by several different mechanisms which include **splitting of the myelin sheath,** accumulation of extracellular fluid, swelling of cellular (e.g., astrocytic, neuronal) processes, and axonal injury (e.g., Wallerian degeneration) when swollen axons are no longer detectable within distended spaces.

Gross lesions in brain range from no gross lesions to swelling, oedema, and paleness of the white matter, and dilation of the ventricles. **Microscopically,** the lesion is characterized by empty spaces of different sizes within the white matter. Ultrastructurally, there is splitting or separation of the myelin sheath with the formation of large intra-myelinic spaces. In some cases, myelin formation is deficient.

Some species affected **dogs, cats,** and **cattle**. An autosomal recessive mode of transmission has been reported for some forms of the disease. A form of the disease described in **calves** called **'maple syrup urine disease'** is due to a branched chain keto acid decarboxylase deficiency, resulting in an increased concentration of the branched chain amino acids valine, isoleucine, and leucine in the serum, plasma, CSF, and **urine.** The unique odour associated with urine of affected animals is caused by the amino acid **isoleucine. Calves** are affected within 2 days of birth with a severe generalized CNS disorder characterized by dullness and weakness that progresses to recumbency (lying down position) and opisthotonus (position of the body in which head, neck, and spine are arched backward). **Mechanism** which causes status spongiosus (splitting of the myelin sheath) involves formation of a toxic metabolite from the oxidative decarboxylation of alpha-keto acids.

Circulatory Disturbances

Extracellular oedema (vasogenic and hydrostatic) due to inflammation, neoplasms, trauma, and hydrocephalus can cause **degeneration of myelin sheath.**

Physical Disturbances

Physical compression of CNS tissue, which can result from various causes, can also cause **demyelination. Mechanisms** include compression on myelin sheaths and oligodendroglia, as well as interference with circulation resulting in CNS tissue ischaemia.

Infectious Diseases
(Confirmed or Suspected of Being Caused by Viruses)

Progressive Multifocal Leuko-Encephalopathy

Some viruses have the ability to cause demyelination within the CNS by directly infecting and destroying oligodendroglia. One of these diseases (**progressive multifocal leuko-encephalopathy**) which occurs in **human beings** and **monkeys,** is caused by the JC (human) or SV40 (monkey) strain of **papovavirus.** The disease has been associated with immunosuppression.

Canine Distemper

Canine distemper is one of the most important diseases of dogs. It is caused by a **morbillivirus** and has a worldwide distribution. In addition to the **dog, fox, wolf, panda, lions, tigers,** and **leopards** are also susceptible to canine viral infection. **Morbilliviruses** other than canine distemper virus (CDV) include measles virus, rinderpest virus, and peste- des-petits-ruminants virus.

Lesions of canine distemper do not always occur from direct viral infection, but may involve other factors (e.g., immunological and possibly toxic). **The virus is pantropic** (i.e., having an affinity for many tissues or cells), but has a **particular affinity for lymphoid and epithelial tissues** (e.g., lungs, gastrointestinal tract, urinary tract, skin) and the CNS (including the optic nerve) and eye. Lymphoid depletion and necrosis can cause **immunosuppression,** affecting both the humoral and cell-mediated responses, making the animal less able to fight the primary viral as well as secondary bacterial infections.

Following **infection through the respiratory tract,** the virus infects **macrophages** and **monocytes** present in or on the respiratory epithelium and tonsils. After a brief replication, virus spreads through lymph and blood to other lymphoid tissues, where additional replication takes place. The initial replication and spread are followed by cell-associated (monocytic) or non-cell associated haematogenous **spread of the virus to epithelial tissues and to the CNS about 8 to 9 days after infection.** It is at this stage of the infection that the host's immune response decides the outcome of the disease. **First,** the animal may die from an acute severe infection with unrestricted spread of the virus throughout the body. **Death generally results from** secondary bacterial infection or severe involvement of the CNS. **A second type** of infection is characterized by a more delayed progression of the disease accompanied by an immune response. **Finally,** some dogs recover from the infection and remain clinically normal.

Neurological signs include convulsions, myoclonus (a sudden spasm of the muscles), tremor, disturbances in voluntary movement, circling, hyperaesthesia (increased sensitivity to stimulation, particularly to touch), paralysis, and blindness.

Initial natural infection of CNS was believed to occur by the haematogenous route. However, more recent evidence indicates entry and spread by the cerebrospinal fluid (CSF), within infected mammalian cells. It is during this period that a **pronounced immunosuppression** occurs due to **lymphotropism** of the canine distemper virus. The early stage of demyelination, which is non-inflammatory, coincides with replication of the virus in the white matter, particularly in astrocytes. In addition to demyelination, there is status spongiosus, astrocytic hypertrophy and hyperplasia, reduced number of oligodendroglia, and neuronal degeneration. **Inclusion bodies (cytoplasmic, nuclear, or both)** are seen, particularly in astrocytes, which are important target cells for the distemper virus. However, they are also seen in ependymal cells and sometimes in neurons. The earliest evidence of **myelin injury** is a **ballooning change** resulting from a split in the myelin sheath, or more degenerative changes including axon swelling. This lesion is associated with astroglial and microglial proliferation. This initial injury of the myelin sheath is followed by a progressive removal of compact myelin sheaths by phagocytic microglial cells (that infiltrate the myelin lamellae) and variable axonal necrosis. A late stage of demyelination, which indicates affected animal's improved immune status, is more pronounced and is characterized by non-suppurative inflammation (perivascular cuffing, leptomeningitis, and choroiditis) and also can be accompanied by tissue degeneration and accumulation of **'gitter cells'** (macrophages).

Of the above lesions affecting the white matter, **status spongiosus** (empty spaces in the white matter) and **demyelination** (uniformly pale-stained areas of the white matter) require some clarification. **Status spongiosus** can occur in several different disease processes (mentioned under 'spongy degeneration'). Demyelination (primary demyelination) refers to loss of the myelin sheath and is characterized microscopically by a uniform decrease, or an absence of, myelin staining with many of the axons remaining intact. Such affected areas appear pale pink following haematoxylin eosin staining. Status spongiosus occurs within areas that are demyelinated or myelinated.

Lesions mainly occur in the cerebellum (medullary area, folial white matter, and sub-pial white matter) and cerebellar peduncles (with both white and sometimes grey matter involvement of the pons). **Lesions** also occur in medulla oblongata, cerebrum (both white and grey matter), optic nerves, optic tracts, spinal cord, and meninges.

The **pathogenesis of demyelination** in canine distemper infection is not completely understood and appears to result from damage to oligodendroglia.

Old-Dog Encephalitis

Old-dog encephalitis is a rare condition seen in mature adult dogs and is associated with clinical signs of dementia (disorder of behaviour and intellectual function). **Lesions** are mainly in the cerebral hemispheres and brain stem. **Microscopic lesions** are characterized by non-suppurative encephalitis with lympho-plasmacytic (lymphocytes and plasma cells) perivascular cuffing, leptomeningitis, and neuronal degeneration. Nuclear and cytoplasmic inclusions, **positive for canine distemper viral antigen**, have been detected in neurons and astrocytes in the cerebral cortex, thalamus, and brain stem, but in contrast to distemper, not in the cerebellum. Demyelination also occurs but is not prominent.

The **mechanisms** involved in the development of the lesions are not known, but it is believed that the disease occurs from a persistent infection with replication of a defective form of canine distemper virus.

Visna

Visna (which means 'wasting') is a slowly progressive, transmissible **disease of sheep.** The disease is caused by a strain of the ovine maedi-visna virus (MVV) complex, one of the eight basic **lenti-** (slow) **viruses.** A different strain of the same virus causes a lymphocytic interstitial pneumonia called **'maedi'.** Visna was originally described in Iceland. **CNS signs** include an abnormal hind limb gait that progresses to incoordination and rear limb paresis over a period of weeks or months.

Early lesions affect grey and white matter of the brain and central canal of the spinal cord. The lesions include non-suppurative encephalomyelitis accompanied by pleocytosis (presence of more than normal number of cells in cerebrospinal fluid), oedema, parenchymal necrosis, astrocytosis, and non-suppurative leptomeningitis. Degeneration of myelin sheaths also occurs and is usually accompanied by axonal degeneration. Neural cell bodies and oligodendroglia are normal.

In recent years understanding of the **factors associated with infection** and **mechanism involved in the development of the lesion,** has improved. Visna is a persistent viral disease and results from the ability of the virus to form **provirus** (integration of viral and host genome). **The virus can also change its antigenic characteristics (antigenic drift),** which enables it to avoid the effects of the host's immune response. Although the visna virus (and other **lentiviruses**) can infect pro-monocytes and monocytes in the bone marrow and blood, viral replication is restricted in these cells where it remains as **provirus DNA** until maturation and differentiation to **macrophages, where primary replication occurs.** However, the visna virus can also be present in oligodendrocytes and astrocytes located in foci of demyelination.

It appears that virus enters in these cells through close contact with infected monocytes. The primary demyelination which occurs during the late stages of the disease process (6 months to 8 years after infection) occurs from oligodendroglial cell infection. The **main sources of virus excretion** are udder and lungs (mainly as cell-associated virus), and transmission occurs readily **between the dam and lamb** through milk and **between confined individuals,** through respiratory secretions. The maedi-visna virus (MVV) has also been detected in semen of infected rams.

No profound immune deficiency occurs with MVV infections, as is the case with immunodeficiency lentiviral infections which infect CD4+ T-lymphocytes. However, secondary infections can still accompany MVV infection.

Caprine Leuko-Encephalomyelitis-Arthritis
(Caprine Arthritis Encephalitis, CAE)

This disease was first described in the United States and since has been recorded in other parts of the world, including India. The infection is readily transmitted by colostrum and milk following birth, or by direct contact. **A close relationship exists between maedi-visna viruses (MVVs) of sheep and the caprine arthritis encephalitis (CAE) virus,** but there are **genomic differences between them**. As with MVV infection of sheep, **CAE viral infection is also a lymphoproliferative disease** with a tropism for the macrophage which acts as a carrier of the virus.

The pattern of disease is age dependent. Neurological signs are usually seen in **young kids** 2 to 4 months of age, but unlike visna in **sheep**, there is a more rapid progression and quadriplegia develops within weeks to months. As with visna, affected **goats** have pleocytosis. **Gross lesions** in the nervous system include foci of necrosis and inflammation sometimes in the brain but usually in the spinal cord. **Microscopic lesions** are similar to those of visna (non-suppurative encephalomyelitis), but can be more severe. Non-neural lesions include interstitial pneumonia and moderate severity in some kids.

In adult goats, the primary target tissue is **synovium** (synovial membrane) of the joints. Those animals which survive the initial infection develop **lymphoproliferative synovitis** and **arthritis**. Pneumonia, lymphocytic mastitis, and encephalomyelitis also occur in adult animals.

Immune-Mediated Disorders

This category of demyelinating disease involves the development of type IV hypersensitivity. The best example in this group is an experimental model called **'experimental allergic encephalomyelitis (EAE)'**. EAE is produced by inducing a hypersensitivity to **myelin** or, more specifically, to **myelin basic protein**. If appropriate laboratory animals are injected with white matter or myelin basic protein, **they become paralyzed** after 2-3 weeks. Lesions are characterized by accumulation of lymphocytes and macrophages. A similar process, called **'post-vaccinal encephalomyelitis'**, occurs sometimes when human rabies vaccine contained CNS tissue. A third situation in which this type of demyelination occurs follows infection with certain viruses (e.g., rubeola) in human beings. This disease, which is rare, is called **'post-infectious encephalomyelitis'**. It is characterized by development of lesions in the CNS similar to those of EAE. **Such a naturally occurring process is not commonly seen in animals.**

Neurodegenerative Diseases

There is no clear-cut classification of the neurodegenerative diseases. Many of the diseases described here have a **familial** or **hereditary** basis and a specific pattern of degeneration in the CNS. Others have a fairly similar pattern of CNS damage, but the **cause is unknown.**

Primary Neuronal Degenerations

These are those diseases which are characterized by degeneration, necrosis, and loss of specific neuronal populations. Although these diseases in human beings and animals usually have a genetic basis, the pathogenesis for most remains unknown. **Primary neuronal degenerations include:**

1. Multisystem Neuronal Degeneration

These diseases have been described in various breeds of **dogs** and affect connected neural systems, an example being **striatonigral** (basal nuclei and substantia nigra) and **cerebello-olivary** (cerebellar cortex and caudal olivary nucleus) **degeneration in the Kerry blue terrier dogs.** This **hereditary disease** is characterized clinically by rear limb ataxia, tremors and hypermetria (a form of ataxia) of front and rear limbs. **Gross lesions** include a slight reduction in the size of cerebellum and narrowing of cerebellar folia. **Microscopic lesions** are degeneration and loss of cerebellar Purkinje and granule cells, followed by neuronal loss.

Another example of multisystem neuronal degeneration is the one that **occurs in the red-haired cocker spaniel breed of dogs.** It is suspected of being inherited. **Clinical signs** include progressive ataxia and mental deterioration.

A third example of multisystem neuronal degeneration can be given **from the disease that occurs in the Cairn terrier breed of dogs.** It is also suspected of being inherited. There is onset of progressive cerebellar ataxia, spastic paresis, and collapse. Widespread neuronal chromatolysis affecting multiple neuronal systems is observed in the central and peripheral nervous system.

2. Primary Cerebellar Degeneration

Depending on the degree of maturation of the cerebellum at the time of birth in various species, clinical signs in **cattle** and **sheep** affected with **'neonatal syndromes'** appear immediately after birth. In the **dogs,** clinical signs are delayed until the pups are able to walk. Hereditary transmission is known or suspected in some cases.

Animals with **'postnatal cerebellar syndromes'** are normal at birth or at the time they are able to walk. Onset of ataxia and various other clinical signs due to cerebellar disease begins **weeks or months after a period of apparently normal development. Grossly,** cerebellum can be normal or reduced in size and atrophic. **Microscopically,** lesions are similar to those that occur in the neonatal syndromes with loss of Purkinje cells, neuronal depletion in the granular layer, and astrogliosis in the molecular layer.

3. Brain Stem and Spinal Syndromes

Diseases associated with axonal swellings in the neuraxis (i.e., central nervous system) have been called **'neuraxonal dystrophy'.** As stated earlier, axonal degeneration can occur in diseases caused by vitamin E deficiency. However, included here are those diseases which have a species and breed association and occur early in life, usually before one year of life. **Clinical signs** vary and include gait abnormalities, dysmetria (disturbance of the power to control movement in muscular action) or hypermetria (a form of ataxia), or other cerebellar signs. **Lesions** differ in severity and distribution but are characterized by **axonal swellings in various nuclei** (often sensory) in the brain stem, cerebellum, and spinal cord. The disease has been described in **cats, dogs, and horses.**

4. Spinal Cord-Motor Neuron Disease

These diseases are characterized clinically by severe muscular weakness and widespread muscular atrophy. Onset of disease in different species is early in life, and a hereditary basis is often suspected. **Lesions** include degeneration and loss of motor neurons in ventral horns of the spinal cord and axonal degeneration in the ventral spinal nerve rootlets and peripheral nerves.

The disease known as **'shaker calf syndrome'** is a motor neuron disease. The disorder occurs in **newborn calves** and is characterized clinically by **shaking of the head, body, and tail.** All segments of the spinal cord are severely affected.

Spongy Degeneration

See 'Disorders of Myelin Formation and Maintenance'.

Mitochondrial Encephalopathies

In humans, various encephalopathies and myopathic syndromes (i.e., affecting muscles) due to **point mutations in mitochondrial DNA** are grouped together under the acronyms **MELAS** (mitochondrial encephalopathy, lactic acidosis, stroke-like episodes) and **MERRF** (myoclonus epilepsy, ragged red fibres). The diseases have different clinical signs and lesions.

Diseases that might be classified as **mitochondrial encephalopathies are not well characterized in animals.** Despite this, diseases reported in **cattle** and **dogs**, could represent mitochondrial disorders. The main features of the diseases include ataxia and other motor disturbances. Characteristics of these diseases in both humans and animals are symmetrical bilateral involvement of the neuraxis (i.e., central nervous system) and lesions of status spongiosus with progression to cavitation or necrosis.

Degenerative Leukomyelopathies (White Matter of Spinal Cord)

Diseases with degeneration of mainly spinal cord white matter have been described in **domestic animals.** These can be inherited or have familial predisposition. **Paresis and ataxia are the main clinical findings.** The leukomyelopathies are characterized by **axonal degeneration with secondary changes in myelin sheaths and myelin loss.** These diseases have been described in **dogs, cattle, and horses.** ·

Inflammation of the CNS

Infectious agents can spread to the CNS in four ways:

1. **Haematogenously**. Mostly they may spread in a cell-associated state (e.g., with monocytes), or in a cell-unassociated state,

2. By **movement within the axoplasm** of peripheral axons,

3. **From the olfactory mucosa** that contains receptor cells whose processes synapse within the CNS and by direct spread from the nasal sub-mucosa into the CSF through focally exposed subarachnoid space, and

4. **By direct spread.** Direct spread of infection can occur from trauma (skull or vertebral fracture), various para-cranial and para-vertebral infections associated with inner ear infection, vertebral osteomyelitis, and following docking of lambs. **Within the CNS, infectious agents can spread in the interstitium and within neurons and neuroglia** through the infected leukocytes that enter from the circulation, and in the CFS.

Four commonly occurring changes that characterize inflammation of CNS include:

1. **Leptomeningitis** (inflammation of pia mater and arachnoid together),

2. **Perivascular cuffing**,

3. **Microgliosis**, and

4. **Neuronal degeneration**

Although less common but important other lesions include **ganglioneuritis** (e.g., in rabies), **vasculitis, necrosis** (e.g., in pseudorabies of pigs), and demyelination (e.g., in canine distemper).

The type of inflammatory response can vary with the cause. A simple guideline (there are always exceptions) which compares the type of inflammation with different aetiological agents is as follows: **suppurative** or **purulent response** can be due to several species of **bacteria; non-suppurative** (lymphocytic, monocytic [macrophage], plasmacytic) response can be due to **viruses** and certain other infectious agents (e.g., **protozoa** such as *Toxoplasma gondii*) and **parasitic infestations**; and **granulomatous response** can be due to **fungi** and **some bacteria** (e.g., **Mycobacteria** species).

Viral Infections

Rabies

Rabies virus is one of the most neurotropic of all viruses infecting mammals. Gross lesions of the infected central nervous tissue are often **absent. Microscopic lesions** are typically non-suppurative and include leptomeningitis and perivascular cuffing with lymphocytes, macrophages, and plasma cells; microgliosis (sometimes prominent); neuronal degeneration (usually not severe); and ganglioneuritis.

Neurons may also contain **intra-cytoplasmic inclusions (Negri bodies)**. Also, some species (e.g., **dogs**) have a tendency to develop a more severe inflammatory reaction than others (e.g., **cattle**), in which little if any inflammation may occur. Non-neural lesions include non-suppurative sialitis (inflammation of a salivary gland) accompanied by necrosis and presence of **Negri bodies** (e.g., **dog**) in salivary epithelial cells.

Negri body formation within neurons of the CNS and even in the peripheral ganglia has long been characteristic feature of rabies infection, although it is not detected in all cases. The **inclusions** are **intra-cytoplasmic** and initially develop as an **aggregation of strands of viral nucleocapsid**, which quickly change into an ill-defined granular matrix. **Mature rabies virions**, which bud from the endoplasmic reticulum, can also be seen around the periphery of the matrix. **With time, Negri body becomes larger and detectable by light microscope. In H and E-stained sections, Negri body**, which is **eosinophilic**, has one or more small, light clear areas called **inner bodies** which form as a result of invagination of cytoplasmic components (that includes virions) into the matrix of the inclusion. Inclusions which do not contain inner bodies are called 'Lyssa bodies', but **are actually Negri bodies without cytoplasmic indentation.** Also, both fixed viruses (adapted to the CNS by passage) and **street viruses** (which produce the naturally occurring disease) produce the same ultrastructural features, but fixed virus strains usually cause severe neuronal degeneration that prevents the development, and thus the detection, of Negri bodies. **Negri bodies** also occur more frequently in large neurons (e.g., pyramidal neurons of the hippocampus and large neurons of the medulla oblongata) than in smaller ones. Moreover, inclusions are usually present in neurons not located in areas of inflammation.

A spongiform lesion, which is similar to the characteristic of several spongiform encephalopathies (see 'prion infections', 'scrapie'), is present in naturally occurring rabies in **fox, horse, cow, cat,** and **sheep**. The lesion occurs in the neuropil (network of interwoven dendrites and axons and of neuroglial cells) of the grey matter (mainly thalamus and cerebral cortex), initially as **intra-cytoplasmic membrane-bound vacuoles in neuronal dendrites** (less commonly in axons and astrocytes). The **vacuoles** enlarge, compress surrounding tissue, and ultimately rupture with formation of a tissue space. Although the **mechanism** responsible for the development of this lesion is not known, it is thought to result from **an indirect effect of the rabies virus** on neural tissue (possibly involving a change in neurotransmitter metabolism).

Rabies is usually transmitted by a bite from an infected animal. Respiratory infection is extremely rare and may occur following exposure to virus in **bat caves** and from **accidental human laboratory exposure.** The mechanism for spread of rabies virus from the inoculation site (for example, rear leg of an animal) to the CNS is as follows: The virus first enters into the peripheral nerve terminals or local skeletal muscle myocytes or both at the site of inoculation. The virus is taken up by both **axon terminals** and **myocytes** following a large inoculation dose. If the virus directly enters peripheral nerve terminals, the **incubation period** is short regardless of whether muscle cells are infected. With increasingly lower doses of virus, however, there is a greater possibility that **virus will enter nerve terminals or myocytes, but not both.** This situation can result in a **short incubation period** if virus directly enters nerve terminals as described above or could result in a more prolonged incubation period if there was initial infection and retention of virus in myocytes before its release and uptake by nerve terminals. **Virus replication** within infected monocytes has been suggested, but the specific degree to which this can occur remains to be clarified. **Virus moves from the periphery to the CNS by axoplasmic transport through sensory or motor nerves. With sensory axons,** the first cell bodies to be met following inoculation of a rear leg would be the sensory dorsal root ganglia or the dorsal horn of the spinal cord; **for motor neurons,** the cell bodies of the ventral lower motor neurons or those in autonomic ganglia are the ones initially infected. It is not known whether viral infection and replication in neurons of dorsal root ganglia are essential for infection of the CNS. **Virus then moves into the spinal cord and spreads to the brain.**

Recent experimental results have clarified the mechanism by which the virus spreads within the CNS. Following axoplasmic spread of virus from an inoculated rear leg to neurons of the segments of the spinal cord (e.g., L2 and L3), **rapid spread of infection to the brain occurs through long ascending fibre tracts**, bypassing the grey matter of the rostral spinal cord. This early spread of the virus explains how induction of the behavioural changes occurs before there is sufficiently severe injury to cause paralysis, and allows spread of infection before there is time for a significant immune response. **Spread of infection within the neurons of CNS** occurs through both **anterograde** (moving anteriorly) and **retrograde** (moving backward) **axoplasmic flow,** with corresponding **neuron-to-neuron spread by axosomatic-axodendritic** (i.e., between axon of one neuron and the cell body of another; and between axon of one neuron and dendrites of another) and **somatoaxonal-dendroaxonal transfer of infection** (i.e., between the body of one neuron and axon of another; and between dendrites of one neuron and axon of another). The latter type of trans-synaptic spread can occur by budding of developing virions from the neuronal cytoplasm (cell body or dendrite) into a synapsing axon. Trans-synaptic spread can also occur in the form of bare viral **nucleocapsid (ribonucleoprotein-transcriptase complexes)** in the absence of complete virion.

As indicated, viral spread within the CNS can be quite rapid, and **although neurons are the cells mainly affected, occasional and slight infection can also involve leptomeninges, ependyma, oligodendroglia, and astrocytes.** During the spread of virus, there is simultaneous centrifugal movement of virus peripherally from the CNS through axons, which results in infection of various tissues including the oral cavity and the saliva. **During centrifugal spread,** there is also infection of neurons of dorsal root ganglia with widespread involvement of ganglia occurring terminally. Affected ganglia have a moderate to severe non-suppurative inflammatory response that may be accompanied by neuronal degeneration. An important feature is that infection of nervous (i.e., limbic system, which includes hippocampus and dentate gyrus) and non-nervous tissues (salivary glands) occur at the same time. **This provides affected animals with necessary virus inoculum in the saliva to transmit the disease.**

The **clinical signs** in domestic animals are similar with some differences between species. **Clinical disease in the dog** occurs in **three phases: prodromal, excitatory, and paralytic.** In the **prodromal phase,** which lasts 2 to 3 days, the animal has a change in temperament. **Furious rabies** refers to animals in which the excitatory phase is predominant and **dumb rabies** to animals in which excitatory phase is extremely short or absent and the disease progresses quickly to paralytic phase. **Cattle usually have the furious form of rabies,** and animals are **restless and aggressive.** Other signs in cattle include bellowing, general straining, tenesmus, and signs of sexual excitement followed by **paralysis and death. Mules, sheep, and pigs** usually have the excitatory form of rabies. **Horses** can have early **signs** which are **atypical for a neurological disease** but terminally tend to have the furious-violent form.

When conducting a postmortem on animal suspected of having rabies it is important to remember:

1. To provide adequate protection to the person conducting the postmortem, and

2. To collect the proper CNS tissues (cerebral hemisphere which includes hippocampus, cerebellum and medulla, and optionally spinal cord) for histopatholgy and examination by immunofluorescence and sometimes mouse inoculation.

Pseudorabies (Aujeszky's disease)

Several species of domestic and wild animals are susceptible to infection with pseudorabies virus. **The disease is usually fatal in species other than the pigs.** Although **pigs** (particularly young, suckling ones) can die from infection, **most mature pigs remain persistently infected and act as carriers.**

Gross lesions in pigs occur in several non-neural tissues including organs of the respiratory system, lymphoid system, digestive tract, and reproductive tract. Focal tissue necrosis also occurs (e.g., liver, spleen, adrenal glands), particularly in **young suckling pigs,** and mortality in such animals can be high. **The CNS is free from gross lesions except for leptomeningeal congestion. Microscopic lesions in pigs** are characterized by a **non-suppurative meningo-encephalomyelitis** with ganglioneuritis. Injury to CNS tissue can be severe, with neuronal degeneration and parenchymal necrosis. **Intranuclear inclusion bodies** are not usually detected in **pigs** but can be present in neurons, astrocytes, oligodendroglia, and endothelial cells.

The **route of infection in pigs is intranasal** (by direct contact or through contaminated air), followed by replication of the virus in the upper respiratory tract. The virus then travels to the tonsil and lymph nodes by way of the lymph vessels. Following replication in the nasopharynx, **virus invades sensory nerve endings** (e.g., bipolar olfactory cells and other nerve terminals) and is then **transported in axoplasm** through the trigeminal ganglion and olfactory bulb **to the brain**. The virus can also spread trans-synaptically. Recently it has been shown that some strains produce lesions in the gastrointestinal tract and myenteric plexuses (i.e., enteric plexuses within the muscular layer), suggesting that infection may spread from the intestinal mucosa of the CNS through autonomic nerves. **In latently infected pigs,** the oro-nasal epithelium can be recurrently infected by virus spreading from the nervous system, followed by its excretion in oro-nasal fluid. The virus can also spread haematogenously, although in low titre, to other tissues of the body. Cellular attachment, entry, and cell-to-cell spread of the virus is mediated by glycoprotein projections that extend from the surface of the viral particle.

Infection of secondary host, namely, cattle, sheep, dogs, and cats involves direct or indirect contact with pigs. Infection can also occur by ingestion, inhalation, and wound infection. **Dogs** and **cats** usually become infected by ingesting organs from **pigs** that contain pseudorabies virus. The **pathogenesis** involves axonal spread to the CNS and is similar to that of pigs, with lesions that include non-suppurative encephalomyelitis accompanied by ganglioneuritis. **Intranuclear inclusion bodies,** either eosinophilic or basophilic, have been described in neurons of the brain.

Equine Herpesvirus 1 Infection

Equine herpesvirus 1 (EHV-1), an alpha-herpesvirus, is an important cause of **abortion in horses and perinatal foal infection and death.** In addition to myeloencephalitis (inflammation of spinal cord and brain), EHV-1 can also cause **rhinopneumonitis.**

The **neurologic form** of EHV-1 infection affects other equidae including **zebra** in addition to the **horse,** but is relatively uncommon compared with the incidence of abortion and upper respiratory tract disease caused by EHV-1. The neurologic disease may accompany or follow outbreaks of respiratory disease or abortions.

The **characteristic lesion in the** CNS caused by EHV-1 infection **is a vasculitis** (affecting arterioles, capillaries, and venules) accompanied by thrombosis and focal parenchymal necrosis (infarction). **Lesions** occur in both grey and white matter of the spinal cord, medulla oblongata, mesencephalon, diencephalon, and cerebral cortex. **The endothelium is the site of involvement,** with intimal and medial degeneration, haemorrhage, thrombosis, escape of plasma proteins into the perivascular space, neuronal degeneration (e.g., axonal swelling with ballooning of the myelin sheath and degeneration of the cell body), and mononuclear cellular cuffing. Other lesions include vasculitis in non-neural tissues including the endometrium, nasal cavity, lungs, hypophysis and skeletal muscle.

The disease begins with infection of the respiratory mucosa. The virus replicates in the epithelium of the respiratory or intestinal tracts following infection. **Intranuclear inclusions** occur in the nasal mucosa. Infection of mononuclear leukocytes (mainly T-lymphocytes) then occurs and is followed by **cell-mediated viraemia.** The **virus**, which is **endotheliotropic**, even though infection of neurons and astrocytes occurs, localizes in small arteries and capillaries of the CNS and some other tissues following direct spread from the circulating infected cells. Inflammation of the vascular wall results in vasculitis, thrombosis, and infection of the neural tissue supplied by thrombosed vessel. Latent infection of the trigeminal ganglion and lymphoid tissues can also occur.

EHV-1 does not appear to be neurotropic, which is in contrast to some herpesvirus encephalitides (pleural of 'encephalitis') of other species in which the virus replicates in neurons (e.g., herpes simplex virus infection in **human**, infectious bovine rhinotracheitis viral infection in **calves**, and pseudorabies viral infection in **pigs**). In addition to vasculitis as the main lesion, the infection in **horse** also differs from most other herpetic infections of the CNS in being mainly a disease of the adult (although young animals can be affected).

Bovine Malignant Catarrhal Fever

Malignant catarrhal fever is **a highly fatal disease of cattle and other ruminants** including **buffalo, deer,** and **antelope** and **can involve several animals in a herd.** It is usually a sporadic disease. The primary target tissues are lymphoid organs, epithelial tissues (particularly respiratory and gastrointestinal tracts), and the vasculature, but the kidneys, liver, eyes, joints, and CNS are also affected in some **cattle.**

Two general types of disease occur, the **sheep-associated** and **wildebeest-derived forms.** The **causative agents** are **herpesviruses.** The disease occurring outside Africa, caused by **ovine herpesvirus 2 (OHV-2),** usually involves close contact of **carrier sheep** with susceptible ruminants. **In Africa,** and sometimes in wildlife outside Africa, the source of infection (named '**alcelaphine herpesvirus-1** or **AHV-1**) is the **wildebeest.**

Gross lesions of the CNS include congestion and cloudiness of the meninges. **Microscopically,** the lesion is a non-suppurative meningo-encephalomyelitis which may be associated with vasculitis. Lymphocytic perivascular cuffing and varying degrees of necrotizing vasculitis occur in all parts of the **brain** and sometimes in the spinal cord, usually involving the white matter. Other lesions in the CNS include neuronal degeneration, microgliosis, leptomeningitis, haemorrhage, choroiditis, necrosis of ependymal cells and ganglioneuritis.

Infectious Bovine Rhinotracheitis Virus-Induced Encephalitis in Cattle

Infectious bovine rhinotracheitis, caused by **bovine herpesvirus type 1 (BHV-1),** is best known as an **infection of the respiratory tract of cattle.** **Lesions** involve eyes (conjunctivitis), and tissues of the reproductive, alimentary, integumentary, and nervous systems. Although BHV-1 sometimes causes a non-suppurative meningo-encephalitis mainly in **young cattle, two** recently isolated **variants of BHV-1** have a particular tropism for the CNS and cause outbreaks of disease in **young cattle.** Infection of the respiratory and genital tracts (with abortion) can also occur.

Gross lesions are non-specific and include meningeal congestion and petechiation of the brain. **Microscopic lesions** consist of non-suppurative meningo-encephalitis. Other changes include vasculitis, focal malacia, neuronal degeneration, and presence of **intranuclear inclusions in neurons and astrocytes.**

Enterovirus-Induced Porcine Polioencephalomyelitis

Several diseases of **pigs,** such as Teschen disease, Talfan disease and others, caused by **porcine enteroviruses,** are characterized by **polioencephalomyelitis** (inflammation of the grey matter of brain and spinal cord). As stated, **Teschen disease** is caused by porcine enterovirus (serotypes 2 and 3). **Clinical signs in** different diseases vary in severity from death of affected animals **(Teschen disease)** to less severe disease with signs of fever, diarrhoea, and paralysis (most severe in the hind legs) in **pigs.**

No gross lesions are detectable. All forms of the disease are **characterized microscopically** by non-suppurative polioencephalomyelitis. The sequence of changes in neurons includes acute swelling, central chromatolysis, necrosis, neuronophagia, and axonal degeneration.

Natural infection occurs by the oral route and is followed by viral localization and replication in the tonsil and infected tract (mainly ileum, large intestine, and mesenteric lymph nodes). Following replication in the intestine, virus travels haematogenously to the brain and spreads into the parenchyma.

Haemagglutinating Encephalomyelitis Viral Infection of Pigs

This is a **disease of nursing pigs** characterized by high morbidity, vomiting, anorexia, constipation, and severe progressive emaciation. The aetiological agent is a **coronavirus.**

Gross lesions include cachexia and enlargement of the abdomen caused by gaseous distension of the stomach and intestines. **Microscopic lesions** occur in the respiratory tract, stomach, and central and peripheral nervous systems. Lesions in the CNS, which are most pronounced in the grey matter are characterized by a non-suppurative meningo-encephalomyelitis and neuronal degeneration.

Infection by the oro-nasal route is followed by replication of the virus in epithelial cells of the nasal mucosa, tonsils, lungs, and small intestine. After local replication, the virus spreads to the CNS by the peripheral nerves to the spinal cord. Viral antigen is restricted to the cytoplasm of neurons. The **vomiting** associated with the disease results from altered function of neurons (gastric intramural plexuses) secondary to viral infection.

Borna Disease

Borna disease, an **equine disease**, named after Borna, a town in Germany, is an **encephalomyelitis** caused by **an unusual enveloped RNA virus** that replicates in the nucleus and has no cytopathic effect. Borna virus has been classified as the first type of a new virus family, Bornaviridae.

The natural infection has a broad host range and has been reported to occur most frequently in **horses** and **sheep**, but also occurs in **cattle, goats, cats, dogs,** rodents, rabbit, deer, llamas, hippopotamus, ostriches, **monkeys,** and **human beings.** Borna disease has a long incubation period from weeks to several months.

Borna disease virus infection in **horses** was originally thought to result in a high mortality, 80% to 100%. More recent evidence indicates that most of the infected animals are either asymptomatic or have mild clinical disease associated with behavioural changes, and is followed by recovery.

There are no important gross lesions. Microscopic lesions, which are limited to the nervous system, consist of a non-suppurative encephalomyelitis and neuronal degeneration. **Lesions** are mostly confined to the grey matter, although white matter can be affected. **Marked inflammation also occurs in the hippocampus.** Inflammation of the meninges and spinal cord is usually mild. Small, round to oval, **eosinophilic intranuclear inclusions** occur in neurons of the brain, hippocampus, and cerebrospinal ganglia.

Borna disease virus is highly neurotropic, similar to the rabies virus, and is transported to the CNS from the periphery intra-axonally. Non-neuronal infection of **astrocytes,** oligodendroglia, ependyma, choroid plexus epithelial cells and Schwann cells occurs and contributes to virus replication (e.g., astrocytes and Schwann cells). After reaching the CNS, virus spreads intra-axonally and trans-synaptically as described for rabies virus. The specific lesions that develop in the CNS appear to depend on a **viral-induced cell-mediated immune mechanism.** Antibody to Borna disease does not appear to play any significant role in the disease process.

Equine Encephalomyelitis

Infection of horses with Eastern, Western, or Venezuelan equine encephalomyelitis (EEE, WEE, VEE) viruses **produces a range of clinical disease.** The viruses are members of the genus **Alphavirus. Besides horses,** Eastern encephalomyelitis has also been reported in **cattle** and **pigs.**

Lesions of the CNS caused by all three viruses are similar, but there are some differences. **Gross lesions** include cerebral hyperaemia, oedema, petechiation, focal necrosis, and leptomeningeal oedema. **Microscopic lesions** are most important in the grey matter of the brain and spinal cord and are characterized by perivascular cuffing (with lymphocytes, macrophages, and neutrophils), neutrophilic infiltration of the grey matter parenchyma, microgliosis, neuronal degeneration, focal parenchymal (cortical) necrosis, perivascular oedema and haemorrhage, necrotizing vasculitis, thrombosis, and leptomeningitis.

Following infection (by mosquito), the circulating virus first infects several tissues haematogenously. These include bone marrow, lymphoreticular tissue, muscle, and connective tissue. In some tissues (e.g., lymphoid and myeloid [bone marrow]), there may be cellular depletion, necrosis, or both. A **second viraemia** results in haematogenous infection of the CNS. Viruses replicate in endothelial cells before entering the nervous system and infecting neurons, for which they have affinity. Viruses of this group (e.g., VEE virus) can be associated with changes in the metabolism of neurotransmitters of CNS which are responsible for certain clinical signs.

Japanese Encephalitis

Japanese encephalitis is an important disease in **human beings, but infection also occurs in animals (horses, pigs, cattle,** and **sheep).** The disease occurs in India. The causative virus is a **flavivirus** and is transmitted by mosquitoes, mainly, **Culex.** In nature, infection is maintained in a cycle involving vector mosquitoes, birds, and mammals (e. g., **pigs).**

Young pigs may have **signs,** but detectable illness is not seen in adult or pregnant pigs. However, foetal infection during pregnancy can result in mummification and **stillbirth of foetuses, or the birth of weak live pigs** with nervous signs accompanied by non-suppurative encephalitis and neuronal degeneration.

Outbreaks of meningo-encephalomyelitis in horses have been reported. **Young or immature horses are more susceptible** to infection than older animals. Lesions are limited to the nervous system. **Grossly,** they include leptomeningeal congestion, hyperaemia, and haemorrhage within brain and spinal cord. **Microscopic lesions** are characterized by an early leptomeningitis and encephalitis in which neutrophils predominate. This is followed by non-suppurative inflammation, neuronal degeneration, focal haemorrhage, and focal necrosis. **Neurons are the target cell.**

The lesions are distributed diffusely throughout the nervous system but affect the grey matter more than the white matter.

Louping Ill

Louping ill is tick-transmitted **sheep encephalomyelitis. It is mainly a disease of sheep** but also affects **cattle, horses, pigs, goats, dogs, deer,** and **human beings**. It is caused by a **flavivirus**. The disease occurs in British Isles and Norway.

No significant gross lesions are present. Microscopic lesions are characterized by a meningo-encephalomyelitis which is mainly non-suppurative, although neutrophils can be present. The most consistent and pronounced lesions are inflammation and degeneration of Purkinje cells. They occur in the cerebellar cortex and are partially responsible for **clinical signs (peculiar leaping gait)** shown by affected ataxic animals. Prominent lesions also occur in the medulla oblongata and spinal cord. No inflammation of spinal ganglia occurs, but inflammation has been detected in peripheral (e.g., sciatic) nerves.

Following infection by the tick *Ixodes ricinus*, the virus replicates in the lymphoid tissues (e.g., lymph nodes and spleen) resulting in the development of **viraemia**. Infection of the CNS (mainly of neurons) occurs haematogenously. Excretion of the **virus in milk of infected ewes** and **goats** has been reported. It has been suggested that transmission by ingestion may be important in sucking kids.

Swine Fever (Hog Cholera)

This disease of **pigs** is caused by a **pestivirus. Lesions of the acute disease**, which occur due to tropism of the virus for vascular endothelium with subsequent haemorrhage, are present in many organs. These include kidneys, intestinal serosa, lymph nodes, spleen, liver, bone marrow, lungs, skin, heart, stomach, gallbladder, and CNS. **Microscopic lesions** of CNS are characterized by swelling, proliferation, and necrosis of endothelium; microgliosis; neuronal degeneration; choroiditis; and leptomeningitis. **Lesions occur in both grey and white matter** and are most prominent in the **brain stem** (medulla oblongata, pons) and thalamus but also occur in the cerebrum, cerebellum, and spinal cord.

Infection under natural conditions occurs by oro-nasal route. The virus initially infects epithelial cells of the tonsillar crypts and surrounding lymphoid tissue, and then spreads to draining lymph nodes where it replicates. The spread continues through the circulation (in association with mononuclear cells, e.g., lymphocytes) to the spleen, bone marrow, visceral lymph nodes, and lymphoid tissue of the intestinal tract, where high titres are reached. Target cells for virus replication include endothelial cells, lymphoid cells and macrophages, and epithelial cells. Haematogenous spread of the virus throughout the infected pig (including the CNS) is usually completed in 5 to 6 days.

Feline Infectious Peritonitis

Feline infectious peritonitis (FIP) of cats is caused by a **coronavirus**. It is mainly a disease of the **domestic cats**, although wild felidae can be affected. It usually occurs sporadically in cats of all ages, but is more common in younger cats, and is **clinically important** because it can result in **death**. The **disease occurs in two forms**: (1) **effusive (wet)** or (2) **non-effusive (dry)**.

The **basic lesion in both forms** is a **pyogranulomatous inflammation**. Initially, there is vasculitis followed by vascular necrosis and infarction. The **effusive form** is characterized by serositis, accumulation of fluid in the abdominal and thoracic cavities, and inflammation of visceral tissue. **Lesions** of the **non-effusive form** include leptomeningitis, focal encephalomyelitis and ophthalmitis. However, involvement of other tissues, such as kidneys, hepatic and mesenteric lymph nodes, and less commonly serosa and other abdominal organs, can occur.

There are **two feline coronaviruses: feline enteric coronavirus (FECV)** and **feline infectious peritonitis virus (FIPV)** which cause FECV and FIP infections, respectively. The viruses for each infection are antigenically and morphologically indistinguishable. Currently they are considered to represent avirulent (FECV) and virulent (FIPV) strains of the same basic feline coronavirus. Following ingestion, FECV infects and replicates in small intestinal epithelium **and usually is an unimportant infection.**

The **FIP virus (FIPV) enters into the cat mainly by ingestion** following faecal contamination. However, transmission by direct inoculation (cat bites, licking open wounds, etc.) and rarely in utero have been reported. Following infection, virus replicates in macrophages which spread the virus to other tissues of the body (e.g., liver, visceral peritoneum and pleura, and meninges and ependyma of the brain and spinal cord).

Following spread of the virus in the body, the development of the disease depends on the type and degree of immunity that develops. If there is development of strong cell-mediated immunity, virus is contained, with resistance to the disease. **Humoral immunity by itself is not protective.** On the other hand, can actually increase development of the disease (the effusive form of FIP) by **two mechanisms:** The **first** involves development of **virus-antibody-complement complexes** which particularly accumulate in the same areas as infected macrophages (around small blood vessels), resulting in inflammation and vascular injury accompanied by effusion of large amounts of fluid. The **second mechanism** involves a process called antibody-dependent enhancement (shown experimentally) which involves uptake of **virus-antibody-complement complexes** by macrophages followed by significant viral replication. The heavily infected macrophages, with frequent perivascular location, release **cytokines** that cause **vascular damage** which leads to leakage of significant amounts of fluid.

Non-effusive FIP is thought to occur when partial cell-mediated immunity develops and represents **an intermediate stage between non-protective humoral immunity alone and protective cellular immunity.**

Prion Infections

'Prions' are the most recent addition to the class of infectious agents causing diseases in domestic animals and humans. **Prion is a proteinaceous infective particle.** Recent work has revealed that prion is a heavily glycosylated specific protein (a polypeptide) of 30 kilodaltons (30-kD), called **'prion protein (PrP)'. Prions lack nucleic acid (RNA or DNA),** and also do not produce any inflammatory or immune reaction in the host. Unlike conventional viruses, prions are unusually resistant to many chemical agents, including formalin, chloroform and ether, also to heat, ultraviolet and ionizing radiation, ultrasonication, proteases and nucleases. For his discovery of prions, in 1997, Dr. Stanley Prusiner, Professor of Biochemistry at the University of California, San Francisco was awarded the Nobel Prize for Medicine. The diseases caused by prions are called **'prion diseases'.** Both, in domestic animals and humans, prions cause a group of diseases known as **'transmissible spongiform encephalopathies (TSEs)".**

Transmissible Spongiform Encephalopathies (TSEs)

These diseases are so named because they are all characterized microscopically by a spongiform change in the grey matter of brain (encephalopathy), and are caused by transmissible agents (**prions**). The **spongiform change** is characterized by the development of vacuoles or empty spaces (**vacuolation**) both in the neurons and the neuropil (i.e., complex network of the cytoplasmic processes of neurons and neuroglia in the grey matter). Thus, transmissible spongiform encephalopathies are **'prion diseases'** that constitute a distinct group of neurodegenerative disorders.

Scrapie is the original and **typical example of 'transmissible spongiform encephalopathies (TSEs)'.** The group initially included the animal diseases **scrapie, transmissible mink encephalopathy** (scrapie infection of mink), **transmissible feline encephalopathy,** and **chronic wasting disease** of mule deer and elk. **Human diseases** have included **kuru** (associated with cannibalism), **Creutzfeldt-Jacob disease,** and Gerstmann-Sträussler-Scheinker syndrome. **More recent additions** to this group include **a variant form of Creutzfeldt-Jacob disease and fatal familial insomnia in human beings** and bovine spongiform encephalopathy (BSE).

Since prion diseases are the most recent additions to the list of diseases occurring in domestic animals, the two most important, namely, **scrapie and bovine spongiform encephalopathy, are discussed at some length.**

Scrapie

Scrapie is the oldest of prion diseases. It is best known as **a degenerative disease** that **affects the CNS of sheep** and was recognized in Great Britain (in 1732) and other countries of Western Europe more than 250 years ago. Although scrapie is best known as a disease of **sheep**, it also occurs in **goats**. The name is derived from almost continuous **scraping** (rubbing) of the skin against any stationary objects because of intense pruritus (severe itching) the animal suffers, which often results in loss of wool in sheep. **Scrapie is the most intensely studied prion disease.**

Incubation period

The incubation period **is long (2 years or more),** restricting the clinical disease to **adult sheep.**

Aetiology

The current belief is that the agent is a proteinaceous infective particle **(prion)**. It is a heavily glycosylated specific protein (a polypeptide) of 30 kilodaltons called '**prion protein (PrP)**'. Prions contain no nucleic acid (RNA or DNA), and also do not produce any inflammatory or immune reaction in the host. Immune B-cell and T-cell functions are intact.

Transmission

The principal means of **transmission is from infected ewes to their lambs** early in life. The placenta is infectious. Thus, prenatal transmission may also be important. Owing to the resistance of prions to physical and chemical agents, environmental contamination probably persists for long periods.

Clinical Signs

The disease progresses relentlessly with **early signs** of changes in behaviour or temperament. The eyes have a wild and fixed expression. Pupils are dilated. The sheep may hold its head down and move it rapidly from side to side or up and down. Its movements are aimless. The animal usually grinds its teeth. This is followed by scratching, **scraping**, and rubbing against fixed objects because of pruritus. Incoordination may be followed by paralysis and inability to stand. Other signs include weight loss (despite retention of appetite), biting of the feet and limbs, lip smacking (i.e., to close and open lips noisily in rapid succession), gait abnormalities, trembling (when suddenly stressed), recumbency (lying down position), **and eventually death after 1 to 6 months or longer.**

Pathogenesis

Following oral infection at an early age, there is **an extremely long eclipse phase** (about one year) before the infectious agent can be detected in infected animals. At this time the agent occurs in low titres in the tonsil, supra-pharyngeal (medial retro-pharyngeal) lymph node, and lymphoid tissue of the intestine. Infection then spreads to regional lymph nodes and eventually to other lymph nodes and the spleen. Other extra-neural tissues are not significantly affected.

The agent continues to replicate in the extra-intestinal and intestinal lymphoid tissues for many months, **or even a year or more, before it reaches the CNS, which is the .target organ.** It has been suggested that CNS in sheep is infected by haematogenous spread. However, **axonal spread** has been suggested as a mechanism of spread. The infectious agent first appears in the CNS, initially in the medulla oblongata and diencephalons, **when infected sheep are clinically normal.** It then spreads to other parts of the CNS and replicates to titres greater than those in non-neural tissues. Infection in non-neural tissues remains, where moderate titres persist until death of the animal. **Classical disease usually occurs when sheep are 3 to 4 years of age,** when high concentrations of the agent are present in the CNS, especially in the diencephalons, brain stem, cerebellar cortex, spinal cord, and sometimes cerebral cortex. **The pathogenesis of the natural disease in goats is similar to that in sheep.**

Molecular Mechanisms of Pathogenesis

Molecular mechanisms in the pathogenesis of the disease involve conversion of **normal animal protein (PrP)** in the CNS, slowly and progressively, **to an abnormal form (PrP^{sc}) and this causes development of the disease.** The normal protein (PrP) occurs naturally in the brains of animals and humans. It is found predominantly on the outer surface of neurons, attached by a glycosylphosphatidyl inositol (GPI) anchor. Its function is not clearly understood, but in experimental models it appears to play a role in protecting cells and helping them respond to oxygen deficiency. Because they lack nucleic acid, prions cannot reproduce, but they replicate by stimulating normal cellular prion to fold into the abnormal form (PrP^{sc}). Normally, prions are harmless, but when they are misshapen, they produce disease.

Infectious prions are the modified form of a normal structural protein found in the mammalian nervous system. The **normal prion protein** is designated by the abbreviation PrP^c. It is a 30kD (kilodalton), membrane-associated protein encoded by a gene on chromosome 20. **However, function of normal prion protein remains unknown.**

Prion-associated diseases develop when PrP^c undergoes a conformational (structural) change to form a structurally abnormal protein known as PrP^{sc}. The 'sc' designation is derived from the sheep disease 'scrapie'. Once present, PrP^{sc} is capable of inducing other **normal PrP^c molecules** to undergo conformational change to the PrP^{sc} **form, resulting in the generation of extremely large numbers of abnormal molecules.** The polypeptide chains of PrP^c and PrP^{sc} are exactly similar in their chemical composition, **but differ in their three-dimensional conformations.** The infectious agent causing BSE is a conformational isomer of the normal host protein PrP^c. Both PrP isoforms are encoded by the same gene, exhibit the same amino acid sequence but differ in conformation. PrP^c is rich in alpha helices, whereas the **PrP^{sc} has much fewer alpha helices and many more beta sheets.** BSE can arise in animals that carry an allele which causes previously normal protein molecules to contort (twist or bend) by themselves from an alpha helical arrangement to a beta-pleated sheet, which is the disease-causing shape of the protein. **This structural change is the fundamental event in the pathogenesis of prion disease.**

All proteins are long molecules folded up into particular shapes. Proteins cannot perform their intended function until amino acids fold into a specific three-dimensional shape. The shape a particular protein assumes is determined by the sequence of its amino acids. Most proteins fold spontaneously. But some proteins do not fold as intended. **A prion protein is folded differently from the normal protein. In fact, it is misfolded. Moreover, they enter into the brain cells and force normal proteins to fold in the same abnormal way.** When this happens, the proteins, which are normally in the liquid form, begin to solidify within the brain cells. The abnormal prion accumulates in the cells of the nervous system, causing nervous symptoms and finally death. When the infected cells die, the defective prions are released into normal tissue and go on to infect more cells. Ultimately, large clusters of cells die, **leaving the brain filled with microscopic holes.** This is a prolonged process, and symptoms of the disease may not appear for years. **The process, by which the prion recruits normal prion protein (PrP^c) to convert it to the disease-causing form (PrP^{sc}), remains unknown.**

The normal prion protein consists of **a number of flexible coils called alpha helices.** In the abnormal form of the protein, **some of these helices are stretched out into flat structures called beta sheets.** The normal protein is broken down by cellular enzymes called **proteases**, but the abnormal protein shape is resistant to these enzymes. As a result, as prions replicate, they are not broken down by proteases **and accumulate in brain tissue. The accumulation of prions in the brain causes neuronal cells to die, and a type of protein called amyloid accumulates in plaques, or flat areas, and causes degeneration of brain tissue.** Recent research suggests prions disrupt the normal cell process of protein recycling. This causes a buildup of faulty proteins and death of the cell. **The destruction of neural cells (neurons) causes tiny holes in the brain tissue** and a sponge-like appearance under the microscope. This has given rise to the term **spongiform disease.**

Lesions

Grossly, sheep and **goats** have loss of body condition and skin lesions which occur from pruritus. Except an increase in cerebrospinal fluid, **no gross lesions of the nervous system are detectable.**

Microscopic lesions in **sheep** and **goats** are limited to the CNS and are usually present in the diencephalons, brain stem, and cerebellum (cortex and deep nuclei), with variable lesions in corpus striatum and spinal cord. Except for minor changes, the cerebral cortex is unaffected. **The characteristic lesions include** neuronal degeneration, astrocytosis, and variable **spongiosis. The spongiosis is characterized by prominent neuronal and neuropil vacuolation, usually affecting**

the grey matter (Fig. 41). The type of neuronal degeneration can vary and is usually characterized by shrinkage with increased basophilia and **cytoplasmic vacuolation** (Fig. 41), although other changes (e.g., central chromatolysis and ischaemic cell change) variably occur. Astrocytosis in affected areas of brain, including cerebellar cortex, can be severe. Pronounced hypertrophy and hyperplasia of astrocytes are characteristic of scrapie (Fig. 42A, B). Whether astrocytic reaction is a primary or secondary response has not been clarified. An abnormal protein **(prion amyloid protein)** first accumulates in **astroglial cells** in the brain during scrapie infection. It means that this cell is the primary site of replication. The spongiform change tends to affect the grey matter, and greater severity of this lesion has been associated with long incubation periods. The lesion when it occurs in the grey matter, results from dilation of neuronal processes. However, other causes including vacuolation of neuronal and astroglial perikarya (i.e., in their cell bodies), swelling of astrocytic processes, dilatation of the periaxonal space, and splitting of myelin sheaths have been reported. Another lesion that occurs variably in experimentally infected animals and **with other**

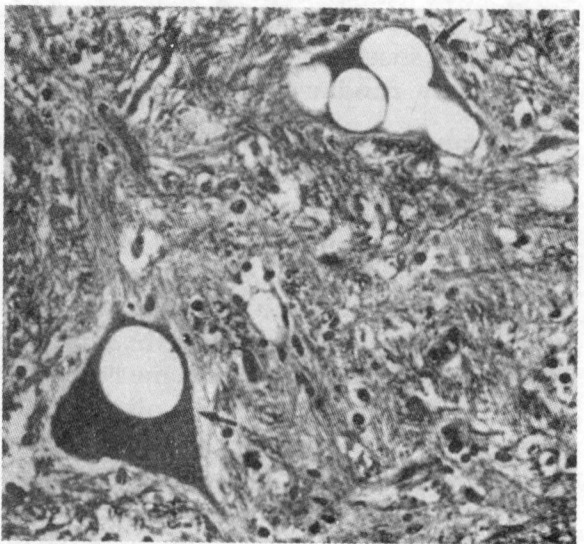

Fig. 41. Brain, medulla oblongata; cow. Bovine spongiform encephalopathy. There is prominent vacuolation of two neuronal cell bodies (arrows). H & E stain.

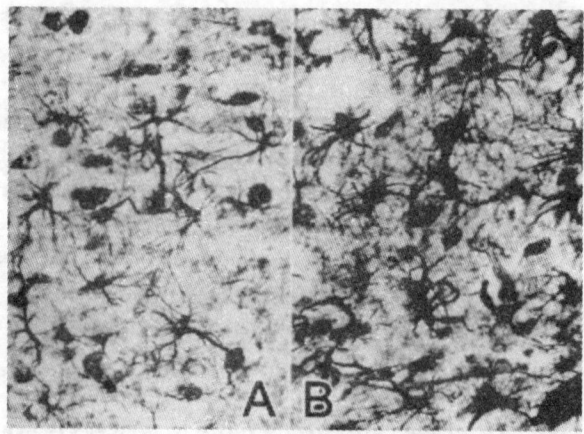

Fig. 42. Brain, medulla oblongata; mouse. A. Normal brain. Compare the size, shape and density of normal astrocytes with **B. Scrapie.** Pronounced hypertrophy and hyperplasia of astrocytes are characteristic of scrapie. Cajal's gold sublimate impregnation.

TSEs is **amyloid plaque formation. Cerebrovascular amyloidosis** also has been detected in scrapie-infected sheep. **Microscopic lesions similar to those of scrapie occur in the grey matter of the brain stem in cattle with BSE.**

Diagnosis

Diagnosis is made on the basis of clinical signs, and confirmed by microscopic examination of the brain and spinal cord. Specific diagnosis is now possible with antisera against purified prion protein, or scrapie-associated fibril protein, either on extracts of brain or on reaction with tissue. More recently, **immunohistochemistry** has been used to detect the infectious agent.

Bovine Spongiform Encephalopathy

Bovine spongiform encephalopathy (BSE) is a degenerative disease of the central nervous system (CNS) in cattle, which is **always fatal**. Commonly known as **'mad cow disease'**, BSE is a recent edition to the group of diseases, described earlier, as **'transmissible spongiform encephalopathies (TSE)'.**

Bovine spongiform encephalopathy was originally identified and confirmed as a prion disease in British diary herds in November 1986, but probably existed there as early as April 1985. **This disease was subsequently confirmed in cattle** in Northern Ireland, in the Channel Isles, Isle of Man, the Republic of Ireland, Belgium, France, Luxembourg, The Netherlands, Portugal, and Switzerland. **BSE has also been detected in cattle imported from the United Kingdom to** Canada, Denmark, Falkland Islands, Germany, Italy, and Oman. The bovine agent has also experimentally produced disease in **pigs**, but only following the use of highly infectious inoculum given simultaneously by multiple routes. Also, **a BSE-like encephalopathy** has been identified in Great Britain in the **domestic cat (feline spongiform encephalopathy)** and **several zoo ruminants. In naturally infected cattle,** the BSE agent (prion) has been identified in the brain, spinal cord, retina, lymphoid tissue, bone marrow, and trigeminal and dorsal root ganglia of **experimentally infected calves.**

Epidemiology

In the early 1980s, in Britain, there was an increase in the use of protein derived from ruminants, as a cheaper source of protein for cattle feed. This was done following an increase in the world prices of protein supplements, such as fish meal and soyabeans. The epidemiological evidence strongly indicates that disease was caused initially, during the early 1980s, by the **feeding of rations containing sheep meat-and-bone meal (MBM) supplements to cattle, contaminated with the scrapie agent (a prion).** This abnormal protein (prion) **can withstand extremely high temperatures** and does not get destroyed during the rendering (treatment) procedure. **Prions are not destroyed at 135° C for 18 minutes and resist treatment at 600° C dry heat.** It appears this happened because of a change from high temperature rendering (treatment) of sheep carcass material to low temperature continuous rendering. This changed process, introduced in the 1980s, **appears to have been less efficient in inactivating the scrapie agent.** When meat-and-bone meals processed in this manner were fed to cattle as part of their concentrate ration, **the agent got introduced into cattle.** The epidemic then became amplified by the subsequent recycling through meat-and-bone meal of infected cattle within the cattle population. Cases of BSE have occurred in a number of other countries as a result of the export of infected cattle or infected MBM from Great Britain.

So far no case of BSE has been reported in India. However, in view of the safety of our dairy herds and the human health significance of BSE, the disease requires constant monitoring and surveillance, since one introduced, it would be an extremely difficult task to get rid of it.

Transmission

BSE is not contagious by direct contact. **It is transmissible orally** and parenterally.

Pathogenesis

Resistance of prion infectivity to protease digestion allows a significant proportion of the infectious agent to survive passage through the digestive tract. It is not clear how prions pass through the intestinal mucosa. It is believed that, after oral uptake, prions may penetrate the intestinal mucosa through **M cells** (which are portals of entry for antigens and pathogens) and reach **Peyer's patches** as well as the **enteric nervous system**. Depending on the host, other lymphoreticular tissues, in particular the spleen, but not lymph nodes, are sites in which prions replicate and accumulate. This is the case in sheep scrapie, **but not BSE in cattle.** From the lymphoreticular system and possibly from other sites, **prions proceed along the peripheral nervous system to finally reach the brain**, either directly via the vagus nerve or via the spinal cord, under involvement of the sympathetic nervous system.

Molecular Mechanisms of Pathogenesis

For this, refer to **molecular mechanisms of pathogenesis**, discussed under scrapie.

Symptoms

As already stated, **BSE has a very long incubation period** (about 4-5 years), and has an insidious onset. That is, it develops so gradually as to be well established before becoming apparent. The disease advances mercilessly, and there is an invariable progression to death within weeks or months (usually six months). **Clinical signs** include behavioural, gait, and postural abnormalities which usually begin with apprehension, anxiety, and fear. That is, the affected cattle show a variety of nervous signs, mainly changes in behaviour, abnormalities in posture and gait, and extreme sensitivity to sound and touch (hyperaesthesia). **Following the onset of clinical signs, affected cattle lose weight until they die**, or require euthanasia. **This period ranges from 2 weeks to 6 months.** Slaughter of the affected animals becomes necessary because of their unmanageable behaviour, traumatic damage as a result of repeated falling and prolonged recumbency. It is because of this peculiar and uncontrollable behaviour of the affected cow that the disease has been termed **'mad cow disease'**. All cases of the disease in cattle have occurred in **adult animals**, with an age group of 3 to 11 years, but most animals develop clinical signs between 3 and 5 years of age.

Histopathological Findings

There are no gross postmortem changes.

BSE was initially diagnosed in 1986 by **histopathological examination of section of brain.** The characteristic changes comprise discrete ovoid and spherical vacuoles, or microcavities in the neuropil (see Fig. 41 under 'scrapie'). This **spongiosis** (i.e. neuropil vacuolation) is a predominant form of vacuolar change observed, and **is a feature of TSEs.** Subsequently **it was established that the pathognomonic vacuolar changes are consistently present in the brain stem facilitating routine diagnosis of the disease.** Neuronal perikarya and neurites (axons) of certain brain stem nuclei contain **large well-defined intracytoplasmic vacuoles** (Fig 41). These are single or multiple, and sometimes distend the soma to produce ballooned neurons with a narrow rim of cytoplasm. The contents of vacuoles, both in the neuropil and in neurons remain unstained and clear, after histological staining for glycogen in paraffin and for lipids in fixed cryostat sections. A mild gliosis sometimes accompanies the degenerative changes. The changes described in the brains of cattle affected with BSE are clearly pathological, and distinguishable from single large intracytoplasmic vacuoles recognized in healthy cattle. Also now established as an additional diagnostic criterion for the spongiform encephalopathies is the detection by electron microscopy in extracts of affected brain of abnormal fibrils called **'scrapie-associated fibrils'.**

Diagnosis

At present, there is no reliable test to detect the disease in live animals. Diagnosis is based on clinical signs, and confirmed by **characteristic pathological changes found in the brain of affected animals and also by several other tests.** There are no gross postmortem changes. The current diagnostic tests include:

1. **Histopathological examination**: Traditionally, confirmation of BSE is by conventional light microscopy of stained tissue sections. This is the primary laboratory method used to confirm a diagnosis of BSE. The changes in the brain (grey matter) include identification of spongiosis (vacuolation), gliosis, and neuron loss without inflammatory lesions. Preferably whole brain may be taken as soon as possible after death.

2. **Electron microscopic examination**: Examination by transmission electron microscopy for the presence of abnormal disease-specific brain fibrils (**scrapie-associated fibrils, SAFs**). Fresh cervical spinal cord or caudal medulla (3 g) may be taken frozen as soon as possible after death.

3. **Immunohistochemistry:** This is used to detect the disease agent. Because of its sensitivity, **immunohistochemistry of abnormal prion protein (PrP^{sc}) is of great help in the diagnosis.** Immunohistochemical methods are used to identify specific prion protein (PrP) peptide sequences in specific cell types of the brain. However, it requires formalin-fixed material. If this is not available, PrP^{sc} can be detected histochemically in fixed brain samples that may have been previously frozen and used for Western blotting analysis. This is because, **despite damage to the histological structures, PrP^{sc} is still detectable in the fixed-frozen brain sections.**

4. **Western immunoblotting:** This is also used to detect the disease agent. **Western immunoblotting technique** detects bovine disease-specific protease-resistant prion protein (PrP^{sc}) in bovine brain tissue samples.

5. **Serological Tests:** The absence of detectable immune responses in BSE prevents serological tests.

To conclude, currently the only reliable test is histopathological examination of tissues during postmortem examination.

Control

There is at present no specific evidence to suggest BSE is transmitted by contact between cattle, or from mother to offspring. Artificial insemination and embryo transfer do not seem to transmit the BSE agent. Since there is no treatment, control measures should include immediate destruction of affected animals and **ban on the feeding of ruminant tissues to livestock.** Carcasses and all parts from affected cattle must be destroyed.

Other measures include pathological surveillance to occurrence of clinical neurological disease, and safeguards on importation of live ruminant species and their products. There must be **total ban on the importation of live ruminants, and ruminant products, such as meat-and-bone meal, bovine serum,** and embryos from the UK and Europe. Also, government must exercise strict controls on recycling of mammalian protein and on effective identification and tracing of cattle.

In addition, a fairly large number of veterinarians should be trained throughout the country in the diagnosis and recognition of BSE.

Chlamydial Infections

Sporadic Bovine Encephalomyelitis

Chlamydia psittaci and *Chlamydia pecorum* are the two species that cause disease in **domestic animals.** Sporadic bovine encephalomyelitis is uncommon and caused by as yet unclassified chlamydial organism. **Calves** younger than 6 to 12 months of age are most susceptible.

Lesions are serofibrinous polyserositis, arthritis, tenosynovitis, and non-suppurative meningo-encephalitis. **Gross changes** in the CNS, when present, are congestion and oedema of the leptomeninges. **Microscopic lesions** consist of leptomeningeal and perivascular infiltrates of lymphocytes, plasma cells, and a few neutrophils. Leukocytes extend into the adventitia of blood vessels accompanied by endothelial swelling and vasculitis. Other lesions include neuronal and parenchymal necrosis and microgliosis.

Protozoal Infections

Protozoal infections with involvement of CNS occur in a wide variety of animals. **Lesions are similar** and **diagnosis** of infections based on the light microscopic morphology of the different organisms is difficult.

Sarcocystosis

Equine Protozoal Encephalomyelitis

This is caused by *Sarcocystis neurona*. **Clinical infection occurs in horses. Lesions** occur throughout the neuraxis (i.e., CNS), but the spinal cord, particularly the cervical and lumbar intumescences (swellings), are particularly affected. When **gross lesions** are present, they consist of necrotic foci, often with haemorrhage. **Microscopic lesions** include necrosis, axonal swelling, haemorrhage, and accumulation of lymphocytes, macrophages, neutrophils, eosinophils, and a few multinucleated giant cells in perivascular areas and neuropil, or less commonly in leptomeninges. Gemistocytic astrocytosis can be prominent.

In lesions, *S. neurona* is small and crescent-shaped to round, has a well-defined nucleus, and is usually arranged in aggregates. **Organisms can be difficult to detect and occur intracellularly or extracellularly.** The sequence of events in the pathogenesis of the characteristic lesion is: (1) focal parasitic aggregation and replication, (2) inflammation, (3) axonal damage, (4) axonal transection (transverse cut), (5) axonal swelling and degeneration, and (6) Wallerian degeneration

Toxoplasmosis

Toxoplasma gondii can infect a wide variety of animals **as intermediate hosts,** including fish, amphibians, reptiles, birds, **human beings,** and **many other mammals. New World monkeys** (i.e. of western hemisphere) are the **most susceptible,** whereas **Old World monkeys** (of eastern hemisphere), **rats, cattle, and horses are highly resistant. Cats serve both as definitive and intermediate hosts.**

T. gondii **can parasitize a wide variety of cell types in the intermediate hosts** and can cause **lesions** in such tissues as lungs, lymphoid system, liver, heart, skeletal muscle, pancreas, intestine, eyes, and nervous system. **In the CNS, gross lesions** include haemorrhage, haemorrhagic infarcts, ventricular dilation, and oedema of sufficient severity to cause brain displacement and herniation. Early **microscopic** vascular degeneration and oedema are followed by invasion of organisms into the parenchyma with tissue necrosis, and haemorrhage. Perivascular cuffing with mainly mononuclear leukocytes, astrogliosis, and microgliosis; cellular necrosis involving neurons, astrocytes, and oligodendroglia; and leptomeningitis are the other lesions of the disease. **Lesions can involve any area of the neuraxis with predilection for grey or white matter, and radiculitis (inflammation of the spinal nerve roots) can occur.**

Following ingestion, bradyzoites from tissue cysts or sporozoites from oocysts enter interstitial epithelium and multiply. There is active penetration of plasma membranes by organism-secreted lytic products allowing entry into the cell, rather than their uptake by phagocytosis. *T. gondii* then spreads locally, free in lymph or intracellularly in lymphocytes, macrophages, or granulocytes to Peyer's patches, and regional lymph nodes. **Intracellularly organisms multiply** as tachyzoites within a parasitophorus vacuole by repeated cycles of endodyogeny during the early acute stages of infection. Spread to distant organs is through lymph and blood, either as free organisms or intracellularly in lymphocytes, macrophages, or granulocytes. With time, and an increasing antibody response by the host, tachyzoites of *T. gondii* transform into slow-growing bradyzoites that replicate into tissue cysts.

Infection of the CNS occurs haematogenously. Neurons and **astrocytes** are the final target cells. The sequence of events in the **pathogenesis of the characteristic lesions** is similar to that in *S. neurona* infection (see previous section). **In utero infections** in animals and human beings can result in CNS infection. The incidence in sheep foetuses approaches 90%. **In foetal brains,** foci of necrosis are common in the brain stem and are associated with a glial cell response. Also foci of necrosis and mineralization (calcification) occur in cerebro-cortical white matter and are due to foetal hypoxia and ischaemia or hypotension. In older more mature animals, *T. gondii* are associated with immunosuppression such as occurs in concurrent canine distemper virus infection and toxoplasmosis.

Immune-mediated mechanisms are involved in causing vascular injury (type III hypersensitivity) and cellular or tissue necrosis (type IV hypersensitivity). Lysis of infected cells by cytotoxic (CD8+ T-lymphocytes) also could contribute to the tissue damage. **The organism does not produce a cytotoxin.**

Neosporosis

Disease caused by *Neospora caninum* or a **Neospora**-like coccidian occurs in a variety of animals including **dog, cat, cattle, sheep,** and **horse** as well as laboratory rodents. First described as a multisystem infection in the **dog,** the organism has an affinity for the nervous system. The dog is the **definitive host** for the organism but other hosts may exist. The organism has some features similar to *Toxoplasma gondii,* including division of tachyzoites by endodyogeny and having both proliferative (tachyzoites) and tissue cyst phases. However, *N. caninum* does not develop within a parasitophorous vacuole as does *T. gondii.*

Neurological disease is divided into two categories: that occurring **during postnatal life** and that associated with **mid-to late-term abortions.** Postnatal syndromes have been observed in **young and adult dogs** but **horses** are also affected. **In young dogs, clinical signs** are ascending paralysis due to poly-radiculoneuritis (i.e. acute idiopathic polyneuritis) and polymyositis (inflammation of many muscles). **In adult dogs,** lesions are more of CNS involvement complicated by polymyositis, myocarditis, and dermatitis. **In horses,** clinical signs resemble protozoal myelo-encephalitis (inflammation of the spinal cord and brain) caused by *Sarcocystis neurona.* **Lesions in horses** include meningo-encephalomyelitis, vasculitis and necrosis with microgliosis, and perivascular cuffing by macrophages, lymphocytes, plasma cells, or neutrophils. Necrosis can be marked with axons containing swellings located at the periphery of the lesion. Organisms are usually identified in the lesions with routine stains, but immunohistochemistry facilitates their detection and identification. The infection is systemic and lesions can occur in several other tissues.

Abortions due to congenital infections with *N. caninum* or **Neospora**-like organisms occur usually only in **cattle. Dairy herds are most frequently affected.** Cases have been reported in **horses. Abortions** can be mid-gestational to late term. Lesions include placentitis, myocarditis, myositis, and multiple foci of necrosis in the CNS with peripheral gliosis. An infiltration of leukocytes occurs throughout the neuraxis but usually in the brain stem.

Bacterial Infections

Bacterial infections of the CNS in domestic animals are rare. Infection can be haematogenous or occur from penetrating injuries or fractures that disrupt the natural defences provided by the meninges and osseous tissues. Bacteria can also spread from foci of infection in adjacent tissues such as the nasal cavity or inner ear. With one infection, listeric encephalitis, there is evidence of spread through the axons of cranial nerves.

Listeria monocytogenes

Listeriosis is a bacterial infection which has a particular affinity to cause disease in the CNS, mainly in **domestic ruminants.** Infections in **human beings** also occur. **Listeriosis occurs in three forms:** (1) **meningo-encephalitis,** (2) **abortion,** and (3) **septicaemia.** Septicaemia usually develops in young animals from an in utero infection.

Gross lesions are usually absent but leptomeningeal opacity, foci of necrosis in the terminal brain stem, and cloudy CSF have been noted. **Microscopically,** a meningo-encephalitis around the pons and medulla and involving both grey and

377

white matter is characteristic. Small early parenchymal lesions consist of loose clusters of microglia which, with time, enlarge and contain neutrophils. Gradually neutrophils dominate, but in some foci macrophages are the main cell type. Necrosis and accumulation of gitter cells can be prominent in some cases. **Numerous Gram-positive bacilli can be detected in some lesions.** Other changes include neuronal necrosis and leptomeningitis. Leptomeningitis is regularly present and is usually severe with accumulation of macrophages, lymphocytes, plasma cells, and some neutrophils.

L. monocytogenes invades through the mucosa of the oral cavity and into the branches of the trigeminal nerve. Intra-axonal migration to the trigeminal ganglion and brain (medulla) initiates central infection which spreads anteriorly and posteriorly. The **mechanism of tissue injury** is not completely understood. A correlation between the degree of cell-mediated immunity and severity of brain damage indicates **immunological injury**. The organism also produces a **haemolysin (listeriolysin)** which is a virulence factor required for intracellular multiplication.

Haemophilus somnus

H. somnus is a small Gram-negative bacillus and **causes a septicaemic infection in cattle.** It occurs in different clinical manifestations which include pneumonia, polyarthritis, myocarditis, abortion and meningo-encephalitis. The disease occurs in feedlot cattle (i.e., fattened for market) but can occur in other situations. All manifestations, particularly meningo-encephalitis are sporadic with single to many animals in a herd affected. The CNS form of the disease is called '**thrombotic meningo-encephalitis (TME)**'.

Gross lesions in the CNS are foci of haemorrhage and necrosis scattered randomly and seen both externally and on cut surfaces. Lesions are most common in the cerebrum, usually at the cortical-white matter junction (grey matter-white matter interface). Bacteria lodge, adhere, and replicate in these vessels. The spinal cord also has lesions.

Microscopic lesions in all organs including CNS are marked vasculitis and vascular necrosis which are followed by thrombosis and infarction. Colonies of small Gram-negative bacilli are common in thrombi, in and around affected vessels, and, in areas of necrosis.

Bacterial Infections of the CNS in Young Farm Animals

These infections involve *Escherichia coli,* **Stretococcus, Salmonella, Pasteurella,** and **Haemophilus.** In general, these organisms tend to produce fibrino-purulent inflammation of membranous tissues of the body (**neonatal septicaemia**). Leptomeninges, choroid plexus, and ependyma of the CNS, synovium, uvea, and the serosal lining of the body cavities can be affected. **Infections are usually acquired perinatally, and onset is usually within a few days of birth up to 2**

weeks. The route of entry can be oral, intrauterine, umbilical, following surgical procedures (e.g., castration, ear notching), or through the respiratory system.

Gross CNS lesions include congestion, haemorrhage, and diffuse to local cloudiness in the leptomeninges due to accumulation of exudate. **Microscopic lesions** vary according to the organism. With the exception of **Salmonella** sp., the lesions consist of fibrin deposition and an infiltration of mainly neutrophils in the leptomeninges, choroid plexus, and ependymal or sub-ependymal areas of the brain. The lesions can extend into the parenchyma. Vasculitis with thrombosis and haemorrhage can be associated with lesions caused by *Escherichia coli*. Lesions caused by **Salmonella** sp. are not limited to the perinatal period. CNS involvement is usually limited to **foals** and **pigs**. In contrast to the above infections, the leukocyte response has a greater proportion of macrophages and lymphocytes even to the extent the inflammation is termed histiocytic or granulomatous. As in other tissues, vasculitis, thrombosis, necrosis, and haemorrhage usually accompany **Salmonella** infections of the CNS.

Bacterial infection of CNS with visceral involvement occurs **in neonatal pigs.** Several strains of *Streptococcus suis* can cause disease. **Type 1 strains** cause disease in suckling pigs, whereas **type 2 strains** affect older pigs. **Type 2 strain** is the most important serotype. It causes **meningitis** not only in pigs but also in **human beings,** particularly those **working with pigs** or handling porcine tissues. The type of inflammation is fibrino-purulent, and necrotic foci can be found in brain stem (including cerebellum) and anterior spinal cord.

Haemophilus parasuis, **Glasser's disease**, is also a frequent cause of leptomeningitis, polyserositis, and polyarthritis in **pigs**. Again, lesions are fibrino-purulent inflammation and involve leptomeninges, serosal lining of body cavities, and joints.

Brain Abscesses

Cerebral abscesses in animals are usually associated with penetrating wounds including fractures, or spread of infection from adjacent tissues. **Abscesses** of the pituitary fossa occur in **cattle**. Bacteria isolated from the cases include *Pasteurella multocida* and *Actinomyces pyogenes*. The abscess can occur from spread of infection originating in the nasal cavity or sinuses, through direct extension or through the venous circulation. Infection can extend through the infundibular recess of the third ventricle in the ventricular system, resulting in **meningitis** and **empyema**. **Brain abscesses** can also originate in **cattle** and **sheep,** from an extension of otitis interna. These animals often show signs of facial nerve paralysis such as a drooping ear.

Brain abscesses are space-occupying lesions and as such have a very harmful effect on brain function. Depending on size and location, compression of vital structures and brain displacements are two common sequelae.

Mycotic Infections

Cryptococcosis

Cryptococcosis is caused by the fungus *Crytptococcus neoformans*. This infection causes disease which affects several organs, but **mainly CNS**, **nasal passages**, and **lungs**. Infection occurs through the respiratory route with haematogenous spread or direct spread to other tissues. **Two virulence factors** have been shown. **First**, a thick mucopolysaccharide capsule protects the organism from host defences. **Second**, virulent organisms possess a biochemical pathway. This pathway protects the organism from oxidative damage in the brain and presumably the adrenal glands. **Both virulence factors are important for survival of the organism in the host.**

Cryptococcosis with CNS infection occurs in cats, dogs, horses, and cattle. Grossly, the leptomeninges vary from normal to cloudy. **Multiple small cysts** with a gelatinous appearance can be seen in the parenchyma. **Microscopically**, these lesions contain numerous cryptococcal organisms with little or no inflammation.

Parasitic Infestations

Lesions occurring from parasitic infestation of the CNS vary in degree and distribution. **Gross lesions** of haemorrhage, malacia, migratory tracts, or space-occupying cysts occur with the various parasitic stages. **Microscopically**, there is necrosis, haemorrhage and a leukocytic response, with a significant infiltration of **eosinophils**.

Insect Larvae

Among the common larvae are those of *Oestrus ovis* and *Hypoderma bovis*. The larvae of *O. ovis* develop in the nasal cavity of **sheep** but can penetrate into the cranial vault through the ethmoid bone. Larvae of *H. bovis* can enter the spinal canal during their migration in **cattle** and rarely as an aberrant (wandering) parasite in the brain of **horses**. Damage in the CNS due to *H. bovis* in **cattle** is the result of inflammation directed at the degenerating parasites incidental with anthelmintic treatment.

Cestodes

Coenurus cerebralis, the larval form of the **dog** tapeworm *Multiceps multiceps*, usually infests **sheep** and sometimes **other ruminants**. The larval forms reach the CNS haematogenously causing some damage during migration and encysting, **forming space-occupying lesions. Human beings** are the definitive host of *Taenia solium*, **pigs** being the intermediate host. The larval stage, *Cysticercus cellulosae*, generally develops in muscle of the **pig** but can also occur in meninges and brain.

Nematodes

Nematodes cause damage in the brain either from aberrant (abnormal) migration in the definitive host or migration in an aberrant host (i.e., unnatural host). **Larval stages** of the parasite are involved, the exception being *Dirofilaria immitis* where the adult parasite is found. More damage is usually created by migration of the parasites in an aberrant host.

Several nematodes produce lesions in the CNS. **'Setariasis'** affects **goats, sheep**, and **horses**. In India, it is known as **'kumri'** (Hindi = weakness of the loin). The causal parasite is *Setaria digitata*. It affects the **natural hosts cattle** and **buffaloes**, and resides in the abdominal cavity without causing injury. Mosquitoes transmit the larvae. In **unnatural hosts**, such as **goat, sheep**, and **horse**, the parasite passes through the **nervous system**, where it produces lesions.

Larvae of **Strongylus** species (e.g., *Strongylus vulgaris*) can also rarely invade the CNS of the **horse**, and can be one of the common causes of **equine 'cerebrospinal nematodiasis'**.

Neoplasms

Neoplasms of the CNS in animals are not rare as was once believed. At least in the **dog**, neoplasms occur with a frequency and variety which is similar to that in human beings. **Most of the neoplasms described are in the dog and cat, mainly in the older population.** The more common or better-known neoplasms of the CNS in animals are presented.

Primary Neoplasms of Neuronal Cells

Medulloblastoma

This neoplasm has characteristics similar to the less commonly occurring **neuroblastoma**, both originate from cells of the neuronal lineage (common ancestor). However, the cell of origin of medulloblastoma has not been clearly identified, but it is thought that the neoplasm can arise from primitive cells originating in the neuro-epithelial roof of the fourth ventricle that give rise to the external granular cell layer.

In animals, medulloblastoma has been reported in **dogs** and **cattle**, in which young animals of both groups are affected. The neoplasm has also been described in the **cat** and **pig**. It mainly occurs in the **cerebellum of puppies** and **calves** and sometimes also in **adult dogs**. Neoplasm is well circumscribed, soft, grey to pink, and usually does not show haemorrhages, cysts, or necrosis. The growth compresses the fourth ventricle and can cause hydrocephalus. It may metastasize through the CSF in the ventricular and meningeal areas. **Microscopically**, the neoplasm is highly cellular and consists of round to elongated nuclei. The cells are arranged in sheets or broad bands. **Mitoses can be numerous.**

Primary Neoplasms of Neuroglial Cells

Neoplasms of the neuroglial cells are relatively more common in domestic animals and include:

1. Astrocytoma

Astrocytomas occur in **dogs, cats,** and **cattle,** but are **best known in the dog.** It is the **most common neuroglial neoplasm in dogs.** Dogs 5 to 11 years of age are usually affected. Common sites include pyriform lobe, convexity of the cerebral hemisphere, thalamus-hypothalamus, midbrain, cerebellum, and spinal cord.

Grossly, the affected area is enlarged with displacement of normal tissue. In less malignant forms, there is little demarcation between neoplastic and normal tissue. Such neoplasms are solid or firm and grey-white. More rapidly growing neoplasms are better demarcated from adjacent normal tissue and are soft and friable and contain areas of necrosis, haemorrhage, oedema and cavitation (formation of a pathological cavity). **Microscopically,** astrocytomas have been classified according to the degree of cytological malignancy from 1 to 4, or as differentiated or undifferentiated or anaplastic. The undifferentiated forms (grades 3 and 4) are also classified as **glioblastoma** or **glioblastoma multiforme.**

The **more differentiated neoplasms** consist of rather uniform cell type which has loose organization. Cell size varies and cells have distinct ramifying processes. Nuclei vary in size and shape. Cells are arranged around and along blood vessels. Astrocytes have been classified as fibrillary, protoplasmic, and gemistocytic based on cell morphology. **The fibrillary form is the most common.** Cellular pleomorphism can be extreme, and some neoplasms have **giant cells.**

2. Oligodendroglioma

Neoplasms composed of oligodendrocytes usually occur in the **dog,** but cases are also reported in **cats** and **cattle.** Oliogodendroglioma appears to be the most common neuro-ectodermal neoplasm. As with astrocytomas, there is a predilection for **dogs,** and the age range is as mentioned for astrocytomas. Neoplasms occur in all areas of the cerebrum, brainstem, and inter-ventricular septum.

Grossly, oligodendrogliomas are well demarcated from the surrounding tissue. The neoplsms vary in size, are grey to pink-red, and are soft or gelatinous with areas of haemorrhage. **Microscopically,** neoplasms are composed of densely packed cells. Nuclei are hyperchromic, and surrounded by pale or non-staining cytoplasm creating a perinuclear halo. Mitoses are usually uncommon. Degenerative changes include mucoid degeneration, oedema, cavitation, and rarely mineralization. Extensive necrosis is uncommon.

3. Ependymoma

Ependymoma is a less common neoplasm of **dogs, cats, cattle,** and **horses**. Ependymomas have continuity with the ventricular system and usually invade the lateral or, less commonly, third and fourth ventricles. They also occur in the central canal of the spinal cord. The neoplasm can spread within the ventricular system and subarachnoid space. Occurrence of neoplasm in a **cat** as young as 18 months old and in a **calf** 5 months old have been reported.

Grossly, the neoplasm is an invasive and destructive growth into adjacent tissue. It is soft and grey-white to red depending on blood content. Degenerative changes include gelatinous consistency and cavitation. **Microscopically**, ependymomas are highly cellular and well vascularized. Cells have hyperchromatic, round to oval nuclei with scant or undetectable cytoplasm. Cells are arranged in sheets and bands. Haemorrhage, mucinous and cystic degeneration, and capillary proliferation occur. Malignancy is indicated by invasive growth, frequent mitoses, and anaplasia.

Primary Neoplasms of the Choroid Plexus

Choroid Plexus Papilloma and Carcinoma

Choroid plexus papilloma occurs usually in the **dog** but has been reported in the **horse** and **cattle**. In the **dog,** neoplasm usually occurs in the fourth ventricle, but it can also be located in the third and lateral ventricles.

Grossly, the neoplasm is well-defined, expansive, granular to papillary growth which is grey-white to red and compresses the adjacent nervous tissue. Some neoplasms cause hydrocephalus. **Microscopically**, these neoplasms usually resemble choroid plexus and are characterized by an arborizing vascular connective tissue stroma which is covered by cuboidal to columnar epithelial layer. Mitoses are not present in the benign form. The malignant variety, **choroid plexus carcinoma**, is characterized by invasiveness, presence of mitoses, and tendency to spread to brain or spinal cord, or both. Metastasis can occur within the ventricular system, or into the subarachnoid space.

Primary Neoplasms of Mesodermal Tissue

Meningioma

Meningioma is the most common mesodermal neoplasm of the CNS of animals. It occurs usually in the **dog** and **cat** but has been reported in **horses, cattle,** and **sheep**. Most of the meningiomas in **dogs** occur between 7 and 14 years of age and in **cats** 10 years old or older. Sites of occurrence **in the dog** include basal area of the brain, over the convexity of the cerebral hemispheres, the lateral surface of the brain, and surface of the spinal cord. **In the cat,** neoplasm typically occurs in the tela choroidea of the third ventricle over the cerebral hemisphere, over the cerebellum, and rarely at the base of the brain. Occurrence in the meninges of the spinal cord is not common.

Grossly, neoplasms in the **dog** are single and vary in size. The neoplasms are well-defined, vary in shape (spherical, lobulated, or plaque-like), firm, encapsulated, and grey-white. They usually grow by expansion, causing pressure atrophy of the surrounding nervous tissue. They can be invasive, and sometimes there is hyperostosis (hypertrophy) of the overlying bone. **In the cat,** meningiomas vary in size from just detectable to 2 cm in diameter. **Cats,** and sometimes **cattle,** have more than one neoplasm. Other characteristics are similar to those described in the dog.

Microscopically, several patterns of neoplastic cells can occur. The more common pattern is characterized by the formation of nests, islands, or laminated whorls of cells. The cells have large cell bodies with abundant cytoplasm, and elongated, oval, open nuclei with peripherally located chromatin. The centre of whorls can be mineralized material referred to as **'psammoma bodies'.** Degenerative changes include haemorrhage and cavernous vascular formations. Invasive growth occurs but is less common than growth by expansion.

Secondary Neoplasms

Secondary neoplasms of the CNS can occur from growth of the adjacent bone, from direct extension of adjacent neoplasms through the bone or foramina (plural of 'foramen'), or by haematogenous metastasis.

Benign growths include **osteomas, chondromas,** and **osteochondromas,** which can cause compressive injury to the brain and spinal cord. One neoplasm (**multilobular osteoma**), also called **chondroma rodens,** originates from the periosteum of the canine skull. Also, malignant neoplasms near cranium or spinal cord can cause injury by direct invasion. Examples are extracranial **osteosarcoma** and **fibrosarcoma** in the **dog.** Also, **malignant melanoma** of the oral cavity (soft palate) in the **dog** and melanoma involving the paravertebral lymph nodes in the **horse** can invade adjacent CNS tissue. Other examples of direct extension include **lymphosarcoma** affecting the spinal cord in **cattle** (less frequently spinal cord or brain in the **dog and cat**), and carcinomas of the ethmoidal area and nasal cavity.

Neoplasms metastasizing haematogenously also occur and affect the brain more than the spinal cord. **Metastasis** has been most commonly reported in the **dog;** the next most frequent is the **cat.** Of the metastasizing carcinomas, the **mammary gland carcinoma** in the **dog** occurs most frequently, although others have been described. **Haemangiosarcoma** is one of the most common metastasizing sarcomas in the **dog;** others are the mesenchymal component of the **malignant mixed mammary gland tumour,** lymphosarcoma, fibrosarcoma, and malignant melanoma. **In the cat,** neoplasms that metastasize to the CNS include mammary gland carcinoma and lymphosarcoma.

The Peripheral Nervous System

The peripheral nervous system (PNS) is an extension of the CNS, conveying motor impulses from and returning sensory input to the CNS. This is achieved by cranial, peripheral, and autonomic nerves which leave CNS and innervate all tissues of the body.

Peripheral nerves consist of groups of axons, both myelinated and non-myelinated. Transport from the neuron cell body to the distal axon (**anterograde flow**) occurs at fast (400 mm per day) and slow (1 to 4 mm per day) rates. **Retrograde transport** from the distal axon to the cell body progresses at a rate of 200 mm per day.

Schwann cells surround both myelinated and non-myelinated axons and are responsible for formation of the myelin sheaths. Schwann cells are necessary for maintenance of axons and secrete neurotrophic factors that play a role in regeneration. **Axons** are grouped into fascicles (small bundles) along with surrounding tissue fibrils (**endoneurium**) and specialized endoneurial fibroblastic cells with phagocytic properties. Collagen bundles and modified fibroblastic cells called perineurial cells form the **perineurium** which ensheathes individual nerve fascicles. The fibrous **epineurium** is continuous with the dura mater and encloses groups of nerve fascicles.

Diseases of the Peripheral Nervous System

Many disorders affecting the CNS manifest themselves in lesions of the PNS. Despite this, however, **there are certain diseases that primarily affect the PNS.** Diseases of the PNS can show clinically as motor disturbance, sensory deprivation, or a combination of motor and sensory alterations.

Congenital Anomalies

Agenesis and Hypoplasia

These defects are uncommon in domestic animals. Colonic agangliosis or **lethal white foal syndrome** is a disorder involving development of the PNS. It is similar to Hirschsprug's disease in infants. **Affected foals die soon after birth** from functional blockage of the colon due to lack of innervation and normal gut motility. **Microscopically**, the myenteric (i.e. present in the muscular coat) and sub-mucosal autonomic ganglia are absent.

Traumatic Injury

Traumatic peripheral nerve injury is relatively uncommon in animals. It can result from lacerations, violent stretching and tearing, or compression or contusion. Reaction patterns following injury are similar to those in the CNS, **but peripheral nerves have a greater capacity for repair. Three patterns of lesions** have been described: (1) **Mild injury** which leaves axon intact (**neuropraxia**) can result in temporary conduction block but total recovery and function is possible. (2) **More severe damage** that destroys the axon but leaves the connective tissue framework intact (**axonotmesis**) results in Wallerian degeneration distal to the point of injury, but the potential for regeneration and re-innervation is good. (3) Severance (separation) of the nerve with destruction of the supporting framework (**neurotmesis**) results in Wallerian degeneration distal to the injury with the potential for regeneration **but little chance of normal re-innervation.** The pattern of Wallerian degeneration and the reaction of the neuronal cell body to damage of its axon have already been described (see 'neurons, reaction to injury').

Disorders of Myelin Formation and Maintenance

In contrast to the CNS, disorders of myelin formation are rare. Hypomyelination has been described in **dogs.** Clinical signs include a peculiar hopping gait and circular movement of the limbs while walking. Lesions in peripheral nerves include thin myelin sheaths and increased numbers of Schwann cells. **Congenital hypomyelination** has been described in **2-month old lamb** with tremors and incoordination.

In contrast to hypomyelination or disordered myelin formation, **demyelination in the PNS is common.** Myelin loss occurs following axonal degeneration, compressive lesions, is frequent in inflammatory disorders, and demyelination is the primary lesion in some neuropathies. **Schwann cells can proliferate to restore the myelin sheaths.**

Metabolic/Toxic Peripheral Neuropathies

A variety of metabolic disturbances can affect the PNS. These disturbances include inherited lysosomal enzyme deficiencies (see 'inborn errors of metabolism'), endocrine disorders, and certain vitamin deficiencies.

Of the endocrine disorders, hypothyroidism, hyperadrenocorticism, and diabetes mellitus can affect the PNS. **Nutritional neuropathies** are relatively uncommon and involve vitamin A and some of the B vitamins. **Vitamin A deficiency** results indirectly in peripheral neuropathy by affecting bone growth and remodelling. **Vitamin B deficiencies** are mainly diseases of **pigs** and **poultry. In pigs,** deficiency of pantothenic acid causes a sensory neuropathy with axonal degeneration, demyelination, and neuron loss in the dorsal root ganglia. **In poultry,** deficiency of riboflavin causes curled-toe paralysis, which is primarily a demyelinating neuropathy.

A number of toxins can affect the PNS, with or without changes in the CNS. The initial toxic effect can be at the level of the neuron cell body, axon, or myelin sheath.

Degenerative Neuropathies

These are the hereditary, familial, and breed or species-associated syndromes reported in a variety of **domestic animals** which result in degeneration of PNS neurons, or axons, or both. Examples include **primary sensory neuropathies, progressive axonopathy, giant axonal neuropathy,** and **dancing Doberman disease in dogs.**

Inflammatory Neuropathies

Inflammation of the PNS can occur from certain viral (e.g., herpesvirus and rabies), and protozoal infections of the CNS. **Polyradiculoneuritis** (inflammation of many peripheral nerves and dorsal, ventral, or both dorsal and ventral **spinal nerve rootlets),** and to some extent **ganglionitis** (inflammation of spinal ganglia), occur in **toxoplasmosis** and **neosporosis** (see 'protozoal infections in CNS section').

A **chronic polyradiculoneuritis** with **infiltrations of** lymphocytes, plasma cells, or macrophages, demyelination, and axonal degeneration in cranial and **spinal nerve rootlets** has been reported in **dogs** and **cats.** Other inflammatory neuropathies are rare.

Neoplasms of the PNS

These are extremely rare. Only Schwannoma is of importance.

Schwannoma

Terminology used for neoplasms of nerve origin in animals has been quite confusing. For example, the names **Schwannoma, neurofibroma,** and **neurilemmoma** have all been used by different pathologists for the same neoplasm. More recently it has been accepted that the majority of such neoplasms should be designated **schwannomas.** However, designation of the malignant variety of the neoplasm be called **malignant Schwannoma.**

Schwannomas of animals have been best recognized in **dogs** and **cattle,** and less commonly in the **cat. In the dog,** the neoplasm usually affects the cranial nerve (fifth, trigeminal) or spinal nerve roots. Although **Schwannomas of the skin** have been reported, there should be careful interpretation of other neoplasms (e.g., haemangiopericytoma and fibromas) which can have similar morphological features.

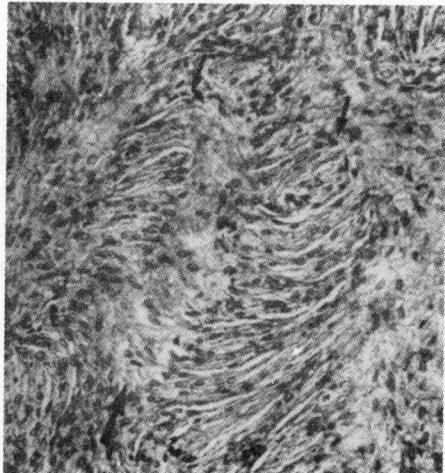

Fig. 43. Skin, right hind limb; cat. Schwannoma. Two bundles of parallel spindle-shaped cells (with nuclei arranged in rows, upper two **small arrows**) separated by strands of their processes (below one **large arrow**) indicate Verocay body formation. H & E stain.

Schwannoma in cattle usually **occurs in mature animals**, although the lesion has been reported in **young calves**, and involves the eighth cranial nerve, brachial plexus, and inter-costal nerves. Also, autonomic nerves of liver, heart, mediastinum, and thorax can be affected. The skin is rarely involved.

Grossly, Schwannomas are nodular or **varicose thickenings along nerve trunks, or nerve roots.** They may be firm or soft (gelatinous) and white or grey in colour. **Schwannomas of the spinal cord nerve roots** may remain inside the dura mater or extend through the vertebral foramina to the exterior. **Microscopically,** the neoplasm consists of spindle-shaped Schwann cells, with poorly defined eosinophilic cytoplasm and basophilic nuclei, which are present in a collagenous stroma. The nuclei of these cells are usually arranged in rows, between which are parallel stacks of their cytoplasmic processes (Fig. 43). In other words, two bundles of parallel spindle-shaped cells (with nuclei arranged in rows) are separated by strands of their processes. Such arrangements are referred to as **'Verocay bodies'**.

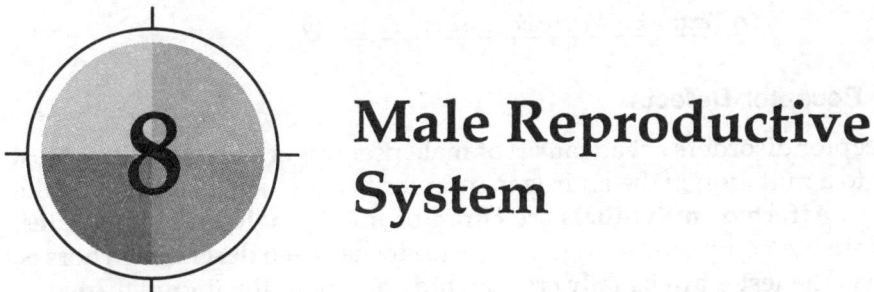

Male Reproductive System

8

Developmental Abnormalities

Intersexes

Abnormalities of Phenotypic Sex

Individuals which are clearly male or female in respect of their chromosomes (XY or XX) and gonads (testes or ovaries), but whose reproductive tract's phenotypic appearance is not clear are called **pseudohermaphrodites.** They can be **male pseudohermaphrodites** or **female pseudohermaphrodites** according to the gonad present. Individuals with both male and female gonadal tissue are called **'hermaphrodites'**. In many cases, the mechanism for abnormal differentiation is unknown.

Three male pseudohermaphrodite syndromes in which the pathogenesis is understood are:

1. Persistent Müllerian Duct Syndrome (PMDS)

This is a **rare disorder of Müllerian-inhibiting substance (MIS) production or function.** MIS is a polypeptide hormone secreted by Sertoli cells. Sertoli cells are present in the seminiferous tubules to which the spermatids become attached, which support, protect and nourish them until they develop into mature spermatozoa. **In animals the syndrome is described in dogs,** with an autosomal recessive mode of inheritance. **Affected dogs** have XY (or XXY) chromosomes, and are externally normal males, with the exception of unilateral or bilateral cryptorchidism. Dogs with unilateral or bilateral scrotal testes can be fertile. However, PMDS-affected dogs are prone to Sertoli cell tumour and pyometra. Testicular abnormalities, such as reduced spermatogenesis, could be due to cryptorchidism.

2. Deficiency of 5-Alpha Reductase Type 2

This is inherited as an autosomal recessive trait in human beings. It has **not yet been recorded in animals,** but is thought to exist. The enzyme converts testosterone to dihydrotestosterone, which is required for the masculization of urogenital sinus, tubercle, and genital swellings.

3. Androgen Receptor Defects

Androgen receptor disorders act as causes of male pseudohermaphroditism. Most cases are due to a mutation in the androgen receptor gene, which is located on the X chromosome. **Affected individuals are chromosomally male and have testes. In domestic animals,** complete androgen insensitivity has been described in horses, cattle, and cats. The testes are usually cryptorchid and are in the inguinal area.

Abnormalities of Gonadal Sex

Hermaphrodites

Hermaphrodites have abnormal gonads, and the gonads possess both testicular and ovarian tissues. There can be separate testis and ovary, or one or both gonads can be mixed. The mixed organ is called an **ovotestis.** Each type of gonadal tissue is well developed and easily seen. **Bilateral hermaphrodites** have an ovotestis on each side, **unilateral hermaphrodites** have an ovotestis on one side, and **lateral hermaphrodites** have a testis on one side and an ovary on the other. The genital tract in hermaphrodites is not clear. **Hermaphrodites occur in dogs, pigs,** and **goat** XX sex reversals and **bovine** freemartin XX/XY chimera. **Sex reversal** is the term used when the gonad is not the type corresponding to the XX or XY chromosomal make-up of the individual. **XX males** have been identified in several species. **XY females** are rare, but they have been identified in **horses** and **human beings.**

Abnormalities of Chromosomal Sex

Sex chromosomes can be abnormal in structure or number. Affected individuals have female phenotype and extremely hypoplastic gonads. A few **cattle** have been identified with an isochromosome Y. Klinefelter's syndrome (XXY) is discussed under testicular hypoplasia.

Testis

Developmental Abnormalities

Descent of the testis into the scrotum is facilitated by **gubernaculum,** a cord of mesenchymal tissue which attaches the developing testis and epididymis to the forming scrotal pouch. The movement of the testis from the inguinal to the scrotal area is **androgen dependent.**

Cryptorchidism

Cryptorchidism is incomplete descent of the testis. In most mammals, the testis normally descends into the scrotum by the time of birth. **Cryptorchidism is usually unilateral than bilateral. Cryptorchidism** is the **most common** disorder of sexual development **in the dog.** It appears to have a genetic basis. **In the horse,** left unilateral crytorchidism predominates over right. This is due to relatively slower rate of descent of the left epididymis and testis and the fact that internal inguinal ring closes at about the same time at birth.

The **gubernaculum may cause cryptorchidism** by its failure to develop, improper position, excessive growth, or failure to regress. **Some other contributory factors** for crytorchidism include testicular hypoplasia, oestrogen exposure in pregnancy, breech labour interfering with blood supply to the testis, and late closing of the umbilicus, delaying the ability to increase abdominal pressure.

Degeneration occurs in the crytorchid testis after puberty. The **testis** is **small** and **fibrotic** and has changes in interstitial collagen deposition, hyaline thickening of the tubular basement membranes, and atrophy of germinal epithelium. **Therefore, only a few spermatogonia remain** along with the normal number of Sertoli cells. Spermatogenesis depends on the relatively cool scrotal temperature. **Apoptosis** (programmed cell death) of germ cells in the higher temperature environment of the abdomen is mediated by the regulatory protein p53. **Leydig cells** (cells constituting the endocrine tissue of the testis, which secrete testosterone) are more numerous than in descended testis.

Cryptorchid testes are much more prone to neoplasms than those placed in the scrotum. This possibility is increased with the extent to which the testis is retained in the abdomen. **In the dog, Sertoli cell tumours** are more likely to occur in the testes present in the abdomen, while **seminomas** develop more commonly in inguinally placed testes. **In men,** undescended testes are prone to develop germ cell neoplasms (seminomas and teratomas). A retained testis enlarged by a neoplasm is prone to torsion.

Hypoplasia

Hypoplasia of the testes is difficult to differentiate from testicular degeneration by morphological features. Testicular hypoplasia or degeneration can occur alone, with or without contributory or influencing factors. Each can also be associated with some other lesion. **Testicular hypoplasia** has been associated with crytorchidism, intersex development, poor general nutrition, zinc deficiency, and **endocrine** and **cytogenetic abnormalities**, that is, abnormalities of chromosomes. Endocrine disturbances causing testicular hypoplasia are related to reduced production of either **luteinizing hormone** by the pituitary gland, which in turn influences testosterone production by Leydig cells, or **follicle-stimulating hormone** by the pituitary gland, which stimulates the nurturing function of the Sertoli cells.

A number of **cytogenetic abnormalities** result in **testicular hypoplasia.** These include **translocations** (attachment of a fragment of one chromosome to a non-homologous chromosome), **mosaics** (individuals having two or more cell lines that are karyotypically or genotypically distinct but are derived from a single zygote), and **non-disjunctions** (failure either of two homologous chromosomes to pass to separate cells during the first meiotic division, or of the two chromatids of a chromosome to pass to separate cells during mitosis or during the second meiotic division. As a result, **one daughter cell has two chromosomes or two chromatids, and the other has none**) causing **polysomies** (an excess of a particular chromosome) **of sex chromosomes.** The best known **example of polysomy** is the XXY karyotype of **Klinefelter's syndrome**, seen in **cats, bulls, dogs, a boar** (male pig), and **a horse. In the cats,** the syndrome is seen in **male cats,** which can be XXY, XX/XXY, or more complex chimeras (individuals with genes of two species) or mosaics with two or more X chromosomes and one or more Y chromosomes.

Hypoplasia of the testes is usually not seen until after puberty. Unilateral hypoplasia is more common than bilateral hypoplasia. Unilateral hypoplasia is difficult to explain because most of the causes act systemically, and therefore, should produce a bilateral effect. The **size** of the **hypoplastic testis** ranges from one quarter of normal to almost normal. **Consistency** is near to normal.

The severity of hypoplasia can be graded histologically by the proportion of hypoplastic tubules scattered through the organ. **Hypoplastic tubules** have a small diameter, are lined by Sertoli cells, stem cells and spermatogonia, have a thickened basement membrane, and are surrounded by collagen. Leydig cells appear proportionately more numerous. **In severe testicular hypoplasia,** most or all of the tubules are abnormal. **In moderate hypoplasia,** in most tubules, when the stage of spermatocyte is reached, the **spermatocytes undergo degeneration**, leaving tubules lined by Sertoli cells with vacuolated cytoplasm. **When hypoplasia is mild,** only a few small tubules are lined mostly by Sertoli cells. Most of the tubules are active, many producing spermatozoa. Mild hypoplasia is difficult to differentiate from testicular degeneration. The number of hypoplastic tubules does not increase with age, **because hypoplastic tubules do not form after puberty.**

Degeneration

Testicular degeneration (testicular atrophy) is a common lesion. Mild degeneration can be detected only microscopically, but when it is severe and chronic, testis is small and firm. **Causes** are many. However, in a particular individual the specific cause is usually not known. **Degeneration** can be **unilateral** or **bilateral**, depending whether the cause is local or systemic. In **young growing males,** the distinction between **testicular degeneration and hypoplasia** is often difficult to make using morphological features. Both lesions are usually present together **because hypoplastic kidneys are prone to degeneration.** Inflammation can also be superimposed on degeneration when the cause is obstruction, resulting in back pressure, rupture of seminiferous tubules, and spermatic granuloma formation. **Recovery** of a testis with degeneration back to normal testis is possible, if the injurious agent is eliminated and damage is not too severe.

Specific causes of degeneration are many. Many agents act through **apoptosis** on germ cells. **Fever** or **local heat** from inflammation on the scrotal skin can injure the testis. **Obstruction** to the flow of spermatozoa causes testicular degeneration. **Obstruction can be due to** developmental anomalies such as local injury or inflammation of the epididymis, or vascular damage from age-related mineralization of the spermatic cord or testicular vessels. Torsion or severe crushing of the spermatic cord can cause obstruction. **Systemic injurious factors include** nutritional deficiency, hormonal aberrations, toxins, and irradiation. **Vitamin A and zinc** are specific nutritional deficiencies. General malnutrition also causes testicular degeneration. **Interference with gonadotropin-releasing hormones,** or luteinizing hormone, or follicle-stimulating hormone can have a damaging effect on the seminiferous epithelium. Such interference could occur, for example, when a neoplasm of the pituitary gland causes local suppression of the pituitary, hypothalamus, or both. **Oestrogen produced by Sertoli cell tumours causes testicular degeneration.** Some drugs, such as amphoteracin B, gentamicin, and chemotherapeutic compounds, cause testicular degeneration.

Of the toxins which cause testicular degeneration, **most damage the spermatogonia and dividing primary spermatocytes,** but some damage later stages spermatocytes and spermatids, or injure Sertoli cells. Degeneration of seminiferous epithelium can be secondary to severe injury of Sertoli cells.

A testis undergoing degeneration is swollen and softer than normal. However, as the degeneration progresses, the testis becomes swollen. After the acute phase, testis becomes **firmer** and has small flecks or large **areas of calcification.** **Microscopically,** tubular degeneration has similar features to that of testicular hypoplasia. Small **seminiferous tubules have a thickened basement membrane,** decreased numbers of seminiferous epithelial cells, and interstitial fibrosis. **Vacuolation of the Sertoli cells** is much more severe in the testis undergoing degeneration than in testicular hypoplasia because of the degeneration of Sertoli cells and loss of germ cells. At the end stage of testicular degeneration, **Sertoli cells** are the only lining cells that remain, but with time, **these also disappear, leaving only the basement membranes. Calcification** can involve intratubular cellular debris, tubular basement membranes, or the interstitium.

Inflammation

Orchitis

Inflammation of the testis is called **orchitis.** It can occur in any species but is **more common in sheep, cattle,** and **pigs.** It is likely that many cases begin as an **epididymitis** (inflammation of epididymis). The infection then spreads up the tubular passages into the testis.

Causes

The **causes** of acute orchitis may be **traumatic** or **infectious. Traumatic orchitis** is common in the **ram** because of the pendulous position of the testes, and their vulnerability to injury. **Infectious orchitis** may result from haematogenous metastasis, or from extension of infection up the genital tract, and through the epididymis, as mentioned earlier.

1. Non-Specific Orchitis

This is a mild, multifocal, subacute, intertubular inflammation of unknown cause which is relatively common in **bulls** and **stallions** (adult male uncastrated horses). **There are no gross lesions. Microscopically,** lymphocytic foci are present between tubules and around vessels. Other forms of orchitis which produce gross lesions are much less common.

2. Intratubular Orchitis

This originates from an infection ascending from the urethra, urinary bladder, ductus deferens, and epididymis. It starts as inflammation in the seminiferous tubules, which then spreads to interstitium. **Intratubular orchitis** appears **grossly** as yellow foci (up to 1 cm) which become firm and white as the lesions become chronic. Initially, the affected tubules have acute inflammatory debris. The lining of the tubule is lost, but the tubular outlines are present. **Spermatic granulomas** can form any time spermatozoa make contact with extratubular tissue. In the centre of these granulomas, spermatozoa can be seen free and within macrophages. Macrophages and lymphocytes infiltrate around the core of spermatozoa and macrophages, and with time, collagen is deposited at the edge of the lesion.

3. Necrotizing Orchitis

This is the most severe form of orchitis. It can begin as an intratubular disease or can originate haematogenously. In some cases, the affected areas are so severely inflamed and the necrosis is so extensive that the original structures form a **caseous mass.** Grey-brown, firm, necrotic debris replaces an irregular, but large portion of the testis. In a few extremely severe cases, a **fistula** develops through the scrotum.

4. Granulomatous Orchitis

This is characterized by the formation of multiple, coalescing, **inflammatory nodules, displacing and replacing parenchyma.** Inflammation of the tunica vaginalis or the epididymis can be secondary to intratubular, necrotizing, or granulomatous orchitis. **Orchitis in bulls** caused by *Brucella abortus* is the most important example of granulomatous orchitis in domestic animals. **It is a haematogenous intratubular orchitis which becomes necrotizing.** Initially, swelling of the testis occurs. **Fibrinous exudate** distends the cavity of the tunica vaginalis. Foci of necrosis of the parenchyma expand and can coalesce so that much of the testis is involved, becoming either liquefied, or caseous and gritty. Any surviving parenchyma becomes densely fibrous. Finally, the testes become small and suspended in abundant fluid or semi-fluid exudate. **Microscopically,** bacteria are seen in small groups in the cytoplasm or in cytoplasmic vacuoles of macrophages in the areas of necrotizing pyogranulomatous inflammation.

Brucella canis causes inflammation of the testis, epididymis, and prostate gland in **dogs**. The bacteria multiply in the cytoplasm of macrophages and epithelial cells in these organs. The heads of agglutinated spermatozoa in the epididymal duct and semen are coated with IgA antibody, considered as anti-spermatozoan autoantibody locally produced. Serum agglutinating antibody is also detectable.

Organisms which commonly cause orchitis in domestic animals are presented in **Table 12**.

Table 12. Common causes of infectious orchitis in domestic animals

Bull	Ram
Actinomyces pyogenes	*Brucella ovis*
Bluetongue virus	*Chlamydia psittaci*
Brucella abortus	*Corynebacterium ovis*
Lumpy skin disease virus	Sheep pox virus
Mycobacterium tuberculosis	
Nocardia asteroides	
Buck	**Boar**
Brucella melitensis	*Brucella suis*
	Burkholderia pseudomallei
	Rubulavirus
Dog	**Stallion**
Brucella canis	Equine infectious anaemia virus
Canine distemper virus	Equine viral arteritis virus
Escherichia coli	*Salmonella abortus equi*
Proteus vulgaris	*Strongylus edentatus*
Burkholderia pseudomallei	

5. Autoimmune Orchitis

Spermatozoa are kept separated within the seminiferous tubules and isolated from the general circulation by Sertoli cells. **More mature stages of spermatogenesis can thus be protected from immune cells and antibody or from toxins.** The **'Sertoli cell barrier' ('blood- testis barrier')** has **two permanent compartments: (1) a basal compartment** bounded by peritubular myeloid cells and Sertoli cells below their tight junctions with associated spermatogonia and preleptotene (pre-prophase) spermatocytes, and (2) **an adluminal** (toward lumen) **compartment** beyond the tight junction between Sertoli cells, with the later stages of spermatogenesis. **Cell surface antigens** undergo many changes during spermatogenesis, and **mature**

sperm cells have a set of surface antigens not present at the time of foetal life when immune self-recognition takes place. Even then, spermatozoa in normal locations are not recognized as foreign by the immune system of the male animal. Isolation of the mature spermatozoa from the immune system is the mechanism believed responsible for their not being treated as foreign, since **lymphocytes have not been identified in the testicular interstitium.** Another theory is that minute amounts of soluble spermatozoan antigen pass into the host through the numerous tight junctions of the Sertoli cells, and this soluble antigen activates suppressor lymphocytes involved in decreasing cytotoxic immune responses.

The **formation of anti-spermatozoan antibodies** in human males is associated with major disruption of the blood-testis barrier. **Antibodies against spermatozoa can form after testicular damage caused by trauma, neoplasms, and infections.** Disruption of the ductus deferens following obstruction or surgical vasectomy allows immune cells and antibody to gain access to spermatozoa. **Antibody attached to the cell surface can interfere with spermatozoan function. Anti-spermatozoan antibodies** have been identified in the seminal fluid or the serum of **stallions** that had low sperm viability following **trauma to the testis.**

If **autoimmune orchitis** occurs in **domestic animals**, the rete testis or efferent ducts are the starting sites for the process. When the disruption of the **blood-testes barrier is so** severe that spermatozoa are outside their normal compartment within the testis, epididymis, ductus deferens, and urethra, **a foreign body granulomatous reaction occurs.**

Hydrocele

Hydrocele is an accumulation of watery fluid in the cavity of the scrotum. The fluid lies among all the layers of tunica vaginalis, and occupies all spaces between the testis and the skin.

Hydrocele sometimes occurs in generalized oedema involving the whole ventral abdominal wall, which is mostly the result of intra-scrotal disorders. These include interference with the return flow of the spermatic veins. **In the majority of cases, however, hydrocele is an inflammatory oedema,** as shown by the higher specific gravity and protein content of the fluid, which make the fluid an exudate and not a transudate. The condition thus is a mild inflammatory disease of the scrotal tissues (with or without testis), and is caused mostly by trauma and sometimes by local infections.

Neoplasms

Testicular neoplasms are common in older dogs, occur in older bulls, and are rare in other species. They can originate from germ cells or from gonadal stroma (Sertoli cells or Leydig cells). Sometimes, neoplasms of testicular mesenchymal structures or metastatic neoplasms are found. The **three common primary testicular**

neoplasms, namely, **seminoma, Leydig cell adenoma,** and **Sertoli cell tumour,** can occur singly or in combination.

Germ Cell Neoplasms

These are **seminoma, teratoma,** and **other less common types.**

Seminomas

These are the **second most common testicular neoplasm in the dog** and the **most common** testicular neoplasm **in the aged stallion.** In other species, these neoplasms are rare. They are **more common in cryptorchid than in descended testes.** Originating from primitive seminiferous tubules, **they do not produce hormones.**

Multicentric origin (i.e., having many centres) within the testes and **local invasiveness** are characteristic. The neoplasm is white, firm, bulging when cut, and has fine fibrous trabeculae (Fig. 44). Microscopically, seminomas have an intratubular and diffuse arrangement of large, polyhedral, clearly demarcated cells with a large nucleus, variable nuclear size, and very little cytoplasm. **Giant cells are sometimes present.** Lymphoid nodules are usually present in seminomas. These neoplasms are rarely malignant.

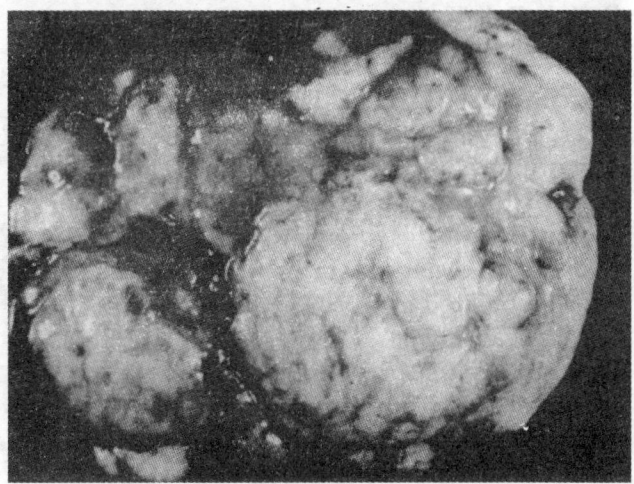

Fig. 44. **Testis; dog. Seminoma.** The neoplasm bulges from the cut surface, is distinct, and is divided by a few fibrous trabeculae.

Teratomas

Teratomas originate from germ cells. **They are uncommon,** but are best known in the **horse,** especially in the cryptorchid testis of the **young horse.** The neoplasm can be large, cystic or polycystic and can contain hair, mucus, bone, or even teeth. **Microscopically,** at least derivatives of two of the three embryonic germ layers (ectoderm, mesoderm, and endoderm) are present. Most teratomas have well-differentiated structures and are **benign.**

Gonadal Stromal Neoplasms

These are **Leydig cell adenoma, Sertoli cell tumour,** and some other less common types.

397

Leydig Cell Tumours

Also called **'interstitial cell tumour'**, these are the most common testicular neoplasms of the **dog** and **bull**. They are rare in **stallion**, in which most cases are in un-descended testes. **Grossly**, the neoplasm is spherical, of yellowish brown to orange colour and well demarcated. **These neoplasms are almost always benign. Microscopically,** cells of the bovine neoplasms vary little, but in the **dog,** the cells can be large, round, polyhedral, or spindle shaped. The cells have abundant cytoplasm, which is often finely vacuolated, and has brown pigment. Although haemorrhage, necrosis, and cyst formation are common, Leydig cell adenomas **are non-invasive.**

Sertoli Cell Tumour

This is the third most common testicular neoplasm of the dog. It is rare in other species, but occurs in **stallions** and **bulls. In the dog,** most of the Sertoli tumours are present in **un-descended testes. Grossly**, the neoplasm is firm, white, lobulated by fibrous bands, and can cause enlargement of the affected testis (Fig. 45). The neoplasm can invade the spermatic cord and metastasize to the local internal iliac lymph node. Metastases beyond the local lymph node are rare. The abundant fibrous connective tissue in Sertoli cell tumours differentiates them from the other two common types of testicular neoplasm.

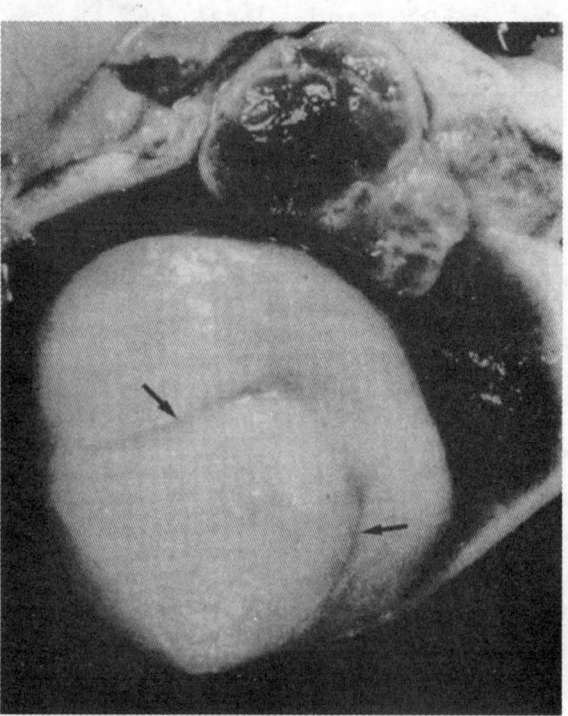

Fig. 45. Testis; dog. Sertoli cell tumour. White bands of fibrous tissue (arrows) dissect through the neoplasm.

Besides local invasion, the other important aspect of Sertoli tumours is that about **a third of them produce oestrogen,** which has a feminizing effect, causing **gynecomastia** (enlargement of the mammary glands). **A serious effect of oestrogen secretion is myelotoxicity,** resulting in non-regenerative anaemia, granulocytopaenia, and thrombocytopaenia. Other effects of oestrogen are induction of hypothyroidism and alopecia, hyperplasia, or squamous metaplasia of the acini of the prostate gland.

Scrotum

Developmental Anomalies

Disturbances in the formative stages can lead to various defects in the scrotum, such as failure of fusion, cleft formation, or bifurcation of the scrotum. Defects can be local, confined to the scrotum and penis, or part of a wider range of defects in an intersex animal.

Dermatitis

Dermatitis of the scrotal skin is common. Usually it is non-specific, the result of trauma, frostbite, or exposure to environmental irritants. Some pathogens have scrotum as a predilection site. These are *Dermatophilus congolensis* and *Besnoitia besnoiti* in the bull, and *Chorioptes ovis* in the ram. The heat generated in scrotal dermatitis can interfere with the thermoregulatory function of the scrotum, causing testicular degeneration.

Neoplasms

Neoplasms which occur in the skin can occur in the scrotum, but are much less common in the scrotal skin. Neoplasms sometimes encountered are mast cell tumours, melanomas, and haemangiomas in the **dog** and papillomas in the **boar**. Vascular abnormalities, which could be haemangiomas, occur on the scrotum of the **dog**. The scrotal veins of **bulls** sometimes become varicose.

Tunica Vaginalis

The term vaginalis is **extension of the peritoneum** that lines the scrotal sac as the parietal layer and covers the testis, epididymis, and spermatic cord as the visceral layer. **The cavity between the two layers is continuous with the peritoneal cavity.** Therefore, tunica vaginalis is prone to all the inflammatory and neoplastic diseases of the peritoneum and peritoneal cavity. However, mesothelioma is the most commonly encountered neoplasm.

Inflammation

Inflammation of the tunica vaginalis as part of a systemic disease will have the characteristics of that disease. Inflammation of tunica vaginalis without initial inflammation of the abdominal peritoneum can have a **non-infectious**, that is, traumatic, **or infectious cause**. The latter can be an extension from an orchitis or epididymitis. Well-known causes are *Brucella ovis* and *Actinobacillus seminis* in **rams**, and trypanosomes in **bulls, rams**, and **male goats. Adhesions** between the parietal and visceral tunica vaginalis are common.

Spermatic Cord

Varicocele

This is **local dilatation of the spermatic vein** in the pampiniform plexus. In the **ram,** it can cause lowered fertility with poor spermatozoan motility, immature spermatozoa in the semen, and **testicular degeneration.** Thrombosis of the affected vessels is common. Varicoceles can cause **enlargement of the scrotum,** even to the extent that the scrotum touches the ground.

Torsion

Torsion of the spermatic cord can occur when the testis is un-descended. Torsion causes vascular occlusion, which may involve the spermatic vein or both the vein and artery, and results in necrosis (**infarction**) of the testis.

Inflammation

Inflammation of the spermatic cord, known as **funiculitis,** occurs after the contamination of a castration wound. Sometimes the lesion is acute and necrotizing, but usually it is **chronic** and a **scirrhous cord** is present. Great enlargement of the distal part of the cord is due to excessive granulation tissue in which numerous small pockets of pus are scattered. **Staphylococci** are usually recovered from the pus in **horses.** The term **'botryomycosis'** has been used for these staphylococcal pyogranulomas. Radiating club-shaped eosinophilic deposits (**Splendore-Hoeppli material**) are present around the central clusters of bacteria.

Funiculitis is caused by *Staphylococcus aureus, Actinomyces pyogenes, Fusobacterium necrophorum, Actinobacillus lignieresii, and Mycobacterium tuberculosis.*

Scirrhous Cord

As stated, **scirrhous cord** is **chronic funiculitis.** The inflammatory process is a **chronic suppurative inflammation.** A gross enlargement of the scrotum and its contents occurs in scirrhous cord. The condition is **excessive granulation formation** on the stump of the cut spermatic cord following castration. The cause is a chronic hyperplastic proliferative inflammation resulting from operative injury and infection. It is common in **pigs** because of their closeness to the soil, their usually unsanitary surroundings, and the crude sort of surgery, which is sometimes performed by the stockmen. The next species usually involved is the **horse** because of the horse's poor resistance to many of the ordinary infections, mainly pyogenic.

The mass of abnormal tissue may attain extreme proportions in a few weeks. **It consists usually of dense fibrous tissue.** It varies in size from a small nodule to masses that weigh as much as 11kg. **Abscesses,** which may perforate to the exterior and then drain through sinus tracts, are usually present in the affected cord and surrounding tissue. The exudate, especially in **pigs**, has a very foul smelling odour.

Epididymis, Ductus Deferens, Ampulla, Seminal Vesicle

The **seminal vesicle** is an outpouching of the ductus deferens. **Cats and dogs lack seminal vesicles.**

Spermatocele

Spermatocele is a local distension of the epididymis, containing accumulated spermatozoa. **Spermatic granulomas** can form in the connective tissues at the rupture site.

Immotile Cilia Syndrome

This is a rare disease described in **humans, dogs,** and **pigs,** and is caused by one or more of several defects in the axoneme of cilia (i.e., the central core of cilia) throughout the body and of the flagellum of spermatozoa. The disease has an autosomal recessive mode of inheritance. The effect on the reproductive system is **immotile or hypomotile spermatozoa** due to flagellar lesions, or to **oligospermia** (subnormal concentration of spermatozoa), or **azoospermia** (no spermatozoa), due to defective cilia in the epididymis and ductus deferens. Female infertility is related to defective function of cilia of the uterine tube.

Inflammation

Any lesion along the length of **epididymis** can cause obstruction to the flow of spermatozoa.

Epididymitis

Epididymitis, inflammation of epididymis, can be focal, multifocal, or diffuse, unilateral or bilateral. **In acute inflammation,** epididymis is soft and swollen; **in chronic inflammation,** it is firm and enlarged because of the deposition of fibrous tissue. Obstruction to the outflow of spermatozoa is one of the causes of **testicular degeneration.** Grossly, testis is atrophic. Focal fibrinous or fibrous adhesions occur between the visceral tunica vaginalis over the epididymis and the parietal tunica vaginalis lining the scrotal sac. If an abscess ruptures into the cavity of the tunica vaginalis, diffuse inflammation of the tunics can result, followed by **adhesions** across the cavity. In some cases, fistulas discharge through the scrotum.

Non-infectious causes of epididymitis include trauma, influx of urine along the ductus deferens, and any lesion in which spermatozoa escape from the lumen of the epididymis. Such escaped spermatozoa incite a foreign body response. **Microscopically,** the lumen has a mixture of inflammatory cells, containing neutrophils, but macrophages are prominent. The lumen also contains desquamated epithelial cells, and intact and fragmented spermatozoa.

Infectious epididymitis occurs from the entry of organisms from the urinary tract rather than from haematogenous spread. *Brucella abortus*, *Actinobacillus seminis*, or *Histophilus ovis* infections in rams produce epithelial hyperplasia, spermatic granuloma and abscesses. Testicular atrophy occurs secondarily. In *Brucella abortus* infection in **bulls**, epididymitis is accompanied by orchitis. Epididymitis occurs in **mature dogs** as a non-specific infection, or as a part of a specific disease such as canine distemper. **Intranuclear** and **intracytoplasmic inclusions** can be found in the epithelial cells of the epididymis in canine distemper. *Brucella canis* infection causes epididymitis, followed by testicular degeneration and atrophy. The lesions are often unilateral.

Seminal Vesiculitis

Seminal vesiculitis is an important problem in the bull because fertility is reduced after the seminal vesicles contribute pus to the semen. Inflamed seminal vesicles are the most common source of inflammatory cells in **bovine semen**. The **cause** is usually infectious. Various organisms including viruses, protozoa, **Chlamydia**, **Mycoplasma, Ureaplasma,** *Brucella abortus*, and other bacteria are involved. The pathogenesis is uncertain.

The **common form** of seminal vesiculitis is a **chronic interstitial inflammation.** The glands are enlarged, firm, and have loss of lobulation. Lymphocytes, plasma cells, macrophages, and a few neutrophils and eosinophils are present in the interstitium. The lumens have neutrophils, desquamated epithelial cells, and debris. The **seminal vesicles in bulls** can be among the organs **involved in** *Brucella abortus* and *Mycobacterium bovis* infections.

Prostate Gland

Most domestic animals have both **prostate** and **bulbo-urethral gland.** The **dog** and **cat**, however, **have only the prostate gland.** Both oestrogens and androgens have trophic action on the prostate gland.

Prostatitis

Prostatitis can be **clinically important** if the gland becomes large enough to cause urinary obstruction. **In the dog,** prostatitis is found in the **old animals,** usually along with hyperplasia, or in young animals without hyperplasia. Prostatitis can be divided into acute, chronic, abscess formation, and specific (*Brucella canis*) forms. Organisms such as *Escherichia coli, Proteus vulgaris,* and others invade from the urethra. Prostate gland may be diffusely or focally involved, swollen, congested, and oedematous. The early **microscopic lesion** is catarrhal inflammation of the acini, expanding later to interstitium, with abscess formation. **The abscesses can persist or are replaced by fibrous tissue.**

Hyperplasia and Metaplasia of the Prostate

Enlargement of the prostate is relatively common in **old dogs.** The dog is the only domestic animal that develops prostatic hyperplasia with age. **Clinical consequences of prostatic hypertrophy** are obstruction and infection of the urinary tract and development of hydronephrosis. Partial obstruction of the rectum causes constipation. Enlargement of the prostate is hormone related, but the precise cause is unknown. Hypertrophy of the gland does not occur in castrated dogs. **Microscopically,** hyperplasia of the fibromuscular stroma occurs along with hyperplasia of the acinar epithelium, often with the formation of papillae. Some acini are distended with fluid and have a flattened epithelium. The presence of dilated cystic acini with attenuated (thin) epithelium is the basis for classifying prostatic hyperplasia as benign complex rather than benign glandular. Increase in size and weight of the prostate are due to increase in interstitial tissues. Increase in the glandular component is due to cystic dilation, not to the volume of glandular epithelium.

Oestrogen-induced hypertrophy of the canine prostate gland, due to the presence of Sertoli cell tumour, also shows squamous metaplasia of acinar epithelium, ducts, and prostatic urethra. Flattened keratinized epithelial cells are desquamated into the acini, and neutrophils and other inflammatory cells are present. **Squamous metaplasia** of the prostate gland in **dogs is not pre-neoplastic.**

Adenocarcinoma of the Prostate Gland

Adenocarcinoma of the prostate gland in the **dog** is the only prostatic neoplasm of importance in domestic animals. **However, it is uncommon.** The cause has not been well defined but appears to be related to abnormal hormonal environment. Some of the clinical signs of prostatic carcinoma are similar to those of prostatic hyperplasia, because of the enlargement of the organ. But, in addition, adenocarcinoma and its metastases cause cachexia and locomotory abnormalities through pressure and invasion of nearby structures, especially bones. **Grossly,** the neoplasm is firm, shows enlargement, and has cystic cavities. **Microscopically,** areas of hyperplasia of epithelial and fibroplasias are present. Prostatic adenocarcinomas can form acini, or single cells can invade the connective tissue. **In dogs,** no specific regions of the prostate have been associated with the development of hyperplasia or metaplasia.

Penis and Prepuce

Developmental Abnormalities

The penis is subject to many abnormalities in size and form. These include congenital absence, hypoplasia, duplication, and directional deviations. **None of these lesions is common.**

Hypoplasia

Hypoplasia of the penis and prepuce can be the result of early castration.

Persistent Frenulum

This is a minor anatomical abnormality rather than a serious defect. Frenulum is the fold under the penis connecting it with the prepuce. Persistent frenulum can have an important harmful effect in limiting the extent to which the penis can be protruded from the sheath, and in causing the erect penis to be curved instead of straight. **Persistent frenulum is important in bulls.**

Hypospadias and Epispadias

These are **malformations of the urethral canal** which create abnormal openings of the urethra on the ventral surface of the penis (**hypospadias**), or on the dorsal surface (**epispadias**). Hypospadias is a mild form of pseudohermaphroditism. Either hypospadias or epispadias can occur in individuals with other malformations incompatible with survival, or they occur alone. They can cause urinary obstruction and also interfere with normal insemination.

Phimosis and Paraphimosis

In men, **phimosis** means inability to retract the prepuce over the penis because of too small preputial opening, and **paraphimosis** is inability to replace the prepuce over the penis because of penile (of penis) swelling. **True congenital phimosis does not occur in animals because of the larger preputial cavity and opening. Inflammatory phimosis in animals** occurs when inflammation causes swelling of the penis or prepuce in which case the penis cannot be extruded from the prepuce.

Inflammation

Inflammation of the glans penis is called **balanitis**, and inflammation of the prepuce is called **posthitis**. Non-specific inflammation of the penis and prepuce (**balano-posthitis**) occurs in a number of situations. A large microbial flora normally inhabits the preputial cavity and can be source of infection causing inflammation secondary to trauma, such as bite wounds in **dogs** and **boars**. Traumatic lesions occur in **bulls** in breeds which have a pendulous sheath easily torn by sticks or other sharp objects. The everted preputial mucosa is subject to injury. In males with phimosis, the initial problem is greatly increased by urination into and **retention of urine in the preputial cavity,** creating an environment for the overgrowth of bacterial organisms. Depending on the cause, balano-posthitis takes **several forms**, which include mild to severe, focal to diffuse, acute to chronic, ulcerative, necrotizing, diphtheritic, catarrhal, or suppurative.

Herpesvirus can cause **balano-posthitis** in several species. Bovine herpesvirus causes balano-posthitis in the .bull, especially of the glans penis. In the pustule stage, **intranuclear inclusion bodies** are present in epithelial cells of the penis and prepuce. **Ulcerative balano-posthitis** with acidophilic intranuclear inclusions has been observed in **goats** caused by caprine herpesvirus infection. Equine herpesvirus 3 is the cause of **equine coital exanthema**, a disease of **stallions** and **mares**. **Canine herpesvirus** causes inflammation at the base of the penis. Resolution of these lesions in the affected species is rapid.

Ovine ulcerative posthitis is caused by urease-producing *Corynebacterium renale*. When urine has a high concentration of urea, it produces ulceration of the prepuce near the orifice. A high-protein diet predisposes to the disease. Lack of testosterone is also involved because the disease occurs mainly in **wethers** (castrated male sheep).

Other organisms which can cause balano-posthitis include *Strongyloides papillosus* in the bull and the larvae of **Habronema** sp. in the **horse**.

Neoplasms

The **penis** and **prepuce** can be involved in metastatic or multicentric neoplasms, such as **mast cell tumour melanoma**, and **lymphosarcoma**. The following are the most important neoplasms of penis and prepuce.

Transmissible Venereal Tumour

This neoplasm of **dog** is of **histiocytic immunophenotype cells.** The primary neoplasm is usually on the external genitalia, **but extra-genital primaries do occur,** as well as **metastatic neoplasms**. In the **male dog,** the neoplasm is found on the penis, mostly on the proximal parts, and usually not on the prepuce. The neoplasm can be single or multiple, a few millimetres to 10 cm in diameter, **with an inflamed, ulcerated, cauliflower-like surface. Microscopically,** the neoplasm is the same as it is in the bitch, composed of sheets of neoplastic cells and minimal stroma. The neoplastic cells are large, uniform, with a large nucleus and nucleolus, indistinct cell outline, and numerous mitotic figures. **Regression and recovery are the rule. The neoplastic cells express major histocompatibility complex class II antigen** and show infiltration of inflammatory cells, including increased numbers of T-lymphocytes during the regression of the tumour. The neoplasm is thought to originate from a **specific genetic alteration of dog histiocytes,** followed by the transmission of abnormal cells from dog to dog. Based on data obtained from immunological, cytogenetic, and nucleotide sequence studies, **the neoplasms are found very similar throughout the world.**

Squamous-Cell Carcinoma

This neoplasm of the penis is **important in the horse,** and to a lesser extent in the **dog. In the horse,** both stallions (uncastrated male horses) and geldings (castrated male horses) have neoplasms, and the common site is the glans penis. Rather than producing a proliferative mass, the neoplasm at this location is invasive, necrotic, and ulcerating. **Microscopically,** the neoplasm is well differentiated, with well-developed **keratin pearls. Metastases** in the inguinal and iliac lymph nodes usually can be found.

Papilloma (or Fibropapilloma)

This neoplasm **occurs on the glans penis of young bulls.** It is believed to be caused by a virus. The single or multiple warty growths have a fibrous core and a papilliferous (bearing papillae) epithelial covering. **Surface ulceration** is usually extensive following spontaneous necrosis or trauma. Larger neoplasms can interfere with breeding or cause phimosis or paraphimosis.

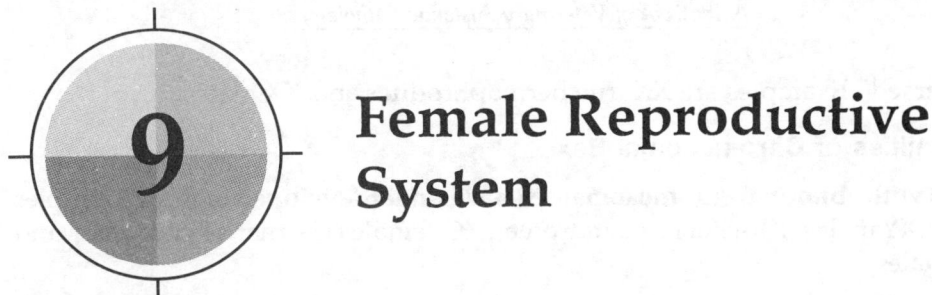

Female Reproductive System

Developmental Anomalies

The **sex of an individual** can be defined at several different levels: **genetic, chromosomal, gonadal, ductal, and phenotypic.** Normal mammalian chromosomal sex is **XX for female** and **XY for male**. On the Y chromosome, a gene (sex-determining region Y) for the testis-determining factor has been identified. The differentiation of a gonad to a testis depends on this gene.

Intersexes

Gonadal sex is based on the histological components of the gonad. The appearance of the external genitalia is the criterion used for determination of **phenotypic sex.** The gender can be uncertain when the various components are of mixed male and female types.

Abnormalities of Phenotypic Sex

Pseudohermaphrodites

Pseudohermaphrodites have the chromosomes and gonads of one sex and the tubular organs modified towards those of the opposite sex. **They are classified according to the gonadal tissue. Female pseudohermaphrodites are rare.** The best known example is the masculinization of female foetuses by sex steroid hormones given to the dam during pregnancy, or shortly before conception.

Aplasia (lack of development) **of a segment of the uterus** can affect the ovaries.

Abnormalities of Gonadal Sex

Hermaphrodites

Hermaphrodites have both ovarian and testicular tissue in their gonads. They may be 'bilateral' or 'unilateral', according to whether a combined organ, called an **ovotestis**, is present on one side or both sides, and 'lateral', with a testis on one side and an ovary on the other. Hermaphrodites have genital tract that cannot be easily classified as male or female. **True hermaphrodites are rare.** In many cases, the mechanism for the development of hermaphrodites is unknown, but the mechanisms for some are known. **Hermaphrodites occur in dogs, pigs, and goats.** Animals in which the gonadal sex does not follow the chromosomal sex are termed 'sex reversed'. Examples are XX true hermaphrodites and XX males.

Abnormalities of Chromosomal Sex

Animals with abnormal chromosomal sex have underdeveloped organs. Examples include XXY males (Klinefelter's syndrome), XO females (Turner's syndrome), and XXX females.

Chimeras and **mosaics** have two or more types of cells, each with a different chromosomal constitution. The cells of a **chimera** come from two different sources (such as from male and female members of a set of twins in the **bovine freemartin**), whereas the cells of a **mosaic** come from the same source. Several cases of **chimeras in dogs** have been described.

The **most common chimera** in the domestic animals is the **freemartin calf**. Placental vascular anastomoses, **which allow exchange of blood between foetuses,** are required for the occurrence of a freemartin. These anastomoses occur usually in the **bovine species**, and less commonly in other ruminants. **The freemartin is the female in a set of male and female twins.** The percentage of male cells in freemartins varies widely. **Müllerian inhibitory substance** from the male twin's testes causes the differentiation of foetal Sertoli cells and seminiferous cord-like structures in the female twin's ovaries. The **ovaries are small,** with reduced number of or **no germ cells,** to organs **partially converted to testes,** or to organs composed entirely of structures resembling seminiferous tubules. **Externally the animal appears female,** but the vestibule and vagina are short, vulva is hypoplastic, and clitoris is enlarged. **The male twin is minimally affected.**

Vagina and Vulva

Cyst

The causes of **cyst formation in the vaginal wall of a cow** include inflammation of the lining of the duct or gland, and hyperoestrogenism, in which oedema due to oestrogen stimulation is prolonged.

Tumefaction

Tumefaction (swelling) of the vulva is normal during oestrus. Excessively large or persistent swelling is abnormal. Abnormal tumefaction occurs in hyperoestrogenism. An example is **poisoning** of **pigs** by the **mycotoxin zearalenone** found in mouldy maize. Other effects of the mycotoxin are precocious mammary development, and tenesmus leading to rectal prolapse.

Inflammation

The vagina and vulva are lined by **stratified squamous epithelium** which is **quite resistant to infection.**

Post-parturient vulvitis and **vaginitis** occur when these organs are lacerated during dystocia and become infected. **Trauma** not related to parturition can also progress similarly. Inflammation of the cervix and posterior vagina following dystocia can have a more serious outcome because of the possible local spread of infection into and through the vaginal wall into the peritoneal cavity.

Granular vulvitis in cows may be associated with **Mycoplasma** and **Ureaplasma** sp. Granular vulvitis in the **acute stage** has a profuse purulent vulvular discharge and hyperaemic vulvular mucosa with raised granules. The disease can become **chronic**. Reduced fertility may occur due to persistence of the organism in the uterus for up to 7 days following contamination of the uterus from the vulvular lesions at breeding.

Infectious pustular vulvovaginitis of cattle is caused by **bovine herpesvirus 1**, which is similar to BHV-1 that is the cause of infectious bovine rhinotracheitis (IBR). Vulvovaginitis is transmitted by coitus and artificial insemination. **Gross lesions** include hyperaemia and oedema of the vagina and vulva, followed by petechial haemorrhages and slight nodularity of the mucosal surfaces. In the later stages, erosion and ulceration of the mucosa are seen. **Microscopically**, the epithelium with eosinophilic intranuclear inclusions undergoes ballooning degeneration followed by necrosis, neutrophil infiltration, and desquamation. The lamina propria is hyperaemic and infiltrated by inflammatory cells, mostly lymphocytes and plasma cells. Resolution of the disease is rapid. Lesions are similar in the penis of affected **bulls**. Caprine herpesvirus 1 causes lesions in **goats** similar to those of bovine vulvovaginitis.

Dourine

Dourine, caused by *Trypanosoma equiperdum*, is a venereal disease of the **horse** and ass. *T. equiperdum* can penetrate the intact vaginal mucosa and multiply locally in the wall before becoming systemic. **Lesions** are found in the skin and nervous system as well as in the **genital tract**. In the male and female external genital organs, the acute lesion is extensive oedema. With time, the areas with oedema become fibrotic. Lymphoid nodules of the genital tract are hyperplastic, and mucosa is ulcerated.

Neoplasms

Transmissible Venereal Tumour (TVT)

This tumour of the **dog** is transmitted by coitus and by the transfer of neoplastic cells. A viral cause has been found. **TVT cells have 50 chromosomes compared with the normal canine number of 78. Both sexes are affected.** The **lesion** begins as a nodule under the genital mucosa. **In the bitch**, it proliferates into the lumen of the vagina and can protrude through the vulva as the ulcerated mass.

Microscopically, the neoplastic cells are large, round, or oval, and uniform in size. Cytoplasm is poorly defined and stains lightly. The number of cells in mitosis is increased. Spontaneous regression of the neoplasm occurs, and neoplasms have multifocal necrosis, infiltration of lymphocytes, and deposition of collagen. A few neoplasms have metastases in other sites.

Squamous-Cell Carcinoma

This neoplasm of the vulva occurs in the **mature cows, ewe,** and the **mare.** Solar radiation is an aetiological factor. Squamous-cell carcinoma originates on the hairless and less pigmented skin of the vulva and has the appearance and behaviour of squamous-cell carcinomas in other sites. The neoplasm metastasizes late in the course of disease to the iliac lymph nodes.

Cervix

Anomalies

In **cows,** some developmental anomalies are restricted to the cervix. These include **hypertrophy** or **hypoplasia** of the whole structure, **aplasia** of one or more of the usual five rugae, tortuosity, and dilation or diverticulum formation of the cervical canal.

Cervicitis

Cervicitis usually occurs as a minor lesion along with more severe endometritis or vaginitis. This distribution is observed in contagious equine metritis, and in postparturient metritis, cervicitis, and vaginitis. Cervicitis can also result from poorly performed traumatic artificial insemination. Inflammatory exudate covers the cervical mucosa and collects in the vagina. Most cases of cervicitis resolve readily.

Neoplastic disease of the cervix in domestic animals is rare.

Uterus

Non-Inflammatory Abnormalities

Torsion

Torsion of the uterus occurs mostly in pregnant animals, mainly in the **cow,** and to a lesser extent in the **bitch** and **mature female cat (queen),** and when the uterus is enlarged by **pyometra** (pus in uterus) or **mucometra** (mucus in uterus). The result of torsion is circulatory damage. The veins, being thinner walled, are compressed and occluded before the arteries. The uterine wall and placenta become congested and oedematous. The foetus dies and mummifies or putrefies. The uterine wall is friable and prone to rupture.

Prolapse

Prolapse of the uterus is important in the **ewe, cow,** and **sow** after parturition. Factors that cause uterine inertia such as prolonged dystocia, hypocalcaemia, and ingestion of oestrogen plants; usually contribute to prolapse of the uterus. Vascular damage, shock, trauma, and infection follow prolapse.

Subinvolution of Placental Sites

Placental sites are those places on the mucosal surface of the uterus where placenta is attached. The placental site is a circular band which is more raised and rough surfaced than a normal placental site at the same time after parturition. **Involution** means shrinking of the uterus to its normal size after parturition.

Subinvolution of placental sites is the longer than normal persistence and deeper than normal penetration of trophoblast-like cells in the uterus after parturition. **In the normal placenta,** trophoblasts are found in the endometrium, but they rapidly degenerate in the postpartum period. **In the bitch,** subinvolution of placental sites is characterized clinically by a bloody vaginal discharge which lasts for weeks or months after parturition. **Grossly,** subinvoluted placental sites are **about twice the size of normal sites** for the same time after parturition. **The mucosal surface of each site is a raised, rough, irregular, grey to brown plaque. Microscopically,** the superficial part of the plaque near the lumen is composed of cell debris, haematoma, thrombus, and regenerating endometrium. In the deeper part of the site, the changes are collagen deposition, haemorrhage, and distension, and decreased density of endometrial glands. **Trophoblast-like cells** are more numerous in subinvolution sites than in the normal placental sites. The cells invade the myometrium and penetrate the full thickness of the wall **and perforate the uterus.**

Endometrial Atrophy

This is due to loss of ovarian function secondary to hypopituitarism, because endometrial atrophy of old age is not seen in domestic animals. **In the mare,** diffuse endometrial atrophy occurs in anoestrus and is due to ovarian inactivity of debility. **In the mare,** the longitudinal folds in atrophic areas are indistinct, and **in the cows,** the caruncles are flattened.

Endometrial Hyperplasia

This is **an important lesion in the ewe and bitches,** and also occurs in the **cow, cat,** and **sow,** but is **rare in the mare.** It is caused by **prolonged hyperoestrogenism.** Ingested clover is the source of oestrogen in the **ewe;** cystic follicles, granulosa cell tumours, and oestrogens from plants are the causes in **cow;** and mycotoxin zearalenone from mouldy feed is a cause in the **sow. In the bitch,** endometrial hyperplasia occurs under the influence of progesterone, but with priming by oestrogen from the ovaries. In the queen (female cat), strong association has been found between endothelial hyperplasia and actively secreting corpora lutea. It may also be due to chronic stimulation of the endometrium by oestrogen.

When the condition progresses to the stage of cystic endometrial hyperplasia, the lesion is easily recognized at postmortem examination. Endometrial cysts are filled with clear fluid in **ewe** and **bitch**. Because of the local influence of progesterone in the **bitch** and **queen, infection can be superimposed,** resulting in cystic hyperplastic endometritis. **Microscopically,** there is an increase in the size and number of glands. **Bitches** and **queens** may develop **endometritis** and then **pyometra,** and in some cases, **endometrial polyps.** In all species, cystic lesions are probably irreversible. **In ewes,** endometrial hyperplasia results in reduced fertility, dystocia, and uterine prolapse. Even when non-pregnant, **ewes** have mammary gland enlargement. **Endometrial hyperplasia is not precancerous in domestic animals, as it can be in women.**

Mucometra

Mucometra is accumulation of mucus in the uterine lumen. The **cause is congenital** or **acquired obstruction** of the outflow of mucus initially produced in normal amounts. However, mucometra can be due to the production of excessive amounts of mucus in cases of hyperoestrogenism.

Adenomyosis and Endometriosis

Adenomyosis and endometriosis are of importance only in **monkeys.** However, adenomyosis is sometimes seen in domestic animals, namely, **queen, cow,** and **bitch,** and is the result of prolonged oestrogen stimulation. **Adenomyosis** is the presence of nests of endometrium within the myometrium, and is not of much importance in domestic animals which do not menstruate. **Endometriosis** is the presence of endometrial glands or stroma in locations outside the uterus, such as the ovary, mesometrium, and peritoneum. The mechanism for development of endometriosis is unknown.

Inflammation

Most uterine infections begin in the endometrium, and are due to introduction of **semen contaminated with bacteria** or to metabolic disturbances that favour an environment for bacteria in pregnancy, parturition, or postpartum involution. **Resistance of the uterus to infection depends on** humoral and cellular immune mechanisms, by the hormonal environment, and by physical factors.

Humoral and Cellular Immune Mechanisms

Following infection, changes in the uterus include hyperaemia and rapid entry of oedema fluid in the uterine wall and lumen. **Accumulation of neutrophils** from the blood occurs in response to chemotactic substances released by **bacteria** and to

leukotriene B4 released from endometrium and leukocytes. Neutrophils infiltrate the endometrium and enter uterine lumen and contribute more amount of leukotriene B4, providing additional chemotactic stimuli. **Neutrophils** release substances that are toxic to gametes (sperm and ovum) and embryos. **Complement activation,** directly by bacteria by the alternate pathway or by specific antibody by the classical pathway, can eliminate bacteria either by lysis following attack on their membranes or by phagocytosis increased by opsonization. Leakage of serum into the uterine lumen from the inflamed endometrium contributes to the antibody content of the uterine fluid. **Opsonization of bacteria by antibodies, especially IgG, promotes their more efficient phagocytosis by neutrophils and macrophages.**

The role of immunoglobulins in protecting the female genital tract has been **best studied in mare. IgG and IgA** predominate in urine secretions in the mare, but IgM is just present. Immunoglobulins in the uterine lumen are produced by cells in the endometrium, rather than being derived from the blood. **Local uterine immunity is better developed in the mare than other species.** Concentrations of luminal immunoglobulins and immunoglobulin-containing cells of the endometrium are not influenced by the stage of the oestrus cycle. However, recent demonstration of greater concentrations of IgA and IgG **in the uterine secretions of mares** more susceptible to infection has led to the belief **that immunoglobulins play only a minor role in the defence of the uterus against infections.**

Locally produced IgA is not directly bactericidal and neither acts as an opsonin nor as a macrophage activator. It can, however, interfere with the attachment of bacteria to mucosa and can activate complement through the alternate pathway.

Hormonal Influences

Infections of the uterus are more easily overcome at oestrus than at other stages of the cycle. This is because of the better drainage through an open cervix under oestrogen stimulation and to the increase in leukocytes in the uterine wall at oestrus. **Leukocytic phagocytosis** is either unchanged or increased under the influence of oestrogen, but neutrophil activity is reduced under the influence of progesterone. Generally, uterus is more susceptible to infection during the progestational phase of the oestrus cycle **because progesterone reduces the migration of blood neutrophils and reduces phagocytosis and killing of bacteria by uterine neutrophils.** The mechanism of how sex hormones influence neutrophils is unknown, and receptors for sex hormones have not been demonstrated. **The non-pregnant uterus is highly resistant to infection.**

Prostaglandins are normally produced by endometrium. The epithelium secretes most of **PGF** and the endometrial stroma most of **PGE.** In **most species (except dog, cat,** and **monkeys)** prostaglandins are responsible for lysis of the corpus luteum. **In acute inflammation,** prostaglandin production by the endometrium is increased, by the release by arachidonic acid from the phospholipids of cell membranes. Under these circumstances, lysis of the corpus luteum occurs sooner. When chronic inflammation progresses to the stage of epithelial and mucosal surface loss, production of prostaglandins is decreased and corpus luteum persists.

Conformation

Conformation of the external genitalia is the physical factor which is important in uterine infections. **In the mare,** most of the vulva is higher than the floor of the pelvic canal, and the vulva tends to suck the air and contaminants, including faeces, into vagina or even into the uterus. **Urine can collect in the vagina of mares** with defective function of the muscles of the vestibule and vulva. When contamination and collection of urine occur, vestibule and vagina get inflamed. The cervix and uterus either become inflamed from direct contact with environmental organisms, or from local spread of the inflammation.

Organisms which cause inflammation of the uterus can enter through the vulva (**ascending infection**), or can arrive through the blood (**haematogenous infection**). Ascending infections occur at breeding and parturition, whereas haematogenous infections are mostly specific infections, such as *Brucella abortus* or bovine viral diarrhoea virus infection in **cows** that occur during pregnancy. A few specific organisms, such as *Streptococus equi* in the mare, are ascending infections, but most ascending infections are due to a mixture of organisms. Organisms which cause placentitis, foetal infection, and abortion, usually also spread and cause inflammation of the endometrial component of the placenta. **In those species** with a zonary (**dog, cat**) or cotyledonary (**ruminant**) rather than a diffuse placenta (**horse, pig**), endometritis extends beyond the boundaries of the part of the endometrium making close contact with the foetal part of the placenta. **Postpartum metritis** occurs to some extent even after a normal pregnancy and parturition, but metritis is particularly common and more severe following an abnormal parturition. **Lochia,** the debris which is discharged from the uterus for a short time after parturition, is **an excellent nutrient medium for bacterial growth.**

Endometritis

Endometritis is inflammation limited to the endometrium. Almost all uterine infections begin as endometritis. The mucosa is swollen and has a rough surface, usually with adherent shreds of fibrin and necrotic debris. **Microscopically,** neutrophils are found in the stroma and in the glands, with desquamation of a few surface epithelial cells to severe necrosis of the endometrium. Mild lesions resolve completely. **Severe acute endometritis** usually becomes **chronic** and the necrotic endometrium is replaced by granulation tissue devoid of glands and ultimately by fibrous tissue.

Persistent endometritis is a problem in mares. Affected animals are unable to resolve the acute endometritis which usually follows mating. **This persistence**

appears to be due to defects in both cellular and humoral response to infectious agents.

Metritis

Metritis is inflammation of all layers of the uterine wall. In the acute stage, serosa is finely granular, and has petechial haemorhages and fine adhering strands of fibrin. **Microscopically**, sub-serosal tissue and muscle layers are oedematous and infiltrated by neutrophils. Endometritis is present.

Pyometra

Pyometra occurs as **a sequel to endometritis or metritis.** It is an **acute** or **chronic** infection of the uterus with **accumulation of pus in the lumen** as the result of a closed cervix. The closure of the cervix is not always complete and some discharge occurs. In some cases, obstruction of the cervix is mechanical, but most cases are caused by a functional obstruction of the cervix under the influence of progesterone produced by the retained corpus luteum. **In the cow**, persistence of the corpus luteum is usually secondary to a pathological process in the uterus. **In the bitch** and **queen**, most cases of pyometra are the result of bacterial infection secondary to the endometrial hyperplasia, and most occur during pseudopregnancy. The colour and consistency of the exudate vary with the infecting bacteria. Exudate is viscid (thick and sticky) and brown with *Escherichia coli* infection and creamy yellow with streptococcal infection. The uterus can be greatly distended. **Grossly**, necrotic, ulcerated, and haemorrhagic areas are present in the uterine mucosa, as well as dry, white, thickened cystic areas. **Microscopically**, the dry white areas show hyperplasia and squamous metaplasia of surface epithelium, common in chronic inflammation of any mucous membrane, and the cystic areas are due to cystic endometrial hyperplasia.

Neoplasms

Uterine neoplasms are not common in domestic animals. The primary neoplasms that do occur are **carcinoma in the cow** and **leiomyoma in the bitch.** **Lymphosarcoma in the cow** is the most common metastatic neoplasm.

Leiomyomas in the bitch are multiple neoplasms, not only in the uterus, but also in the cervix and vagina, and are associated with endometrial hyperplasia, follicular cysts, or mammary gland neoplasms. Oestrogens have a role in producing these neoplasms in the bitch. **In other species, these neoplasms are rare.** The neoplasms are well demarcated but not capsulated, are spherical, and vary greatly in size. Some luminal neoplasms in the vagina are pedunculated and liable to trauma and torsion.

Carcinoma of the endometrium is rare in domestic animals. However, **in the cow,** the early carcinoma is found in the endocrine glands of the horns and less often in the body of the uterus. As it increases in size, the neoplasms thicken the uterine wall. Deposition of large amounts of fibrous tissue makes the neoplasm firm. The neoplasms can be small or involve a large area of the uterine wall. **Microscopically,** the neoplasm is easily differentiated from normal endometrium by the increased size, pleomorphism, and the accompanying scirrhous reaction (i.e., deposition of the fibrous tissue). **Metastases** occur in the regional lymph nodes, lungs, and seed the serosal surfaces of the abdomen.

Lymphosarcoma in the cow is caused by the **bovine leukaemia retrovirus** and usually affects heart, abomasum, lymph nodes, and **uterus. In the uterus,** infiltration of neoplastic cells can be focal or multifocal. Affected areas are light yellow, centrally necrotic, and replace any or all layers of the uterine wall. In such **cows,** vaginal lesions are multiple, small, often haemorrhagic, but non-ulcerated nodules. **An extensively involved uterus can support pregnancy even to an advanced stage.**

Placenta and Foetus

Non-Inflammatory Diseases

Retention of Foetal Membranes

Retention of foetal membranes, for longer than normal after parturition, is common especially in the cow. In the cows, membranes are considered retained, if not expelled by 12 hours after parturition. The **cause** of retention is **uncertain,** but infectious, nutritional, hormonal, circulatory, hereditary, and weather factors have been suggested. The membranes act as nutrient medium for the growth of contaminant bacteria and for the development of severe endometritis from the transient mild post-parturient endometritis.

Twinning of the Mare

Twinning in the mare is the most common non-infectious cause of abortion. Aborted twin foetuses usually appear to have died at different times. **Death is** due to **placental insufficiency.**

Endometrial Fibrosis

In the mare, endometrial fibrosis is usually the result of previous endometritis. It reduces the area of the endometrium available for formation of a diffuse placenta. Chorionic villi do not develop where there is no endometrium. **In large areas of endometrial fibrosis,** chorion does not develop microcotyledons and their villa. **Severely affected mares** become pregnant, but do not carry the foetus to term because the functional area of the placenta is too small.

Premature Placental Separation

This has been described in **mare,** and occurs in two forms. **One form** occurs around the time of parturition. The **other form** occurs some time before parturition.

416

Prematurely detached areas become brown and dehydrated.

Torsion of the Umbilical Cord

This is a cause of abortion in mare. In torsion, the cord is long, excessively twisted, and the twists are difficult to undo. The cord is oedematous and haemorrhagic, and congested. Lesser degrees of torsion occur without seriously affecting the umbilical blood vessels and killing the foetus.

Hydramnios and Hydrallantois

These terms refer to **excessive accumulation of fluid in the amniotic and allantoic sacs, respectively.** These lesions occur in the **cow**, are **rare**, and usually do not occur together. **Abortion** or **dystocia** follow, with a dead and sometimes **small anasarcous** and **ascitic foetus**.

Embryonic and Foetal Death

Regardless of the source of hormones responsible for maintaining pregnancy in large animals, embryonic or foetal death permits the release of **PGF 2-alpha and expulsion of the embryo or foetus. In animals** as well as **human beings,** many of the embryos die because of **chromosomal abnormalities.**

Mummification

Mummification is an outcome of foetal death. Rather than being expelled soon after death the **foetus** is retained and dehydrates to **become a firm, dry mass,** coloured brown to black by degraded haemoglobin, and consists of leathery skin enclosing harder parts of the foetus. The **cause of death** can be infectious or non-infectious. The situations in which mummification usually occurs are in twin pregnancy in the **mare** and in parvovirus infection in the **sow**

Maceration

Maceration (softening) of the dead foetus requires the presence of **bacterial organisms** in the uterus. These bacteria could be those that caused the foetal death, or putrefactive organisms that entered the uterus through the cervix after the death of the foetus. **Endometritis** or **pyometra** is present.

Abortion

Abortion in domestic animals **is expulsion of the foetus** before the development is sufficiently advanced to allow survival. **An aborted foetus can be alive or dead at the time of abortion, but most are dead. Stillbirth** is delivery of a dead foetus at a stage of development at which it should have been viable. **Uterine infections produce a range of effects from foetal mummification, abortion, or stillbirth** to the birth of a live, but sick, foetus.

Foetal Anomalies

These can take many forms. They include aplasia or hypoplasia of the adrenal glands; displacement, dysgenesis (defective development), or absence of the pituitary gland; anencephaly (absence of the brain); hydrocephalus, hydrops foetus, and arthrogryposis. All these conditions directly influence the reproductive process by causing problems at parturition.

Inflammatory Diseases

Bacterial Causes

Bacteria causing inflammation of the placenta and foetus are numerous. Almost any organism which causes **septicaemia** can infect the uterus, but here only those organisms are discussed which target the placenta or foetus, or both. The **route of infection** of the uterus and foetus is usually **haematogenous**, after the organisms have entered the dam either through the digestive or genital tract. For some diseases, method of spread can be either **venereal** or by **ingestion. In the mare,** most placental pathogens enter the pregnant uterus through the cervix.

Campylobacter foetus var. *venerealis* can be a long-term **inhabitant** of the exterior of the **bovine penis** and the **preputial cavity.** It is transmitted venereally and can survive for some time on the vaginal mucosa, but the **cow** must become pregnant for it to establish in the uterus. **Embryonic** or **early foetal death** is the most common manifestation of **campylobacteriosis.** Usually the only clinical abnormalities are irregular oestrus cycle or the return of oestrus of an animal thought to be pregnant. **Cows** become resistant to subsequent infections by the bacteria. **Gross** and **microscopic lesions** in placenta are similar to those described in brucellosis (discussed next), that is, oedema of the inter-cotyledonary chorioallantois and necrosis of cotyledons with microscopic inflammation of both, but are less severe and with fewer organisms in the desquamated chorionic epithelial cells. **Foetal lesions are non-specific.**

Campylobacter foetus subsp. *foetus* and *Campylobacter jejuni* are mainly intestinal inhabitants and cause similar lesions in **sheep.** The organisms are transmitted by ingestion and abortions occur in outbreaks. Infection of the pregnant uterus results in **late-term abortion** or the birth of live, but sick lambs. The **placentitis** is characterized by an oedematous inter-cotyledonary chorioallantois and yellow cotyledons. **Grossly,** the foetuses may have multiple yellow areas of liver necrosis. **Microscopically,** chorioallantois is infiltrated by a mixture of cells, mainly neutrophils. **Campylobacter** organisms are abundant among the inflammatory cells.

Brucella abortus **in cattle is ingested with feed** contaminated by an infected aborted foetus or placenta. The initial lesion is a persistent naso-pharygeal lymphadenitis. Bacteria are released into the blood in waves causing **bacteraemia**. Bacteria then localize in the spleen, lymph nodes, mammary glands, testes, accessory male glands and joint capsules, bursae, and tendon sheaths. **Brucella** organisms are removed from most organs, but a small focus of infection usually persists in some organs. **The pregnant uterus is particularly susceptible to infection.** With time, the uterine disease process becomes chronic, eventually resolving after abortion or parturition. **Gross lesions** in the placenta are oedema of the inter-cotyledonary chorioallantois which is opaque with a leathery texture, light brown exudate on the chorionic surface, and necrosis of the cotyledons. The foetal lesions are non-specific. **Microscopic lesions** include inflammation with oedema and infiltration of mononuclear cells and a few neutrophils both in the inter-cotyledonary chorion and the chorionic villi. A striking feature is the presence of numerous coccobacilli in the chorionic epithelial cells. **In ruminants,** *B. abortus* moves from the maternal circulation into the haematomas that occur at the tips of the maternal septa within the placentome. **Most foetuses have pneumonia** that ranges from minimal to severe. **Microscopically,** granulomas that include multinucleate giant cells occur in various organs such as liver, spleen, and lymph nodes.

Brucella canis is acquired by the **dog** either by ingestion or venereally. Both sexes have lymphadenitis, especially of the nodes of the head and neck, and bacteraemia. **Lesions** are epididymitis and testicular degeneration in **male dogs** and **females** have placentitis and foetal endocarditis, pneumonia, and hepatitis. **Microscopically,** chorionic epithelial cells are packed with **Brucella** organisms. Other foetal lesions include renal haemorrhage, subacute infection of the pelvic connective tissue, and lymphadenitis.

Brucella ovis in **sheep** is transmitted venereally from a **ram** with epididymitis shedding large numbers of organisms in the semen. **Gross lesions** in placenta are similar to those produced by *Brucella abortus* in **cattle**. Foetal lesions at postmortem are non-specific. **Microscopically,** large numbers of coccobacilli are found in chorionic epithelial cells. **Lesions in the foetus** are pneumonia, lymphadenitis, and interstitial nephritis. *Brucella melitensis* infection in **sheep** and **goats** occurs mainly in Mediterranean countries. The infection has a septicaemic phase, but infection is localized in the mammary gland and pregnant uterus. **Goats have more severe febrile disease and more severe mastitis than in sheep.**

Brucella suis causes a disease in **pigs** which differs in several ways from brucellosis in ruminants. The **lesions** are more widespread and have a **predilection for bones and joints. Necrosis** and **caseation** occurs in many lesions. Pregnancy is not a requirement for endometritis in **pigs**. Miliary granulomas in the endometrium are mixed with multiple hyperplastic lymphoid nodules. Endometrial glands become distended with mucus and leukocytes and the surface epithelium is partly desquamated and has focal squamous metaplasia.

Enzootic Abortion in Ewes

This is caused by *Chlamydophila psittaci,* producing **late-term abortions in ewes.** The disease occurs in Britain and United States. Transmission is oral and **ewes** seem to be immune to re-infection after the first abortion. **Microscopically**, the chorioallantois is infiltrated by neutrophils. The organisms distend the chorionic cells, but are difficult to visualize without special stains.

Leptospirosis

Leptospirosis can cause **abortion**. A large percentage of **cattle** and **pigs** are infected, **but most animals do not show clinical signs.** Several different serovars are associated with abortion, especially *Leptospira interrogans* serovar *hardjo* in **cattle** and serovar *pomona* in **pigs. In adult animals,** the organisms localize in the kidneys after the septicaemic phase. **Pregnant sows** and **cows** abort weeks after the septicaemic phase, usually in the last trimester. Placental lesions are usually limited to oedema. **Foetal lesions are usually mild.** Some dead foetuses expelled near term without extensive autolysis have gross lesions of ascites and fibrinous peritonitis. **Microscopic lesions** include subacute interstitial nephritis and subacute necrotizing hepatitis.

Listeriosis

Listeriosis is caused by *Listeria monocytogenes*. It causes sporadic abortions in **cattle, sheep,** and **goats,** and outbreaks of abortions in **sheep.** Listerial **abortions occur in last trimester of pregnancy.** Some aborting dams are septicaemic and have endometritis. The **placental lesions** include severe diffuse necrotizing and suppurative inflammation of both cotyledons and the inter-cotyledonary areas. **Microscopically,** there is severe inflammation of the mesenchyme (embryonic connective tissue) of the villi and the inter-cotyledonary chorion. Chorionic epithelial cells, especially in the areas between the villi, are filled with **Gram-positive listerial bacilli.**

Other Bacterial Causes

Organisms which cause bacteraemia in adult animals are capable of causing lesions in the placenta and foetus. Thus, in **cattle,** bacteria such as **Salmonella** and **Pasteurella** sp. and *Haemophilus somnus* are potential causes of placentitis, foetal inflammatory lesions, and abortion. **In pigs,** various **Streptococcus** sp. can cause similar lesions. **Ureaplasmas** can cause abortion in **cattle.**

Various bacterial organisms can cause abortion in the mare. Haemolytic streptococci are usually recovered from foetal organs, placentas, and uterine discharges. Other commonly encountered organisms are *E. coli* and **Pseudomonas, Klebsiella,** and **Staphylococcus** sp. Although some infections are haematogenous, the **ascending route of infection,** through the cervix, is the most common. Affected parts of the placenta are oedematous and covered by small amounts of fibrino-necrotic exudate. **Gross foetal lesions** are enlarged liver and increased abdominal and thoracic fluid. **Microscopically,** lesions are moderately severe subacute inflammation of the stroma of the chorionic microcotyledons and desquamation of chorionic epithelium.

Fungal Causes

Aspergillus and phycomycetes cause **sporadic abortions** in **cows** and **mares**. **In cows,** the organisms spread to the placenta haematogenously. **In the mare,** the fungi enter through the cervix. In the affected bovine placenta, cotyledons are enlarged and the inter-cotyledonary chorioallantois becomes leathery and covered with a brown exudate. Thus, the gross appearance of the placenta is similar to that of placenta in bovine brucellosis. Affected areas of equine chrioallantois are initially thickened, and later, shrunken and friable. In both **cows** and **mare**, the amnion has thick, white or yellow, leathery areas. **Microscopically,** the lesions include inflammatory cell infiltration of allantoamnionic and chorionic mesenchyme and desquamation of chorionic epithelium. **Lesions in the foetuses** are confined to the skin and include subacute dermatitis and hyperkeratosis. **Fungal hyphae,** septate in the case of **Aspergillus** and non-septate in the case of phycomycetes, are abundant in the lesions of the placenta and skin of the foetus.

Viral Causes

Herpesviruses are **well established causes of outbreaks of abortion in cows** (infectious bovine rhinotracheitis virus), **mares** (equine herpesvirus 1), and **sows** (pseudorabies virus, Suid herpesvirus 1), and have been also described in **goats** (caprine herpesvirus 1), and **dogs** (canine herpesvirus 1). Generally, **lesions in the affected foetuses** are lymphoid necrosis in spleen, thymus, and lymph nodes and multiple small foci of necrosis, mild acute inflammation, and **intranuclear inclusion bodies** in parenchymal cells in a number of organs, especially liver, lungs, and adrenal glands. Pulmonary lesions usually include hyperplasia, focal necrosis, and desquamation of bronchial epithelium. Placenta may be oedematous. Only in the **sow** inflammation and inclusion bodies are easily observed in the chorion.

Equine herpesvirus 1 (EHV-1) is **an economically important abortigenic** (causing abortion) **herpesvirus.** Virus infection of uterine endothelial cells has a major role in the pathogenesis of abortion. **Damage to the endothelial cells** results in thromboses, accompanied by perivascular infiltration of lymphocytes, neutrophils, and monocytes and perivascular oedema and subsequent **infarction of the endometrium.** The fluid that escapes through the damaged endometrium causes separation of the maternal and foetal layers of the placenta and this separation allows virus from maternal leukocytes and lysed endothelial cells to enter the foetus. Foetal endothelial cells and the cells of a number of organs are targets for the virus.

In the cow, virus has an affinity for the endometrium. Infectious bovine rhinotracheitis virus (bovine herpesvirus 1) produces an **acute necrotizing endometritis** in the **cow. Microscopically,** the lesions range from mild lymphocytic endometritis to severe diffuse necrotizing metritis.

Pestiviruses in **cattle** (bovine viral diarrhoea virus), **sheep** (border disease virus), and **pigs** (swine fever virus/hog cholera virus) **can cause foetal death** of malformation. **In the mare,** equine viral arteritis virus causes abortion. The mechanism is foetal anoxia due to compression of uterine blood vessels by virus-induced myometritis.

Porcine parvovirus is an important cause of embryonic and foetal loss and causes death and mummification of several litters. **Pig foetuses** have widespread necrotizing lesions, along with inflammation and **inclusion bodies**, especially in the liver, lungs, kidneys, and cerebellum.

Trans-placental infection of pig with porcine reproductive and respiratory syndrome virus, an arterivirus, causes haemorrhage in the umbilical cord as a result of necrotizing arteritis. **Gross lesions** include ascites, hydrothorax, and oedema of perirenal tissue, and mesentery. **Microscopically,** mild to moderate arteritis occurs in lungs, heart, and kidneys. Alveolar septa in the lungs are thickened by mononuclear cell accumulation and proliferation of type 2 pneumocytes.

Akabane virus and **Cache Valley virus** are bunyaviruses which cause **foetal infection** and **abortion** in **sheep** and **other ruminants**. The virus produces a number of **lesions in the developing foetal nervous system** including hydranencephaly, microencephaly, cerebellar hypoplasia, and loss of spinal cord ventral horn neurons. The loss of ventral horn neurons causes **denervation muscle atrophy**. Atrophy and myositis cause **arthrogryposis** (fixation of limb joints) and **skeletal deformities** such as torticollis and scoliosis.

Protozoal Diseases

Toxoplasma gondii is **an important cause of abortion in ewes.** The organism has a **cat-sheep life cycle,** with contamination of **sheep** feed by cat faeces and the ingestion of sheep foetal membranes by **cats. Gross lesions** in the foetal membranes include oedema of the inter-cotyledonary chorioallantois and white 1 to 2 mm foci in the cotyledons. **Microscopically,** the cotyledonary lesions consist of chorionic epithelial hypertrophy and hyperplasia with toxoplasma organisms within chorionic epithelial cells.

Neospora caninum has come to be known as a cause of **abortion in cows.** Foetuses are of 3 to 9 months gestation and have no gross lesions. **In the brain,** multiple foci of necrosis or proliferated microglial cells are usually seen near capillaries with hyperplastic endothelium. **Groups of** *N. caninum* in these foci are either extracellular or occur in neuronal cells or endothelial cells. In the heart, lesions include subacute multifocal epicarditis, myocarditis, and endocarditis. Protozoal organisms are present either in myofibres or endothelial cells.

Tritrichomonas foetus in **cattle** is another protozoal organism which can cause **abortion**. Mild placentitis, with no foetal lesion, is present. Endometritis can be severe, and pyometra may occur. Infiltration of endometrium with mononuclear cells is moderate to severe. Lymphoid nodules and secondary follicles develop. These are the sites of local production of IgA. The standard method of diagnosis is the demonstration of protozoa in the contents of the foetal stomach.

Uterine Tubes

Most lesions of the uterine tubes are **secondary to lesions elsewhere in the reproductive tract**. In **dogs** and **cats**, lesions of the uterine tubes do not affect reproductive performance.

Hydrosalpinx is distension of the uterine tubes by clear fluid. It may be **congenital** or **acquired**, and is caused by mechanical or functional obstruction of the lumen. The obstruction can be at either end of an uterine tube. The distension can be uniform or irregular. The wall is thin, and the tube increases in length. Multi-loculated cysts (i.e. having many compartments) are numerous in the mucosa. The **congenital type** results from segmental aplasia (lack of development) of the uterine tube as present in freemartins. The **acquired type** is secondary to trauma or chronic inflammation. Acute inflammation causes pyometra rather than hydrosalpinx. **Hydrosalpinx** and **pyometra** are common cause of **sterility in pigs**.

Salpingitis results from spread of infection from the uterus to the uterine tubes and is usually bilateral. **Gross lesions** are few, except some hyperaemia and thickening of the mucosa. However, even very mild inflammation can reduce **fertility**. **Microscopically,** the inflammation ranges from mild to severe and from acute to chronic. When severe, salpingitis involves other parts of the mucosa and sometimes the muscular layer. Exudate is present in the lumen. With time, adhesions form between the denuded areas and adjacent mucosa becomes cystic, or is replaced by granulation tissue.

Pyosalpinx, collection of pus in the uterine tubes, has similar pathogenesis as salpingitis. **Grossly,** pus accumulates in the lumen. **Microscopically,** numerous neutrophils are present along with other inflammatory cells, both within mucosa and in mucosal cysts. Most of the mucosa is lost; some of the epithelium undergoes squamous metaplasia.

Ovary

Developmental Anomalies

Sometimes, **agenesis** (absence) from unknown cause involves one or both ovaries. The reproductive tract can be absent as part of the defect.

Duplication of an ovary is a rare anomaly.

Hypoplasia

Hypoplasia of the ovaries **occurs mostly in cows**. It is usually bilateral but non-symmetrical. The affected ovaries are small, lack follicles or surface scars from ovulation, but sometimes have cysts. **Microscopically,** cortical stroma and ova are absent or poorly developed. **Ovarian hypoplasia does not result in hypoplasia of the remaining female** genital tract. The tract, however, remains infertile after puberty.

Hypoplasia because of genetic and chromosomal abnormalities has been reported in cattle.

Vascular Hamartomas

Vascular hamartomas of the ovary are incidental findings in the **cow, sow,** and **mare**. They occur as a dark red mass on the surface of the ovary and are composed of connective tissue and vascular channels lined by mature endothelial cells.

Cysts

Cysts in the mesovarium near the ovary, called **paraovarian cysts**, originate from either mesonephric or paramesonephric ducts. **These cysts are common in the mare** and can be several centimetres in diameter. **Cysts within the ovary are of three types:** non-gonadal stromal, gonadal stromal, and neoplastic.

Acquired Ovarian Lesions

Oophoritis, inflammation of the ovary, is rare in domestic animal.

Ovarian bursal adhesions vary from thin bands to large sheets of fibrous tissue binding together the walls or crossing the cavity of the **ovarian bursa,** a peritoneal pouch formed around the ovary by the broad ligament and the mesosalpinx. The lesion is often bilateral in **cows** and could result from an ascending uterine infection that follows a retained placenta as a complication of pregnancy. **Physical trauma** from manipulation of the ovary is another possible cause. Bursal adhesions are common in beef heifers.

Lesions Related to Cyclic Changes

Haemorrhages into follicles are sometimes present in **cows,** and haemorrhages into cystic follicles occur sometimes in the **bitch**. Some haemorrhages, usually small and few, occur at the time of ovulation in all species. **The mare is an exception.** Organization of the blood clot can result in adhesions between the ovary and adjacent structures such as fimbriae of the oviduct or ovarian bursa.

Atretic follicles are those which become **arrested at any stage of development and then regress**. Atretic follicles, in most cases, **are normal**. In any oestrus cycle, only one or a small number of follicles mature, while the others undergo atresia at various stages of development. **Follicular atresia is considered abnormal when it is a part of any disease process** that interferes with the release of, or the pituitary response to, gonadotropin-releasing hormone. Development of the follicle can be arrested at any stage, and in time, it degenerates. The follicle either persists as a cyst, or is infiltrated by macrophages, theca cells, and fibrous connective tissue, eventually becoming **a small scar.**

Cystic graafian follicles are important in **cows** and **sows. In dairy cows,** prolongation of the postpartum interval to first oestrus is the main outcome of cystic follicles. **Ovulation does not occur.** Bovine cystic follicles persist for 10 or more days without the formation of a corpus luteum, They develop because of a deficiency of luteinizing hormone (LH). Postpartum uterine infection can cause **cystic ovaries** in **dairy cows. Cystic ovaries** are associated with the recovery of *Escherichia coli* from the uterus and increased concentration of prostaglandin F2alpha metabolites and cortisol. It is believed that bacterial endotoxins, or the prostaglandins produced because of damage caused by endotoxins, stimulate the adrenal cortical secretion of cortisol. Cortisol excess suppresses the preovulatory release of LH, **resulting in the development of cysts.**

Follicular cysts cows can be single or multiple, unilateral or bilateral, and usually thin walled. **Microscopically,** the granulosa cell layer is thicker than normal or is degenerating and eventually becomes a flattened single cell layer with no luteinization. **Follicular cysts can undergo spontaneous regression.** However, cysts that develop after the first postpartum ovulation are replaced by other cystic follicles.

Anovulatory luteinized cyst is caused by delayed or insufficient release of LH. **It occurs in cows and sows** more than in other species. **Ovulation does not occur.** Cystic follicles and luteinized cysts can occur in the same ovary.

Cystic corpus luteum is of uncertain pathogenesis. **In cows,** it must be differentiated from anovulatory luteinized cyst.

Supernumerary follicles are caused **in bovine ovaries** by chorionic gonadotropin or follicle-stimulating hormone used in doses to cause superovulation in preparation for embryo transfer. In these cows, it is not unusual for more than a dozen well-developed follicles or corpora lutea of the same age to be present.

Neoplasms

Germ Cell Neoplasms

In domestic animals, most of the neoplasms of germ cells are **benign** undifferentiated **(dysgerminoma),** or benign with somatic differentiation **(teratoma).**

Dysgerminoma is a rare neoplasm of bitches, sows, cows, and mares composed of cells resembling primitive germ cells. The neoplasm is a solid lobulated mass with areas of haemorrhage and necrosis. It is similar to seminoma in the male. **Mitotic rate is high, but metastases are rare.**

Ovarian teratomas are rare, usually well differentiated, and benign. They originate from totipotential primordial germ cells. Malignant teratomas occur less often, except in the **bitch.**

Gonadal Stromal Neoplasms

Granulosa cell neoplasms are the **most common ovarian neoplasms in large animals.** They are unilateral, smooth surfaced, and round. They can be solid, cystic, or polycystic. **Microscopically,** the granulosa cells are not different from normal granulosa cells and are normally arranged as they would be in normal graafian follicles, that is, in single or multiple rows of round to columnar cells lining fluid-filled spaces. In less differentiated areas, the neoplastic cells are arranged in sheets. **Granulosa cell neoplasms** are often **malignant in the queen** and sometimes in the **bitch,** but in the **cow** and **mare**, sex chord stromal neoplasms are usually benign. **Many stromal neoplasms produce oestrogens or androgens.** The **mare** can have signs of anoestrus, nymphomania (excessive sexual desire in a female), or stallion-like behaviour. The **bitch** has prolonged oestrus as well as cystic endometrial hyperplasia and pyometra, as lesions of progesterone stimulation.

Surface Neoplasms

Neoplasms of the ovarian surface epithelium resemble several neoplasms of the endometrium. This is because ovaries are covered by coelomic epithelium, the same type of tissue that invaginates in early foetal life to form the lining of the reproductive tract. Of the surface neoplasms, the **serous type is the only important one in animals. Serous papillary cystadenoma** and **cystadenocarcinoma** occur commonly in the **bitch.** They originate from the surface epithelium. The neoplasms are usually bilateral. **Malignant forms** spread over the peritoneal surface. **Ascites** results, either from obstruction of the diaphragmatic lymph vessels, which re-absorb peritoneal fluid or from excess fluid secretion by the neoplasm.

Mammary Gland

Inflammation

Mastitis

Inflammation of the **mammary gland** is called **mastitis.** Mastitis in domestic animals is **almost always due to infection by microorganisms.** Because of increased vascular permeability in mastitis, plasma components enter the milk, ionic balance is altered, and the **products of inflammation enter the milk, altering its appearance.** Alveolar epithelium damaged by inflammation secretes less milk. **Thus, bovine mastitis is a cause of great economic loss.** The discussion that follows is that of **mastitis in the cow,** with a brief description on the disease in other animals.

Causes

Most of the organisms responsible for mastitis are bacteria. They can be **divided in three groups:**

1. Those organisms such as *Streptococcus agalactiae, Staphylococcus aureus* and **Mycoplasma** species for which mammary gland is the main site of persistence or reservoir.

2. **Coliform organisms** are in the group which has the environment as reservoir, and

3. An overlap group has members such as *Streptococcus uberis* and *Streptococcus dysgalactiae.*

Cow-to-cow transmission is important for the mammary reservoir group, whereas contamination of the teat end is important for the disease caused by the environmental group. The chances of new mammary gland infections in **dairy cows** caused by the environmental pathogens are greatest during the first and the last 2 weeks of 60-day non-lactating period. **Coliform** and **streptococcal infections** which are established during the non-lactating period from the environment are present at the time of parturition and cause clinical mastitis soon afterward.

Although haematogenous and percutaneous entries are possible, **the usual route is through the opening of the ductus papillaris** in the teat. Ductus papillaris is about 1 cm long keratinized, stratified squamous epithelium-lined duct between the exterior and the lactiferous sinus in the teat. **Bacteria colonizing the lining of the ductus papillaris multiply and persist and later cause intra-mammary infections.**

Non-Immune Defence Mechanisms in the Mammary Gland of the Cow

The **teat orifice** and the **ductus papillaris offer mechanical resistance to the entry of organisms. In cows,** a long ductus protects against mammary gland infection. The **keratin** of the ductus papillaris is protective by having **bactericidal fatty acids,** and by adsorbing bacteria and desquamating when coated with bacteria. Infection and inflammation of the ductus papillaris are rare.

The mammary gland has some intrinsic defence mechanisms which are not immune mediated. Regular milking of the mammary gland is a natural defence mechanism because of the flushing of organisms and products of inflammation from the gland. **Lactoferrin,** the major iron-binding protein of saliva and milk, is a non-specific natural protective factor in milk. **Lactoferrin concentration** is increased in acute mastitis and in the involuting gland. The binding of iron withholds an essential nutrient from pathogenic bacteria and thus has a **bacteriostatic effect.** The **lactoperoxidase-thiocyanate H_2O_2 system** temporarily inhibits some streptococci and coliforms and *Staphylococcus aureus.* **Lactoperoxidase is synthesized by mammary gland epithelium, thiocyanate** is derived from certain green feeds, and H_2O_2 is produced by streptococci or comes from an exogenous source. **Hypothiocyanite** produced by the system damages the inner bacterial membrane **killing the bacteria. Lysozyme,** synthesized locally or from blood, **destroys bacteria** by lysis of cell wall peptidoglycan. Of minor importance is **complement activation** by the alternate pathway in response to the presence of bacterial endotoxin.

Immune-Mediated Defence Mechanisms in the Mammary Gland

The **mechanisms** are divided into **cellular** and **humoral types.**

(i) Cellular Immune Defence Mechanisms

After the epithelial lining, the first elements that bacteria encounter in the cellular defence system are the **cells of the ductus papillaris and the rosette of Furstenberg.** The **rosette** is a circle of cells at the base of the lactiferous sinus in the teat. The rosette area is regarded as the site where the mammary gland proper begins. **The lamina propria of the ductus papillaris and Furstenberg's rosette has greater number of immunoglobulin-bearing leukocytes than parenchymal mammary gland tissue in both uninfected and infected quarters.** The sub-epithelial cells in the lamina propria near Furstenberg's rosette are predominantly **plasma cells,** and the main antibody produced is **IgG1.**

In the mammary gland, **resident macrophages are the detector cells against invading bacteria.** Macrophages are found in the alveoli and the interstitium, as well as in the lamina propria of the lactiferous sinus and interlobular and intralobular lactiferous ducts. **Macrophages are the most numerous cells in normal milk.** In the lactating cow, at least 5, 00,000 phagocytes per millilitre (ml) of milk are needed for defence of the mammary gland against invading bacteria. In the uninfected bovine mammary gland, 50,000 to 2, 00,000 neutrophils and macrophages are found per millilitre in milk, with the macrophages predominating.

Upon stimulation by microorganisms, macrophages in any tissue produce **interleukin-1,** which causes **increased membrane phospholipase activity,** releasing **arachidonic acid,** a substrate for the synthesis of **prostaglandins** and **leukotrienes. Milk macrophages secrete less interleukin-1 than blood macrophages. Leukotriene B4** produced by macrophages in any tissue is a powerful attractant of **neutrophils.** Whether leukotriene B4 is produced by macrophages is not clear.

Neutrophils are the main effector cells in eliminating bacteria from the mammary gland. The main method by which neutrophils kill bacteria is by **phagocytosis** after opsonization by antibody from blood, with or without complement from blood. A method of minor importance is lysis by antibody plus complement.

Recruitment of neutrophils from the blood to infection site is the first step in an inflammatory response. Recruitment is rapid, so that the neutrophils become the dominant cells as early as 2 hours after infection. Cell counts in milk can average 7, 00,000/ml in sub-clinically infected quarters, **and millions of neutrophils per ml are common in clinical infections.** When the neutrophil counts are at a peak **bactericidal activity** per cell is most efficient, by as much as 10,000-fold (times), and phagocytosis at its best. The **source of re-infection** of the mammary gland is **those neutrophils** which are inefficient at killing intracellular bacteria at the time of low cell count. As these cells undergo necrosis and lysis, their previously protected intracellular viable bacteria are released to multiply, and re-infection occurs.

Although **neutrophils** recruited from the blood are so important in fighting the infection in the mammary gland, **they do not kill bacteria as well in milk as they do in blood. Milk seems to be a poor medium for the functioning of neutrophils.** Some possible reasons are absence of glucose in milk for the glycolytic metabolism of neutrophils, decreased amounts of glycogen in milk neutrophils, deficiency of opsonins and complement in milk, coating of the surface of neutrophils with casein, loss of neutrophil pseudopodia caused by phagocytosis of fat, and decrease of hydrolytic enzymes within neutrophils after phagocytosis of casein and fat.

In the first week after parturition, when neutrophils are most needed to deal with mammary gland infections, **bovine blood neutrophils are already defective before they pass into the mammary gland.** They have defective chemokinesis (i.e., defective directional movement towards bacteria) and decreased superoxide anion production, antibody-dependent cell-mediated cytotoxicity, and phagocytosis of bacteria. In the parturient period (at parturition), the concentration of **glucocorticoid is increased.** This means that leukocyte function is less effective, because expression of L-selectin and CD18 on neutrophils is decreased by glucocorticoids. This, in turn, decreases adhesion between blood neutrophils and vascular endothelium and trans-endothelial migration of neutrophils.

The **tumour necrosis factor** (TNF) in mammary gland secretions increases in amount toward the end of gestation. This increase is accompanied by an increase in the number of **macrophages,** the source of TNF. **Bovine neutrophils do not respond to TNF in the same way as do neutrophils of other species.** Cattle treated with TNF have decreased numbers of neutrophils in blood, and exhibit decreased migration and decreased synthesis of reactive oxygen species. The large amount of TNF could contribute to the poor performance of bovine mammary gland neutrophils in the post-parturient period, **leading to establishment of bacteria in the gland.**

Interleukin-1 from mammary gland macrophages stimulates the immune system by activating T and B lymphocytes. Only a few **B-lymphocytes** are present in the mammary gland and milk. T-lymphocytes in normal mammary gland tissue and milk have a large proportion of **CD8$^+$ cells.** The **CD4$^+$/CD8$^+$ ratio is <1, reversed from that in the blood.** The mammary gland thus has selective lymphocyte trafficking, **favouring CD4+ cells**, which have either cytotoxic or suppressor function. CD4$^+$ T-lymphocytes (T-helper), which activate B-lymphocytes, CD8$^+$T-lymphocytes, and macrophages, are less in normal mammary gland tissues and milk. CD8$^+$ T-lymphocytes are found in lactiferous duct and alveolar epithelium, while less numbers of CD4$^+$ lymphocytes and B-cells are in clusters in the connective tissues. In early lactation, the CD8$^+$ lymphocytes in milk function more as suppressor cells (express interleukin- 4) than cytotoxic cells (express interferon-gamma), **but the situation is reversed in mid and late lactation.** Suppressor T-cells control, modulate, or suppress the immune responses, and cytotoxic T-cells act as scavengers, removing damaged mammary cells. **In response to bacterial infection, an influx of CD4$^+$ T-cells occurs in milk,** and these cells ultimately outnumber CD8$^+$ T-lymphocytes.

(ii) Humoral Immune Defence Mechanisms

Antibody concentration in normal bovine milk is small, about 1 mg/ml. **Most IgG is serum derived. IgG$_1$** is selectively transferred into mammary gland secretion and is the **major immunoglobulin class in milk. IgG$_2$** is both serum derived and locally produced by resident plasma cells. **IgA and IgM are synthesized locally in mammary gland. Local production** is caused by stimulation of sub-epithelial leukocytes. Particulate antigens, such as **bacteria,** stimulate an antibody response in the mammary gland of **cow, whereas soluble antigens do not. In colostrum** and in **milk from inflamed mammary glands,** antibody concentration approaches 50 mg/ml. Early in inflammation, **IgG$_1$** and **IgG$_2$** opsonize bacteria to increase phagocytosis by macrophages, but later importance of **IgG$_2$** as an opsonin increases as neutrophils enter the gland. Neutrophils transport **IgG$_2$** to the mammary gland as they move to the site of inflammation. **IgA does not opsonize,** but could prevent bacterial adherence to epithelium, inhibit bacterial multiplication, neutralize leukocyte-inhibiting bacterial toxins, and agglutinate bacteria.

Specific Pathogens in Mastitis

Streptococcal Mastitis

Streptococcus agalactiae is an important pathogen of the bovine mammary gland. Resistance of cows to mastitis caused by this organism decreases with age. **The mammary gland is the only organ affected by this organism.** *S. agalactiae* does not remain long in the environment. However, once a **cow** is infected, the organism persists in the lactiferous sinus, multiplies, increases its virulence, and invades tissue. The initial response is interstitial oedema and influx of neutrophils in the interstitium and alveoli. The alveolar epithelium undergoes either hyperplasia or vacuolation, and then is desquamated. Macrophages quickly infiltrate into the alveoli, and fibrosis obliterates the lumen of these alveoli. Oedema, cellular infiltration, and fibrosis are the lesions found in the infected and adjacent alveoli. This increases the pressure within the lobule and within adjacent lobules. The **increased pressure causes** stagnation of milk flow, initiating premature involution of a portion of the gland. After the acute phase, periductal fibrosis occurs and granulation tissue replaces part of the normal cuboidal to columnar epithelium of smaller ducts. **Fibrous polyps can completely obstruct milk flow.** Restoration of ductal epithelium can occur after the granulation tissue has matured and contracted.

The **gross appearance** of mammary gland with mastitis caused by *S. agalactiae* depends on the stage of the disease. **Usually more than one quarter is involved.** In the acute stage, hyperaemia involves the mucosa of the sinuses. **Milk quality is altered, and the milk is transformed into pus.** The areas of parenchymal oedema and cellular infiltrations are grey and swollen. Groups of alveoli in which the secretion is retained because of the obstruction of the duct by granulation tissue resemble **small abscesses.**

Staphylococcal Mastitis

Staphylococcus aureus isolates obtained from the bovine mammary gland range from **non-pathogenic** to **highly pathogenic.** Products released by staphylococci during their growth and the ability of the organisms to adhere to epithelial surfaces are important **virulence factors. The severest form of staphylococcal mastitis is the gangrenous form,** usually seen soon after parturition. Severe acute inflammation, with classical **heat, redness, swelling,** and **pain** progresses to necrosis. Affected necrotic area is cold, of blue-black colour, and shows exudation fluid and crepitation.

Microscopically, during the first 48 hours, the infected tissue has severe interstitial oedema which increases inter-alveolar stromal area and reduces alveolar luminal area. The organism attaches to epithelial cells, causing focal damage, and later can be seen within ductal and alveolar epithelium. Inflammatory cellular response is rapid. Neutrophils are initially in the sub-epithelial tissues of the distal parts of the duct system, then within the epithelium, and later in the interstitial and epithelial tissue of alveoli.

Staphyloccocal mastitis in the less acute form follows a course similar to that of the streptococcal mastitis. Organisms extend along the ducts rapidly and produce acute inflammation in groups of adjacent terminal alveoli. In chronically infected quarters, **macrophages** are the main inflammatory cell in epithelial lining, lumens, and especially, in the glandular interstitium. Lymphocytes also increase in number.

Staphylococcus aureus has a greater tendency than *Streptococcus agalactiae* for invading the interstitial tissue between alveoli. The initial inflammatory reaction is necrotizing, and abscess formation can follow. **Abscesses are scattered, and vary in size from being microscopic to those grossly visible. Sometimes the staphylococcal organisms are surrounded by rosettes of immunoglobulin-containing club-shaped material. The outdated term 'botryomycosis'** was applied to such lesions.

Coliform Mastitis

Coliform mastitis is caused after organisms from the **environment** contaminate the opening of the papillary duct at the end of the teat and ascend the duct. The most common organisms are *Escherichia coli, Enterobacter aerogenes*, and *Klebsiella pneumoniae*. The coliform organisms produce damage through **endotoxin** acting on the blood vessels. In the acute form of the disease,**lesions** are hyperaemia, haemorrhage, and oedema of the affected areas around the lactiferous ducts. The secretion in the lactiferous sinus is cloudy and blood stained and has clumps of fibrin. **Microscopically**, interlobular septa are oedematous. Epithelium of ducts and alveoli is necrotic and very few inflammatory cells are present in the alveoli. **Coliform organisms are numerous in the alveoli.** Large numbers of organisms are phagocytosed by the secretory epithelium. The cow's response to endotoxin is influenced by the stage of the reproductive cycle. **The non-lactating mammary gland is much less sensitive to the effects of endotoxin than the lactating gland.**

Actinomyces pyogenes causes mastitis in lactating, non-lactating, and even immature bovine mammary glands. It is characterized by **abscesses** in the tissue around the large and small lactiferous ducts. **Abscesses** range from those microscopic in size to those grossly visible. **Fistulas** from the abscesses can form at the base of the teat. The wall of the large abscesses is thickened by granulation tissue.

Mycoplasma Mastitis

Mycoplasma mastitis in **cows** occurs in herds in which the conventional forms of the bacterial mastitis have been eliminated. Several mycoplasmas can cause bovine mastitis, but *Mycoplasma bovis* is the most prevalent. It tends to involve the whole gland, with marked purulent exudate in the early stages. Affected quarters are enlarged, firm, light brown, and have a nodular parenchyma. **Abscesses** can be up to 10 cm in diameter. Exudation of **neutrophils** in the lobular interstitium and alveoli is intense. The exudate changes with chronicity to include mononuclear cells. Early changes are followed by hyperplasia of alveolar and ductal epithelium, and the metaplasia of the epithelial lining. Aggregates of lymphocytes occur in the lobular interstitium. **Interstitial fibrosis** and **lobular atrophy** are seen in the late stages.

Tuberculous Mastitis

Tuberculous mastitis occurs in three forms: (1) **miliary**, (2) **organ**, and (3) **caseous**. All fórms involve the lactiferous ducts. The **miliary form** has multiple nodules less than 1 cm in diameter. The **organ form** has larger nodules, whereas **caseous tuberculosis form** has large irregular **caseous areas. In the cow**, *Mycobacterium bovis* arrives at the mammary gland **haematogenously** from organs with previously established tubercles. In most cases, the first lesions are in the interalveolar and interlobular connective tissue which later spread to the ducts. **Most cases are of the organ type,** but a few are of the **miliary type,** which occurs with the massive release of organisms into an organ. Cases of the **caseous type** occur when the immune response of the organ to the bacteria is especially suppressed. **Microscopically, the miliary type** consists of **classical tubercles,** with **central caseation** surrounded by a zone of epithelioid macrophages and multinucleate giant cells, bounded by lymphocytes and fibrous tissue. In the more common organ type, the same cellular elements are present but are not organized into tubercles.

Iatrogenic Granulomatous Mastitis

This has been reported in the **cow** when drugs for mastitis treatment are introduced through the teat and are contaminated with *Nocardia asteroides*, *Cryptococcus neoformans*, and **Mycobacterium** sp. other than *M. bovis*, or **Candida** sp. **Nocardiosis** can also be spontaneous mammary gland disease, from organisms normally resident in the soil. **Clinical signs** of the disease are systemic illness and the presence of discharging sinuses from the mammary gland through the skin. An udder affected with **cryptococcal mastitis** has the same yellow gelatinous material that is typical of cryptococcal lesions elsewhere.

Non-Bovine Mastitis

Progressive pneumonia can cause **mastitis in sheep.** Clinical signs and gross lesions are mostly absent, but microscopic lesions include diffuse interstitial accumulation of lymphocytes and focal degeneration of ductal epithelium in the mammary gland. **In more severe cases,** lesions include periductal lymphoid nodules with germinal centres and hyperplasia, vacuolation, and focal necrosis of overlying epithelium. The mammary gland is highly susceptible to non-oncogenic **lentivirus** and spread of the virus is facilitated through the milk.

Caprine arthritis-encephalitis virus, a closely related lentivirus found in **goats,** is associated with diffuse and nodular infiltration of lymphocytes and a few macrophages around ducts in the mammary gland. In this disease also, **mammary gland is an important target organ** and allows transmission of the virus through the colostrum from doe (female goat) to kid (young goat).

Mycoplasma agalactiae causes **mastitis in sheep** and **goats** in Mediterranean countries and in the United States. In the systemic disease, localization of inflammation occurs in the joints and eyes as well as the **mammary gland.** The glands are firm, swollen, and have thick yellow secretions.

Pasteurella haemolytica causes **mastitis in lactating ewes,** and sometimes also causes rhinitis and pneumonia in their lambs. The acute phase is characterized by swelling of the mammary gland and by a watery secretion instead of milk. If the disease is not fatal, **abscess formation** is followed by sloughing of the affected side of the gland.

Coliform mastitis plays an important role in the clinical syndrome of **mastitis-metritis-agalactia** in **sows**.

Mastitis is not common in dogs and cats. When it does occur, it is an extension from minor lesions of the nipples, or to be superimposed on mammary hyperplasia or neoplasia. The organisms mostly involved are streptococci and staphylococci, which in the acute phase tend to cause suppurative or necrotizing inflammation, respectively.

Hyperplasia

Hyperplasia of mammary gland is **important only in dogs**. It occurs in **two forms**, in **older dogs**:

1. **Cystic glandular hyperplasia (fibrocystic disease):** This is characterized by dilated cysts and acini in a dense fibrous connective tissue containing mononuclear leukocytes. The cause is unknown.

2. **Lobular hyperplasia:** This is characterized by nodules of acinar and ductular tissues, with or without an increase in connective tissue.

Neoplasms

Neoplasms of the mammary gland are **most important in dogs**. They also occur in **cats**, but much less frequently than in dogs. **In the dog**, neoplasms of the mammary gland are second in frequency only to neoplasms of the skin. Interestingly, **in cattle, mammary neoplasms are practically unknown. In dogs**, they are **most common in older female dogs** and are rarely seen in males. The inguinal lymph nodes are often affected and multiple neoplasms are common. Hormones play some role in their pathogenesis, as the incidence is considerably lower in bitches spayed (ovaries surgically removed) at an early age. **In cats** also, mammary neoplasms are most frequent in older individuals. No hormonal influence has been identified in cats.

Adenoma

These are **of two types**:

1. **Intraductal adenomas (intraductal papillomas)** are composed of well differentiated papillary growth within a dilated, or cystic interlobular duct. They are usually single, roughly spherical lesions projecting into a duct. The neoplastic cells are cuboidal and form a single row of cells on a core of connective tissue. If the cells pile up, the neoplasms could be potentially malignant.

2. **Acinar adenomas** originate from acinar epithelium, or small intralobular ducts. They are well circumscribed nodules. The cells closely resemble normal acinar epithelium, and usually there is little connective tissue.

Adenocarcinoma

Adenocarcinomas originate from epithelial lining the interlobular ducts, or acinar and intralobular ductal epithelial cells. **They are of different types:**

Papillary adenocarcinomas originate from the epithelial lining interlobular or major ducts. When present within a duct, they are called **'intraductal papillary adenocarcinomas'.** They grow as papillary projections. The cells are pleomorphic and anaplastic. Their characteristic feature is invasion. Groups of cells can be seen extending into lymphatics. If the neoplastic tubules are cystic, the tumour is called **'papillary cystadenocarcinoma'.**

Tubular adenocarcinomas also originate from interlobular or major ducts, but their mode of growth is not papillary. **These are the most common form of adenocarcinomas of the mammary gland in dogs. Microscopically,** they are characterized by uniformly sized tubules lined by single or multi-layered cuboidal or columnar epithelial cells.

Lobular (acinar) adenocarcinomas resemble tubular adenocarcinomas, but the glands more closely resemble acini rather than tubules, and the neoplastic cells are smaller. **Scirrhous adenocarcinomas** may be of tubular or papillary type, but are accompanied by a marked fibroblastic proliferation which differentiates to mature collagenous connective tissue.

Mixed Neoplasms

These neoplasms contain neoplastic proliferation of both **epithelial** and **mesenchymal tissue. They are the most common mammary neoplasm in the dog. In the cat,** they are rare, but not non-existent. The neoplasm consists of the glandular tissue, myxomatous connective tissue, cartilage, and bone. Any one of the tissues can constitute the major part of the primary neoplasm, or of its metastases. Thus, tumours consisting mainly of cartilage or bone are not rare. **All mixed neoplasms are potentially malignant.** The epithelial or mesenchymal elements can be invasive, and resemble typical adenocarcinoma, osteosarcoma, chondrosarcoma etc.

Sarcomas

Osteosarcomas, chondrosarcomas, fibrosarcomas, and liposarcomas are not uncommon in the mammary gland of the **dog,** but **rare in all other species.**

Muscle

Several aspects of normal muscle fibre morphology and physiology are important in the understanding of muscle pathology. **Structural** and **physiological features** of skeletal muscles determine much of its response to injury.

Structural Features

Although **muscle cells** are usually called **muscle fibres** or **myofibres**, they are in fact multinucleated cells of considerable length, which in some animals may approach one metre. This feature has an important effect on the **process of regeneration**. Under favourable conditions, muscle cells are able to restore themselves after a segment has become necrotic. **Segmental necrosis (segmentation/fragmentation)** is a common reaction of a myofibre to a wide variety of insults. Also the physiological features of a muscle fibre, namely, its rate of contraction and type of metabolism (oxidative, anaerobic, or mixed), are determined not by the muscle cell itself **but by the neuron responsible for its innervation, the ventral horn, or the brain stem motor neurons** (Fig. 46). This fact is important in evaluating histological changes in muscle fibres. **Changes in muscle fibres can be divided into two major classes: neuropathic and myopathic. Neuropathic changes** are those that are determined by its nerve supply, for example, atrophy after denervation. **Myopathic changes** or 'myopathy' include those muscle diseases where the primary change takes place in the muscle cell, not in the interstitial tissue and **are not secondary to effects of the nerve supply.** Myopathies include some types of myofibre degeneration, **for example**, metabolic myopathies, muscle dystrophies, myofibre necrosis, and inflammatory conditions **affecting the myofibre itself, not the interstitium.**

In the past, there has been some confusion regarding use of the term **'sarcolemma'.** The word **'sarcolemma'** has been used in three different ways by pathologists: (1) for the **plasmalemma** (i.e., plasma membrane covering a striated muscle fibre), (2) for plasmalemma plus basal lamina, and (3) for the endomysium plus basal lamina. **Electron microscopy has revealed that myofibre's plasmalemma** (plasma membrane) is in close contact with basal lamina (see Fig. 48A) and outside this basal lamina is an interlacing network of fine reticular fibrils that form the endomysium (Fig. 48A). That is, endomysium surrounds each muscle fibre. **The key structure in the 'sarcolemma' is the basal lamina.** Basal lamina is a layer of the basement membrane. In myofibre necrosis, the myofibre's plasmalemma

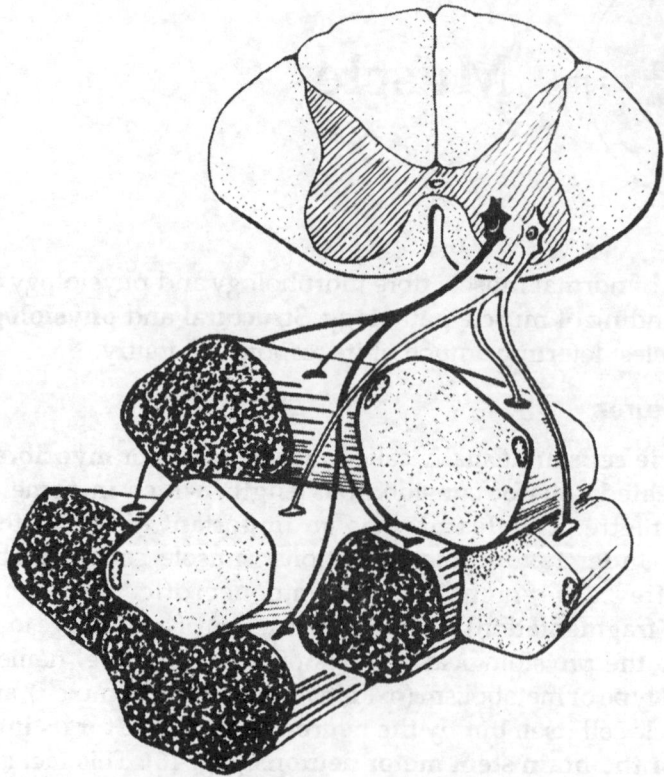

Fig. 46 Schematic diagram of motor unit and muscle fibre types. All myofibres innervated by the one motor neuron are of the same fibre type. Thus, the motor neuron determines whether the myofibres are **type I** (light) or **type II** (dark).

disappears, **but the basal lamina remains** and is the basic component of the 'sarcolemmal tube'. **The basal lamina is resistant to insults that destroy the myofibre.** It can be penetrated by macrophages which enter to remove necrotic debris **and is responsible for orderly regeneration** (see 'regeneration'). In this chapter, the term **'sarcolemmal tube'** is used for the tube formed by the basal lamina.

Physiological Features

Mammalian **muscles are composed of muscle fibres of different contractile properties.** This is based on their three main features: (1) rate of contraction (fast or slow), (2) rate of fatigue (fast or slow), and (3) type of metabolism (oxidative, glycolytic, or mixed). Based on various physiological and histochemical features, **muscle fibres are divided into two types – type I and type II fibres (Table 13).** **Type I fibres** are low in myosin adenosine triphosphatase (ATPase) activity, rich in mitochondria, oxidative in metabolism, slow-contracting, and slow-fatiguing fibres. **Type II fibres** are rich in myosin ATPase, have fewer mitochondria, and are glycolytic, fast-contracting fibres. **Type II fibres are further divided into type IIA and type IIB (Table 13).** Type IIB are the fast-contracting, fast-fatiguing, glycolytic fibres (FF) that depend on glycogen for their energy supply. **Type IIA** are mixed oxidative-glycolytic, and therefore, although fast contracting, are also slow fatiguing (FR). Thus, type IIA fibres are 'intermediate' in the concentration of mitochondria and myosin ATPase activity between type I and type IIB, and are also known as **'intermediate fibres'.**

Type I and type II muscle fibres can be differentiated under the microscope by histochemical methods. **ATPase stains differentiate between type I and type II fibres,** because they produce a 'checker-board-like pattern' (like chess board) of light (type I) and dark (type II) staining fibres (see Fig. 46). This is because, as already stated, type I fibres are low in myosin ATPase (hence lightly stained) and type II are rich in ATPase (hence darkly stained).

Most muscles contain both type I and type II fibres. They are easily demonstrated by the **myosin ATPase reaction** (see Fig. 46). The percentage of each fibre type varies from muscle to muscle and within the same muscle. However, there is some correlation with function. **Type I fibres** (slow contracting, slow fatiguing, oxidative) are in abundance in those muscles whose main function is to maintain posture, support the weight of the animal, and slow locomotion. Muscles that contract quickly, for running very fast, contain more **type IIB fibres.** Muscles that contract slowly and continuously, for example, ruminant's masticatory muscles, contain a high percentage of type I fibres. **Rarely are muscles composed of only one type of fibre,** for example, the vastus intermedius muscle in the leg of sheep is type I. Athletic training causes some type B fibres to be converted to IIA, and this is the basis of the 'training effect'. There are also variations within breeds and differences in the same muscle in different species, for example, **the dog has no type IIB fibres.**

Table 13. Relationship between histochemical and physiological classification of myofibres

	Histochemical Features	Biochemical features	Physiological features
Type I	Low myosin ATPase activity , heavy mitochondrial staining	SO = Slow twitch oxidative	S = Slow contracting
Type IIA	Intermediate ATPase activity, heavy mitochondrial staining	FOG = Fast twitch oxidative- glycolytic	FR = Fast contracting, fatigue resistant
Type IIB	High ATPase activity, light mitochondrial staining	FG = Fast twitch glycolytic-	FF = Fast contracting, fast fatiguing

Examination of Muscles

The most common change in muscle samples submitted for routine histopathological examination is **artefact**. This aspect therefore needs attention, and has been discussed under microscopic examination.

1. Gross Examination

Gross examination includes evaluation of changes in shape, colour, texture, and volume (atrophy or hypertrophy). **Subjective assessment of size and colour of muscles can be misleading.** The variation in the percentage of type I and type II fibres affects muscle's colour. **Type II fibres** are light (called **'white fibres'**; e.g., the pectoral muscles of a chicken). **Type I fibres** are dark (called **'red fibres'**; e.g., the pectoral muscles of a duck). **Muscles** which are formed **of mainly type II fibres** such as semi-membranosus (made up in part of membrane or fascia) and semi-tendinosus (in part having a tendinous structure), **are pale.** On the other hand, **muscles in which type I myofibres predominate,** such as the canine superficial digital flexor and the bovine masseter, **are dark red. Therefore, a pale muscle is not necessarily undergoing degeneration. However, muscles undergoing necrosis are pale,** and these lesions appear as clear streaks or foci, or even involve large areas of a muscle (e.g., an infarction). If necrotic areas **calcify,** they are glistening chalky-white foci or streaks. **Muscles** infiltrated by fat (e.g., steatosis) **are also pale.**

Other discolorations visible grossly are from pigment. The most important pigment is **lipofuscin,** the so-called **'wear-and-tear-pigment'** that accumulates in secondary lysosomes which are later converted into small, compact aggregates known in electron microscopy as **'residual bodies'.** The tendency to store lipofuscin is not the same in all domestic animals. It is **greatest in the skeletal muscles of cattle,** particularly old high-producing dairy cattle. The masseter and diaphragm (two hard-working muscles) are the most commonly affected. **The lesion is of no clinical importance.** Its significance at postmortem in muscles and other organs such as myocardium, neurons, liver, kidney, and adrenal cortex is that it **indicates old age, or of past or present condition of cachexia or starvation.** The characteristic microscopic appearance in skeletal muscle consists of rounded granules of yellow-brown to dark brown pigment at the two poles (ends) of the nucleus of the myofibre.

Sometimes **melanin** discolours the fascial sheaths and epimysium of muscles in the syndrome of **congenital melanosis in calves.** In this, **melanocytes** are present within the fascial sheaths and epimysium. The pigment appears grossly as black foci or streaks. Muscle fibres themselves are unaffected, and the pigmentation has no clinical significance.

Myoglobin may discolour muscles after extensive muscle necrosis, known as **rhabdomyolysis** (discussed below). Damage to the myofibre's cell membrane allows myoglobin to leak into the adjacent tissues. This leakage is seen only if muscle necrosis is extensive and sudden, as in crush injuries or in the early stages of a toxicosis (e.g., monensin poisoning in **horses**). It is actually the result of an acute necrosis. Another cause of localized coloured areas in muscle is from injections of medicines, for example, tetracycline (yellow) and iron dextran (dark brown).

Thus, a complete postmortem includes palpation of and multiple incisions into muscles. Incisions should be less than 1 cm apart in order not to overlook small foci, such as very early lesions in blackquarter (blackleg). **Clinical findings should be used to determine which muscles are most likely to have lesions.**

Microscopic Examination

Muscle is made to contract when stimulated, and if still irritable when placed in fixative, it will contract. This artefactual (not natural) contraction of myofibres varies in severity. Contraction of a certain length of myofibres can result in that segment being **deeply eosinophilic and round in cross section.** Such fibres have been **confused with hyalinized fibres.**

Because contraction artefacts make it difficult to detect lesions at microscopic examination, **their prevention at the time of fixation is important. Contraction depends on two mechanisms:** (1) an energy supply available to the myofibre to allow it to contract, and (2) lack of the restraint of the muscle sample when it is placed in fixative. **If the muscle is depleted of energy (e.g., glycogen) it will not contract in the fixative.** This occurs in muscles from emaciated animals, animals dying of septicaemia, or diseases of long duration, if there is a long delay between death and fixation, or if rigor mortis has passed. **To produce a section best suited for microscopic examination, muscle samples must not twist or contract during fixation.** Both of these are likely to occur in unrestrained muscle samples placed in fixative.

After fixation, both transverse and longitudinal sections should be cut from each muscle for histological examination. Myofibre diameters and the percentage of abnormal myofibres are best evaluated in transverse sections. However, longitudinal sections show the length of changes, such as segmental necrosis and the length of the nuclear rows.

Enzyme Histochemistry

Histological examination of fixed muscles is used routinely for the detection of inflammatory and degenerative changes in muscle. However, **myofibre typing** was done only on frozen sections. **Recently, immuno-histochemical staining of myosin has been developed for demonstration of myofibre types in formalin-fixed muscle.** This is a great advantage because now two samples – one for formalin fixation and the other for freezing – do not have to be taken at the time of postmortem and biopsy. Moreover, the myofibre typing can now be limited to those muscles in which lesions are confirmed microscopically. **Fibre-type staining is absolutely essential for the complete evaluation of muscle.** It is very useful in demonstrating greater involvement of a particular fibre type, as in some muscular dystrophies or neuropathic changes such as those due to denervation and re-innervation, resulting in fibre type grouping.

Rigor Mortis

Immediately after the death of an animal, the muscles are still alive biochemically. However, as energy stores are used a sequence of changes takes place. These result in contraction and stiffening of muscles that fix the positions of joints. This stiffening of muscles in a dead body is known as **'rigor mortis'**. Muscles are affected in a specific sequence: jaws, trunk, and then extremities. Rigor passes off in the same order as onset and does not return. Usually the onset begins 2 to 6 hours after death, reaches a maximum at 24 to 48 hours, and passes off in another 48 hours – **a total of about 4 days. However, rigor mortis varies so much in routine postmortem examination that it has little value in interpretation**. Once the basic mechanism is defined, variations in the rapidity and severity of rigor can be understood.

In muscle contraction, actin and myosin filaments slide past each other powered by myosin heads attached to actin-binding sites. **ATP (adenosine triphosphate) is necessary for muscle relaxation after normal contraction.** Rigor occurs when majority of the myosin heads remain attached to actin-binding sites at the end of the 'power stroke'. ATP can be reconstituted from adenosine diphosphate (ADP). The energy is supplied either by glycolysis or by phosphocreatine. Factors that control the rate of onset of rigor mortis include the **amount of glycogen stores, pH of muscles, and body temperature.** Therefore, if glycogen stores have been reduced by starvation or vigorous muscle contractions, as occurs in animals dying from **tetanus** or **strychnine poisoning** or after being **chased during hunting, onset of rigor is rapid.** However, in cachectic animals with little of no energy stores, rigor may be slight or in extremely emaciated animals, may not even occur at all. Rigor disappears by autolysis or putrefaction (bacterial decomposition). **Thus, the basic factor in the delay in onset and strength of rigor is the energy stores of the muscle in the form of ATP, phosphocreatine, or glycogen at the time of death.** One important effect of rigor is to interfere with the histological examination of muscle.

Response of Muscle to Injury

The response of any organ to injury is the sum total of the responses of each of the tissues or cells that compose it. **Muscle is composed of myofibres** surrounded by blood vessels and fibroblasts (endomysium) and penetrated by blood vessels and nerves. **The cell to respond to injury is the myofibre.** Unfortunately its range of response to injury is extremely limited, and apart from those involving its nerve supply, the main response of the myofibre is **degeneration, necrosis,** and **regeneration**. These responses are the end result of a wide variety of injuries such as **trauma, ischaemia, infarction** (e.g., bluetongue in **sheep** resulting from vasculitis), **metabolic diseases** caused by nutritional deficiencies (e.g., vitamin E, selenium), **toxic myopathies,** and **infections** such as gas gangrene.

Degeneration

The term **'degeneration'** in general pathology means a potentially reversible injury. **In muscle pathology,** it is loosely applied and includes **reversible changes** such as the 'vascular degeneration' caused by hypokalaemia (low potassium levels in the body) and hyperkalaemia (excess of potassium in the blood), autophagic vacuoles, and sometimes, even necrosis. In this chapter, the term is used for changes that may or may not lead to myofibre death, and for some miscellaneous categories, such as **calcification** and **ossification. Thus, the term degeneration includes the following:**

1. **'True degenerations':** cellular swelling, hydropic, vacuolar, granular, and fatty

2. Calcification

3. **Ossification,** and

4. Cyto-architectural changes

1. True Degenerations

When muscle is injured metabolically from a wide variety of causes, the final result is **segmental necrosis (i.e. segmentation or breakdown of a muscle fibre). The muscle** fibres go through a series of degenerations before becoming frankly necrotic, or in some less severely affected fibres, the degenerations may be reversed and the fibre returned to normal. The **earliest detectable change** starts in the individual myofibre as **extremely fine vacuoles** that are hardly visible by light microscope. After hours to a day, these **vacuoles become larger** and are then relatively easy to detect microscopically (Fig. 47). **If the degeneration is not reversed,** the fibre or a

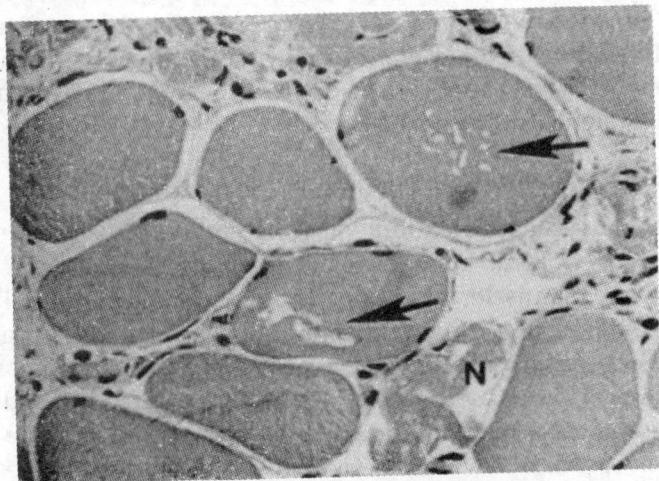

Fig. 47. Muscle; cow. Early **vacuolar degeneration (arrows)** has progressed to segmental necrosis (**N**) in an adjacent myofibre. H & E stain.

segment of it progresses to **floccular, granular, hyaline, and Zenker's degeneration. All these are different stages of necrosis.**

Vacuolar degenerations are caused by swelling of organelles or accumulation of glycogen or fat within the myofibre. If there is a mild damage to the myofibre, **the vacuoles are autophagic.** These phagosomes are membrane-bound vacuoles in which damaged organelles undergo autodigestion by fusion with a lysosome. **Glycogen vacuoles** occur in **Pompe's disease,** or glycogen-storage disease seen in **cattle. Neutral lipid droplets** are present in myofibres in lipid-storage diseases. Both hypokalaemia and hyperkalaemia cause vascular degeneration of myofibres, which can lead to myofibre necrosis.

2. Calcification

The causes of calcification are:

1. Calcification of necrotic muscle fibres,
2. Calcification of fibres in extreme old age,
3. Rare cases of gross calcification of unknown cause of parts or most of a muscle, and
4. Segmental calcification in diseases with defects of the myofibre's plasmalemma, e.g., in canine X-linked muscular dystrophy

Calcification is the next step in the necrosis of individual myofibres and is **prominent in some domestic animals (e.g., sheep).** The deposits may be so dense as to be visible grossly as glistening, chalky-white foci or steaks. Calcification of myofibres is a common finding in small donkeys (burros) over 40 years of age. Gross calcification of a large portion of a muscle is rare. The cause is unknown. **Ingestion of toxic plants** that contain an active vitamin D metabolite (*Solanum malacoxlyn*) causes **widespread calcification** that sometimes includes tendons and ligaments (*C. diurum* in **horses**) but does not involve skeletal muscles.

3. Ossification

In the past, **ossification** was called **myositis ossificans,** which means formation of non-neoplastic bone, cartilage, or both in extra-osseous sites, which may or may not be in muscle. **It is basically a metaplasia to bone.** The disease has been reported in **horses, pigs, dogs, and cats** and is divided into **progressive** and **localized forms.** The **generalized form** is better called **'fibrodysplasia ossificans progressiva',** rather than myositis ossificans progressiva, **because it is a disorder of connective tissue associated with skeletal muscle, and the muscle itself is only secondarily involved.** It has been described in **pigs** and **cats.** The **pig** disease is inherited, but this link has not been proved in **cats. Lesions may replace large portions of the muscle.**

The **microscopic appearance** is of interlacing bundles of dense, fibrous connective tissue, containing dense accumulations of calcium, cartilage, and bone. The hyperplastic connective tissue compresses the adjacent skeletal muscles. This type has been seen in **horses** and **dogs.**

4. Cyto-Architectural Changes

There are a number of 'degenerations' peculiar to myofibres. These include target fibres, central cores, moth-eaten fibres, myofibrillar whorls, tubular aggregates, and nemaline rods. Some of these are visible only in histochemical preparation (e.g., target fibres and in sections treated with oxidative enzyme stains), and in other cases the lesions are visible only by electron microscopy.

Necrosis

Because myofibres are long, **local physical injuries cause necrosis of only a segment.** Toxic, metabolic, and nutritional myopathies also cause **segmental necrosis. Total necrosis of myofibres is rare**, occurring in extensive infarcts, massive trauma, and large burns. **Therefore, segmental myofibre necrosis is present after many different types of injuries.** That is, **segmental necrosis is a type of 'final common pathway'.** This stage of necrosis quickly merges into **regeneration,** described below. Necrotic portions of myofibres have different microscopic appearances. Necrotic portions of the fibre may become **floccular** or **granular** because that portion of the myofibre starts to **break into fragments.** The neighbouring microscopically normal portion of the myofibre may separate from the necrotic segment, forming retraction caps. Sometimes, necrotic segments of myofibres are mineralized.

Once the plasma membrane of the myofibre is damaged or a segment of the myofibre becomes necrotic, some of the contents of the cell leak out and are taken up into the blood. **The concentrations of some of these components in serum are used as an index of the extent of myofibre damage.** The most commonly used is **creatine kinase (CK). Aspartate aminotransferase (AST),** earlier known as serum glutamic-oxaloacetic transaminase (SGOT) is also released, but it is not as specific an indicator of muscle damage **because it is also present in hepatocytes and cardiac myocytes.** Because CK has a low renal threshold, it is quickly excreted in the urine. The half-life of AST in the serum is much longer, however, **and serum AST concentrations remain elevated for several days following muscle injury.** The term 'rhabdomyolysis' was coined to replace myoglobinuria and draw attention to the fact that rhabdomyolysis indicates muscle damage.

Regeneration

Skeletal muscle has great ability to regenerate. Under most favourable conditions, a necrotic segment of a muscle fibre can be repaired so efficiently that it cannot be differentiated from the normal. However, the success of regeneration depends on the **extent and nature of the injury** and also on **whether** the integrity of the **supporting stroma** around the muscle fibre (sarcolemmal tube) **is intact**. It will be helpful first to consider the **sequence of events** that occur under best conditions.

If a portion of the muscle fibre is damaged, for example by a toxin, and the sarcolemmal tube (i.e., basal lamina and endomysium) is intact, **the sequence of events is as described below.** However, some 'stages' overlap with others. **The sequence of events is shown diagrammatically in Fig. 48.**

1. **In the necrotic segment**, the muscle nuclei disappear, and in H & E-stained sections, the **sarcoplasm** (the cytoplasm of muscle cells) and **myofibrils** (contractile filaments found within the cytoplasm of striated muscle cells) become hyalinized (i.e., eosinophilic, amorphous, and homogeneous), indicating the loss of normal myofibrillar structure (Fig. 48B). The necrotic portion may separate from the adjacent viable myofibre during contraction (Figs. 48C and 49A). **In some species, the necrotic fibre may be mineralized.**

2. Within 24 to 48 hours, and usually between 1 and 4 days, **monocytes** emigrate from capillaries, become **macrophages** and enter the necrotic portion of the myofibre (Fig. 48D and 49B). Neutrophils may also be present initially, but they rapidly disappear because they die. As a result, the **satellite cells**, normally located between the basal lamina and the myofibre's plasmalemma (plasma membrane), begin to enlarge (Fig. 48C), become vesicular with prominent nucleoli, and then undergo mitosis.

3. The proliferated **satellite cells** move from the peripheral location to the centre of muscle fibre, among the macrophages (Fig. 48D and 49B).

4. **Macrophages lyse and phagocytose** necrotic debris and form a clear space in the sarcolemmal tube (i.e., between basal lamina and endomysium). At the same time the plasmalemma disappears, and the shape of the sarcolemmal tube is maintained by the basal lamina.

5. **Satellite cells form myoblasts. Myoblasts** are embryonic cells containing myofibrillar protein such as myosin. **Myoblasts form muscle cells.** Myoblasts fuse with one another to form **myotubes**, which are thin, elongated muscle cells with a row of central, closely spaced nuclei. They send out cytoplasmic processes in both directions within the sarcolemmal tube (Fig. 48C). When the processes contact each other or a viable portion of the original muscle fibre, in most cases they fuse. At this stage, the regenerating fibre is characterized by basophilia, internal nuclei that are sometimes in rows, a lack of striations, and a narrower than normal diameter (Fig. 48E and F).

6. **The fibre grows and differentiates.** Its diameter increases, and longitudinal and cross striations appear, indicating the formation of sarcomeres (cross-striation).

7. **Between 1 and 3 weeks after the initial injury, the muscle nuclei** move to the 'sarcolemmal' or peripheral position, that is, the normal position for muscle nuclei in mature mammalian muscle. **However, there are species differences.**

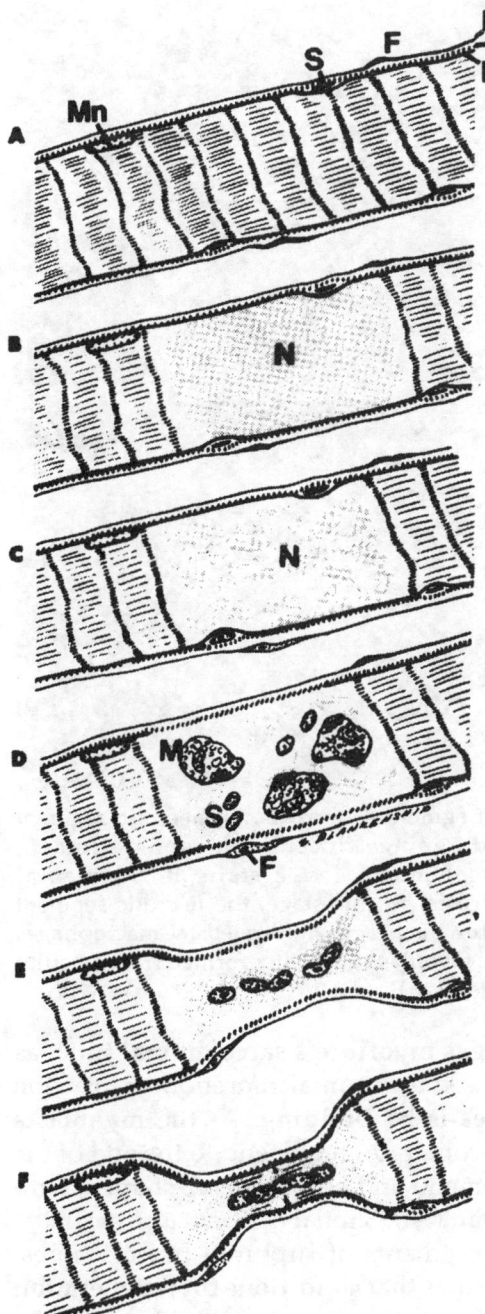

Fig. 48. Diagrammatic representation of segmental myofibre necrosis and regeneration. A. Longitudinal section of **normal muscle fibre**. E, endomysium; F, fibroblast; BL, basal lamina; Pl, plasmalemma; Mn, muscle nucleus; S, satellite cell, which lies between the basal lamina and plasmalemma. **B. Segmental necrosis.** Coagulative necrosis (N). **C. The necrotic segment** of myofibre (N) has become **floccular and detached** from the adjacent viable portion of the myofibre. The **satellite cells** are enlarging. **D.** The necrotic segment of the myofibre has been **invaded by macrophages (M) and satellite cells (S). Satellite cells will develop into myoblasts.** (Myoblasts are embryonic cells which become muscle cells.) The plasmalemma of the necrotic segment has disappeared. **E. Myoblasts have formed a myotube,** which has produced **sarcoplasm**. This extends to meet the viable ends of the myofibre. The integrity of the myofibre is maintained by the sarcolemmal tube formed by the basal lamina and endomysium. **F. Regenerating myofibre.** Note the reduction in myofibre diameter and **central row of nuclei.** There is early formation of sarcomeres (cross-striations), and the plasmalemma has re-formed. **Such fibres stain basophilic with H & E stain.**

The success of regeneration depends on the following:

1. The **presence of an intact basal lamina** to contain and guide the proliferating myotube cells and to keep fibroblasts out.

2. The **availability of viable satellite cells** as a source of nuclei to undergo mitosis to form myonuclei necessary to initiate the production of sarcoplasm. Normal mature myonuclei have lost this ability. Therefore, segmental necrosis in which sarcolemmal tubes are preserved, as in metabolic (nutritional and toxic) myopathies, regenerate very successfully. However, when large areas of satellite cells are killed, for example, by heat or infarction, the situation is very different. **In this case, a return to normal is not possible, and healing is mainly by fibrosis.**

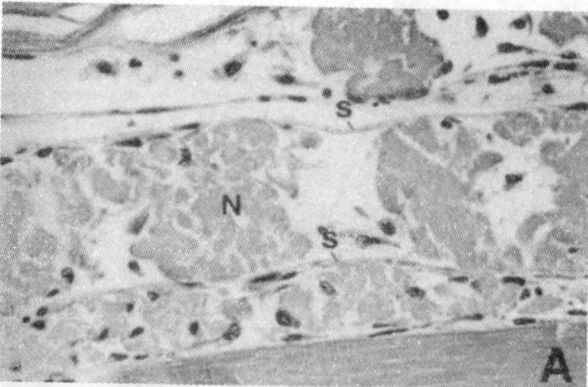

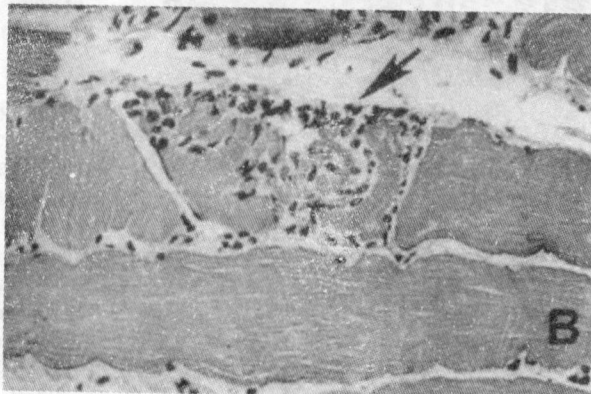

Fig. 49. A. Segmental necrosis. N, necrotic segment undergoing 'floccular' degeneration. S, Sarcolemma. H & E stain. B. Segmental necrosis. At this stage, the necrotic segment (arrow) is heavily infiltrated by **macrophages** and **myoblasts**, the latter **formed from satellite cells**. H & E stain.

Regeneration by Budding

If injury to the muscle is severe and damages myofibre's sarcolemmal tube, as occurs in destructive lesions such as those caused by trauma, infarction, or injection of irritants, **regeneration in those myofibres is by budding.** As the **myoblasts** (embryonic cells which form muscle fibres) proliferate and extend to the end of the ruptured tube, sarcolemma bulges from its cut end and becomes club shaped, with numerous internal nuclei forming **a muscle giant cell.** Similar cells can also originate from satellite cells remaining in scattered fragments of ruptured muscle fibres. Thus, the **presence of muscle giant cells indicates that conditions for regeneration are not favourable.** Myotubes (i.e., developing muscle cells or fibres with a centrally rather than peripherally located nucleus) are able to bridge gaps of 2 to 4 mm, **but longer ones heal by fibrosis, which reduces elasticity and efficiency of muscle contraction.**

Histopathological Interpretation

Segmental necrosis and **regeneration** are the most common result of a wide variety of injuries. Therefore, a histological diagnosis of **'segmental necrosis'** is usually not helpful in deciding the cause of the disease. **However, the usefulness of this histological diagnosis is due to:** (1) difference between lesions confined to one or multiple sites, and of (2) whether lesions were all at one stage, for example, segmental necrosis without macrophages, or at different stages, for example, segmental necrosis and regeneration.

Based on this a concept of **monofocal** (or focal) **versus multifocal** and **monophasic versus multiphasic lesions**, has been introduced. **Monofocal lesions** are those confined to one site and could be the result of a single incident of trauma, such as an intramuscular injection. **Most systemic diseases cause necrosis at multiple sites.** However, the concept of monophasic versus multiphasic is more helpful. If there were only one injury, for example, a single event of extremely strenuous exercise (**exertional myopathy**) or a toxin being fed on one occasion (e.g., a horse eating one dose of monensin), then at postmortem, **all lesions would be at the same stage of necrosis or regeneration.** However, if the injury were ongoing, such as occurs in vitamin E-selenium deficiency or in continuous feeding of a toxin, then new lesions (segmental necrosis) would form at the same time when regeneration was taking place. **In other words, it would be a multiphasic disease.** Using this approach, it is sometimes possible to rule out a diagnosis (e.g.; vitamin E-selenium deficiency is usually multiphasic), **but this is not a hard and fast rule.** In **cattle** with borderline concentration of vitamin E and selenium and on pasture, a sudden stress can cause a monophasic necrosis.

Congenital, Neonatal, and Hereditary Diseases

Muscle is subject to many **hereditary, congenital,** and **neonatal defects (Table 14). These are discussed in some detail under the myopathies of each species of domestic animal.**

Muscular Dystrophy

The **term 'muscular dystrophy' is unclear and rather confusing** in veterinary medicine. It was introduced in human pathology to define a group of inherited progressive muscle diseases. In the 1930s, the term nutritional muscular dystrophy was applied in veterinary medicine to describe nutritional myopathy due to vitamin E deficiency, **which was wrong.** It should have been termed **nutritional myopathy or nutritional myodegeneration. This is because muscular dystrophy is a progressive, hereditary, degenerative disease of skeletal muscles.** The innervation of the affected muscles is intact. It is believed that the **primary defect in muscular dystrophy is in the myofibre itself.** Muscular dystrophies are a subgroup within the inherited diseases of muscle.

Table 14. Confirmed or Suspected Inherited or Congenital Myopathies

Disorder	Species Affected
Myotonia	Horses, goats, dogs, cats
Hyperkalaemia periodic paralysis (HYPP)	Horses
Glycogenoses	Horses, cattle, sheep, cats, dogs
Muscular dystrophy	Sheep, dogs, cats
Malignant hyperthermia	Horses, pigs, dogs
Labrador myopathy	Dogs
Phosphofructokinase deficiency	Dogs
Steatosis	Cattle
Double muscling	Cattle
Diaphragmatic dystrophy	Cattle
Congenital myasthenia gravis	Dog, cats

Muscular dystrophy in animals has been described in **cattle, sheep, dog, cats,** and **chickens. In humans**, the disease is divided into major subtypes based on age of onset, group of muscles affected, histological appearance, and type of inheritance. **As in humans**, muscular dystrophy in animals also preferentially involves certain groups of muscles, and sometimes, a specific fibre type (**type I in sheep**).

Storage Diseases

There are different types of glycogen storage diseases. They depend on which enzyme is deficient. **Those diseases in which glycogen accumulates in muscle** have been described in **horses, cattle, sheep,** and **dogs** (Table 13). Of these, six cause glycogen accumulations in muscle, and of the **glycogenoses**, only types II, III, and VII have been recognized in animals.

Changes in Myofibre Size

Atrophy

The main types of atrophy are:
1. Denervation
2. **Disuse,** and
3. **Malnutrition, cachexia**, and **senility**

Atrophy means either a reduction in the diameter of the muscle as a whole, or in the diameter of a myofibre. **During growth**, additional sarcomeres (the contractile units of a myofibril) are added to increase length, and additional myofilaments are added to increase diameter. **During atrophy**, myofibrils are removed by disintegration, and this results in the sarcolemma being too large. As a result, it is thrown into unnecessary folds. The rate of atrophy depends not only on the lack of use, but also on whether the muscle is still receiving trophic impulses from nerves.

1. Denervation Atrophy

Also known wrongly as **'neurogenic atrophy'**, denervation atrophy is not uncommon in animals. Example includes equine roarers due to damage to the left recurrent laryngeal nerve. **Any interference with the nerve supply to any muscle will result in its atrophy.** Under some circumstances, a major nerve supply can be re-established, thus reversing the atrophy. **Denervation atrophy is rapid,** and more than half the muscle mass of a completely denervated muscle can be lost in a few weeks. **Microscopically,** the loss of a nerve fibre to a muscle results in **atrophy of all myofibres innervated by that nerve.** The change is even more marked when a complete motor unit is denervated. A motor unit consists of either ventral horn or brain motor neuron and all the myofibres innervated by it. **Because the motor neuron decides the histochemical myofibre type in that case all the atrophic myofibres will be of the same histochemical type (type I or type II).**

Following denervation, fibres become smaller in diameter as peripheral myofibrils disintegrate. If an atrophic fibre is surrounded by normal fibres, it may be pressed into an angular shape, the so-called **small, angular fibres** (Fig. 50A and B). However, if atrophic fibres are not compressed, they become **round** in cross section. The most striking change is the increase in the **concentration of myofibre nuclei.** Although myofibrils disappear, muscle nuclei do not disappear at the same rate. Therefore, the end stage of a denervated myofibre is **a cell devoid of myofibrils but consisting of a row of nuclei.** As the muscle fibres atrophy, the fibrous stroma of the endomysium and epimysium (the fibrous sheath around an entire skeletal muscle) becomes more prominent because of condensation rather than

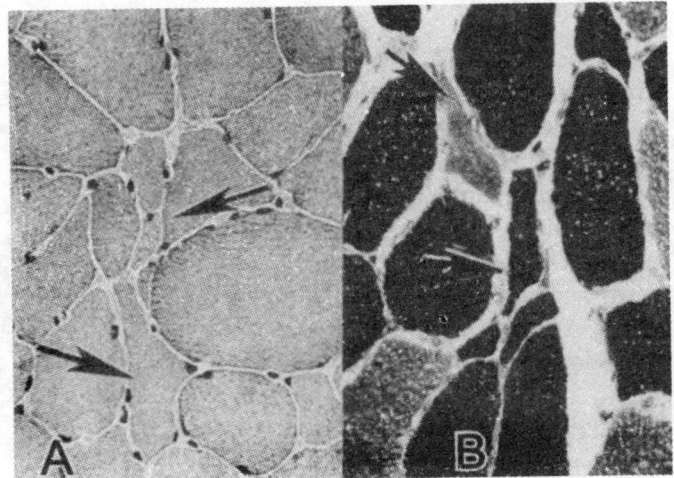

Fig. 50. Muscle, denervation atrophy. A. Early denervation atrophy. Note several small, angular fibres (arrows). H & E Stain. B. Serial section of the same muscle stained with myosin ATPase. The atrophic angular fibres (arrows), type I (light) and type II (dark) are a feature of denervation atrophy.

proliferation. Finally, the contractile elements completely disappear, leaving behind empty spaces surrounded by endomysium. **Eventually, the endomysium becomes compact and the end result is a muscle that consists of only fibrous tissue.** Sometimes, atrophic myofibres disappear, and the space is filled by **adipocytes** (fat cells), which causes the muscle to become larger than normal, a condition called **pseudohypertrophy**.

The extent of changes in the muscle fasciculi (a fasciculus is a small bundle of muscle fibres) depends on how many motor units have been denervated. **If all motor units are affected, then all the muscle will atrophy.** However, if some of the motor units are still intact, then the muscle fasciculi will have **a mixture of atrophic and normal myofibres.**

If the damage is in a single motor unit, then atrophic fibres will be scattered through one or more fasciculi, depending on the number of myofibres innervated by that single neuron and size of the motor unit. The denervating muscle fibres can be re-innervated by sprouting of fibres from adjacent normal nerves. Usually these nerves are from a neuron that innervates a different type of myofibre, and because muscle fibre type is a function of the motor neuron, the newly innervated myofibre takes on the fibre type decided by that neuron. **This process results in a loss of the normal arrangement of type I and II myofibres,** and formation of groups of the same type of fibre adjacent to each other, so-called **'fibre-type grouping'.**

2. Disuse Atrophy

This results in a less rapid atrophy of muscle than that due to denervation. The **cause** can be anything that stops the use of muscle, for example, fractured limbs, failure to use a painful leg, upper motor neuron damage, or recumbency (lying down). The loss of myofibrils resembles that of denervation atrophy, but there are differences. Histochemical examination shows that **type II fibres atrophy faster** (Fig. 51A and B). **Disuse atrophy is reversible** except when atrophy is so severe and prolonged that myofibres are lost.

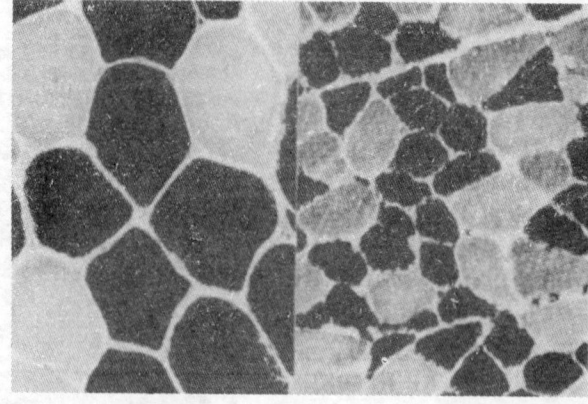

A   **B**

Fig. 51. Muscle, disuse atrophy; dog. A. Normal muscle. B. Same muscle, 60 days after forced disuse. Both **type I (light)** and **type II (dark)** fibres are atrophic, **but the type II fibres are more severely affected.** Myosin ATPase.

3. Atrophy due to Malnutrition, Cachexia, and Senility

In starvation, muscle protein is metabolized to supply the need for nutrients. This type of muscle atrophy occurs gradually, except in cachexia occurring in some febrile diseases. **All muscles of the body are not affected to the same degree.** Unlike in muscles undergoing denervation atrophy, some nuclei in muscles undergoing this type of atrophy disappear as the volume of the myofibre is reduced. **On gross examination,** muscles are swollen, thinner, and darker than normal, and no fat remains. In muscles with **lipofuscinosis,** the brown pigment is concentrated, intensifying the brownish discoloration.

Hypertrophy

This term is used in two ways: (1) for **an increase in the diameter of the muscle as a whole**, and (2) for **an increase in myofibre diameter** even if the muscle diameter is not enlarged. Increase in muscle fibre diameter is caused by an increased workload on those fibres.

Hypertrophy is of two types: (1) **work hypertrophy,** and (2) **compensatory hypertrophy.** **Work hypertrophy** means an increase in normal physiological work, as occurs in muscles during athletic training. **Compensatory hypertrophy,** which is actually a type of work hypertrophy of individual fibres, is in response to an increased load caused by the loss or absence of myofibres in a muscle or by denervation atrophy of adjacent myofibres in a muscle fasciculus. Thus, **compensatory hypertrophy** can be secondary to denervation atrophy, muscular dystrophies, cachectic atrophy, and extensive necrosis in nutritional or toxic myopathies in which muscles have lost many myofibres.

The exact mechanism controlling hypertrophy is unknown. Myofibres are increased in diameter by the addition of myofilaments (ultramicroscopic threadlike structures composing the myofibrils). Fibres undergoing compensatory hypertrophy may enlarge to more than 100 μm in diameter. These large-diameter myofibres may undergo longitudinal fibre splitting. **In histological cross sections of muscles,** these fibres have a characteristic appearance. The myofibre is divided into 2 to 4 segments. These pieces are usually of different sizes but all still lie within the same endomysial tube. Not all longitudinal fibre splitting is due to increased workload. Some is caused by faulty myofibre regeneration with failure of individual myoblasts to fuse completely.

Disturbances of Circulation

Congestion

Passive congestion of muscles due to localized or generalized stasis results in dark red to very dark red muscles.

Ischaemia

Ischaemia is deficiency of blood in a part, usually due to functional constriction or actual obstruction of a blood vessel. **Anaemic animals have pale muscles.** As muscles have relatively small energy stores of glycogen and lipid, these are rapidly exhausted during exercise. **Myofibres are well supplied with capillaries.** The density of capillaries is greater in type I fibres, which depend on aerobic metabolism, than in type II fibres, which are either glycolytic or mixed oxidative-glycolytic.

The basic factor in deciding the effect of ischaemia on muscle is the differential susceptibility of the various cells forming the muscle as a whole. **Myofibres are the most sensitive, satellite cells less sensitive, and fibroblasts the least sensitive to anoxia (total lack of oxygen).** Therefore, infarction of an area of muscle first leads to segmental necrosis, then to death of satellite cells, and finally to the death of all cells, including the stromal cells (Fig. 52). **The loss of satellite cells prevents rapid regeneration.** Since they are not available to form myoblasts, satellite cells have to be recruited from the edges of viable myofibres. Because all cells

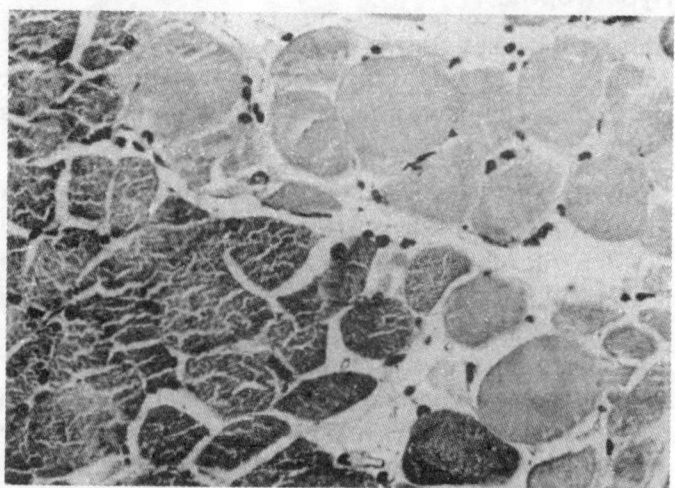

Fig. 52. Muscle. Infarct. Note that in the infarcted area (upper right), all myofibres are necrotic (rounded, hyalinized), and all stromal nuclei are pyknotic, **indicating necrosis.** H & E stain.

in the infarcted muscle die, **healing takes place mostly by fibrosis and scar formation.** Disrupted myofibres at the periphery of the lesion may attempt regeneration by budding.

The basic causes of ischaemia are:

1. Occlusion of the vascular system
2. External pressure on a muscle
3. Swelling of a muscle in a non-expandable compartment

Vascular Occlusion

Muscles have numerous capillary anastomoses and well-developed collateral circulation. **Therefore, infarction from embolism is rare.** Blockage of the iliac arteries by aortic-iliac thrombosis in the **horse** and of the aortic bifurcation by a 'saddle' thromboembolus in the **cat** can cause **ischaemia. In the cat,** the feet may be cool and cyanotic and myofibres may undergo segmental necrosis before the collateral circulation can be established.

Sometimes **in dogs,** *Dirofilaria immitis* (heartworm) may cause proliferative arteritis and thrombosis of the external and internal iliac arteries, and their branches. These lesions produce thromboemboli, some of which cause scattered foci of necrosis (infarcts) in the muscles of the hind limbs. One case of muscle infarction in **sheep** is vasculitis caused by the **bluetongue virus. Grossly,** these infarcts appear as fine grey streaks, and foci or haemorrhages may be so small as not to be visible.

Equine Purpura Haemorrhagica

This is a sporadic non-contagious disease of **horses** (discussed in 'myopathies of the horse'). The **muscle lesions are infarcts** due to vasculitis, believed to be immune-mediated. The disease occurs in **horses** recovering from streptococcal infection such as **strangles.** Muscle infection may be so extensive as to cause **myoglobinuria** (presence of myoglobin in the urine).

The **size of the infarct** depends on the size of the vessel obstructed and the duration. Blockage at capillaries causes segmental necrosis, but when larger arteries are blocked, whole areas of muscle, including the satellite cells, are killed. **Healing is by fibrosis.**

External Pressure on Muscle

Long periods of recumbency (lying down), such as during anaesthesia or in animals unable to rise, or too tightly fitting plaster casts or bandages can put external pressure on muscles. **Post-anaesthesia myopathy** is seen particularly in **horses** anaesthetized for long periods. The basic mechanism is that the pressure in the muscle exceeds the perfusion pressure in the capillaries. Muscle infarction is seen in **cows,** when the weight of the body of the animal in ventral recumbency causes ischaemia of the pectoral muscles and of any muscles of the fore or hind limbs folded under the body. **Ewes** in advanced pregnancy with twins or triplets develop an ischaemic necrosis of the internal abdominal oblique muscle, and this can lead to rupture. **The duration of ischaemia decides the severity of necrosis and the success of regeneration** (see 'necrosis').

Trauma

External trauma to muscles includes bruising (crushing with haemorrhage), laceration (tearing), surgical incisions, burns, gunshot and arrow wounds, and certain injections. Some of these may result in complete or partial **rupture of large muscles. Rupture is common in automobile accidents.** The diaphragm is usually ruptured due to a sudden increase in intra-abdominal pressure. **In racing dogs,** spontaneous rupture of muscles can occur during strenuous exercise. Tearing (**myorrhexis**) of muscle fibres occurs in the adductor muscles of **cattle** in which the legs are stretched across on a slippery floor in opposite directions.

Healing in these traumatic wounds follows the principles of regeneration.**Most of the healing is achieved by budding and fibrosis.** Collagen is not elastic, and therefore, large scars reduce the contractibility of adjacent myofibres.

Thus, in muscle trauma, damage is due to destruction of myofibres, compression of myofibres with destruction of the sarcoplasm, and secondarily from **haemorrhage.** The haemorrhage may increase intramuscular pressure, resulting in ischaemia and later on (infarction).

Myositis

Inflammation of muscle, called **myositis** (plural: myositides) can be caused by a wide variety of agents, that is, bacteria, viruses, protozoa, and helminths, or it can be due to immune-mediated mechanisms.

At times, the term **myositis** has been wrongly applied to certain disorders, such as exertional and masseter (a large muscle that raises the lower jaw) myositis of the jaw. **The two disorders are degenerative myopathies, not inflammatory myopathies.** It is very important to differentiate between **true myositis** and a **degenerative myopathy** in which there is segmental necrosis. In the normal response to necrosis, the necrotic segment is infiltrated by macrophages, which clear the cellular debris. Severe acute necrotizing myopathy may even be accompanied by a certain degree of infiltrating lymphocytes, plasma cells, neutrophils, and even eosinophils. **True myositis occurs when inflammatory cells are directly responsible for initiating and maintaining myofibre injury.**

Bacterial Myositis

Bacteria may cause **suppurative (**pyogenic bacteria), **sero-haemorrhagic** (clostridia), or **granulomatous lesions (Table 15).** Infection may be introduced by direct penetration (wounds or injections), haematogenously, or by spread from an adjacent cellulitis, fasciitis (inflammation of fascia), tendinitis, arthritis, or osteomyelitis.

Table 15. Bacterial and Parasitic Myopathies

Infectious Agent	Species affected
Clostridium sp. causing myositis	Horses, cattle, sheep, goats, pigs
Clostridium botulinum (botulism)	Horses, cattle, sheep, goats
Pyogenic bacteria	Cattle, sheep, goats, pigs
Streptococcus equi	Horses
Sarcocystis sp. Cattle, sheep, goats	
Neosporum caninum	Dogs
Trichinella spiralis	Pigs

Pyogenic bacteria usually cause localized suppuration and myofibre necrosis. This may resolve completely or become localized to form an **abscess,** or in some cases, the infection may spread down the fascial planes. For example, a non-sterile intramuscular injection into the gluteal muscles may cause myositis that extends down the fascial planes of the muscles of the femur and tibia and erupts on the surface through a sinus.

Although the **majority of inflammation** is **serous or sero-purulent** and involve fascial planes, some bacteria extend into and cause necrosis of adjacent muscle fasciculi (a fasciculus is a small bundle of muscle fibres). *Streptococcus equi* **(horses)**, *Arcanobacterium pyogenes* (earlier called *Actinomyces pyogenes*/*Corynebacterium pyogenes* **(cattle** and **sheep),** and *Corynebacterium pseudotuberculosis* **(sheep** and **goats)** are common causes of muscle diseases. *S. equi* in **horses** can also cause myopathy as a result of immune-mediated vasculitis or muscle necrosis and wasting (see 'myopathies of horses'). After bite wounds, **cats** may develop **cellulitis** due to *Pasteurella multocida* that extends into the adjacent muscle. **Clostridia** may produce serous or sero-haemorrhagic cellulitis, or cellulitis and myositis.

Granulomatous Myositis

Granulomatous myositis is characterized by the presence of **single or multiple granulomas (focal granulomatous myositis)** and is relatively rare. It may be caused by *Mycobacterium bovis* **(tuberculosis),** usually in **cattle** and **pigs,** *Actinobacillus lignieresi* **(wooden tongue in cattle),** *Actinomyces bovis*, and *Staphylococcus aureus* **(botryomycosis in horses).** Rarely, infection by **Sarcocystis sp.** may cause a granulomatous myositis of the tongue in **horses.**

Tuberculosis

Lesions are yellowish, variably sized **nodules** with **yellowish caseous contents** usually enclosed in a thick fibrous capsule. **Microscopically,** the lesion is granuloma with central necrosis surrounded by epithelioid and giant cells.

Actinobacillosis

Actinobacillosis (*Actinobacillus lignieresii,* **wooden tongue in cattle**) is usually due to **direct penetration of the tongue by the bacterium,** which produces small, pale granulomas that contain **'sulphur granules'** composed of masses of Gram-negative rods. This disease has also been reported in the tongue and muscles of the rear limbs of a **dog.**

Actinomyces bovis

Actinomyces bovis produces a **granulomatous osteomyelitis** in the mandible or maxilla of **cattle (lumpy jaw).** The lesion may extend into adjacent muscles, including the masseter. **Lesions** have caseous to suppurtaive centres, surrounded by epithelioid cells and giant cells. The central exudate contains 'sulphur granules' in which are present Gram-positive rods and branching filaments.

Botryomycosis

In **horses** and **pigs**, *Staphylococcus aureus* can cause a low-grade, persistent infection that becomes granulomatous. The disease is called **botryomycosis in the horse** and is usually the result of wounds. **Lesions** are fibrous nodules present in the muscles of the head, pectoral region, and less often, back and thighs. **In pigs,** the lesions may be in castration wounds or mammary glands. The **nodules are hard** and have a fibrous capsule that encloses cavity containing yellow-brown pus and granules. **Microscopically,** lesions are **encapsulated granulomas** containing **central 'clubs' colonies** in which there are demonstrable staphylococci. The granulomas can extend peripherally to involve adjacent muscles.

Fungal Granulomatous Myositis

This disease is rare. Sometimes, *Blastomyces dermatitidis* causes lesions in the laryngeal mucosa. These may extend into the adjacent intrinsic muscles of the larynx, causing a **granulomatous myositis**. It is not clear whether the infection is spread haematogenously or by direct penetration of fungi coughed up from the lungs.

Viral Myositis

These are relatively few and include **porcine encephalomyelitis** (causal agent **enterovirus**), **foot-and-mouth disease** (causal agent **aphthovirus**), **bluetongue** (causal agent **orbivirus**), and **Akabane disease** (causal agent **Akabane virus**). **Gross lesions** may or may not be visible, and if present, are small poorly defined foci or streaks. **Muscle lesions** caused by viruses are either infarcts secondary to a vasculitis, as seen in **bluetongue in sheep,** or multifocal necrosis, because of a direct effect of the virus on the myofibres. Multifocal necrosis is seen in infections by different enterovirus (e.g., porcine encephalomyelitis) and foot-and-mouth disease virus.

Porcine Encephalomyelitis

Porcine encephalomyelitis is due to a **coronavirus** of the **Enterovirus** genus. Besides the destruction of neurons, which results in paralysis, **the virus may also cause multifocal necrosis of myofibres**, accompanied by focal interstitial and perivascular infiltrations of lymphocytes, macrophages, and a few neutrophils.

Foot-and-Mouth Disease

The main lesions are **vesicles** in the **skin** and **mucous membranes,** particularly the oral mucosa. Besides these, heart and **skeletal muscles** may have yellow streaks and grey foci. **Microscopically,** these are areas of **segmental myofibre necrosis** accompanied by intense lymphocytic and neutrophilic infiltration.

Akabane Virus

Akabane virus of the family Bunyaviridae can produce **non-suppurative myositis** in the **bovine foetus.**

Bluetongue

Bluetongue, caused by **orbivirus,** is a non-contagious, insect-borne viral disease that causes vasculitis in a wide variety of tissues, particularly the oral mucosa. **Gross lesions in muscles are foci of necrosis (infarction) and haemorrhage.** Depending on the age of the lesions, necrosis, calcification, or regeneration may be present. Because of the size of the infarcts, regeneration is usually by muscle giant cells and fibrosis.

Parasitic Myositis

Parasitic infections of the skeletal muscles in domestic animals are **not common.** The most important have been listed in Table 14. Most diseases are of not much economic importance, except *Trichinella spiralis* in **pigs** (see 'myopathies of pigs').

Ancylostoma caninum Larva Migrans

The larval forms of *A. caninum* migrate in the body, and on entering muscles of paratenic hosts, development is arrested. The larvae cause **inflammation** and **myonecrosis.** As they continue to migrate, they leave a track of segmentally necrotic myofibres and inflammation.

Visceral Larva Migrans

This is invasion and migration into any tissue of the animal body by nematode larvae. *Toxocara canis* larvae migrate through many tissues of the **dog.** Some larvae are arrested, and **granulomas** form around them. These have been found in a wide variety of tissues, including kidneys, liver, lung, myocardium, and **skeletal muscle.** The lesion in a muscle is a **focal granulomatous myositis.** The larvae and granulomas lie between myofibres.

Dirofilaria immitis

In dogs, larvae of this nematode may be present in the external and internal iliac arteries and their branches. Thromboemboli and parasites may cause multiple infarcts in the muscles of the hind limbs.

Cysticercosis

A **cysticercus** is a larva with a solid caudal portion and a bladder-like proximal portion. It is the **intermediate stage in the life cycle of several tapeworms.** *Taenia solium* and *Taenia saginata*, both tapeworms of **human beings,** have a cysticercus stage in the **pig** (*Cysticercus cellulosae*) and **cattle** (*Cysticercus bovis*), respectively.

The cysticerci lodge in the heart, masseter, and tongue, where they appear as small white or grey cysts. **Microscopically**, there is displacement of myofibres by the cyst but **little myositis**. There may be a few lymphocytes, macrophages, and eosinophils around the cyst, which lies in the interstitial tissue, not in the myofibre. With time, the immunological system of the host kills the cysticercus. *C. cellulosae* in **pigs** may become calcified. *Cysticercus ovis* in the heart and shoulder muscles of **sheep** and **goats** is the intermediate stage of *Taenia ovis*, a tapeworm of **dogs**.

Myopathies of the Domestic Animals

These are discussed species-wise, because this is the way diseases are dealt with clinically. The same disease may occur in different species. Various **nutritional, toxic, metabolic, endocrine** and **electrolyte myopathies** in different species are presented in **Table 16** and **17**.

Table 16. Nutritional and toxic myopathies

Disorder	Species Affected	Cause
Nutritional myopathy	Horses, cattle, sheep, goats pigs	Selenium, or vitamin E deficiency
Ionophore toxicity	Horses, cattle, sheep, goats, pigs	Monensin, other ionophores used as feed additives
Plant toxicity	Horses, cattle, sheep, goats, pigs	*Cassia occidentalis*, other toxic plants

Table 17. Myopathies due to metabolic, endocrine, and electrolyte abnormalities

Disorder	Species Affected
Hypokalaemia	Cattle, cats
Hypophosphataemia	Cattle
Hypernatraemia	Cats
Mitochondrial defects	Dogs, horses
Hypothyroidism	Dogs
Hypercortisolism	Dogs

Myopathies of Cattle

Bacterial and Parasitic Myopathies

Clostridial Myositis (Blackquarter, Blackleg)

Blackquarter (BQ) is economically an extremely important disease of **cattle** and **sheep** in India. It is caused by *Clostridium chauvoei*, a spore-forming, Gram-negative anaerobic bacillus. **The most common manifestation is acute death. Signs**

before death are those of toxaemia, heat, swelling, crepitus (crackling sound), and dysfunction of the affected muscle group, and fever and anorexia.

C. chauvoei are found in the soil, and following ingestion can cross the epithelial mucosa, enter bloodstream, and are carried to **skeletal muscle.** The **spores** lie dormant **until local trauma to the muscle,** usually from bruising during handling in a chute (restrainer, crate) or from trauma in crowded feeding, **results in hypoxia.** The resultant anaerobic conditions allow the **spores** to **activate, proliferate,** and **produce toxins.** These cause capillary damage, haemorrhage, oedema, and necrosis of myofibres. **Locally extensive haemorrhage and oedema, usually with crepitus due to gas bubbles, are seen in affected muscles and in overlying fascia and subcutaneous tissue.** Necrotic muscle fibres appear dark-red to red-black and may be wet and exudative (early lesions) or dry (later lesions). Cardiac muscles may also be involved. **A characteristic odour of rancid butter due to butyric acid is typically found.** In other parts of the body, haemorrhages and oedema may be seen associated with toxaemia. Because of the high fever, affected carcasses autolyze rapidly. **Microscopically,** locally extensive areas of muscle fibres undergoing

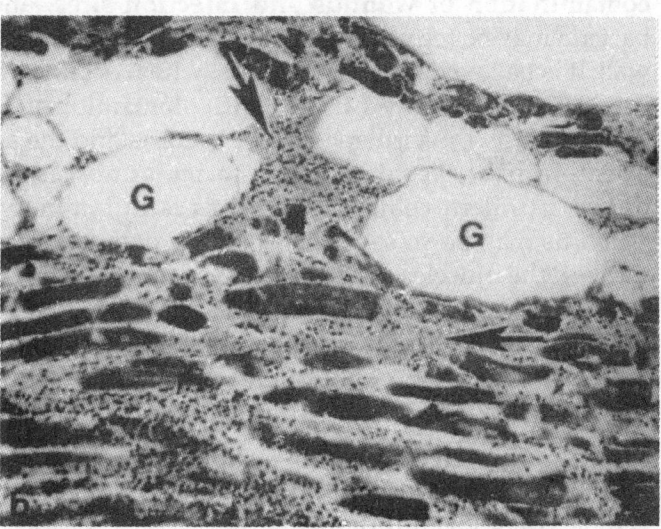

Fig. 53. Muscle; cow. Blackquarter. Early stage. Serohaemorrhagic exudate (arrows) and gas bubbles (G) separate myofibres. H & E stain.

coagulation necrosis and fragmentation, and interstitial oedema and haemorrhage are seen. **Gas bubbles are typical** (Fig. 53). **Gram-positive bacilli** resembling *C. chauvoei* may or may not be seen in the affected muscle.

Isolation of *C. chauvoei* on anaerobic media is useful for confirmation of blackquarter. However, this gives results only when typical gross and microscopic findings are present, **because this bacterium can be cultured from unaffected muscle that harbours dormant spores.** The vaccination history is also important. The unvaccinated or poorly vaccinated animals in situations in which muscle trauma is possible are most at risk. There is no effective treatment for cattle with BQ, and death occurs rapidly. Prevention is the best treatment. Vaccination against clostridial toxins and maintenance of a safe and hygienic environment are very important.

Clostridium botulinum (Botulism)

Botulism occurs in cattle, and clinical signs and pathogenesis are similar to that in the **horse** (see 'botulism' in myopathies of the horse). **Cattle**, however, are much more resistant to botulism than horses.

Pyogenic Bacteria

Cattle are prone to develop abscesses caused by pyogenic bacteria, usually *Arcanobacterium (Actinomyces) pyogenes.* Abscesses in muscle occur usually in the hind leg. Swelling and lameness of the affected limbs are seen.

A. pyogenes is found everywhere. It **infects muscle by two routes:** (1) by **direct contamination of wounds and injection sites,** and (2) **haematogenously.** The bacteria may be found within the reproductive tract of **cows** and within the ruminal wall. It is believed that bacteraemia, which occurs after parturition or disruption of ruminal wall integrity, can result in colonization of damaged muscle. **Lesions** vary depending on the virulence of the bacteria and the age of the lesions. They vary in extent, from **encapsulated intramuscular abscesses** near the site of injection, to diffuse purulent cellulitis (cellulitis is inflammation of the connective tissue). Cellulitis may be so severe that it may extend from the muscles over the sacrum through the muscles on the lateral aspect of the thigh and over the tibia and to the hock. **Grossly,** the **encapsulated abscesses** are filled with thick, yellow-green, foul-smelling **pus.** The cellulitis, actually fasciitis (inflammation of fascia), extends into the nearby myofibres resulting in **myonecrosis** and **subsequent replacement by fibrous tissue.**

The **colour of the exudate** is characteristic, and Gram-positive to Gram-variable coccobacilli may be seen within tissue sections. *A. pyogenes* is readily isolated on aerobic bacterial culture media.

Protozoal Myopathies

Intra-cytoplasmic protozoal cysts of **Sarcocystis** sp. are common incidental findings in **skeletal and cardiac myofibres of cattle.** Being **intracellular,** they are protected from the host's defence mechanisms, and therefore, there is no inflammatory response or reaction by the myofibre. This protozoal organism is a stage of an intestinal coccidium of carnivores that uses birds, reptiles, rodents, pigs, and herbivores as an intermediate host. Ingestion of oocysts by an intermediate host releases sporozoites that invade tissues, **including muscle.** Massive exposure may result in fever, anorexia, and progressive wasting, but this is uncommon. **Usually, Sarcocystis infection is diagnosed as an incidental finding at postmortem or during meat processing.** If the cyst wall breaks down, a focus of myofibre necrosis and later granuloma formation occurs.

Nutritional and Toxic Myopathies

Nutritional Myopathies

Like horses, **calves** and **young cattle** are susceptible to nutritional myopathy due to **selenium** or **vitamin E deficiency**. However, profound involvement of temporal and masseter muscles (maxillary myositis) that occurs in **horses** is **not seen in young cattle**.

Congenital or Inherited Myopathies

Steatosis

This disease occurs in **cattle**. Also called **'lipomatosis'**, steatosis is usually seen as an **incidental finding either at postmortem or at slaughter**. It occurs due to defective muscle development, in which large areas of myofibres are replaced by adipocytes (fat cells). **Lesions** are bilaterally symmetrical; the most severely affected are those of the back and loin. **Severely affected muscles are composed entirely of fat,** whereas less severely affected muscles may appear streaked or partially replaced by fat. **Microscopically,** the space normally occupied by myofibres is filled with mature adipocytes.

Diagnosis is easily made on gross examination, and can be confirmed by microscopic examination, especially in frozen sections stained for fat, with oil-red O or Sudan black.

Glycogenoses

Carbohydrate metabolic defects affect skeletal muscle by interfering with muscle energy metabolism. **This results in abnormal storage of glycogen.** Many disorders of carbohydrate metabolism have been identified in **human**, and an increasing number of **inherited glycogenoses** are being recognized **in animals**.

Acid Maltase Deficiency (Glycogenosis type II, Pompe's Disease)

This disease has been described in **cattle**. **Affected cattle** show **clinical signs of weakness at 3 to 7 months of age** and **die as a result of respiratory and cardiac failure.** The disorder is **inherited** as an autosomal recessive trait. The enzyme defect results in blockage of the glycolytic metabolic pathway and in cellular dysfunction which is mostly seen in skeletal muscle, Purkinje cells of the heart, and neurons.

There are no noticeable changes in the skeletal and cardiac muscle. Also, no gross lesions are seen in the nervous system. **On microscopic examination,** affected myofibres, cardiac myocytes, and neurons are **filled with vacuoles containing glycogen (vacuolar myopathy** and **neuropathy)**, which can be demonstrated by PAS staining. **Glycogen accumulation in skeletal myofibres is segmental,** whereas in neurons it is diffuse. Both degeneration and regeneration of skeletal muscle fibres are present. **Diagnosis** of a glycogenosis can be made by characteristic clinical and microscopic findings.

Myophosphorylase Deficiency (Glycogenosis type V, McArdle's Disease)

This disorder has been identified in **cattle. Clinical signs** of exercise intolerance are recognized at an early age. If forced to exercise, affected cattle become recumbent (lie down) for up to 10 minutes. Myophosphorylase deficiency is **an autosomal recessive disorder** similar to acid maltase deficiency, **but involves only skeletal muscle.** No specific findings are seen at postmortem. **Microscopic findings** in skeletal muscle are similar to those of acid maltase deficiency. **Cardiac myocytes and neurons do not store glycogen. Diagnosis** is based on characteristic clinical and microscopic findings.

Metabolic Myopathies

Hypokalaemic Myopathy

In this condition, a history of **ketosis** occurring within a month of parturition is common. **Affected cows are very weak** and become recumbent and unable to support the weight of their heads. **Serum concentration of potassium is low.**

Hypokalaemia (low potassium levels in the blood) can be due to anorexia. Glucocorticoids with high mineralocorticoid activities used to treat ketosis or intravenously administered glucose or insulin may cause severe hypokalaemia. **Decreased muscle potassium interferes with normal muscle cell function, and can lead to myofibre necrosis.** No specific findings are present at postmortem examination.

Other Metabolic Myopathies

Both **hypocalcaemia** and **hypophosphataemia** can result in severe muscle weakness and recumbemcy in **cattle.** Significant changes are not seen in affected muscles.

Ischaemic myopathy: Ischaemic muscle necrosis due to recumbency is common in **cattle** and is similar to that seen in **horses.**

Myopathies of Small Ruminants

Bacterial and Parasitic Myopathies

Myositis due to *Clostridium chauvoei* (Blackquarter, Blackleg)

This disease sometimes occurs in **sheep** and **goats** and is similar to the disease in **cattle.**

Clostridium botulinum (Botulism)

Botulism also occurs in **small ruminants** and is similar to the disease in **cattle**.

Parasitic Myopathy

Intra-cytoplasmic cysts of **Sarcocystis** sp. are commonly found in the skeletal and cardiac muscle fibres of **sheep** and **goats** as **an incidental finding,** similar to that in cattle. **In goats,** massive infection with **Sarcocystis** may result in lymphoid necrosis, with inflammation involving heart, skeletal muscle, lungs, liver, blood vessels, and the brain and spinal cord.

Nutritional and Toxic Myopathies

Nutritional Myopathy

Young goats and **sheep** are susceptible to **degenerative myopathy** associated with selenium or vitamin E deficiency. The disease in these species is similar to the disease seen in **young cattle.**

Inherited or Congenital Myopathies

Myotonia in Goats

Myotonia is a disorder of muscle characterized by increased muscular irritability and contractility with decreased power of relaxation. **Affected goats develop severe muscle spasms** in response to sudden voluntary effort, starting at about two weeks of age. Attacks of myotonia can last from 5 to 20 seconds and are characterized by **generalized stiffness. Goats** often fall over. Severity of signs varies.

Myotonia in goats is inherited as an autosomal dominant trait. The clinical severity varies due to increased severity in homozygotes compared to heterozygotes. **There are no gross pathological findings. Diagnosis** is based on characteristic clinical signs.

Congenital Muscular Dystrophy in Sheep

Muscular dystrophy in sheep is a progressive disorder seen in **Merino sheep in Australia. Clinical signs** of **neuromuscular weakness** occur as early as one month of age and are characterized by **a stiff gait and exercise intolerance.** The underlying defect in ovine progressive muscular dystrophy is not known. The disease is inherited as an autosomal recessive trait. **Diagnosis** is based on characteristic clinical and microscopic findings.

Glycogenosis

A **glycogen storage myopathy** due to myophosphorylase deficiency has been identified in **sheep in Australia,** and is similar to the disease in **cattle.**

Myopathies of the Horse

Bacterial and Parasitic Myopathies

Clostridial Myositis (Malignant Oedema)

Clostridial myositis (malignant oedema) in the **horse** can be caused by infection with *Clostridium perfringens, C. septicum,* or *C. chauvoei.* These are large Gram-positive anaerobic bacilli. **Clinical signs** are acute onset of heat, swelling, and pain within a muscle group and adjacent fascia, with concurrent fever, depression, dehydration, and anorexia. **Death** from toxaemia/septicaemia usually occurs within 48 hours. **Clostridium** sp. form **spores** within the soil and can contaminate deep, penetrating wounds, such as injection or puncture wounds. **Under anaerobic conditions clostridia proliferate and produce toxins** that damage blood vessels, resulting in haemorrhage and oedema, and cause necrosis of adjacent muscle fibres. **Affected muscle** and adjacent fascia are **swollen and often haemorrhagic, with oedema, necrosis, and gas.** Blood vessels are necrotic, but vasculitis is not seen. Gram-positive bacilli **Clostridium** sp, are usually demonstrable within affected tissue.

Diagnosis can be made based on typical history and gross and microscopic findings. Cytological examination of aspirates of affected muscle reveals Gram-positive bacilli in some cases. **Clostridium** sp. may be identified by culture on anaerobic media or by fluorescent antibody testing.

Clostridium botulinum (Botulism)

Botulism is not due to infection with *C. botulinum,* a Gram-positive anaerobic bacillus, **but due to the effect of its toxin.** Toxin can be ingested whole or produced in the intestine, or rarely at the sites of wounds contaminated by *C. botulinum.* **Horses are extremely sensitive to botulinum toxins.** Severe generalized flaccid paralysis is the characteristic feature of botulism. **Clinical signs** are acute and progress rapidly, usually resulting in recumbency. Dysphagia (difficulty in swallowing) and tongue weakness are common findings which help to differentiate botulism from other neuromuscular diseases causing recumbency.

C. botulinum bacteria are found within the gastrointestinal tract of many animals and their spores are in soil. Preformed toxin in the contaminated feed can be ingested to cause botulism in **adult horses.** Wound infection is an uncommon cause of botulism. **No specific gross or microscopic changes are present in horses dying from botulism.** However, aspiration pneumonia due to dysphagia can occur.

Streptococcus-Associated Myopathy

In this disease, the muscle **damage** is not caused by direct infection of the muscles, but **by an immune response to the streptococcus. Affected horses** are weak, depressed, or become recumbent, with myoglobinuria. **Circulating immune complexes** composed of IgA antibodies and streptococcal M antigen deposit in small vessels. **This leads to vasculitis and vascular wall necrosis**, with resultant haemorrhage and infarction of myofibres. Vasculitis, the diagnostic feature, results in infarction with large areas of coagulative necrosis in muscle. Streptococcal organisms are not present within affected muscle. **Because this is an immune-complex disorder, bacterial cultures of affected muscle do not show *S. equi***, but this organism may be cultured from other affected tissues, especially lymph nodes.

Streptococcus-Associated Muscle Atrophy

A condition of severe and rapid **generalized muscle atrophy** has been seen in **young horses** exposed to *S. equi*.

Protozoal Myopathy

Protozoa (**Sarcocystis** sp.) are common **incidental findings in equine skeletal and cardiac muscle**. The protozoa are **in cysts in the myofibre** and are therefore protected from the body's defences. As a result, there is no inflammatory response.

Nutritional and Toxic Myopathies

Nutritional Myopathy

Foals and **young adult horses** are susceptible to nutritional myopathy due to **deficiency of selenium**, or less commonly **vitamin E. Affected foals** show generalized weakness. Their tongue and pharyngeal muscles may be weak, leading to weak suckling. **Affected young adult horses** usually show involvement of the temporal and masseter muscles ('**maxillary myositis**'), with swelling and stiffness of the jaw muscles and defective mastication. Involvement of pharyngeal muscles may result in dysphagia.

Oxidative injury to actively contracting muscle fibres occurs as a result of **lack of selenium** (a vital component of the antioxidant enzyme glutathione peroxidase) **or vitamin E.** Muscles of the affected **foals** appear pale, usually in a patchy distribution. The most severely affected muscles are those that have the highest workload (e.g., cervical muscles, limb muscles, tongue, masticatory muscles). The **gross appearance** depends on the extent of the **necrosis** and the stage. In early stages, yellow and white streaks are present, and later pale, chalk white streaks appear. The **lesions in muscles** are those of **multifocal, multiphasic segmental necrosis.**

Toxic Myopathies – Ionophore Toxicity

Ionophores such as salinomycin, monensin, narasin, and lasalocid are usually added to **chicken** and **ruminant feeds** for their antibiotic and growth-enhancing effects. **Horses are extremely sensitive to ionophore toxicity and succumb to very small doses.** These may be present as contaminants within horse feed, or the horse may be accidently fed ionophore-containing feeds **intended for other domestic animals.** Most of the available information is on monensin toxicity. After ingestion of monensin, acute death, usually within 2-3 days, occurs from cardiovascular collapse and shock. **Death** is due to cardiac muscle necrosis or in case of recumbency for weeks or months, to cardiac fibrosis.

Inherited or Congenital Myopathies

Myotonia

Congenital or **early-onset myotonia** is seen in **horses.** Affected horses are extremely exercise intolerant, and show stiffness of gait. No specific gross lesions are present except prominent hypertrophied muscles.

Hyperkalaemic Periodic Paralysis (HYPP)

This disease is inherited as an autosomal dominant disease. **Affected foals** usually have a laryngeal muscle dysfunction that results in laryngospasm and laboured breathing. **Affected horses** usually have well-defined muscle groups. Attacks of muscle trembling, followed by weakness and often collapse, are the most common clinical signs. Affected horses may appear normal for many years, may have multiple episodes of collapse, or may die suddenly.

Polysaccharide Storage Myopathy

This disorder is thought to be **inherited**, but the exact mechanism is not clear. **Affected horses** may have a stiff gait, symmetrical muscle atrophy, or generalized weakness. An **underlying carbohydrate metabolic disorder** is suspected to be the cause of the disease.

Glycogen Brancher Enzyme Deficiency

A **congenital lack of the glycolytic enzyme** known as glycogen brancher enzyme occurs in **horses. Affected foals** show cardiac failure at an early age. The exact mode of inheritance is not known.

Other Equine Myopathies

Exertional Rhabdomyolysis

Rhabdomyolysis is disintegration of striated muscle fibres with excretion of myoglobin in the urine. **Equine exertional rhabdomyolysis,** also known as 'azoturia' and 'Monday morning disease' is characterized by sudden onset of stiff gait, reluctance to move, swelling of the affected muscle groups (especially gluteal), sweating, and other signs of discomfort. **Signs may appear during or immediately after exercise.** Electrolyte abnormalities and selenium deficiency have been implicated as causes of exertional rhabdomyolysis in the horse. Abnormal calcium homeostasis within skeletal muscle may also play a role. As muscle necrosis as such is neither painful, nor does it cause muscle swelling, it is suspected that other factors play a role in this disorder in the horse.

Myopathies of the Pig

Bacterial and Parasitic Myopathies

Clostridial Myositis (Blackleg)

Pigs sometimes develop myositis due to *Clostridium chauvoei* infection. The resulting disease is similar to that seen in cattle, sheep, and goats.

Pyogenic Bacteria

Abscesses within muscle and associated fascia due to pyogenic bacteria such as *Arcanobacterium pyogenes* are common in pigs and are similar to those in cattle.

Trichinosis

Infection of pigs by the nematode parasite *Trichinella spiralis* is of major economic importance to the pig industry and poses a health hazard to human beings. No clinical disease occurs in Trichinella infection in pigs

The adult nematode lives in the mucosa of the small intestine. Larvae penetrate the intestinal mucosa and enter bloodstream, from where they enter into the muscle. Larvae invade and encyst within muscle cells. Encysted larvae are not visible grossly, but dead larvae may calcify and may be seen as 0.5 to 1 mm white nodules. Active muscles, such as tongue, masseter, diaphragm, intercostal, laryngeal, and extraocular muscles, are preferentially affected. Focal inflammation consisting of eosinophils, neutrophils, and lymphocytes occurs along with invasion of the muscle by Trichinella larvae. After cyst formation, inflammation is minimal to absent.

Diagnosis is based on identification of the characteristic nematode larvae encysted within muscle fibres. In those cases in which the larvae have died and calcified, a presumptive diagnosis of trichinosis can still be made. Once encysted in the muscle, Trichinella larvae are protected from host immune response and to anthelmintic therapy.

Protozoal Myopathies

Intra-cytoplasmic cysts of Sarcocystis sp. can be found in the skeletal and cardiac muscle fibres of pigs as an incidental finding.

Nutritional and Toxic Myopathies

Nutritional Myopathy

Young pigs are susceptible to dystrophic myopathy due to selenium or vitamin E

deficiency. The resulting disorder is similar to that seen in **calves**.

Congenital and Inherited Myopathies

Splayleg

This **congenital disorder** affects **young piglets** and results in splaying (spreading out wide apart) of limbs to the side (abduction). **Affected animals** drive themselves forward by pushing against the ground with the pelvic limbs. This posture results in progressive flattening of the sternum.

Malignant Hyperthermia ('Porcine Stress Syndrome')

Affected pigs are clinically normal until an episode of **hyperthermia** is triggered by a precipitating factor such as anaesthesia or stress. Episodes consist of **severe muscle rigidity** and **markedly increased body temperature**, and in severe cases, progresses rapidly to **death**. The **disease is inherited** as an autosomal recessive trait.

Myopathies of the Dog

Parasitic

Protozoal Myopathy

The parasitic diseases which affect skeletal muscle in the **dog** are mainly due to **protozoal organisms**. Of these, *Neospora caninum* is the most important. *N. caninum* is a protozoal organism, usually transmitted in utero. **Affected bitches are chronic carriers of the organism**. Both, peripheral nervous system and the **skeletal muscle** are affected by organisms. They preferentially involve the ventral spinal roots. **Damage to these roots results in denervation atrophy of muscles.** Affected muscles are markedly atrophied, firm, and pale. **Signs** of progressive neuromuscular weakness, most marked in the pelvic limbs, begin in the affected **pups** several weeks of age.

Scattered foci of inflammation associated with segmental myofibre necrosis are usually seen **within skeletal muscle**, and intra-cytoplasmic protozoal cysts may be present. Also, these organisms damage the ventral roots and cause denervation atrophy of affected myofibres. As nerve fibres in the ventral root that supply both type I and type II myofibres are damaged, both these myofibre types are denervated.

Congenital or Inherited Myopathies

X-Linked Muscular Dystrophy (Duchenne type)

This disorder **occurs in several breeds of dogs**. This canine disorder is similar to Duchenne muscular dystrophy of **man**. **Affected dogs are always males (X-linked)**.

Severely affected pups may develop a rapidly progressive weakness and **die within the first few days of life.** In **less severely affected dogs,** clinical signs are a stiff gait and exercise intolerance beginning at 8 to 12 weeks of age, followed by progressive weakness and muscle atrophy. Weakness of the tongue, jaw, and pharyngeal muscles results in difficulty with prehension and swallowing of food. As stated, **this disorder is inherited as an X-linked recessive trait,** being non-clinical in carrier females. The underlying defect is the lack of a cytoskeletal protein known as **'dystrophin',** the absence of which makes skeletal muscle fibres susceptible to repeated bouts of necrosis and regeneration after exercise. **Death in older animals** is due to either aspiration pneumonia secondary to dysphagia (difficulty in swallowing), or to progressive cardiac failure. **However, affected dogs may survive for many years.**

Labrador Retriever Myopathy

Affected Labrador retrievers develop signs of neuromuscular weakness within the first 6 months of life. **Exercise intolerance** leads to collapse during prolonged exercise. **Affected dogs usually do not develop normal musculature.** Attacks of collapse can be precipitated by exposure to cold as well as by exercise. The **disorder is inherited** as an autosomal recessive trait.

Congenital Myotonia

Both sexes of **dogs** are affected, and **pups** may begin to show signs of stiff gait as early as 6 weeks of age. **Affected dogs** move with splayed (spread out wide apart), stiff thoracic limbs. During severe attacks, **dogs** may fall over, and laryngospasm may result in transient dyspnoea and even cyanosis. Available evidence supports an autosomal recessive inheritance of myotonia.

Endocrine Myopathies

Hypothyroidism

Signs of neuromuscular dysfunction due to hypothyroidism include generalized weakness, muscle atrophy, and megaoesophagus. Because of its role in muscle metabolism, decreased thyroid hormone causes **skeletal myofibre weakness and atrophy.** Hypothyroidism may also cause peripheral neuropathy. Damage to motor nerves may cause denervation atrophy and contribute to the neuromuscular weakness. **Overall muscle atrophy may be seen.** The thyroid glands may be bilaterally atrophied.

Myopathy Due to Excessive Corticosteroids (Hypercortisolism)

This disorder may be due to **increased adrenocortical cortisol production** or to **administration of exogenous corticosteroids. Clinical findings** may be very similar to those in hypothyroidism. **Overall muscle atrophy may be seen.** Adrenal glands may have bilateral cortical atrophy due to exogenous corticosteroid administration or may be hypertrophied because of stimulation from a pituitary tumour. Findings in affected muscle and peripheral nerves are similar to those seen in **hypothyroid myopathy.**

Immune-Mediated Myopathies

Polymyositis

This is a generalized inflammatory myopathy. It may have an **acute** and rapidly progressive onset **or a slow onset of muscle atrophy** and generalized weakness. Respiratory muscle involvement can occur, and if severe, may cause respiratory distress. **Polymyositis is due to an immune-mediated inflammation that attacks components of the skeletal myofibres, and results in myofibre necrosis. Overall muscle atrophy may be the only finding.**

Masticatory Muscle Myositis (Eosinophilic Myositis, Atrophic Myositis)

Severe, acute cases have bilateral swelling of the temporal and masseter muscles, pain, and inability to fully open the jaw. **Affected dogs** may have difficulty in holding food. Pain may or may not be present. The degree and nature of inflammation varies. In acute cases infiltrates of lymphocytes and plasma cells, **sometimes with numerous eosinophils are present.** Neutrophils are much less common. Inflammation is associated with myofibre necrosis.

Disorders of the Neuromuscular Junction

Myasthenia Gravis

Typical signs are collapse in an adult dog, and normal gait and strength after rest. **Clinical signs** can, however, vary. In most cases, myasthenia gravis is **an acquired disease,** the circulating antibodies being directed at the **acetylcholine receptors** of the neuromuscular junction. In some cases, myasthenia gravis may be associated with· thymoma, or less commonly thymic hyperplasia. **Congenital myasthenia gravis** is due to abnormal development of the neuromuscular junction and is **inherited as an autosomal recessive trait.** No findings are seen at postmortem examination, and no abnormalities in muscle are seen on light microscopic examination.

Myopathies of the Cat

Inherited or Congenital Myopathies

X-Linked Muscular Dystrophy (Duchenne-Type Muscular Dystrophy)

Affected cats develop a progressive, persistent stiff gait associated with marked muscular hypertrophy. They have difficulty in jumping and lying down. Dystrophic cats lack the muscle cytoskeletal protein **dystrophin**, which is also the cause of Duchenne dystrophy in **boys** and X-linked muscle dystrophy in the **dog**.

Congenital Myotonia

Cats with congenital myotonia have similar signs to those of dystrophic cats. **A stiff gait is most obvious.** The pathogenesis of feline myotonia is not known.

Myopathies Due to Electrolyte Abnormalities

Hypokalaemic and Hypernatraemic Myopathy

Hypokalaemia is abnormally low **potassium** levels in the blood, which may lead to neuromuscular disorder. **Hypernatraemia** is an excess of **sodium** in the blood.

Affected cats show severe generalized weakness, with ventriflexion of the neck (i.e., towards the body or ventral surface). The **cause** of the weakness myofibre necrosis is complex and involves abnormal skeletal muscle energy metabolism. **Hypokalaemia** may be due to decreased dietary intake or increased urinary excretion of potassium, and in **cats** it is usually a result of chronic renal disease. No specific gross pathological findings are present, except in cats with hypokalaemia due to chronic renal disease, in which kidneys are small and fibrotic.

Disorders of the Neuromuscular Junction

Myasthenia Gravis

Feline acquired and congenital myasthenia gravis are similar to those disorders in dog, but occur less commonly.

Neoplasms

Neoplasms of muscle can originate from any component of muscle, namely, myofibres, mesenchymal tissue such as fibrous, myxomatous, or adipose tissue; blood vessels; or nerve sheaths. However, **neoplasms of skeletal muscle – benign, malignant, or metastatic – are rare in domestic animals.** Most of the benign muscle tumours, **rhabdomyomas** in the **pig, cattle,** and **sheep,** have been cardiac, but laryngeal rhabdomyomas are recognized in the **dog. Grossly,** the tumours are un-capsulated and lobulated. **Microscopically,** they are composed of large granular cells that stain positively for myoglobin and desmin by immunoperoxidase techniques.

Rhabdomyosarcomas are rare. Most cases have been in **dogs. These tumours are usually highly malignant and metastasize either through the lymphatic or venous routes.** Therefore, metastases appear in lymph nodes, lungs, and spleen, and also in heart and skeletal muscles. **Grossly,** they are pink un-encapsulated masses. The **microscopic appearance** varies greatly. In some neoplasms, cells have characteristic cross-striations, whereas others are composed of undifferentiated cells with no visible striations.

Muscles can also be invaded locally by **carcinomas** and **sarcomas** as they proliferate and increase in size. For example, in the **dog**, squamous-cell carcinomas of the vulva may extend into the pelvic musculature. Bovine mammary adenocarcinomas and mast cell tumours sometimes extend into the adjacent cutaneous muscle.

Infiltrative lipomas are tumours of mature adipocytes in **dogs**. They are usually deep in the subcutis or muscles. **Grossly**, muscles are soft, and muscle fasciculi (small bundles of muscle fibres) are separated by yellow fat. **Microscopically**, the mass consists of well-differentiated adipose cells.

Rarely, skeletal muscle is invaded by local mesenchymal tumours such as **haemangiosarcomas, fibrosarcomas,** and **myxosarcomas** that have originated either in adjacent tissue or in the muscle's stroma. **Tumours metastatic to muscle are rare**, but malignant lymphoma, haemangiosarcoma, pulmonary adenocarcinoma, and pulmonary squamous-cell carcinoma have occurred **in the dog.**

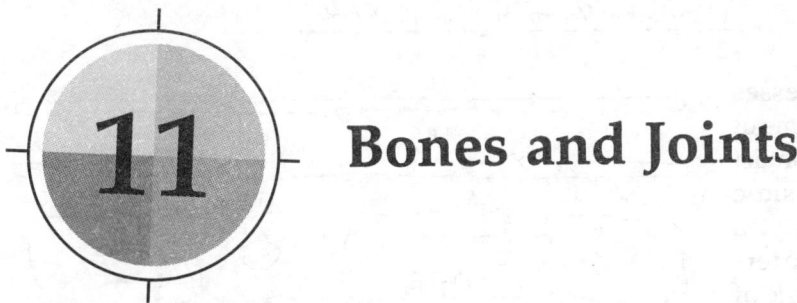

11 Bones and Joints

Diseases of Bone

Normal Structure and Function

Structure and function of the bone can be discussed at the **cellular, tissue,** and **organ levels.** First, normal structure and function are briefly reviewed at the **cellular level** and also include **bone matrix** and **mineral.** Cells involved in the structural integrity of bone are **osteoblasts, osteocytes,** and **osteoclasts.**

1. Bone at the Cellular Level

Osteoblasts

Osteoblasts are mesenchymal cells and originate from marrow stromal stem cells. **Osteoblasts cover bone-forming surfaces and are responsible for production of bone matrix** (i.e. the intercellular substance of bone, consisting of collagenous fibres, ground substance, and inorganic salts, also called **osteoid) and initiation of matrix mineralization.** When **active, osteoblasts** are plump (full and rounded), cuboidal cells with abundant basophilic cytoplasm (rich in rough endoplasmic reticulum) (Fig. 54) **Inactive osteoblasts** have little cytoplasm because of the reduction in the amount of rough endoplasmic reticulum and Golgi apparatus involved in matrix synthesis and secretion. **Osteoblasts send thin,**

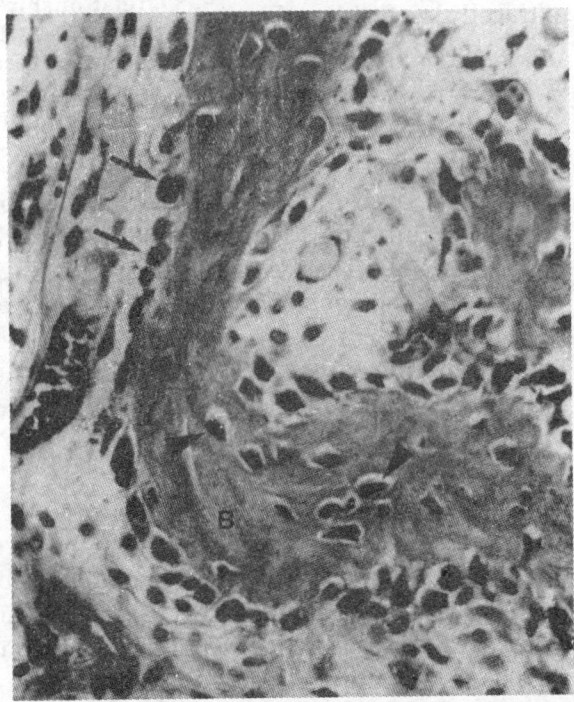

Fig. 54. **Bone. Repair of bone (B) at a fracture site.** Bone surfaces are covered by plump (full and rounded) **osteoblasts** (arrows). Large irregularly arranged **osteocytes** (arrowheads) are located in lacunae and are surrounded by osteoid with coarsely bundled collagen. H & E stain.

cytoplasmic processes into the matrix. Some of these processes contact similar cytoplasmic extensions of **osteocytes** (Fig. 54). This interconnecting network of osteoblasts and osteocytes forms a functional membrane. This membrane separates the extracellular fluid bathing bone surfaces from the general extracellular fluid and regulates the flow of calcium and phosphate ions to and from the bone fluid compartment (bone tissue fluid; see Fig. 55).

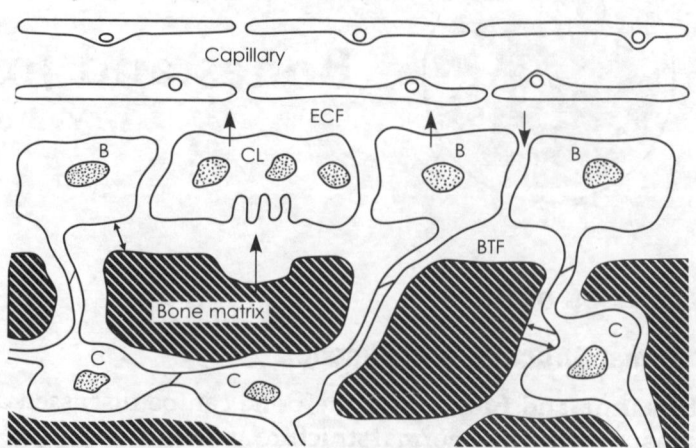

Fig. 55. Diagram of calcium movement (arrows) and relationships of osteoblasts **B**, osteocytes **C**, and osteoclasts **CL** to blood vessels, extracellular fluid **ECF**, and bone tissue fluid **BTF** compartment.

For calcium to get into the bone, calcium passes between osteoblasts. To get out of the bone an intracellular pump (within osteoblasts) moves calcium outward across the cell membrane to the general extracellular fluid compartment (Fig. 55). **Osteoblast membranes are rich in alkaline phosphatase.** The function of this enzyme in the osteoblast is uncertain, but could play a role in mineralization and in pumping calcium across cellular membranes. **Osteoblasts have receptors for parathyroid hormone (PTH).** Activation of these receptors increases the activity of the osteoblast calcium pump and **initiates bone resorption (bone loss or removal) by osteoclasts.**

Osteocytes

Osteocytes are **those osteoblasts which have been surrounded by mineralized bone matrix.** They occupy small spaces in the bone called **lacunae** (singular: lacuna) (Fig. 54), and make contact with osteoblasts and other osteocytesby means of long cytoplasmic processes (Fig. 55) that pass through thin tunnels (**canaliculi;** singular: canaliculus) in mineralized bone matrix.

Osteoclasts

Osteoclasts are multinucleated cells responsible for bone resorption (loss, removal) (Fig. 56). They are **derived from haematopoietic stem cells.** They have abundant eosinophilic cytoplasm, which has a special brush border near the bone surface undergoing resorption. **Osteoclasts resorb (remove) bone in two stages:** (1) First, the **mineral** is dissolved by secretion of hydrogen ions through **a proton**

pump located in the brush border. The hydrogen ions are derived from **carbolic acid** produced within the osteoblast from water and carbon dioxide by the enzyme **carbonic anhydrase**, and (2) second, the **collagen** of the matrix **is cleaved** (split) into polypeptide fragments **by proteinases** released from the numerous lysosomes in the osteoclast and secreted through the brush border. The concavity in the bone created by resorption is called a **Howship's lacuna.**

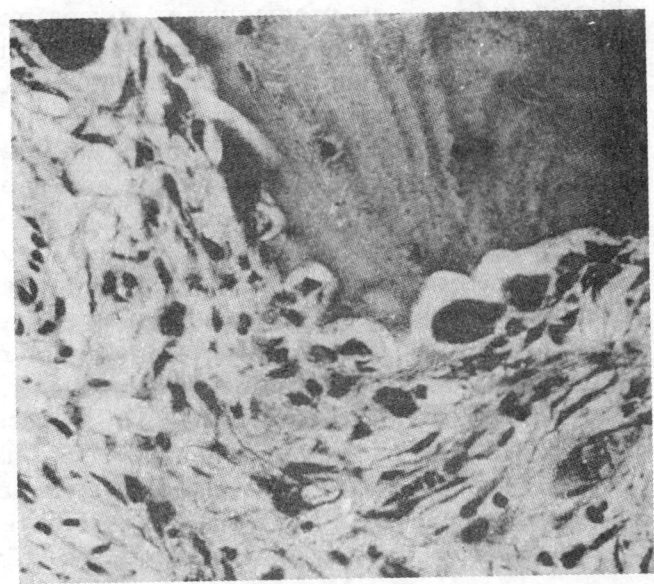

Fig. 56. Bone undergoing osteoclastic resorption in an area of necrosis. Multinucleated osteoblasts with abundant cytoplasm are seen near the bone surface undergoing resorption. The activity of **osteoblasts** results in an irregular (resorbed) bone surface. The resorption cavities are called **Howship's lacunae.**

Parathyroid hormone (PTH) is a stimulator of osteoclastic bone resorption. In response to PTH, osteoclasts increase in number, and their brush borders become more abundant. However, osteoclasts do not have receptors for PTH and that osteoblasts, which do have receptors for PTH, actually initiate the resorption process by signalling to osteoclast precursors and preparing the bone surface for osteoclast attachment. **In response to PTH, osteoblasts contract and expose bone surfaces to which the osteoclasts can attach.**

Calcitonin (a hormone secreted by C cells of the thyroid gland, which lowers calcium and phosphorus concentration in plasma and inhibits bone resorption) **is an inhibitor of osteoclasts. Osteoclasts have receptors for calcitonin** and respond to this hormone by involuting (i.e. turning inward) their brush border and detaching from the bone surface. The stimuli for **osteoclastic bone resorption** in disease processes are under the influence of cytokines (e.g., **interleukin 1 (IL-1), IL-6, tumour necrosis factor (TNF)** and **prostaglandins** released not only from inflammatory cells such as the macrophage, but also from a great variety of hyperplastic, neoplastic, and degenerated tissues.

Bone at the Matrix and Mineral Level

Interstitiun (interstitial tissue) provides strength to the bone. **It consists of a mineralized matrix. Bone matrix** consists of **type I collagen** and **ground substance,** which includes water, proteoglycans, glycosaminoglycans, non-collagenous proteins, and lipases. **Type I collagen** is secreted by osteoblasts and assembled into fibrils, which are embedded in the ground substance and then mineralized. **Type I collagen** is composed of three inter-twined amino acid chains. Unique to these chains is the **hydroxylated form of the amino acid proline (hydroxyproline)**. Type I collagen molecules have **extensive cross-linkages** among the amino acid chains within the molecule and between the molecules. The cross-linkages contribute to the **strength and insolubility** of the fibrous component of the bone matrix. **The collagen content of bone and its lamellar arrangement give bone its strength. The mineral content gives bone its hardness.** The **ground substance** of the bone also synthesized by osteoblasts, consists of **non-collagenous proteins, proteoglycans,** and **lipids.** Among the non-collagenous proteins are enzymes that function in degradation of collagen (e.g., **collagenases**) in bone resorption and can destroy inhibitors of mineralization (e.g., pyrophosphatases). Other non-collagenous proteins in the matrix can function as **adhesion molecules.** They bind cells to cells, cells to matrix, and mineral to matrix. Examples are **osteonectin** and **osteocalcin.** The role of proteoglycans in bone matrix is uncertain.

Bone mineral in fully mineralized bone is about 65% of the bone by weight and consists of calcium, phosphorus, carbonate, magnesium, sodium, manganese, zinc, copper, and fluoride. **The production of osteoid (un-mineralized organic matrix) by osteoblasts is followed by a period of maturation. Then mineral is deposited at the exchange of water.** The process of mineralization is gradual and might not be complete for several months.

2. Bone as a Tissue

Bone is organized into **osteons** or **Haversian systems** in the compact bone of the cortex and in subchondral bone of large animals. **Haversian** or **compact bone** is made up of numerous **osteons.** The **osteonal system** provides channels for the vascular supply to the thick bone of the cortex. In contrast to the compact bone of the cortex and the subchondral bone plates, the **bone in the medullary cavity** is in the form of anastomosing plates or rods and is called **cancellous, trabecular,** or **spongy bone.** These bones are not arranged into osteons, as in cortical bone. Bones produced in response to injury, inflammation, or neoplasia and the bone of the primary trabeculae and early foetus is called **woven bone** and is usually referred to as **reactive bone formation.** In **woven bone,** collagen fibres are haphazardly arranged, and **this bone is of inferior strength** when compared to lamellar bone.

Bone undergoes constant replacement called 'remodelling'. Old bone is resorbed and replaced by new. This turnover of old bones to new bone is necessary for repair of accumulated microscopic injury (**microfractures**). **In normal bone remodelling,** less bone is replaced than removed. This is one of the causes of reduced bone mass in aged animals. **In disease states,** such as **hyperthyroidism,** resorption is usually increased and formation decreased. This leaves a significant net negative bone balance. The remodelling unit of cortical bone is called the **osteon**, and for trabecular bone, it is called the **basic structural unit**.

The term **'modelling'** is used to describe **change of the shape or contour of a bone** in response to normal growth, altered mechanical use, or disease. In modelling, bone surfaces can undergo formation or resorption. This process allows the bone to change its shape or size. **Both modelling and remodelling** are under programmed genetic control but can be markedly changed by disease and changes in the use of the bone.

3. Bone as an Organ

Individual bones of the skeleton differ in the manner of their formation, growth, structure, and function. Flat bones of the skull develop by the process of **intramembranous ossification,** in which mesenchymal cells differentiate into osteoblasts and **produce bone directly.** Cartilage precursors are not involved. Most bones develop from cartilaginous models by the process of **endochondral ossification.**

The **long leg bones** and the vertebral bodies are divided into: (1) **epiphyses,** (2) **metaphyseal growth plates (physes),** (3) **metaphyses,** and (4) **diaphyses** (Fig. 57). The **epiphysis** is cartilaginous in the foetus, with ossification beginning centrally. Growth of the epiphysis also contributes to the overall length of the bone, and is achieved by endochondral ossification.

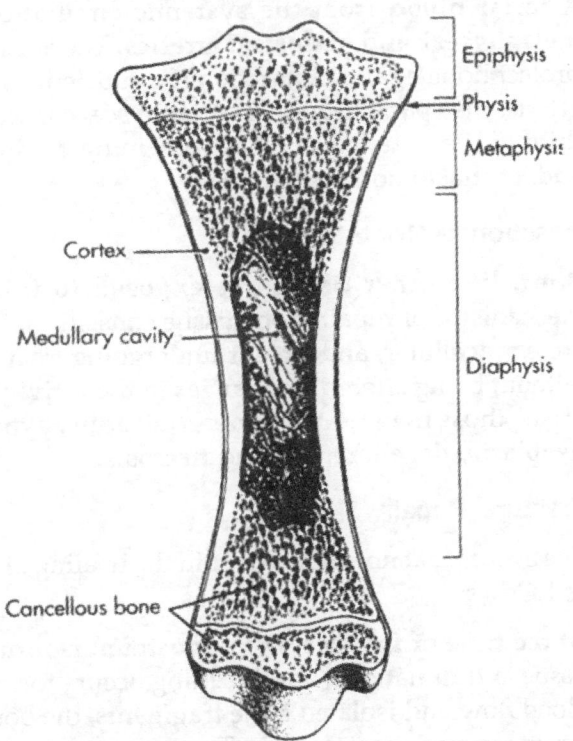

The **metaphyseal growth plate, or physis,** consists of hyaline cartilage. The **cartilage is divided into resting or reserve zone, a proliferative zone,** and a **hypertrophic zone.** The **resting or reserve zone** serves as

Fig. 57. Diagram showing the anatomical components of a long bone.

a source of cells for the proliferating zone where cells multiply, accumulate glycogen,

479

produce matrix, and become arranged in longitudinal columns. The proliferation of cells results in the overall lengthening of the bone. In the **hypertrophic zone**, chondrocytes secrete macromolecules that modify the matrix to allow capillary invasion, initiate matrix mineralization, and finally these chondrocytes undergo apoptosis. **Calcification** begins in the longitudinal section of cartilaginous matrix between columns of chondrocytes.

Growth plates are thickest when growth is most rapid. The plate becomes thin and is entirely replaced by bone at skeletal maturity. One end of the **metaphysis** is bordered by the calcified cartilage of the physis and the other by **diaphysis** (central shaft of the bone- see Fig. 57). The **diaphysis** or **shaft** of the bone has a thick cortex. In adult animals, the medullary cavity of the diaphysis has few trabeculae and contains mostly fatty marrow. Except for articular surfaces, the surfaces of bones are covered by **periosteum.**

Blood Supply to Bone

Arterial blood from the systemic circulation enters bone through **nutrient**, **metaphyseal**, and **periosteal arteries.** The anastomoses among these three arteries protect bone against infarction if a nutrient artery is obstructed. Small periosteal arteries also pass through the diaphyseal cortex, and can supply one quarter to one third of the outer cortex. The remaining cortex is supplied by the nutrient artery and its anastomotic branches.

Reaction of Bone to Injury

Bone, like other tissues, is exposed to injury. It has its own reaction and mechanisms of repair. Bone tissue consists mainly of mineral and collagen, which are extracellular, and except undergoing fracture, they cannot respond to injury without being altered by changes in the activity of bone cells. As with **cells** in any organ, those **in bone can undergo atrophy, hypertrophy, hyperplasia, metaplasia, neoplasia, degeneration, and necrosis.**

Fracture Repair

The events that normally occur in the healing of a closed fracture of a long bone are as follows:

At the time of fracture, the periosteum is torn, the fragments are displaced, soft tissue is traumatized, and bleeding occurs forming **haematoma.** Due to damaged blood flow and isolated bone fragments, the bone at the broken ends and marrow tissue can undergo **necrosis.** The **haematoma** and **tissue necrosis** are important in **callus formation. Growth factors** are released by macrophages and platelets in the blood clot. These growth factors are important in stimulating proliferation of repair tissue (**woven bone**). **Mesenchymal cells**, derived from periosteum, endosteum, and medullary cavity proliferate in the haematoma to form a loose collagenous tissue. These cells mature into **osteoblast** and later produce woven bone. **The term 'callus' refers to an un-organized meshwork of woven bone formed after fracture.** It can be external (that formed by the periosteum) or internal (that formed between the ends of the fragments and in the medullary cavity). The **'primary callus'** bridges the gap, encircles the fracture site, and stabilizes the area. In time, woven bone at the fracture site is replaced by stronger, mature lamellar bone (**'secondary callus'**).

Callus may have hyaline cartilage. Cartilage doesnot provide as strong a callus as woven bone. However, it eventually undergoes **endochondral ossification**, and therefore, ultimately contributesto the formation of the bony callus. **In addition to an adequate blood supply, stability of the bone fragments is of chief importance in fracture repair.** Mechanical tension and compression at the fracture site influence the reparative process. Minimal movement of the bone edges in contact with one another (**slight compression**) and good blood supply favour direct bone formation with minimal periosteal cells. Excessive movement and tension favour the development of fibrous tissue. **Excessive fibrous tissue** between bone ends in a fracture might result in non-union. With time, the bony ends of the non-union can become smooth and move in a pocket of fibrous tissue and cartilage to form a **false joint** or **pseudoarthrosis**. Other factors that can interfere with the normal repair process include malnutrition, bacterial osteomyelitis, and the interposition of large fragments of necrotic bone, muscle, or other soft tissue that might lead to **delayed union or non-union.**

Abnormalities of Growth and Development

The development and growth of bone are very complex. Therefore, a number of errors occur during the maturation of the skeleton.

The **physis (growth plate)** is a fragile structure whose activity and shape are affected by its blood supply. In case of nutrient deficiencies, such as occur in debilitating disease or general malnutrition, the growth plate becomes narrow (growth is retarded). Weakening or destruction of the **matrix** of the physeal cartilage as occurs in hypervitaminosis A and in manganese deficiency can lead to premature closure of growth plates. **If the entire plate is affected, no further longitudinal growth is possible.**

A number of abnormalities in development are characterized by defective cartilage development and are classified as **chondrodysplasias**. The affected animals are short-legged, and the dwarfism varies in severity. **Table 18** presents definitions of terms commonly used in describing **abnormal skeletal developments.**

Table 18. Terms used in describing skeletal abnormalities

Term	Definition
Amelia	Absence of a limb or limbs
Dysplasia	Abnormalities of development
Dystrophy	A disorder originating from faulty or defective nutrition
Hemimelia	Absence of a longitudinal segment of a limb
Kyphoscoliosis	Abnormal dorsal and lateral curvature of the spine
Kyphosis	Abnormal dorsal curvature of the spine
Lordosis	Abnormal ventral curvature of the spine
Phocomelia	Hypoplasia of limbs, hands, and feet attached directly to the body
Scoliosis	Lateral deviation or curvature of the spine
Spondylo	Denotes a relationship to a vertebra, or to the vertebral column
Syndactyly	Fusion of adjacent digits
Synostosis	Osseous union of bones which is normally distinct

Achondroplasia

This is an inherited disease of cattle. The affected homozygous foetus is usually aborted during the 4th to 6th months of pregnancy. The prognathia (abnormal jaw), domed skull, and shortened legs are responsible for the name **'bull-dog calf'** given to the affected foetus. Other features include anasarca, phocomelia (hypoplasia of limbs), protruding tongue, and abnormal growth of metaphyseal growth plate.

Osteopetrosis

This is an osteosclerotic (increased bone mass) disease that occurs in dogs, sheep, horses, and cattle. The basis of the disease is the failure of osteoclasts to resorb and shape (model) the primary trabeculae. **As a result**, spicules of bone with central core of calcified cartilage fill the medullary cavity. This process affects all bones which develop in a cartilaginous model. Affected bones are dense and have no medullary cavity.

Congenital Cortical Hyperostosis

This **disease of newborn pigs** is characterized by new periosteal bone formation on major long bones. Affected limbs are thickened by oedema and by spicules of bone that form on the periosteal surfaces of the metaphysis and diaphysis. **Piglets** are stillborn or die shortly after birth because of other defects.

Osteogenesis Imperfecta

This is **an osteopaenic (reduced bone mass) disease** described in **calves, lambs,** and **puppies**. It involves bones, dentin, and tendons. **Clinically,** affected animals may have multiple fractures, joint laxity, and defective dentin.

Angular Limb Deformity

This term refers to **lateral deviation of the distal portion of a limb.** It can be present at birth or can be acquired later in life. **Causative factors** include malposition of the foetus in uterus, excessive joint laxity, hypothyroidism, trauma, poor conformation, over-nutrition (consumption of excess proteins and calories), and defective endochondral ossification of epiphyses.

Metabolic Bone Diseases

These systemic skeletal diseases are usually of nutritional, endocrine, or toxic origin. Structural abnormalities occur in both growing and adult skeleton during normal modelling and re-modellling. Metabolic bone diseases are often called 'osteodystrophy'. **Osteodystrophy** is a general term and means **defective bone formation.** The **typical metabolic osteodystrophies** are: **(1) osteoporosis, (2) rickets and osteomalacia,** and **(3) fibrous osteodystrophy.**

1. Osteoporosis

Osteoporosis refers to the **clinical disease of bone pain** and **fracture** due to reduction in bone density/mass. When there is reduced bone mass but no clinical disease, the term **'osteopaenia'** is used. **In both osteoporosis and osteopaenia, the cortical bone is reduced in thickness and increased in porosity.** Trabeculae become thinner, fewer in number, and develop perforations within the plates. The medullary cavity becomes enlarged due to endochondral resorption of cortical bone. **The end result is a bone that lacks strength and is more easily fractured. In growing animals,** osteoporosis is **reversible. In adults,** once trabecular bone is lost, it **cannot be reformed.**

Some of the **causes include** calcium deficiency, starvation, physical inactivity, and the administration of glucocorticoids. **Calcium deficiency** can result in **hypocalcaemia** which is compensated by increased parathyroid hormone output and increased resorption. **Starvation** and **malnutrition** can result in arrested growth and osteoporosis due to reduced bone formation and because of protein and mineral deficiency. **Reduced physical activity (disuse** or **immobilization osteoporosis)** causes increased bone resorption and decreased bone formation. Loss of bone mass in long-term paralysis or immobilization is not necessarily progressive, because the skeleton stabilizes at a new (reduced) level.

Rickets and Osteomalacia

Rickets is a disease of **immature skeleton** and **osteomalacia** of **mature skeleton.** However, both are characterized by **failure of mineralization.** This leads to **bone**

deformities and **fractures. In the growing animal, rickets** is a disease of bone and cartilage undergoing endochondral ossification. **In the adult, osteomalacia** is a disease only of bone, mostly caused by the deficiency of vitamin D or phosphorus. However, failure of mineralization and osteomalacia can occur in **chronic renal disease** and in chronic fluorosis. Phosphorus-deficient animals usually have reduced feed intake, are unthrifty, and have defective reproductive performance. The **microscopic lesions of rickets** point to generalized failure of mineralization of growth plate cartilage and bone, as well as disorganization of chondrocytes in the growth plate. **Endochondral ossification** requires an orderly sequence of events finally resulting in mineralization of the physis, apoptosis of chondrocytes, and vascular invasion of cartilage from the underlying bone. If any one of these events does not occur, the cartilage is not removed and replaced by bone. **In rickets, the growth plates are thickened because of failure to mineralize.**

In mammals, when mineralization of the cartilage matrix does not occur, blood vessels with accompanying chondroclasts do not invade the physis. Since the ability of the chondrocytes to proliferate and undergo hypertrophy is particularly retained in rickets, the **growth plate thickens** because production of the cartilage is normal but removal is reduced. **Metaphyses** have excess of **osteoid (un-mineralized matrix)**, islands of surviving chondrocytes and fibrous tissue. Osteoclasts are not able to adhere to osteoid. Therefore, since osteoid cannot be resorbed, it accumulates and wide layers of osteoid occur on bone-forming surfaces. **Hypocalcaemia** can develop in a vitamin D deficiency, and lesions of secondary hyperparathyroidism **(fibrous osteodystrophy)** can also occur. **Grossly,** bones of the rachitic skeleton are deformed, break easily because of reduced mineralization, and are enlarged or 'flared' at the metaphyses of the long bones and ribs. The flared metaphyses indicate thickening of the physis and failure of the normal modelling of the metaphysis, because the poorly mineralized matrix cannot be resorbed.

Osteomalacia is the disease of the mature skeleton. It develops over time in the new bone formed in the process of skeletal remodelling. **The disease is similar to rickets, but** because the physes are absent, **there are no physeal lesions** in the adult skeleton. **Microscopically,** wide layers of un-mineralized osteoid are formed. **Clinically,** affected animals have bone pain, fractures, and deformities such as kyphosis and scoliosis.

Fibrous Osteodystrophy (Osteodystrophia Fibrosa)

As already stated, **osteodystrophy** means defective bone formation. The term **'fibrous osteodystrophy'** describes the skeletal lesions which occur from **increased widespread osteoclastic resorption of bone and its replacement by fibrous tissue that occur in primary, secondary, and pseudo-hyperparathyroidism.** Weakening of bone leads to lameness, fractures, and deformities. **In domestic animals, primary hyperparathyroidism,** such as in cases of functional parathyroid adenoma, parathyroid carcinoma, or idiopathic bilateral parathyroid hyperplasia, **is rare.** **Secondary hyperparathyroidism is more common** and can be **either nutritional or renal** in origin (**nutritional** or **renal fibrous osteodystrophy**).

Nutritional hyperparathyroidism is caused by dietary factors which decrease concentration of serum ionized calcium to which parathyroid glands respond by increased output of parathyroid hormone (PTH). It is more common in young, growing animals that are fed **rations deficient in calcium** and have a **relative excess of phosphorus.** Un-supplemented cereal grain rations fed to **pigs,** all-meat diets fed to **dogs** and **cats,** and bran fed to **horses** are example of **low-calcium-high phosphorus diets** that can **cause secondary hyperparathyroidism,** and eventually, **fibrous osteodystrophy.** Increased concentration of dietary phosphorus is important in the development of fibrous osteodystrophy, due to **interference with the intestinal absorption of calcium.**

Lesions begin with osteoclastic resorption of cancellous and endocortical bone, along with the proliferation of fibrous tissue near endosteal and trabecular surfaces. **In advanced disease,** entire cortices can be replaced by reactive woven bone and fibrous tissue. The lesions are in response to **increased concentration of PTH** rather than to the dietary effect of affected serum electrolytes. Sometimes, the **proliferation of fibrous tissue is excessive** and associated with increased external dimension of the bone. This process is more common in maxilla and mandible and may reflect the response of the weakened bones to the intense mechanical stress of mastication. Bones affected with fibrous osteodystrophy can fracture, their articular surfaces collapse, and some such as the vertebrae and ribs are deformed.

Clinical signs vary from a **mild lameness to multiple fractures** resulting in an inability to stand. Growth plates are normal in fibrous osteodystrophy unless there is an accompanying vitamin D deficiency, in which case young animals have superimposed lesions of rickets.

Renal Fibrous Osteodystrophy

This is a general term which refers to the skeletal lesions that develop secondary to chronic, severe renal disease. **Osteomalacia** and **fibrous osteodystrophy** can occur as separate diseases or in combination as a result of **chronic renal disease** in **human beings.** Fibrous osteodystrophy, which is sometimes complicated by osteomalacia, occurs in **dog,** the animal most commonly affected by **renal osteodystrophy. Dogs** can have **bone pain (lameness)** and loss of teeth and deformity of the maxilla or mandible due to the osteoclastic resorption of bone and replacement by fibrous tissue.

The **pathogenesis** of renal osteodystrophy **is complex,** and may vary depending on the nature and extent of the renal disease and the availability to dietary vitamin D. **Loss of glomerular function,** inability to excrete phosphate, inadequate production of 1, 25-dihydroxyvitamin D by the kidneys, and acidosis are important in the development of renal osteodystrophy. Phosphate retention because of decreased renal excretion causes hyperphosphataemia. As calcium and phosphorus product exceed solubility, **calcium is precipitated in soft tissue resulting in hypocalcaemia.** This hypocalcaemia stimulates PTH output with subsequent fibrous osteodystrophy. The reduced production of 1, 25-dihydroxyvitamin D by the diseased kidneys, together with defective mineralization due to the acidosis of uraemia, leads to development of **osteomalacia.**

Toxic Osteodystrophies

 A number of substances are toxic to bone and growth cartilage. Lesions which occur are described as toxic osteodystrophies. For example, a portion of the ingested **lead** can be bound to the mineral of bone and physeal cartilage undergoing mineralization. **In young animals**, the region of lead deposition can be seen radiographically as a transverse band of increased density in the metaphysis parallel to the physis. This **'lead line'** (a growth retardation lattice) is not due to lead itself, which is present in very small amounts, **but to lead-induced malfunction of osteoclasts.**

Chronic hypervitaminosis D can produce bone lesions of **osteosclerosis**. In acute, massive exposures, death is due to **hypercalcaemia** and widespread soft tissue mineralization. Bone lesions are not present. In long-term intake of smaller doses, the **persistent hypercalcaemia** causes chronic lowering of PTH and increase in calcitonin. This combination stops bone resorption. In addition, vitamin D has a direct stimulatory effect on osteoblasts. The inhibition of bone resorption and stimulation of bone formation result in a denser skeleton. **The matrix produced in hypervitaminosis D is usually abnormal.**

Aseptic Necrosis of Bone

In domestic animals, aseptic necrosis of bone is associated with **intramedullary neoplasms and various non-neoplastic lesions.** Decreased venous outflow from the bone and increased bone marrow pressure are important factors in the **pathogenesis of ischaemic or aseptic necrosis of the bone.** The **gross appearance** of necrotic bone varies. Large areas of necrotic cortical bone have a dry, chalky appearance. **Microscopically,** the main feature of bone necrosis is **cell death and loss of osteocytes from their lacunae.**

In the **femoral heads** of young and small breed **dogs,** aseptic necrosis is associated with clinical signs because of the collapse of the articular cartilage due to resorption of the necrotic subchondral bone that occurs late in the course of the disease.

Inflammation of the Bone

Osteitis

Inflammation of bone is called **osteitis, periostitis** if periosteum is involved, and osteomyelitis if the medullary cavity of the bone is involved. Osteitis is often a painful process causing extreme weakness of the affected animal. **Osteitis is usually caused by bacteria,** although viral, fungal, and protozoal agents can be involved. *Actinomyces pyogenes* and other pyogenic bacteria are common causes of suppurative osteomyelitis in **farm animals.** *Staphylococcus intermedius* is the most common cause of osteomyelitis in the **dog. Osteomyelitis** is usually a chronic process caused by necrosis and removal of bone and by the compensatory production of new bone. The two processes usually proceed simultaneously over a long period.

Bacteria can be introduced by a number of routes directly into the bone at the time of a compound fracture. Infection can extend directly from surrounding tissues, as in sinusitis, periodontitis, or otitis media, or more commonly, osteomyelitis may occur as **an extension from suppurative arthritis.** Suppurative arthritis can cause destruction of articular cartilage, which allows direct extension of the inflammation into subchondral bone.

Haematogenous osteomyelitis can begin in any capillary bed where bacteria lodge and survive. However, in practice, it occurs mostly in **young animals** and is localized in the metaphyseal area of the long bones and vertebrae **where capillaries make sharp bends to join medullary veins.** No vascular anastomoses are present in this region, and thrombosis of these capillaries results in bone **infarction** which is **a predisposing factor for bacterial localization. The exudate,** in bacterial infection in domestic animals, **is typically purulent.** Exudate accumulates in the medullary cavity and spreads. The increased intramedullary pressure compresses vessels causing **thrombosis** and **infarction** of intramedullay fat, bone marrow, and bone. **In areas of inflammation,** bone resorption is mediated by osteoclasts stimulated by prostaglandins and cytokines released by local tissue and inflammatory cells. Reduced blood flow through large vessels also promotes osteoclastic bone resorption. Lack of drainage and persistence of bacteria in areas of necrotic bone are responsible for chronicity of the process. **Bacteria can persist for years in cavities and areas of necrosis.** Inflammation can spread in the medullary cavity, penetrate into and through cortical bone, and damage the periosteum where it further disrupts the blood supply to the bone. Other sequelae of osteomyelitis include extension of inflammation to adjacent bone, haematogenous spread to other bones and soft tissues, and fractures.

Sometimes, fragments of dead bone become isolated from their blood supply and are surrounded by a pool of exudate (**bone sequestrum**). These isolated fragments of bone (**sequestra**) and exudate can become surrounded by a dense collar of reactive bone (the **involucrum**). Sequestra can persist for long periods and interfere with repair.

Haematogenous bacterial osteomyelitis is uncommon in dogs and cats, but it is **common in farm animals.** For example, haematogenous vertebral osteomyelitis caused by *Actinomyces pyogenes* is a common cause of posterior weakness or paralysis in **pigs**.

Mandibular Osteomyelitis and Periostitis

This disease, caused by *Actinomyces bovis,* occurs in **cattle**. Trauma to oral mucosa and eruption of teeth allow the organisms to enter the osseous tissues of the mandible, **where chronic pyogranulomatous inflammation develops.** The affected mandible is enlarged. Teeth can loosen and fall out. **Fungi** and **viruses** can also cause disease in bone.

Hypertrophic Osteodystrophy

Also called **'metaphyseal osteopathy'**, this is a disease of **young, growing dogs** of the large breed. The **lesions** are those of suppurative and fibrinous osteomyelitis of the metaphysis. **The cause and pathogenesis are unknown,** and infectious agents have not been isolated.

Non-Neoplastic Proliferative and Cystic Lesions

These lesions vary widely in their cause, structure, and effect on the host. New (reactive) bone formation (usually excessive) also occurs in fracture repair, in chronic osteomyelitis, and in degenerate joint disease in the form of periarticular osteophytes. The term **exostosis** or **osteophyte** refers to a nodular, benign, bony growth projecting outward from the surface of a bone. An **enthesophyte** is an osteophyte at the insertion of a ligament or tendon. **Hyperostosis** means that the dimension (thickening) of the bone has increased. An **enostosis** is a bony growth within the medullar cavity. It can result in disappearance of the marrow cavity. **All the above are non-neoplastic proliferative lesions in which growth is rarely continuous.** Non-neoplastic proliferative lesions should not be mistaken for skeleton neoplasms.

Hypertrophic Osteopathy
(Hypertrophic Pulmonary Osteopathy)

This condition occurs in **humans** and in **domestic animals, dog** being the most commonly affected animal. The disease is characterized by progressive, bilateral, periosteal, new bone formation in the diaphyseal regions of the distal limbs. The term **'pulmonary'** is included because most cases have intrathoracic neoplasms or inflammation.

Osteochondromas
(Multiple Cartilaginous Exostoses)

Osteochondromas occur in **dogs** and **horses. It is a defect in skeletal development rather than a true neoplasm.** This condition is **inherited** and **lesions appear soon after birth.** Osteochondromas project from bony surfaces as masses which are located near physes. They originate from long bones, ribs, vertebrae, scapulas, and bone of the pelvis, and can be numerous. **Clinically,** they might interfere mechanically with the action of tendons and ligaments, act as space-occupying masses, and they **can undergo malignant transformation and give rise to chondrosarcomas.** Osteochondromas in **cats** develop in mature animals and affect long bones less commonly. Osteochondromas in **cats**, like those in **horses** and **dogs**, can undergo neoplastic transformation.

Fibrous Dysplasia

This is an uncommon lesion. It has been found at various sites (skull, mandible, and long bones) in **young animals.** It could be a developmental defect and can be single or multiple. The pre-existing bone is replaced by an expanding mass of fibro-osseous tissue which can weaken the cortex and enlarge shape of the bone. The **lesion** is firm, usually mineralized, and can have multiple cysts filled with blood-tinged fluid. **Microscopically,** well-differentiated fibrous tissue has trabeculae of woven bone. **Osteoblasts** are not present on the trabecular surfaces, a feature helpful to differentiate this lesion from **ossifying fibroma.**

Bone Cysts

These are classified as sub-chondral, simple, or aneurysmal. **Sub-chondral cysts** are sequelae to osteochondrosis and degenerative joint disease. **Simple bone cysts** may contain clear, colourless, serum-like fluid, or the exudate may be markedly serosanguinous. The **cause** of **simple** and **aneurysmal bone cysts** is **unknown.** They could be consequences of ischaemic necrosis, haemorrhage, or congenital or acquired vascular malformations.

Neoplasms of Bone

1. Primary Neoplasms

Benign neoplasms originating in the connective tissue of bone are not common in animals.

Ossifying Fibromas

These are **uncommon** and occur as **large, heavily mineralized nodules** in the maxillae and mandibles of **horses** and **cattle.** Although considered benign, they can destroy adjacent cortical and trabecular bone by expansion. **Microscopically,** they are composed of fibrous tissue with scattered spicules of woven bone covered by osteoblasts.

Fibrosarcomas

These are **malignant neoplasms of fibroblasts** which produce collagenous connective tissue, but not bone or cartilage. **Central fibrosarcomas** originate from fibrous tissue within the medullary cavity, whereas **periosteal fibrosarcomas** originate from periosteal connective tissue. Central fibrosarcomas must be differentiated from osteosarcoma. **Grossly,** fibrosarcomas are grey-white, fill part of the medullary cavity, and replace cancellous and cortical bone.

Chondromas

These are **benign neoplasms of hyaline cartilage**. They are **uncommon neoplasms** of **dogs, cats,** and **sheep** and usually originate from flat bones. Chondromas are **multilobulated** and have a blue-white cut surface. They enlarge slowly, but can cause thinning of underlying bone. **Microscopically,** they are composed of multiple lobules of well-differentiated hyaline cartilage. They are difficult to differentiate from low-grade, well-differentiated chondrosarcomas. Chondromas which originate in the medullary cavity are called **enchondromas.**

Chondrosarcomas

These are **malignant neoplasms** in which neoplastic cells **produce cartilaginous matrix, but never osteoid or bone**. They are most common in mature **dogs of the large breeds** and in **sheep. In sheep,** they originate from the ribs and sternum, and **in dogs,** from the nasal bones, ribs, and pelvis. In general, chondrosarcomas usually originate in the flat bones of the skeleton. However, most originate in the medullary cavity and destroy pre-existing bone. With time, they become large and lobulated with grey or blue-white cut surface. Some neoplasms are gelatinous on sectioning, and some have large areas of haemorrhage and necrosis. **Microscopically,** the range of differentiation of neoplastic cells is wide. Some neoplasms are well differentiated and difficult to distinguish from chondroma. Other neoplasms are composed of **highly neoplastic cells** and have only a few areas in which differentiation into chondrocytes and chondroid matrix is noticeable. Chondrosarcomas have a **longer clinical course,** grow more slowly, and develop metastases later **than** osteosarcomas.

Osteomas

These are uncommon **benign neoplasms** which usually originate from **bones of the head.** They occur as single, dense mass that projects from the surface of the bone. They do not destroy adjacent bone. Their growth is slow. **Microscopically,** they are covered by periosteum and are composed of **cancellous bone**. Trabeculae are lined by osteoblasts and osteoclasts. The inter-tubular spaces contain delicate fibrous tissue, adipocytes, and haemopoietic tissue.

Osteosarcomas

These are **malignant neoplasms** in which neoplastic cells **form bone, osteoid, or both.** They can be classified as: (1) **simple,** when bone is formed in a collagenous matrix, (2) **compound,** when both bone and cartilage are present, and (3)

pleomorphic, that is, anaplastic, with only small islands of osteoid. **Classification** is also based **on cell type and activity** (osteoblastic, chondroblastic, or fibroblastic), on **radiographic appearance** (lytic, sclerotic, or mixed), **or origin** (central, juxtacortical, or periosteal). **Microscopically,** these neoplasms are composed of osteoblasts, osteoid, and large cystic, blood-filled cavities lined by malignant osteoblasts.

Osteosarcomas are common neoplasms, comprising about 80% of all the primary bone neoplasms in the **dog.** They usually originate at metaphyses (distal radius, distal tibia, and proximal humerus are the most common sites). Growth of the neoplasm is usually rapid and painful. **Grossly,** central osteosarcomas have a greywhite appearance and contain variable amounts of mineralized bone. Large areas of infarction and irregular areas of haemorrhage are common in rapidly growing intramedullary neoplasms. Cortical bone is usually destroyed, and neoplstic cells penetrate and weaken the periosteum and can extend outwardly as an irregular lobulated mass. **Microscopically,** variable amounts of woven bone or osteoid are produced by the neoplastic osteoblasts. **Osteosarcomas in the dogs** are characterized by local invasion. **Pulmonary metastasis is common** Metastasis can be widespread and can involve both soft tissues and other bones.

The **cause** of osteosarcomas is **largely unknown.**

Secondary Neoplasms of Bone

In humans, 60% of cancer patients have skeletal metastases at autopsy. These are mainly in red bone marrow, where the vascular sinusoidal system traps the circulating malignant cells. **In animals, the true incidence of skeletal metastases is unknown.** Metastatic neoplasms can be associated with pain, hypercalcaemia, lysis of bone, fracture, and reactive new bone formation. **In dogs,** rib shafts, vertebral bodies, and humeral and femoral metaphyses are common sites of metastases. **In cats,** skeletal metastases are rare.

Diseases of Joints

Reactions to Injury

Articular cartilage has a limited response against injury and minimal capacity for repair. Superficial injuries to articular cartilage neither heal nor necessarily progress further. However, progress can occur when there is sclerosis (stiffening/hardening) of sub-chondral bone. Repair by the formation of hyaline cartilage is uncommon. Injury to articular cartilage is not painful unless the synovium or subchondral bone is invaded. **Having no blood supply, articular cartilage does not participate in the inflammatory response.**

Sterile injury to cartilage can occur from trauma, joint instability, or lubrication failure because of changes in synovial fluid and synovial membrane. **Destruction**

491

of articular cartilage in response to sterile injury and infectious inflammation is mediated by **enzymatic digestion of matrix** and **failure of matrix production** by degenerated or necrotic chondrocytes. **Lysosomal enzymes (collagenase, cathepsins, elastase, arylsulphatase)** and **neutral proteases,** which are capable of degrading proteoglycans or collagen, can be derived from inflammatory cells, synovial lining cells, and chondrocytes. **Matrix metalloproteinases (gelatinases, collagenases, and stromalysins)** capable of matrix digestion are present in the **matrix in an inactive form.** They can be activated by products of degenerating or reactive chondrocytes and inflammatory cells. Intra-articular **prostaglandin** and **nitric oxide** concentrations are increased in degenerative and inflammatory joint disease.

Prostaglandins and **nitric oxide** inhibit proteoglycan synthesis in synovium and chondrocytes. **This reduction in proteoglycans content can lead to degeneration and loss of the cartilage.** Interleukin 1 (IL-1) is a cytokine secreted by activated macrophages. It promotes secretion of prostaglandins, nitric oxide, and neutral proteases from synovial fibroblasts and chondrocytes. Release of **tumour necrosis factor (TNF)** from macrophages in joints has effects similar to IL-1. That is, it decreases matrix synthesis and increases matrix destruction. **Cytokines** and **growth factors** that are anabolic to cartilage include IL-6, **transforming growth factor-beta,** and **insulin-like growth factor.**

Loss of proteoglycans from cartilage alters the hydraulic permeability of the cartilage. This leads to interference with joint lubrication and causes further mechanically induced injury to the cartilage. Loss of proteoglycans and inadequate lubrication of the articular surface causes disruption of collagen fibres on the surface of articular cartilage. Affected areas of cartilage are yellow-brown and have a slightly roughened appearance. **As more proteoglycans are lost,** the collagen fibres condense, and fraying of surface collagen fibres (i.e., becoming thin and worn out) extends as multiple vertical clefts (fibrillation). **Fibrillation is accompanied by loss of surface cartilage (erosion) and thinning of the articular cartilage.** This is followed by necrosis of individual chondrocytes, making cartilage hypocellular. In response to fibrillation, erosion, and necrosis of chondrocytes, remaining chondrocytes undergo regenerative hyperplasia, but the ability of chondrocytes in the adult to divide is limited and the regenerative attempt is ineffective. **Loss of articular cartilage may become complete with exposure of subchondral bone (ulceration).** Continued rubbing on subchondral bone causes it to become dense, polished, and ivory-like (**eburnation**). In Latin, 'ebur' means ivory.

Degenerative changes in articular cartilage are accompanied by the formation of **periarticular osteophytes** and secondary synovial inflammation and hyperplasia. Synovitis is characterized by the presence of plasma cells, lymphocytes, and macrophages in the synovial membrane, and by hyperplasia and hypertrophy of synovial lining cells. **Osteophytes** do not grow continuously, but once formed they persist as multiple periarticular spurs of bone which cause joint enlargement.

The synovial membrane usually responds to injury by villous hypertrophy and hyperplasia, hypertrophy and hyperplasia of synoviocytes, and pannus formation. Pannus is a fibrovascular and histiocytic tissue which originates from the synovial membrane and spreads over adjacent cartilage as a membrane. Pannus is usually formed only as a response of synovium (synovial membrane) to inflammation and is rare in degenerative joint disease even with secondary inflammation. Villous hypertrophy occurs with and without synovitis. Fragments of articular cartilage can adhere to the synovium. Larger pieces and detached cartilage can float free and survive as 'joint mice' in the synovial fluid.

Pannus can develop in chronic infectious non-suppurative synovitis and in some immune-mediated diseases, such as rheumatoid arthritis. In pannus, tissue histiocytes and monocytes of bone marrow origin transform into macrophages, and they, along with collagenases from fibroblasts, cause lysis of cartilage. As the pannus spreads, the underlying cartilage is destroyed. In time, if both opposing cartilaginous surfaces are involved, the fibrous tissue can unite the surfaces, causing fibrous ankylosis (immobilization) of the joint.

Abnormalities of Growth and Development

Congenital malformation of articular surfaces or fusion of joints is uncommon. The term 'arthrogryposis', refers to persistent congenital flexure (bending) or contraction of a joint.

Hip Dysplasia

Hip dysplasia occurs in dogs and cattle. In the dog, it is an inherited problem. The lesions are not present at birth, but can be well advanced by 1 year of age. Joint laxity (i.e. slackness or displacement in the motion of a joint) leads to subluxation (dislocation) and subsequent abnormal modelling of the acetabulum. Hip dysplasia, which might be inherited, also occurs in bulls. Affected animals have shallow acetabula, joint laxity, and instability, which lead to degenerative joint disease early in life.

Inflammation

Arthritis

The term arthritis means inflammation of a joint (of intra-articular structures), while the term synovitis inflammation of the synovium (synovial membrane). Arthritis is characterized by the presence of inflammatory cells in the synovial membrane. The nature of the inflammatory process is reflected by the volume and character of the exudate in the joint fluid. Joint diseases are classified as inflammatory and non-inflammatory.

Arthritis can be **classified according to cause, duration,** and **nature of the exudate produced (serous, fibrinous, purulent, lymphoplasmacytic).** The term **'arthropathy'** refers to any joint disease. Like osteomyelitis, arthritis can be a serious threat to the well-being of an animal. It is painful and can lead to permanent deformity and crippling. **Synovitis** can be due to infectious agents, presence of foreign material such as urates in gout, or to trauma to intra-articular structures, or it can be immune mediated. **Chronicity** can be due to an inability of the animal to remove the causative agent or substance, repeated trauma, persistence of bacterial, or continuing autoimmune-mediated inflammation. Substances associated with inflammation that contribute to joint injury include **prostaglandins, cytokines, leukotrienes, lysosomal enzymes, free radicals, nitric oxide, neuropeptides,** and **products of the activated coagulation, kinin, complement, and fibrinolytic systems in synovial fluid.**

Bacterial Arthritis

Bacterial arthritis is uncommon in dogs and cats, but is **common in cattle, pigs, and sheep,** where it is usually of haematogenous origin and polyarticular (affecting many joints). Neonatal bacteraemia secondary to omphalitis or oral entry usually causes **polyarthritis in lambs, calves, piglets,** and **foals.** Bacteria can also reach a joint by direct introduction, as in puncture wound, by extension from adjacent bone. **Bacterial osteomyelitis** can extend through the metaphyseal cortex into the joint, or **epiphyseal osteomyelitis** can lyse (cause necrosis) directly through articular cartilage. **The duration of bacterial arthritis varies.** Some organisms are rapidly removed and synovitis is short-lived. In other cases, bacteria can persist, and the inflammatory process can become chronic. Recently it has been explained how an arthritis which begins as an infectious process may persist as a sterile immune-mediated arthritis and that an infection elsewhere in the body can result in sterile immune-mediated arthritis through antigenic molecular mimicry (**reactive arthritis**).

The extent and mechanism of cartilaginous destruction differ in fibrinous and purulent arthritis. Acute fibrinous arthritis is characterized by **deposition of fibrin** within the synovial membrane and on the surface of intra-articular structures. The process can resolve (restore to the normal state) with complete **fibrinolysis** and **repair** without residual effects. However, if deposits of fibrin are extensive, they are invaded and replaced by fibrous tissue, **leading to restricted articular movement.** Fibrinous arthritis of long duration is usually accompanied by marked villous hypertrophy, lymphoplasmacytic synovial inflammation, pannus formation, and progressive destruction of cartilage. **In summary, articular cartilage can remain intact in fibrinous arthritis unless destroyed by pannus.**

An example of chronic fibrinous arthritis is that caused in **pigs** by *Erysipelothrix rhusiopathiae* septicaemia. Survivors have lesions secondary to localization of *E.*

rhusiopathiae in the skin, **synovial joints**, valvular endocardium, or intervertebral disks. **Chronic painful polyarthritis is a common result.** At first, arthritis is fibrinous, and later, it is lymphoproliferative with marked villous hypertrophy of the synovial membrane. **Pannus** formation, accompanied by destruction of articular cartilage and fibrous ankylosis of joints, can occur. Localization of the organism in the inter-vertebral disks is common and leads to inflammation and destruction of the vertebral disks, followed by fibrous replacement of the vertebral disks and surrounding structures (**disco-spondylitis**).

In contrast, purulent arthritis is accompanied by progressive and usually extensive lysis (necrosis) of the articular cartilage, the process usually extending into adjacent subchondral bone. Proteolytic enzymes derived from large numbers of **neutrophils** present in the joint are responsible. *Arcanobacterium pyogenes* is a **common cause of purulent arthritis in cattle and pigs.**

Many different infectious agents cause arthritis in animals. For example, *Escherichia coli* and streptococci cause septicaemia in **neonatal calves** and **piglets** and **localize in joints,** meninges, and sometimes, serosal surfaces. Usually synovitis is serofibrinous and becomes more purulent with time. *Haemophilus parasuis* causes Glasser's disease in **pigs** 8 to 16 weeks of age. **Lesions** consist of fibrinous polyserositis (general inflammation of serous membranes, with effusion), polyarthritis, and meningitis. Acute serofibrinous polyarthritis occurs in **cattle** dying from thromboembolic meningo-encephalitis caused by *Haemophilus somnus*. *Mycoplasma bovis* causes fibrinous arthritis in **cattle**, and the disease is characterized by lameness and swelling of the large synovial joints of the limbs which contain large volumes of serofibrinous exudate. *Mycoplasma hyosynoviae* causes polyarthritis in **older pigs**. The caprine arthritis-encephalitis virus (a retrovirus) causes chronic arthritis in **older goats**. The disease is characterized by lameness, carpal hygromas (an accumulation of fluid), and distension of the larger synovial joints

Arthritis in the dog is classified as erosive or non-erosive. Rheumatoid arthritis in **dog** is an **uncommon**, chronic, erosive polyarthritis which resembles the disease in humans. The **cause** in both is unknown, although it is clear that the process is immune mediated (involves both humoral and cell-mediated immunity). **Antibodies (rheumatoid factor)** of the IgG or IgM class are produced in response to an unknown stimulus. **Immune complexes are ingested by neutrophils.** These cells release **lysosomal enzymes**, which sustain the inflammatory reaction and damage intra-articular structures. In addition, rheumatoid arthritis also has characteristically **excessive pannus formation. In dogs,** rheumatoid arthritis is characterized by progressive lameness involving the peripheral joints of the limbs. **Grossly,** the lesions consist of marked villous hypertrophy of the synovial membrane, erosion of cartilage, pannus formation, formation of periarticular osteophytes, and when severe, fibrous ankylosis of affected joints. **Microscopically,**

changes in the joint are hyperplasia of synovial lining cells and infiltration of large numbers of plasma cells and lymphocytes in the synovium. Large numbers of neutrophils are present in the joint fluid.

Chronic non-erosive arthritis occurs in dogs with systemic lupus erythemtosus. Such **dogs** have anaemia, thrombocytopaenia, polymyositis, or glomerulonephritis. Non-erosive polyarthritis also occurs in **dogs** in chronic disease processes such as pyometra or otitis externa. **Immune complexes** can localize in synovium and cause **synovitis**. In these diseases, villous hypertrophy is minimal, **pannus formation does not occur**, and there is no destruction of articular cartilage. The exudate in the synovial fluid is neutrophilic.

Crystal-induced synovitis and degeneration of articular cartilage occur in **gout** when urate crystals are deposited in and around joints where they produce an acute or chronic inflammatory reaction. **Gout** occurs in species which do not have the enzyme **uricase** (humans, **birds**, reptiles). Deposits of urate, called **tophi**, are white, caseous, and periarticular and can be large enough to be visible grossly. Periarticular and synovial deposits of calcium pyrophosphate (**pseudogout** or **calcium pyrophosphate deposition disease**) and calcium phosphate (**calcium phosphate deposition disease**) have been reported as a **cause of synovitis and lameness in dogs and monkeys.** Single or multiple joints may be involved.

Degenerative Joint Disease

Degenerative joint disease (osteoarthritis, osteoarthrosis) is a disease of synovial joints which occurs in all animals. It is **a destructive disease of articular cartilage** characterized by a sequence of changes beginning with fibrillation and progressing to erosion and ulceration of articular cartilage and formation of periarticular osteophytes. It can be monoarticular or polyarticular, can occur in immature or mature animals, and can be symptomatic or represent an incidental finding. **Affected animals** have joint enlargement and deformity, pain, and articular malfunction. The aetio-pathogenesis of degenerative joint disease is incompletely understood.

Initial changes can be due to traumatic injury to articular cartilage, inflammation of the synovium, or increased stiffness of the subchondral bone. Degenerative joint disease usually progresses to sclerosis (stiffness) of the subchondral bone. This stiffness predisposes the cartilage to mechanical damage. The early biochemical change in articular cartilage is **loss of proteoglycan aggregates,** which leads to improper binding of water and a net increase in the water content of the cartilage. The increased water and its improper binding lead to softening (**chondromalacia**). Core proteins of proteoglycan aggregates are susceptible to the action of neutral proteoglycanases, which are increased in early degenerative joint disease. **Continued proteoglycan loss interferes with joint lubrication** and allows collagen fibres which were previously separated by a hydrated gel (proteoglycans and water) to collapse on each other. Weight bearing on these collapsed fibres causes **fissuring (fibrillation)**. This fibrillated surface with reduced proteoglycan content is prone to physical wear and progressive **loss (erosion) of cartilage.** Finally, complete cartilage loss (ulceration) exposes the underlying subchondral bone. With use of the joint, the subchondral bone becomes smooth and hard (**eburnation** and **sclerosis**). **Periarticular osteophytes** are a prominent feature, and synovitis characterized by villous hypertrophy and infiltration of lymphocytes, plasma cells, and macrophages are usually present.

Synovitis in degenerative joint disease is secondary to release of inflammatory mediators by injured chondrocytes and from synovial macrophages that have phagocytized cartilaginous breakdown products. **Proteases** and **cytokines** released by cells of the inflamed synovium cause more joint damage in the responses of cartilage to injury. **Grossly**, degenerated cartilage is often yellow or yellow brown. **Lesions** can be diffuse but are usually focal. In hinge-type joints, they can occur as linear grooves.

Age-related degeneration of articular cartilage is common in all species, and is not of much clinical importance. **Lesions** are of great importance when they occur at an early age and progress rapidly. Some of the **causative factors** include repeated trauma to articular cartilage, abnormalities in conformation, and joint instability. Also, degeneration of cartilage occurs secondary to inflammatory arthritis.

Osteochondrosis

Osteochondroses are **a heterogeneous group of lesions in growth cartilage of young animals.** They are **characterized by focal or multiple failure (or delay) of endochondral ossification.** Therefore, osteochondrosis involves metaphyseal growth plate and the articular-epiphyseal cartilage complex. The **lesions** are common and have different clinical manifestations in **pigs, dogs, horses, cattle,** and **poultry.** Surprisingly, the disease does not occur in **cat.** The important gross lesion is retention of growth cartilage due to its failure to become mineralized and replaced by a bone (**a failure of endochondral ossification**). **Grossly,** the retained cartilage is white and firm (similar to hyaline cartilage). **Microscopically**, these areas are composed of hypertrophic chondrocytes without evidence of mineralization or vascular invasion.

The **cause** of osteochondrosis is **unknown.**

Epiphysiolysis

Epiphysiolysis is separation of the epiphysis from the metaphyseal bone. It involves some degree of trauma in the metaphyseal growth plate. The **femoral head** can be involved in market-weight **pigs** and in **young gilts** (young female pigs).

Degeneration of Inter-vertebral Disks

Degeneration of inter-vertebral disks is usually an age-related phenomenon in many species. In general, loss of water and proteoglycans, reduced cellularity, and an increase in collagen content of the **nucleus pulposus** (a semifluid mass of elastic fibres forming centre of an inter-vertebral disk) occur. The degenerative changes are caused by various metabolic and mechanical insults which lead to **breakdown of proteoglycan aggregates** in the nucleus pulposus and **to degenerative changes** in annulus fibrosus (fibrous ring of inter-vertebral disk). Changes in structure of the nucleus pulposus, along with a weakened annulus, lead to **tears** or **fissures** in the annulus which allow **bulging** or **herniation** of the nucleus pulposus material.

Neoplasms of Joints

Synovial cell sarcoma is a malignancy of synovial origin. A benign counterpart is not recognized. **Synovial cell sarcomas are rare** and found usually in **dogs**.

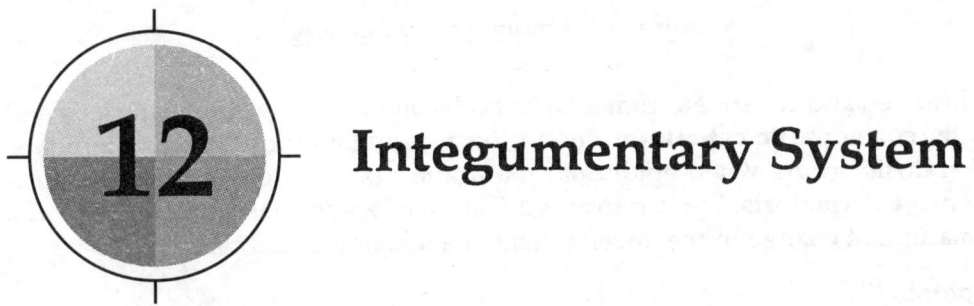

Integumentary System

Response to Injury

A large number of **exogenous** and **endogenous factors** can **cause significant skin changes. Exogenous factors include** infectious, physical, nutritional, chemical, allergic, and actinic (pertaining to rays of light beyond the violet end of the spectrum). **Endogenous factors include** hereditary, congenital, hormonal, metabolic, immunological, internal disease, age-related, and emotional. **Responses to injury are characterized by changes in the epidermis, dermis, adnexa, and panniculus (subcutaneous fat).**

Epidermis

Alterations in Epidermal Growth or Differentiation

Hyperkeratosis

Hyperkeratosis is an increase in the thickness of the stratum corneum. It occurs in two forms. In orthokeratotic hyperkeratosis (also called hyperkeratosis) the cells are anuclear (without nucleus), and in **parakeratotic hyperkeratosis (also called parakeratosis),** the cells have nuclei. Both hyperkeratosis and parakeratosis are common non-specific responses to chronic stimuli (e.g., superficial trauma, inflammation), and also occur in certain diseases. **Hyperkeratosis** occurs in ichthyosis (see 'ichthyosis') and vitamin A deficiency. **Diffuse parakeratosis** occurs in zinc-responsive dermatosis. Dermatosis is any skin disease, especially one not characterized by inflammation. **Hyperkeratosis** is associated with an increased thickness of the granular cell layer (**hypergranulosis**), and parakeratosis is associated with a decreased thickness of the granular cell layer (**hypogranulosis**).

Hyperplasia

Hyperplasia of the epidermis is an increase in the cells in the epidermis, mostly in the stratum spinosum, and is referred to as **acanthosis**. Hyperplasia is a response common in a number of chronic stimuli and occurs in a variety of types.

Dyskeratosis

Dyskeratosis is premature keratinization of cells in the viable layers of the epidermis. Dyskeratotic keratinocytes (epidermal cells which synthesize keratin) are shrunken and separated from adjacent cells and have a pyknotic nucleus and brightly **eosinophilic cytoplasm** due to the accumulation of **keratin filaments**. Dyskeratosis occurs when epidermal maturation is deranged such as in **zinc-responsive dermatosis**. Dyskeratosis is a feature of epidermal dysplasia seen as **a pre-malignant change** in the development of a squamous-cell carcinoma.

Apoptosis

Apoptosis is a programmed cell death. Apoptotic keratinocytes have morphological features similar to dyskeratotic cells. **Apoptotic cells are phagocytosed by adjacent keratinocytes.** Phagocytosis before cell's disintegration prevents the development of an acute inflammatory response, which would otherwise occur if cell's constituents are released. **Therefore, the process of apoptosis is significantly different from necrosis.** In necrosis, lysis occurs releasing cell's contents into the extracellular space. Apoptosis is seen in diseases such as lupus erythematosus and erythema multiforme.

Necrosis

Necrosis is death of cells and is characterized by nuclear pyknosis, karyorrhexis or karyolysis, organelle swelling, plasma membrane rupture, and release of cytoplasmic elements into extracellular space accompanied by acute inflammatory response. **Causes** of epidermal necrosis include physical injury (lacerations, thermal burns), chemical injury (irritant contact dermatitis), and ischaemic injury (vasculitis, thromboembolism).

Atrophy

Atrophy is a decrease in the number and size of the cells in the epidermis. It occurs as a result of sublethal cell injury. **Cutaneous atrophy** occurs in response to hormonal imbalances, such as hyperadrenocorticism in **dogs** and **cats**, partial ischaemia, and severe malnutrition.

Alterations in Epidermal Cell Adhesion

Oedema

Oedema may occur **intercellularly** or **intracellularly**. **Intercellular oedema** is called **spongiosis**. This is because when intercellular spaces widen with fluid, the epidermis develops a **'spongy'** (sponge-like) appearance. Severe intercellular oedema results in the formation of **spongiotic vesicles** and is common in inflammatory dermatoses. **Intracellular oedema** results in **cellular swelling**. If the swelling is severe, the swollen cells may burst, forming **microvesicles** supported by the cell walls of the ruptured cells. This type of epidermal damage is called **'reticular degeneration'**. When intracellular oedema is limited to the basal layer of the epidermis, it is called **'hydropic degeneration'** or **'vacuolar degeneration'** and may result in the formation of intrabasilar vesicles.

Hydropic degeneration is a consequence of **damage to basal keratinocytes.** As a result, basal keratinocytes are unable to maintain normal homeostasis and fluid accumulates within the cells. Examples include lupus erythematosus, dermatomyositis, and drug eruptions.

Ballooning degeneration is a form of intracellular oedema of cells in more superficial layers of the epidermis. It is characterized by swollen cells losing their intercellular attachments and the formation of a **vesicle.** Viruses that infect epidermis such as **pox viruses** cause lysis of cytoplasmic keratin and a build-up of excessive fluid, resulting in ballooning degeneration.

Acantholysis

Acantholysis is **loss of cohesion between keratinocytes** due to the breakdown of intercellular bridges through immune destruction, such as in pemphigus (type II cytotoxic hypersensitivity), or due to neutrophilic enzymatic destruction, seen in superficial pyoderma (any purulent skin disease). Fluid accumulating between the separated layers forms a **vesicle.**

Vesicles

Vesicles are fluid-filled cavities within or under the epidermis. They are generally 5 mm or smaller, and **bullae** are greater than 5 mm. These lesions develop in any layer of the dermis, or under the dermis. **Vesicles** may form from acantholysis, epidermal or dermal oedema, degeneration of basal cells and keratinocytes, or other processes such as frictional trauma and burns. The level of vesicles or bullae formation within the epidermis may involve certain diseases. For example, **intraepidermal vesicles** may occur in viral infections, intrabasilar vesicles in lupus erythematosus, and sub-epidermal vesicles in thermal burns.

Inflammatory Lesions of the Epidermis

Exocytosis

Exocytosis is migration of leukocytes into the epidermis. It is common in inflammation and is usually accompanied by spongiosis (intercellular oedema). The type of leukocyte may indicate the disease process present. For example, eosinophils may be numerous in ectoparasitism. Lymphocytic infiltrations into the epidermis are usually seen in immune-mediated diseases such as lupus erythematosus. Malignant lymphoma affecting the skin is characterized by intraepidermal lymphocytes. Erythrocytes may also be present in the dermis, usually in trauma, circulating disturbances such as marked vasodilation, and vasculitis.

Pustules

Pustules (microabscesses) are vesicles filled with inflammatory cells. They vary in inflammatory cell content and location in the epidermis. The **pustules of superficial bacterial infections** usually **contain degenerate neutrophils** and **coccoid bacteria** and are often located under the stratum corneum.

Crusts

Crusts are dried exudates on the epidermal surface. They indicate a previous exudative process.

Alterations in Epidermal Pigmentation

These include **hyperpigmentation, hypopigmentation,** and **pigmentary incontinence. Melanin** is produced by **melanocytes** located in the stratum basale of the epidermis, the external root sheath of hair matrix of follicles, and perivascularly, in the dermis. **Melanocytes have surface receptors for hormones,** such as melanocyte-stimulating hormone, and these hormones regulate melanogenesis. Other factors which influence the amount of melanin in the skin are genes, age, temperature, and inflammation.

Hyperpigmentation

This results **from an increased production of melanin** from existing melanocytes, or an increase in the number of melanocytes. Most hyperpigmentation results from increased production of melanin from existing melanocytes. Examples of epidermal hyperpigmentation by increased production of melanin include chronic inflammatory diseases and some of the endocrine dermatoses. Dermatosis is a skin disease, especially one **not** characterized by inflammation.

Hypopigmentation

This may be congenital or hereditary and develops because of a lack of melanocytes, failure of melanocytes to produce melanin, or failure of transfer of melanin to epidermal cells. Hypopigmentation may also occur from loss of existing melanin or melanocytes (**depigmentation**). Because **copper** is a component of **tyrosinase,** production of melanin pigment depends on copper, and **copper deficiency may result in reduced pigmentation.**

Pigmentary Incontinence

This refers to **loss of melanin pigment from the basal layer of the epidermis** due to damage to the cells of the basal layer and accumulations of the pigment in the macrophages in the upper dermis. Pigmentary incontinence maybe a non-specific lesion associated with inflammation. **Leukotrichia** and **leukoderma** refer to decreased pigmentation of **hair** and **skin**, respectively.

Dermis

Alterations in Growth or Development

Atrophy

Atrophy is a decrease in the quantity of collagen fibrils and fibroblasts in the dermis. This results in a decrease in the thickness of the dermis. The **causes** include catabolic diseases associated with protein degradation, such as hyperadrenocorticism in **dogs** and **cats**, and starvation.

Fibroplasia

Fibroplasia (formation of fibrous tissue) develops in response to various injuries, particularly ulceration. It consists of proliferation of fibroblasts and newly formed collagen fibrils. **Fibrosis** refers to gradual deposition and maturation of collagen to form a **scar. During fibrosis**, collagen production increases and the fibroblasts and vessels decrease resulting in less cellular, dense collagen bundles (e.g., scar), which grossly appears white and glistening.

Collagen Dysplasia

This is usually **an inherited abnormality of collagen** resulting in decreased tensile strength and increased stretchability. The skin tears with minor trauma and heals by formation of scars.

Solar Elastosis

This is caused by chronic exposure of the skin to the ultraviolet light rays of the sunlight. It is most prominent in the **horse.**

Degenerative Disorders of the Dermis

Collagen degeneration is characterized by increased granularity and eosinophilic staining intensity. It develops in disorders associated with infiltrates of eosinophils and eosinophil degranulation, such as reactions to insect bites, mast cell tumours, and eosinophilic granulomas.

Collagen lysis is dissolution (liquefaction) of collagen fibrils and develops following ischaemia and in microbial and parasitic infections.

Disorders characterized by Deposits in the Dermis

Amyloid is **a protein** which may be **deposited in the dermis** either as a primary event of unknown cause, or secondary to chronic infection, tissue destruction, or plasma cell neoplasms. **Microscopically,** amyloid consists of amorphous eosinophilic material.

Mucin is a normal component of the ground substance of the dermis. It consists of protein bound to hyaluronic acid and may be deposited in increased quantity in focal areas or diffusely. Because hyaluronic acid has a great affinity for binding water, the skin in cases of **mucinosis** has a thick, puffy (swollen and soft) appearance. **In cases of severe mucinosis,** the skin, when pricked with a needle, may exude mucin (a stringy fluid material). In histological sections, much of the water is lost and mucin appears as fine amphophilic (staining with either acid or basic dyes) granules or fibrils separated by dermal collagen. **Examples** of disorders with dermal mucin deposition are called **myxoedema** in hypothyroidism, and **mucinosis** in the **dog.**

Calcium deposits in the dermis may be due to alteration in dermal collagen (**dystrophic calcification**). They may also develop in association with abnormal metabolism of calcium, phosphorus, and vitamin D (**metastatic calcification**), or for unknown reasons (**idiopathic calcification**). Calcification results in **increased basophilia in stained sections.** Calcium deposits produce a **granulomatous inflammatory response,** a foreign body reaction to the deposits.

Inflammatory Disorders of the Dermis

Dermatitis

Dermatitis, inflammation of the skin, begins with hyperaemia, oedema, and migration of leukocytes. The inflammatory response to different stimuli can be quite similar. However, the distribution and types of leukocytes usually develop into certain patterns which suggest a pathogenesis. Patterns include perivascular, interface, nodular, or diffuse. The types of cells in the inflammatory infiltrates also vary. Perivascular and eosinophilic dermatitis is suggestive of lupus erythematosus, and nodular and granulomatous dermatitis indicate a prolonged cell-mediated response usually associated with persistent infection with acid-fast bacteria or fungi. Thus, patterns of inflammation and cellular composition of infiltrates are useful in microscopic diagnosis.

Adnexa

Adnexa refer to appendages or accessory structures of an organ. **In the case of skin,** adnexa include **hair follicles** and **glands.**

Atrophy refers to gradual reduction (involution) in size and may be **physiological** and **pathological. Causes** include hormonal abnormalities, nutritional abnormalities, insufficient blood supply, inflammation, and general state of health including stressful events or systemic illness. Damage to germinal epithelium can result in destruction or **total loss of the adnexa with replacement by a scar. Examples include** severe inflammation, thermal burns, thrombosis causing infarction, and severe physical trauma.

Hypertrophy is an increase in the unit size of a structure or an individual cell.

Follicular hypertrophy, that is, follicles are longer and wider than normal, occurs secondary to repeated surface trauma in acral lick dermatitis.

Hyperplasia is an increase in the number of cells in a structure. **Enlargement of adnexa,** a common response to injury, usually involves both hypertrophy and hyperplasia. It is observed in **sebaceous** and **apocrine gland** (i.e. sweat gland) **hyperplasia** associated with chronic allergic dermatitis.

Follicular dysplasia is incomplete or abnormal development of follicles and hair shafts. Microscopic features vary, but include **an abnormally formed follicle,** which produces an abnormal hair shaft, resulting in reduced or absent hair coat.

Inflammatory Disorders of the Adnexa, Vessels, and Panniculus

Folliculitis

Folliculitis is inflammation of a hair follicle. Folliculitis occurs in different forms which include **perifolliculitis, mural folliculitis, bulbitis,** and **luminal folliculitis.**

Perifolliculitis refers to inflammation around, but not involving the hair follicle. Perifolliculitis is not specific for any category of disease. **Mural folliculitis** refers to inflammation limited to the wall of the follicle. **Bulbitis** refers to inflammation involving the deepest part of the hair follicle, the **bulb. Luminal folliculitis** refers to inflammation involving the lumen and usually the wall of the hair follicle and is mostly due to parasites (**Demodex**), bacteria (staphylococci), or dermatophytes (**Microsporum, Trichophyton**). **Luminal folliculitis can weaken the follicular wall leading to rupture, known as furunculosis.**

Sebaceous adenitis is a specific inflammatory reaction of sebaceous glands. It occurs in **dogs** and rarely in **cats.** Lesions are characterized by accumulation of lymphocytes around sebaceous ducts. Fully developed lesions consist of lymphocytes, neutrophils, and macrophages which replace sebaceous glands. **Chronic lesions have total loss of sebaceous glands and scarring.**

Hidradenitis is **inflammation of apocrine glands (sweat glands).** It is seen in suppurative and granulomatous inflammation.

Vasculitis is inflammation of vessels. It may be the result of infectious agents, immunological injury, toxins, disseminated intravascular coagulation, or may be idiopathic. The species most commonly affected with vasculitis are the **horse** and **dog.**

Panniculitis is inflammation of the subcutaneous adipose tissue. It can be **caused by** infectious agents (bacteria, fungi), immune-mediated disorders (systemic lupus erythematosus), physical injury (trauma, injection of irritant material, foreign bodies), nutritional disorders (vitamin E deficiency), pancreatic disease (pancreatitis, pancreatic carcinoma), and may be of undetermined cause (idiopathic).

Congenital and Hereditay Diseases

The term 'congenital' and 'hereditary' are not synonymous. Congenital lesions develop in the foetus (in utero), are present at birth, and have a variety of causes. An example is hypotrichosis in the foetus (less hair than normal) associated with dietary iodine deficiency in mother. **Inherited conditions are transmitted genetically.** They are not always manifested phenotypically in utero or at birth, but may develop later in life. An example is **familial canine dermatomyositis,** which may not develop until 8 weeks of age or later.

Acanthosis Nigricans

This condition has been described in **young dogs.** The disease is manifested by bilateral axillary hyperpigmentation, lichenification (thickening of the skin with increase in skin creases), and alopecia (hair loss). **Microscopically,** the epidermis is thickened mainly by acanthosis. Hyperkeratosis and focal parakeratosis are accompanied by increased melanin pigment in the epidermis.

Alopecia and Hypotrichosis

Alopecia or **atrichia** refer to absence of hair from the skin where hair is usually present, and **hypotrichosis** refers to less than the normal amount of hair. These conditions have been reported in most species of domestic animals. Degree, location, and age of onset of hairlessness vary. In some cases alopecia or hypotrichosis is not due to an absence or reduction in the number of hair follicles, but a failure of hair growth or failure to maintain hair within follicles caused by an abnormality of the hair follicles (**follicular dysplasia**).

Collagen Dysplasia

Collagen dysplasia occurs in **most domestic animals** and comprises a clinically, genetically, and biochemically heterogeneous group of diseases. In each, the skin tears easily, and is loose, but the severity of these lesions varies among species.

Epidermolysis Bullosa (Red Foot Disease)

Epidermolysis refers to a group of diseases resulting in development of **cutaneous blisters (bullae).** Animals affected with the disease usually die because of their inability to obtain nourishment, and secondary infection leading to bacteraemia. **Epidermolysis bullosa** has been reported in some breeds of **sheep, horses, cattle,** and **dogs.**

Epitheliogenesis Imperfecta (Aplasia Cutis)

Epitheliogenesis imperfecta results from the **failure of the squamous epithelium of skin, adnexa, and oral mucosa to develop completely.** The disease has been **reported in** most domestic animals.

Hypertrichosis

Hypertrichosis is excessive growth of hair. It may be **congenital** or **hereditary**. The exact mechanism controlling the excessive growth of primary follicles is unknown.

Ichthyosis

Ichthyosis is an inherited skin disease mainly in **dogs** and **cattle**. It has also been reported in **pigs**. The skin is thickened by marked hyperkeratosis and may crack into plates **resembling fish scales**, thus the origin of the name (G. ichthyo = fish). **The basic defect is increased adherence of keratinocytes, which prevents normal desquamation. In cattle, two forms** of the disease occur: (1) **Ichthyosis foetalis:** This is **lethal,** and most **calves** are stillborn or die within days of birth. **Grossly** and **microscopically** the skin is alopecic and covered by thick keratinized plaques **separated by fissures.** Fissuring of the skin leads to exudation of proteins and fluids with common secondary bacterial and fungal infection often leading to death. (2) **Ichthyosis congenita:** This is the **less severe form**. The lesions in **calves** are mild.

Pityriasis Rosea

This **disorder of suckling and young pigs** is inherited. **Lesions** develop on the abdomen, groin, and thigh and begin as **small papules** covered by brown crusts. Lesions are of not much significance.

Lethal Acrodermatitis of Dogs

Lethal acrodermatitis is an inherited disease of defective zinc metabolism in dogs. Most affected dogs are dead by 15 months of age, usually due to bronchopneumonia. Skin lesions develop between the digits and on footpads. **Microscopically,** the main lesion is extensive diffuse parakeratotic hyperkeratosis with accompanying acanthosis. **Dogs** do not respond to oral or parenteral zinc supplementation.

Environmentally Related Diseases

Actinic Rays

Actinic rays are those rays of light beyond the violet end of the spectrum **which produce chemical effects. Sunlight** is composed of **visible** (400 to 700 nm), **ultraviolet** (100 to 400 nm), and **infrared** (700 to 20,000 nm) **light rays. The portion of the ultraviolet (UV) light most damaging to the skin is ultraviolet B (UVB)** and is in the range of 290 to 320 nm wavelength. However, **photodynamic chemicals,** if present in the skin, can chemically react with longer wavelengths causing cutaneous damage (**photosensitization, phototoxicity**).

Solar Dermatosis and Neoplasms

The **damage to skin by UV light** can be **acute (sunburns)** or **chronic (solar dermatosis, neoplasia)**. One of the important alterations caused by exposure to UV light rays is the formation of thymidine dimers between pyrimidine bases of DNA. The damage can be easily and accurately repaired before the cell undergoes mitosis by an enzyme system that removes the damaged area and synthesizes a new strand of DNA. **However, if the cell undergoes mitosis before the damage is repaired,** a gap in the DNA strand is left at the location of the thymidine dimer. The gap is repaired by a post-replication repair method that is thought to be error prone and **may lead to mutations and the development of neoplasms.** Factors that irritate the skin and increase the rate of cell division increase the number of cells repaired by the post-replication repair method, and therefore, may enhance development of neoplasms. UV radiation may also alter immunological reactivity by inducing suppressor T-cells, which favour growth of neoplastic cells. **Pre-neoplastic and neoplastcic lesions are common alterations in chronically solar-damaged** skin in domestic animals.

Solar Dermatitis

The lesions of sunburn occur in all domestic animals. The lesions have been described in **cats, dogs, pigs,** and **goats. Grossly,** lesions begin as erythema, scaling, and crusting. After years of exposure, skin becomes wrinkled and thickened and **squamous-cell carcinoma** may develop. **Haemangiomas** and **haemangiosarcomas** have developed in **dogs** and **horses** in the non-pigmented conjunctiva and in the skin of **dogs** and **horses.**

Photosensitization

Photosensitization occurs when long-wavelength UV, or less frequently visible light, is absorbed by a **photodynamic chemical in the skin,** or by a complex of photodynamic molecule and a biological substrate. **The photodynamic substances activated by light of the appropriate wavelength cause direct tissue damage by producing radial oxygen products and inflammatory mediators.** The photodynamic agent may enter the dermis through the systemic circulation or through direct contact.

Photosensitization can occur in several forms:

1. **Primary photosensitization:** This is usually due to ingestion of **preformed photodynamic substances** contained in a variety of plants, or fungal-contaminated plants. Administration of phenothiazine, tetracycline, thiazides, or sulphonamides may also cause primary photosensitization.

2. **Abnormal porphyrin metabolism:** Photosensitization may also develop because of abnormal porphyrin metabolism. **These diseases are usually inherited as an enzyme deficiency** resulting in abnormal synthesis of photody-

namic agents including uroporphyrin and coproporphyrin. **Examples include** bovine congenital porphyria and bovine erythropoietic (haematopoietic) protoporphyria.

3. **Hepatogenous (secondary) photosensitization:** This is due to hepatic disease that damages excretion of phylloerythrin, a product of chlorophyll formed in the alimentary tract. Hepatogenous photosensitization can occur secondary to inherited hepatic defects, biliary obstruction, or as a result of hepatic injury from a variety of sources.

Grossly, lesions in photosensitization are located on areas of the body with non-pigmented skin and hair, and on parts of the body exposed to the sun, such as the muzzle, coronary band, cannon, and pastern in **horses. In cattle,** lesions occur on the teats, udder, perineum, and muzzle. **In sheep,** lesions occur on the pinnae, eyelids, face, muzzle, and coronary bands. **Sheep** may have **extensive oedema on the head** resulting in such names as **'swollen head'** and **'facial head'.** Lesions initially are erythema, necrosis, and sloughing of necrotic tissues. **Microscopic lesions** include necrotic keratinocytes, epidermal degeneration, and sub-epidermal vesiculation.

Photoenhanced Dermatoses

Immune-mediated cutaneous disorders which are intensified by exposure to UV radiation include lupus erythematosus, dermatomyositis, and pemphigus erythematosus. Cytokines liberated from keratinocytes play a role in photo-enhancement.

Chemical Injury

Chemical injuries of the skin are due to local application to the skin, and from absorption of chemicals from the gastrointestinal tract and distribution to the skin.

Contact Dermatitis

Contact dermatitis is seen in **two forms:** (1) One is **immunologically mediated** (see 'allergic contact dermatitis'), and (2) the other is due to **direct damage** by the irritant substances. Most cases of contact dermatitis are non-immunological and are due to direct contact with substances such as body or wound secretions. Contact dermatitis has been described in **dogs, cats,** and **horses. Grossly, erythemic patches** and **papules,** and rarely, vesicles develop. **Microscopically,** lesions consist of spongiotic dermatitis, neutrophilic vesico-pustules, and superficial perivascular neutrophilic inflammation.

Ergot

Ergot poisoning occurs when animals ingest seed heads of grasses and grains which have been infected by the fungus *Claviceps purpurea,* which had produced toxic alkaloids. The alkaloids, particularly **ergotamine,** cause arteriolar vasoconstriction and damage capillary endothelium, leading to perivascular oedema and thrombosis resulting in tissue ischaemia (**infarction**). The species commonly poisoned are **cattle** fed contaminated grain and grazing pastures infected with the alkaloid producing fungus. **Lesions** develop after about one week of consumption and include swelling and redness of extremities, particularly of the hind legs. **Tips of pinnae and tail are affected with dry gangrene (infarction) and may slough.**

Fescue

Fescue poisoning occurs from excessive consumption of the plant *Festuca arudinacea*. It develops after 2 weeks of ingestion and consists of necrosis (**dry gangrene**) of distal extremities with lesions similar to those of ergot poisoning.

Selenium

Selenium toxicity occurs worldwide. Selenium poisoning occurs after ingestion of plants which have accumulated toxic concentrations of selenium, or with over dosage of a selenium supplement. Some plants selectively accumulate selenium, regardless of soil selenium content called '**selective or oblige accumulators'.** They require selenium for growth. They are generally not palatable and are eaten only when other plants are unavailable. Many other plants (**facultative accumulators**) do not require selenium for growth, but accumulate toxic concentrations of selenium if grown in soil with high selenium concentration. **Such plants are commonly eaten by animals and usually are the cause of poisoning.** Susceptibility to selenium poisoning varies with species, dosage, diet, and other factors. **In acute poisoning,** signs indicate involvement of many organs. Animals with **chronic selenium intoxication** are emaciated, have poor quality hair coat, and partial alopecia. **Horses** lose long hair of the mane and tail, develop hoof deformities, and shed the hooves. The mechanism of action is not completely understood.

Physical Injury

Acral Lick Dermatitis

Acral lick dermatitis (lick granuloma, neurodermatitis) is a relatively common dermatitis usually of an extremity (acral = extremity) in **dogs** due to persistent licking and chewing. Usually a single lesion occurs in carpal, metacarpal, metatarsal, tibial, or radial areas. **Grossly,** lesions are circumscribed, hairless, and sometimes ulcerated. **Microscopically,** hyperkeratosis and marked hyperplasia involve the epidermal and follicular epithelium. Ulcers may be present. The dermis is thickened by collagenous fibres and certain perivascular and periadnexal plasma cell accumulations and hyperplastic sebaceous glands. Some cases are complicated by secondary bacterial folliculitis and furunculosis.

Feline Psychogenic Alopecia

Psychogenic alopecia occurs in cats of the more emotional breeds and is multi-factorial. The alopecia is associated with **persistent licking due to hypersensitivity**. Endocrine associated alopecia is rare in the **cat**.

Callus

A callus is a raised, irregular, plaque-like area of cutaneous thickening which develops due to friction, usually over pressure points on bony prominences or on the sternum. **Callosities** can develop in all domestic animals, but are particularly common in **dogs and in pigs kept on concrete or other hard flooring with adequate bedding**. Secondary folliculitis, furunculosis, and ulceration may develop. **Microscopically**, the epidermis and follicular epithelium are thickened by hyperkeratosis and acanthosis.

Injection Site Reactions

Injection of vaccines or drugs into the subcutis can result in **granulomatous nodules** in the panniculus, particularly in **dogs** and **cats**. These granulomas have central foreign and necrotic material bordered by macrophages and multinucleated giant cells and surrounded by a zone of granulation tissue, eosinophils, and perivascular lymphocytes, which with time form lymphoid follicles.

Intertrigo (Skin Fold Dermatitis)

Intertrigo is dermatitis which develops **due to friction between apposing skin surfaces**, for example, adjacent folds. Intertrigo and bacterial growth develop secondary to irritation from skin friction and moisture from tears, saliva, cutaneous glandular secretions, or urine. **Gross lesions** consist of erythema, oedema, and crusting.

Pyotraumatic Dermatitis (Acute Moist Dermatitis)

This dermatitis is **especially common in dogs**, and is secondary to irritation mainly due to self-inflicted trauma of biting or scratching because of pain and itching. Irritants include allergies, parasites, matted hair, and irritant chemicals. **Dogs with long hair and dense undercoat are predisposed.** Lesions develop usually in hot humid weather. **Grossly**, lesions are hairless, red, moist, and exude fluid. **Microscopically, dogs** have superficial erosive to ulcerative exudative dermatitis, or a deeper suppurative folliculitis.

Radiation

Highly proliferative cells, such as those of the **anagen hair matrix** (i.e., the first phase of the hair cycle, during which synthesis of hair takes place) are most susceptible to radiation-induced damage. The earliest lesion is **erythema**. Oedema, epidermal blistering, ulceration, and hair loss may occur. Lesions may resolve or become permanent depending on the degree of damage. **Squamous-cell carcinomas** may develop in some sites of severe radiation damage.

Temperature Extremes

Extremes in temperature such as **excessive and prolonged cold** can cause injury. Exposure to more severe and persistent cold temperature causes vasoconstriction, increased blood viscosity, and tissue anoxia. **Lesions** are located in the extremities such as the ear tips of **cats**, scrotum of **dogs** and **bulls**, and ear tips, tail, and teats of **cattle**. Grossly, lesions consist of **gangrene** and **sloughing** of necrotic tissue.

Lesions due to excessive heat (**burns**) occur from exposure to liquids, flames, friction, electricity, heating pads, and lightning. **Burns** are classified as **partial** and **full-thickness**, or **first, second,** and **third-degree burns. In full-thickness burns,** complete destruction of the entire skin and dermal appendages occurs. **Partial-thickness** burns have preservation of some part of the epidermis or dermal appendages from which epithelial regeneration may occur. These lesions are less severe. **Grossly, lesions are erythema, oedema, and vesicle formation. Microscopically,** partial-thickness burns have coagulative necrosis of the epidermis, sub-epithelial vesicles, necrosis of superficial portions of follicles and sebaceous glands, and degeneration of the sub-epidermal collagen. In more severe burns the necrosis may extend to the panniculus. Secondary infection is characterized by accumulation of large numbers of neutrophils.

Snake and Spider Bites

Snake bites are most common on the extremities of large animals and cause swelling, erythema, and oedema that may be followed by necrosis and sloughing of tissue and death of the animal. **Spider bites** are found on the face and legs. **Lesions** are characterized by erythema and swelling followed, in severe cases, by necrosis and ulceration.

Infectious Causes of Skin Disease

Skin infections occur when there is disruption in the defence mechanisms of the skin. Defence mechanisms include a physical barrier (hair coat, pigment, stratum corneum), **a chemical barrier** (fatty acids, complement, immunoglobulins), and a microbial barrier (resident **microbial** flora such as **Micrococcus** sp., coagulase-negative staphylococci). **Predisposing factors** include those factors which harm the epidermal integrity such as friction, trauma, excessive moisture, dirt, matted hair, chemical irritants, freezing and burning, irradiation, and parasitic infestation. Factors that damage host's immune function such inadequate nutrition may also contribute.

Poxviruses

Poxviruses are DNA epitheliotropic viruses. They infect most domestic animals and birds. **Dogs and cats are rarely infected with poxviruses.** However, infection with contagious ecthyma (parapoxvirus) has been reported in **dogs. Lesions** develop following viral invasion of epithelium, by ischaemic necrosis due to vascular injury, and by stimulation of host cell DNA resulting in the formation of epidermal hyperplasia. The severity of pox viral infection varies in part due to the localized or systemic nature of the infection, and in some cases to **secondary infections.** Skin lesions sequentially consist of **macule, papule, vesicle, umbilicated pustule, crust, and scar.** Sheeppox and goatpox are the most pathogenic poxviruses. Infection causes significant mortality, especially in young animals due to systemic disease.

Contagious Ecthyma (Contagious Pustular Dermatitis, Orf, Sore Mouth)

Contagious ecthyma is a common **localized infection** of **young sheep** and **goats** caused by a parapoxvirus. Less commonly, **human beings, cattle,** and **dogs** are infected. Morbidity in **lambs** is usually severe and, although **mortality** is usually low, it can approach **15% in lambs. Lesions** begin with abrasions caused by pasture grasses or forage at commissures of the mouth and then spread to the lips, oral mucosa, eyelids, and feet. Lambs may infect teats of ewes, and the lesions may spread to the skin of the udder (Fig. 58). The disease is of economic importance due to weight loss in lambs which are

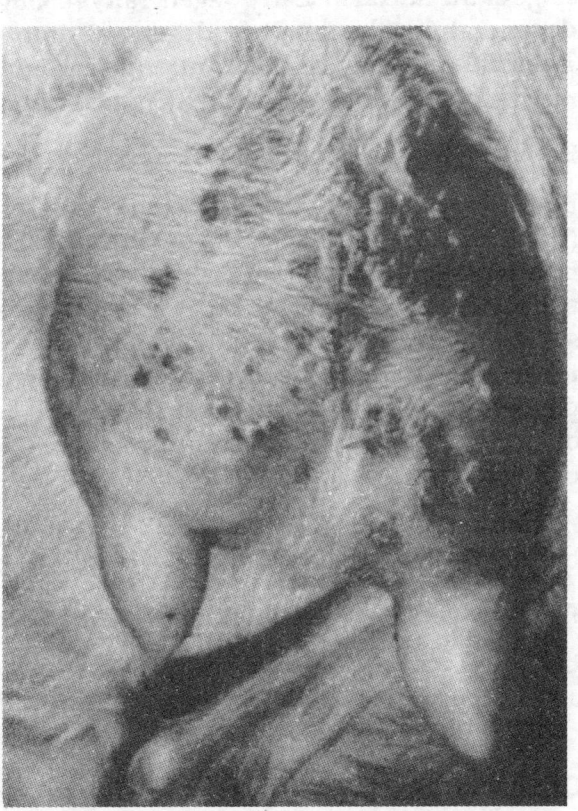

Fig. 58. Skin, udder; goat; Contagious ecthyma. The lesions consist of pustules and crusts. Pustules are short-lived and rapidly develop into crusts.

reluctant to eat because of oral and perioral lesions. **Gross and microscopic lesions** are similar to the typical poxvirus lesions, except that the vesicle stage is very brief. The ulcer and crust stages are clinically prominent, and **lesions are essentially proliferative. Inclusion bodies** are only briefly detectable.

Herpesviruses

Herpesviruses are DNA viruses. They are **rarely associated with skin lesions.** Skin lesions develop in association with non-dermatotropic herpesviruses such as infectious bovine rhinotracheitis (bovine herpesvirus-1) and equine coital exanthema (equine herpesvirus-3). Skin lesions have been rarely reported in **cats** with feline herpesvirus-1 infection. Two important dermatotropic herpesvirus infections are bovine herpesvirus-2 and bovine herpesvirus-4. Herpesviruses may be latent, and lesions can recur at times of stress. **Gross lesions consist of vesicles that rupture to form ulcers which are covered by crusts. Microscopic lesions** depend on the stage of the infection. Early degenerative changes include **ballooning** and **reticular degeneration**, the result of degeneration of epidermal cells and acantholysis. Syncytial cells may be seen. **Intranuclear inclusions** develop, but because of the rapidly developing necrosis, may not be found except at the margins of ulcers.

Bovine Herpes Mammillitis Virus

Bovine herpesvirus-2, **a dermatotropic virus,** may cause a more **generalized disease (pseudo-lumpy skin disease), or a localized infection of the teat (mammillitis is** inflammation of the nipple), called **'bovine herpes mammillitis'.** Localized infection usually occurs in **lactating dairy cows,** but may develop in **pregnant heifers and suckling calves.** Trauma is involved in the pathogenesis as normal skin is resistant to viral penetration. The disease is of economic importance due to decreased milk production and secondary bacterial mastitis.**Lesions** develop in the teats and skin of the nearby udder, or sometimes, perineum. **Suckling calves** may develop lesions on the muzzle.

Bovine herpes mammary pustular dermatitis: Bovine herpesvirus-4 causes a similar but milder disease than the localized form of bovine herpesvirus-2.

Feline Ulcerative Facial Dermatitis and Stomatitis

Ulcerative facial dermatitis associated with necrosis, eosinophilic inflammation, and **herpesvirus inclusion bodies** within epithelial cells has been reported in the **cats.** Feline herpesvirus-1 was identified in lesions by polymerase chain reaction.

Other Viruses

Skin lesions are seen in **foot-and-mouth disease** (picornavirus), **vesicular stomatitis** (rhabdovirus), **swine vesicular disease** (picornavirus), and **vesicular exanthema** (calicivirus). Both **feline leukaemia virus** and **feline immunodeficiency virus,** because of their immunosuppressive capabilities, can predispose to chronic skin infection including abscesses. Rarely, feline calicivirus has been involved as a cause of cutaneous lesion.

Bacterial Infections

Bacterial infections of skin are called 'pyodermas'. They may be superficial or deep. Pyodermas are among the most common lesions of the skin in dogs, but are uncommon in cats and other domestic animals.

Superficial Bacterial Infections (Superficial Pyoderma)

These infections involve the epidermis including that of the hair follicles. They usually heal without scarring, and generally, the regional lymph nodes are not affected. Grossly, the lesions are erythema, alopecia, papules and pustules, and crusts. Microscopically, the patterns include intra-epidermal pustular dermatitis and superficial suppurative folliculitis. Although bacteria are the cause of the lesions, they are not always microscopically demonstrable.

Superficial Pustular Dermatitis (Impetigo)

This infection is observed in dogs, cats, piglets, cows, does (female goats), and ewes. It is caused by coagulase-positive Staphylococcus sp. In cows, does, and ewes, lesions are mainly on the udder. In kittens, neck and shoulders are affected. Streptococcus sp. and Pasteurella sp. are the most common bacterial isolates. Gross lesions consist of pustules which develop into crusts. The microscopic lesion is a non-follicular neutrophilic sub-corneal pustule.

Dermatophilosis (Streptothricosis)

Dermatophilosis is caused by *Dermatophilus congolensis*. It is characterized by skin lesions in cattle, sheep, and horses more often than dogs, cats, pigs, and goats. Lesions develop on the dorsum of back and extremities. The bacteria stimulate an acute inflammatory response in which neutrophils migrate from superficial vessels into the dermis and through the epidermis to form microabscesses. Grossly, lesions consist of papules, pustules, and thick crusts that may coalesce and mat the hair or wool. The microscopic lesions are those of hyperplastic superficial perivascular dermatitis.

Exudative Epidermitis of Pigs (Greasy Pig Disease)

This infection is caused by *Staphylococcus hyicus*. It is an acute, often fatal dermatitis of neonatal piglets and mild disease in older piglets. Dermatitis and brownish exudate develop around the eyes, pinnae, snout, chin, legs, and spreads to the ventral thorax and abdomen. Grossly, the epidermis is thickened with scaling. Microscopically, lesions are those of sub-corneal pustular dermatitis with extension to the hair follicle, resulting in superficial suppurative folliculitis.

Deep Bacterial Infections (Deep Pyodermas)

These infections are less common than superficial infections and occur usually in dogs. These infections cause folliculitis, which may develop into furunculosis.

Deep bacterial infections usually heal with scarring and generally involve regional lymph nodes. **Grossly,** the lesions depend on age and state, and include papules, pustules, alopecia, nodules, abscesses, ulcers, fistulas, and haemorrhagic bullae. The **microscopic patterns** include pyogranulomatous folliculitis and furunculosis, nodular to diffuse dermatitis and panniculitis. Bacteria isolated include **Staphylococcus** sp., **Streptococcus** sp., *Corynebacterium pseudotuberculosis*, **Pasteurella** sp., and *Escherichia coli*. *Staphylococcus intermedius* is the primary pathogen of canine skin.

Staphylococcal Folliculitis and Furunculosis

These conditions are **most common in dogs,** but frequently also affect **horse, goat,** and **sheep,** and rarely **cow, cat,** and **pig. In dogs,** lesions are localized or generalized and occur on the muzzle, nose, pressure points, inter-digital areas, and chin. In other species, they occur on different parts of the body. **Microscopic lesions** include suppurative folliculitis.

Subcutaneous Abscesses

These are **localized collections of purulent exudate** in the dermis and subcutis. **Abscesses are common in cats.** Bacteria involved include *Pasteurella multocida*, Fusobacterium sp., beta-haemolytic streptococci, and **Bacteroides** sp.

Bacterial Granulomatous Dermatitis

This dermatitis is associated with traumatic introduction of bacteria which are generally **saprophytes of low virulence. Grossly,** lesions are diffuse or nodular and may ulcerate and drain to the skin surface by fistulas. **Microscopically,** collections of macrophages with or without giant cells are present.

Microbial organisms produce **granulomatous to pyogranulomatous lesions** in many species including **cattle, pigs, dogs,** and **cats.** Skin lesions are usually caused by *Mycobacterium lepraemurium* (**feline leprosy**). Skin infections with *M. tuberculosis, M. bovis,* or *M. avium* are rare.

Botryomycosis

This term refers to a **granulomatous dermatitis** caused usually by *Staphylococcus aureus*, which form yellow 'sulphur granules'. The granules consist centrally of bacterial colonies surrounded by radiating club-shaped bodies of homogeneous eosinophilic material. The material, considered antigen-antibody complexes, is called **Splendore-Hoeppli material.**

Digital Infections of Ruminants (Bacterial Pododermatitis)

Infections of the digits of **cattle** and **sheep** are usually mixed bacterial infections. These are separated into **two groups:** (1) **contagious footrot,** and (2) **necrobacillosis**

of the foot. Contagious footrot is caused mostly by *Bateroides nodosus* acting synergistically with *Fusobacterium necrophorum*. **Necrobacillosis of the foot** is caused mainly by *F. necrophorum* with other bacteria, including *Bacteroides melaninogenicus* in **cattle.**

Contagious footrot in **sheep** occurs when moisture and trauma damage the inter-digital epidermis and allow colonization by a variety of microorganisms from skin or faeces, including *F. necrophorum*. Lesions are inter-digital, affect both digits, and consist of red, moist, and swollen eroded skin. The inflammation spreads and results in separation of the hoof. In chronic infections, hooves may become long and misshapen. **Footrot in cattle is similar to footrot in sheep.**

Necrobacillosis of the foot of sheep includes **inter-digital dermatitis** and **foot abscesses.** Inter-digital dermatitis is an acute necrotizing dermatitis. **Foot abscesses** include heel abscesses **(infective bulbar necrosis)** and toe abscesses **(lamellar abscesses).** In addition to *F. necrophorum, Arcanobacterium pyogenes* (*Actinomyces pyogenes*) may be isolated from the lesions.

Necrobacillosis (foul in the foot) of **cattle** occurs secondary to trauma and is caused by *F. necrophorum.* The condition is associated with lameness and is characterized by an inter-digital dermatitis and cellulitis.

Systemic Bacterial Infections

Systemic salmonellosis may cause cyanosis of the external ears and abdomen. Cutaneous lesions associated with *Erysipelothrix rhusiopathiae* (**erysipelas**) in **pigs** consist of square to rhomboidal (i.e. having a flat shape with four straight sides of equal length), firm, raised, pink to dark purple areas (Fig. 59) and are due to vasculitis, thrombosis, and ischaemia (infarction). **Bacterial infections** may also develop from direct extension of bacterial infections of deeper tissues such as **clostridial myositis** and **cellulitis.**

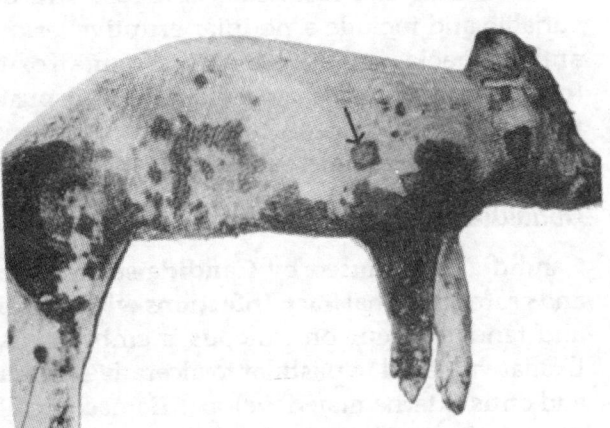

Fig. 59. **Skin; pig. Erysipelas.** Rhomboidal lesions (arrow) are present in the skin. The lesions are due to vasculitis, which has caused infarction.

Fungal (Mycotic) Infection

Mycotic infections are classified into **four categories: superficial, cutaneous, subcutaneous,** and **systemic.**

1. Superficial Mycoses

These are **infections restricted to the stratum corneum or hair with minimal or no tissue reaction.**

2. Cutaneous Mycoses

These are **infections of keratinized tissues** including **hair, feathers, nails, and epidermis.** The fungi are usually restricted to the keratinized layer, but tissue destruction and host response may be extensive. **Infections in animals include dermatophytosis, and cutaneous candidiasis.**

Dermatophytoses are fungal infections of the skin, hair, and nails of animals caused by a group of related fungi known as **dermatophytes.** Pathogenic genera include **Epidermophyton, Microsporum,** and **Trichophyton. Dermatophytosis is** the **most important cutaneous (superficial) mycosis,** and is common in **human beings** and **animals,** especially **cats.** Dermatophytoses are more contagious than other fungal infections.

Dermatophytes invade keratinized tissues (stratum corneum, hair shafts, and nails) by producing proteolytic enzymes, which help in penetration. The fungal products and cytokines released from the damaged keratinocytes result in **epidermal hyperplasia** (hyperkeratosis, parakeratosis, and acanthosis) and inflammation (**superficial perivascular dermatitis**). Bacterial infection increases the severity of the folliculitis and furunculosis. **Gross and microscopic lesions** may be highly variable and include a nodular eruptive lesion, a granulomatous nodular lesion, and alopecia in haired skin, to malformed, broken or sloughed nails (**onychomycosis**). Follicular papules and pustules may be present. **Microscopic patterns** include perifolliculitis, or furunculosis, as well as epidermal hyperplasia with intra-corneal microabscesses.

Candidiasis

Candidiasis is caused by **Candida** sp. which are normal inhabitants of the skin and gastrointestinal tract. **Infections with Candida sp. are rare in domestic animals** and tend to occur on mucous membranes and at mucocutaneous junctions. Exudative, papular, pustular to ulcerative dermatitis of the lips (**cheilitis**), stomatitis, and otitis externa may develop. **Microscopically,** lesions are in the epidermis and consist of spongiotic neutrophilic pustular inflammation with parakeratosis and ulceration with organisms present in the superficial exudate.

3. Subcutaneous Mycoses

These mycoses are **caused by fungi that invade skin and subcutaneous tissues** after traumatic introduction. Some infections remain localized, but others spread to the lymph vessels. **Subcutaneous mycoses include** eumycotic mycetomas, dermatophytic pseudomycetoma, subcutaneous zygomycosis, subcutaneous phaeohyphomycosis, sporotrichosis, and pythiosis (not a true fungus).

Eumycotic mycetomas occur mostly in **horses** and **dogs**, and are rare fungal infections resulting in tumour-like enlargements which consist of **granulomatous inflammation**. Fungi included are *Curvularia geniculata*, and of the genera **Madurella** and **Acremonium**.

Dermatophytic pseudomycetoma is a rare deep dermal and subcutaneous infection by *Microsporum canis* in **cats**. **Gross lesions** are similar to other subcutaneous mycoses.

Phaeohyphomycosis is a mycotic infection caused by **species of pigmented fungi** of a variety of genera. Subcutaneous phaeohyphomycosis **occurs in cats, cattle, horses,** and rarely, **dogs**.

Sporotrichosis is caused by *Sporothrix schenckii*. It is a rare mycosis that occurs in **horses, mules, cattle, cats,** and **dogs**. Cutaneous nodules ulcerate and fistulae may develop at sites of traumatic introduction and along lymph vessels **(lymphangitis)**, but visceral spread is uncommon. The exudate containing organisms is infectious to human beings if introduced into skin wounds.

Zygomycosis (phycomycosis) and **oomycosis (pythiosis)** are skin infections with hyphae or hyphal-like structures. These are caused by two classes of organisms: zygomycetes and oomycetes. The infections are characterized by proliferative, sometimes destructive, erythematous nodular lesions that ulcerate and drain. **Microscopically**, hyphae or hyphal-like structures are present in areas of eosinophilic to pyogranulomatous inflammation.

4. Systemic Mycoses

The lungs are the main route of entry and infection in the systemic mycoses, but cutaneous and subcutaneous infections can occur as part of the disseminated disease or by introduction of fungi by trauma. **Systemic mycoses include** blastomycosis, coccidioidomycosis, cryptococcosis, and histoplasmosis. **Grossly**, one or more nodular areas may ulcerate and have draining fistulas. **Microscopically**, the lesions are **granulomas** or **pyogranulomas**.

Parasitic Infections

Ectoparasites include **mites** and **ticks** (which have 8 legs), and **lice, fleas,** and **flies** (which have 6 legs). The presence of these ectoparasites is called **infestation**. **Endoparasites** causing skin lesions include **nematodes, trematodes,** and **protozoa,** and their presence is called an **infection**.

Mites

Mites cause serious skin lesions in domestic animals.

Demodicosis is caused by host-specific mites. It is a major problem in **dogs**, but is uncommon in other animals. **Demodex mites** live in the **lumens of hair follicles or sebaceous glands. Canine demodicosis** is caused by *D. canis* and occurs in **two forms: localized** and **generalized.** Grossly, localized form shows one to several small scaly, erythematous, alopecic areas on the face and forelegs. **Generalized demodicosis** usually involves large areas of body. **Lesions** consist of larger patches of erythema, alopecia, scales, and crusts. **Microscopic lesions** include epidermal hyperkeratosis, lymphoplasmacytic perifolliculitis, focal mild degeneration of follicular basal cells, and intraluminal mites. Sebaceous inflammation may also occur.

In cats, demodicosis is rare. Lesions are usually localized. **Demodicosis** in **cattle** and **goats** is of little clinical importance.

Scabies is caused by *Sarcoptes scabiei.* It is a highly contagious mite and is the **most important ectoparasite of pigs,** is common in **dogs,** and is rare in **horses, cattle, sheep, goats,** and **cats.** The mites burrow in tunnels in the stratum corneum and cause intense pruritus (itching) due to hypersensitivity reactions. Lesions occur in ears, head, and neck, and may become generalized. **Gross lesions** include erythematous macules, (discoloured spots in the skin), papules, pustules, crusts, and excoriations, **Microscopically,** lesions consist of superficial perivascular dermatitis with eosinophils, mast cells, and lymphocytes. Chronic lesions are associated with epidermal acanthosis, hyperkeratosis, parakeratosis, crusting, and perivascular dermatitis with eosinophils, mast cells, and lymphocytes.

Notoedric mite infestation is caused by *Notoedres cati* in **cats.** It is a rare but highly contagious, pruritic disease characterized initially by an erythematous papular rash followed by scales, crusts, and alopecia. **Microscopic lesions** consist of epidermal hyperplasia, mild spongiosis, crusts, and superficial perivascular dermatitis with eosinophils. **Otodectic mite infestation** caused by *Otodectes cynotis* occurs in the external ear canals of carnivores.

Psoroptic mite infestation in **sheep, cattle, horses, goats,** and **other animals** is caused by several species of host specific mites. *Psoroptes cuniculi* occurs in **horses, goats,** and **sheep. Psoroptes equi** infests the base of the mane and tail and skin under the forelock of **horses.** *Psoroptes ovis* causes serious disease in **cattle** and **sheep,** producing parasitic lesions of thickened skin and dry scales and crusts. **In sheep,** psoroptic mite infestation is called 'sheep scab'. The **microscopic lesion** is a spongiotic, hyperplastic, or exudative superficial perivascular dermatitis with eosinophils.

Chorioptic mite infestation occurs in **cattle, horses, goats,** and **sheep.** Mites on the skin produce **gross lesions** of erythematous, papular, crusted, scaly, hairless, thickened skin on the lower limbs, scrotum, tail, udder, and thigh of **cattle;** lower limbs of **horses;** and lower limbs, hindquarters, and abdomen of **goats.**

Ticks

Ticks, both **soft** (argasid) and **hard** (ixodid), cause injury by **loss of blood** (producing anaemia), by **irritation** due to bites, by hypersensitivity reactions, by causing tick paralysis and toxicosis, and by predisposing to secondary bacterial disease and myiasis (discussed later). **Gross lesions** consist of focal erosions, erythema, and crusted ulcers with alopecia and nodules in some animals. **Microscopic lesions** include epidermal and dermal necrosis and perivascular to diffuse inflammation. The exudate is composed of eosinophils, macrophages, and lymphocytes. Some lesions are granulomas (**arthropod bite granuloma**).

Lice

Pediculosis, or infestation with lice, causes anaemia, weakness, damage to hair and wool, and discomfort. Pediculosis is more common in winter when temperatures are cooler and the wool or hair coat is longer. Infestations are relatively host specific, and spread by direct contact. **Gross lesions** consist of papules, crusts, and lice and eggs are visible in the lesions.

Fleas

Flea infestation is a problem mainly in **dogs** and **cats**. Fleas cause **severe skin irritation** due to frequent biting and release of enzymes, anticoagulants, and histamine-like substances, hypersensitivity reactions to saliva, and trauma from scratching and biting. Severe infestations may cause blood loss (**anaemia**) especially in puppies, kittens, or small debilitated adults. **Lesions** consist of multiple red papules. *Ctenocephalides felis* is the most common flea causing infestation in **dogs** and **cats**, and it also transmits *Dipylidium caninum*.

Flies

Reactions to the bites of flies vary and include irritation, anaemia, direct toxicity, and hypersensitivity. **Biting flies** include *Haematobia irritans* (horn fly), *Stomoxys calcitrans* (stable fly), and horse flies, black flies, biting gnats, and mosquitoes. **Lesions of biting flies** are due to local irritation and include wheals and papules. Such lesions may persist with hair loss, scales, haemorrhagic crusts, and erythema. **Microscopic lesions** associated with fly bites include dermal haemorrhage and oedema with a central area of epidermal necrosis.

Myiasis is **infestation of tissues by the larvae of flies** with two wings and occurs in most areas of the body soiled by urine, faeces, or bodily secretions. **Grossly,** matted hair or wool and multiple irregular cutaneous holes or ulcers with an offensive odour are observed. **Death may occur and is due to septicaemia or toxaemia.**

In hypodermic myiasis, larvae of *Hypoderma lineatum* and *H. bovis* penetrate the skin of the legs of **cattle**, and sometimes **horses**. The larvae may be found in many areas of the body. **Microscopically,** these larvae are present in a cavity filled with fibrin and a few eosinophils and bordered by granulation tissue containing clusters of eosinophils.

Screwworm myiasis is caused by **Cochliomyia** sp. and **Chrysomyia** sp. and is an important disease in domestic animals. Screwworm flies deposit larvae in wounds or near mucocutaneous junctions of living animals. The larvae penetrate and feed on tissues liquefied by secretions of proteolytic enzymes. **Grossly,** foul-smelling wounds contain larvae and shreds of tissue. **Death may occur in untreated animals.**

Helminths

Skin infections with helminths are usually not life threatening. Infections are due to migration of helminth larvae which as adults live in non-cutaneous sites, or by filarial infections (**filarial dermatitis**) in which adults or microfilaria spend some time in skin and subcutis.

Hookworm dermatitis is due to **Ancylostoma** or **Uncinaria** larvae. Red papules with alopecic areas occur on the feet of **dogs.** Footpads may become soft, the keratinized portion may separate, and secondary bacterial dermatitis and paronychia (inflammation surrounding nail) may develop.

Cutaneous habronemiasis (summer sores) occurs in **horses** and is caused by infection with the larvae of **Habronema** sp., or **Draschia** sp. deposited on the skin by house or stable flies. **Lesions** occur on legs. **Grossly,** single or multiple, proliferative, ulcerated red to brown, tumourous masses are present. The **microscopic lesion** is a nodular dermatitis with eosinophils, giant cells bordering larvae or necrotic debris. Granulation tissue infiltrated by neutrophils is present on the ulcerated surface.

Onchocerciasis is a filarial dermatitis mainly affecting horses. Microfilaria may be present without significant dermal inflammation. Adult parasites are present in nodules in connective tissues, and microfilariae are present in the dermis. **In horses,** lesions develop on the head, neck, forelimbs, ventral thorax, and abdomen. **Gross lesions** consist of alopecia, erythema, scaling, crusting, and pigmentary changes. **Microscopic skin lesions** vary from no changes to superficial and deep perivascular dermatitis with eosinophils, lymphocytes, and microfilariae.

Stephanofilariasis, a filarial dermatitis of cattle, buffalo, and **goats,** is transmitted by flies and caused by six species of parasites of the genus **Stephanofilaria.** *S. stilesi* occurs in **cattle** and causes lesions along the ventral midline which consist of small circular patches with moist hairs, foci of epidermal haemorrhage, and serum exudation. Such foci expand and coalesce into a large area. **Microscopic lesions** are superficial and deep perivascular dermatitis with eosinophils, epidermal hyperkeratosis, parakeratosis, acanthosis, with spongiosis, eosinophilic microabscesses, and crust. Adult parasites and microfilaria may be seen.

Protozoa

Cutaneous protozoal infections may develop as part of systemic infections, mainly with **Leishmania**

Immunological Skin Diseases

General

Immunological diseases can be either **hypersensitivity (allergic)** or **autoimmune**. **Hypersensitivity** is a mild to severe reaction which develops in response to normally harmless foreign compounds including antiserum, hormones, pollen, and insect venoms. **Autoimmune diseases** develop when **antibodies or T-cells react against self-antigens.** Four basic immune reactions, type I II, III, and IV mediate the tissue damage in hypersensitivity and autoimmune diseases. **Hypersensitivity reactions are common in dogs and horses,** less common in **cats,** and are uncommon in food animal. **Autoimmune diseases with cutaneous manifestations are uncommon in domestic animals.**

Mechanisms of Tissue Damage

Type I Reactions

These inflammatory reactions are mediated by preformed or newly synthesized pharmacologically active substances. These are released by **mast cells** and **basophils** following reaction between antigen and specific antibody (usually IgE) bound to receptors on the membrane of the mast cells or basophils. Preformed substances released from mast cells include **histamine, factors chemotactic for eosinophils and neutrophils, prostaglandins, serine esterases,** and **tumour necrosis factor-alpha.** Substances synthesized on mast cell stimulation include **leukotrienes, cytokines,** and **platelet-activating factor.**

Type II Reactions

These reactions **depend on IgG or IgM antibodies** formed against either normal or altered cell membrane antigens. Cell damage occurs by complement fixation, antibody-dependent cell-mediated cytotoxicity, or antibody-directed cellular dysfunction.

Type III Reactions

These reactions are **mediated by immune complexes** formed in the circulation or in tissues. Immune complexes are often deposited in vessel walls and result in complement fixation and in the generation of cytokines and leukotactic factors, leading to **vasculitis.**

Type IV Reactions

These are mediated by sensitized CD4+ (helper) T-cells in the case of delayed-type hypersensitivity, or by CD8+ (cytotoxic) T-cells in the case of cellular cytotoxicity.

Hypersensitivity Reactions

Atopy

Atopy (atopic dermatitis, allergic inhalant dermatitis) is an example of **type I hypersensitivity reaction.** The skin is the major target organ in **dogs, cats,** and **horses**. The route of allergen exposure is considered respiratory but absorption through the skin may also occur, at least in **dogs. Atopy is the second most common hypersensitivity dermatitis in dogs** and accounts for 8% to 10% of canine skin disorders. The **main clinical sign** of atopy is **pruritus** (itching), and **in dogs,** it is usually manifested by face rubbing and foot licking. The clinical sign in **cats** and **horses** differ. **Microscopically,** there is hyperplastic superficial perivascular dermatitis with mixed populations of mast cells, mononuclear cells, and eosinophils.

Flea Bite Hypersensitivity

This is **the most common hypersensitivity dermatitis in dogs and cats. It results from flea bites and includes types I and type IV reactions.** It is pruritic, and skin lesions occur mainly along the dorsal lumbo-sacral area, ventral abdomen, thighs, flanks, and **in cats,** around the neck. **Grossly,** there is a papular dermatitis. **Microscopically,** lesions are characterized by hyperplastic superficial perivascular dermatitis with oedema, mast cells, basophils, lymphocytes, histiocytes, and eosinophils.

Culicoides Hypersensitivity

This is **common pruritic dermatitis in horses,** caused mainly by **type I and type IV hypersensitivity reactions** to salivary antigens from bites of Culicoides sp. Gross lesions initially are papules, but later pustules and nodules may develop. **Microscopic lesions** include superficial and deep perivascular dermatitis with numerous eosinophils.

Allergic Contact Dermatitis

This is an example of a type IV hypersensitivity reaction. The lesions are pruritic, resulting in self-inflicted trauma. **Grossly,** erythema, papules with or without vesicles, and exudation develop into crusts. **Microscopic lesions** include spongiotic superficial perivascular dermatitis with mononuclear cells, and when chronic, epithelial hyperplasia. Some cases have many eosinophils including eosinophilic epidermal pustules.

Hypersensitivity Reactions to Drugs

Hypersensitivity reactions to drugs are uncommon in dogs and cats, are rare in other domestic animals, and may result from any of the four types of hypersensitivity reactions. The drugs most commonly associated with hypersensitivity reactions include penicillin and trimethoprim-potentiated sulphonamides, but many drugs may cause a hypersensitivity reaction. **Gross and microscopic lesions** are highly variable.

Autoimmune Reactions

Diseases Characterized by Vesicles or Bullae as the Primary Lesion

Pemphigus

This group of diseases is caused by production of autoantibodies against proteins responsible for keratinocyte cell-to-cell adhesion (**desmosomes**) or cell-to-substrate adhesion (**hemi-desmosomes**). **Vesicles** or **bullae** form within epidermis or at the basement membrane.

Pemphigus foliaceus is the most common and milder form of pemphigus. It has been reported in the **dog, cat, horse,** and **goat. Autoantibodies are formed against protein components of the desmosomes. In the dog,** vesicles and pustules may be localized (muzzle, pinnae, footpads, coronary band) or generalized. **Pemphigus erythematosus is a mild form of pemphigus foliaceus** with lesions restricted to the face and pinnae.

Pemphigus vulgaris is a **very severe form of pemphigus** and has been reported in the **dog, cat,** and **horse. In the dog,** autoantibodies are formed against desmoglein 3, one of the prominent desmosomal proteins of basal epithelial cells. **Microscopic lesions** consist of **suprabasilar vesicle and superficial perivascular to interface** dermatitis. Vesicles or secondary erosions and ulcers are found in the oral cavity, at mucocutaneous junctions, and skin subject to mechanical stress such as in the axilla or groin.

Bullous pemphigoid is characterized by **autoantibodies directed against the hemi-desmosomal proteins,** BPAGI and BPAGII, and more rarely to **desmoplakin.** The location and character of clinical lesions are similar to pemphigus vulgaris. The condition has been reported in **dog** and **horse.**

Lupus erythematosus occurs in **two forms: systemic and discoid. Systemic lupus erythematosus is** a multi-organ disease of **dogs** and rarely **cats** and **horses.** Immune complexes form by antigen-antibody binding and are deposited in a variety of tissues, including skin, and result in a type III hypersensitivity response. **Skin lesions** may be **localized** or **generalized,** usually involve the face, pinnae, oral mucosae, and distal extremities, and consist of erythema, depigmentation, alopecia, scaling, crusting, and ulceration. **Microscopic lesions** include lymphohistiocytic dermatitis.

Discoid lupus erythematosus is relatively common and is a mild variant of systemic lupus erythematosus in which **there is no involvement of other organs and the antinuclear antibody titre is negative. Lesions** consist of erythema, depigmentation, scaling, erosion, ulceration, and crusting. **Microscopic lesions** include dermatitis often with many lymphocytes, plasma cells, and basal cell degeneration.

Dermatomyositis is an inherited disease of **dogs**. Dermatomyositis may develop in **puppies**, with **lesions** of vesicular dermatitis of face, lips, and external ears, and distal extremities. **Myositis** and **atrophy** of muscles of mastication, distal extremities, and sometimes oesophagus, develop after the dermatitis. **Immune complexes appear to play a role in lesion development.** The disease varies in severity.

Erythema multiforme (EM) and toxic epidermal necrolysis (TEN) are two rare diseases **affecting the skin** and possibly mucous membranes. Both conditions occur as **adverse drug reactions.** EM has been reported in **dogs, cats, horses,** and **cattle** and is characterized clinically by circular areas of erythema. Papules, vesicles, ulcers, and erosions may also be seen. **TEN** is seen mainly in **dogs** and **cats** and is often considered a more severe form of EM.

Metabolic Skin Diseases

Cutaneous endocrine disorders are due to imbalances in hormones and usually are manifested as non-pruritic, bilaterally symmetrical alopecia. The lesions are referred to as 'endocrine alopecia'.

Hypothyroidism

Deficiency of thyroid hormone is the most common endocrine disorder in dogs. A number of systemic and cutaneous signs and lesions occur from thyroid hormone deficiency. **Gross lesions** consist of endocrine alopecia that develops over the trunk and neck. **Microscopic lesions** include those of endocrine alopecia. Acanthosis of epidermis may be seen, and in some animals there is an increase in dermal mucin (**myxoedema**), which results in dermal thickening.

Hyperadrenocoticism (Hyperglucocorticoidism)

This condition results in skin lesions mainly in **dogs** and **cats. In dogs,** cutaneous lesions include endocrine alopecia. **Dystrophic calcification** of the dermis of the back, inguinal, and axillary areas may occur in **dogs (calcinosis cutis).** Grossly, lesions of calcinosis cutis are firm, thickened, sometimes gritty, often ulcerated, and alopecic. **In cats,** the skin becomes extremely fragile and may tear with normal handling.

Hyperoestrogenism

This may develop in **both male and female dogs. In females,** oestrogen may be secreted by ovarian cysts, rarely an ovarian neoplasm, or be due to oestrogen administration. **In males,** increased serum concentrations of oestrogen are usually derived from a functional testicular Sertoli cell neoplasm. In addition to endocrine alopecia, **female dogs** have an enlarged vulva and abnormalities of the oestrus cycle. **Male dogs** may have gynecomastia, pendulous prepuce, or an enlarged prostate due to squamous metaplasia of prostatic ducts. **Cutaneous microscopic lesions** include hyperkeratosis, and follicular dilation with keratin.

Nutritional Skin Diseases

Zinc Deficiency

Zinc deficiency occurs mainly in **pigs** and **dogs,** and is of less importance in **ruminants.** It results from diets containing high concentrations of phytic acid (binds zinc), low concentration of zinc, or high concentration of calcium. The **lesions** are circumscribed, reddened papules and plaques, scales, and thick crusts and fissures along the ventral abdomen and medial thighs. **Microscopically,** the lesions are parakeratosis, and acanthosis, Secondary bacterial invasion results in pustular dermatitis and folliculitis.

Zinc deficiency in ruminants has been reported in **cattle, sheep,** and **goats. Skin lesions** include alopecia, scaling, and crusting of the skin of the face, neck, distal extremities, and muco-cutaneous junctions. **Microscopically,** the lesions consist of parakeratosis, and in some cases, hyperkeratosis.

Copper Deficiency

Copper is an essential **component of tyrosinase.** Deficient animals develop **depigmented hair or wool. Cattle** may develop depigmented hair around the eyes. The coat colour also may change from black to reddish brown. **In sheep,** the wool becomes straight (loss of ridges or crimps).

Vitamin E Deficiency

Cats with vitamin E deficiency or fed diets with an excess of dietary fatty acids may develop **steatitis** (inflammation of the adipose tissue). **Grossly,** the subcutaneous tissue contains firm, nodular, yellow to orange masses.**Microscopic lesions** are lobular to diffuse panniculitis (inflammation of subcutaneous adipose tissue) with early lesions of fat necrosis, oedema, and infiltrates of neutrophils. Granulomatous inflammation follows rapidly and is composed of macrophages and multi-nucleated giant cells.

Vitamin A Deficiency

This is a rare disorder occurring mainly **in dogs. Gross lesions** are most prominent in thoracic and abdominal skin. They consist of generalized scaling. **Microscopic lesions** are marked dilation of follicles with keratin.

Disorders of Epidermal Growth or Differentiation

Primary Idiopathic Seborrhoea

This is **a disorder of cornification**. Seborrhoea is a non-specific term for clinical signs of scaling, crusting, and greasiness. **Seborrhoea** occurs most commonly in **dogs** and less commonly in **horses** and **cats. Clinically two forms** occur: **a dry form (seborrhoea sicca)** with dry skin and white to grey scales that exfoliate, or **a greasy form (seborrhoea oleosa)** with scaling and excessive brown to yellow lipids that adhere to the skin and hair. **Microscopic lesions** include hyperkeratosis of the epidermis and follicular epithelium. The dermal papillae are oedematous and congested.

Secondary seborrhoea is not a primary disorder of cornification. However, it clinically resembles the primary cornification disorders, and thus needs to be differentiated from them. The **lesions** of secondary seborrhoea resolve completely if the underlying disease is eliminated. **Microscopic changes** include epidermal and follicular hyperkeratosis with or without parakeratosis.

Sebaceous Adenitis

This **is inflammation of sebaceous glands,** and is probably immune-mediated. It **occurs usually in dogs.** Lesions can be diffuse or multifocal and annular (ring-shaped). **Microscopic lesions** include inflammation of the sebaceous glands, and in some cases, hyperkeratosis.

Disorders of Pigmentation

Hypopigmentation

Disorders associated with reduced pigment may be **inherited** or **acquired**, involve skin or hair, be generalized or localized, idiopathic or associated with other diseases. Terms used for this disorder include **leukoderma** and **vitiligo** for loss of pigment in the skin, **leukotrichia** for loss of pigment of the hair, **hypopigmentation** or **incomplete albinism** for generalized less than normal amount of pigment in the skin or hair, and **albinism** for a hereditary lack of pigment.

Hyperpigmentation

This may occur from inflammation, irritation, and metabolic disorders. Therefore, it is **seen in all species with epidermal melanin pigment**. Hyperpigmentation is also a feature of benign and malignant masses (lentigines, melanocytic neoplasms, and pigmented basal neoplasms). **Lentigines** (plural of lentigo) are rare, non-neoplastic, well-circumscribed, macular to slightly raised plaques characterized by irregular epidermal hyperplasia, hyperpigmentation, and increased numbers of pigmented melanocytes. **Lentigines** are usually multifocal and **have been described in dogs and cats.**

Disorders of Unknown Pathogenesis (Idiopathic Disorders)

Disorders characterized by Infiltrates of Eosinophils

Eosinophilic plaques are common lesions of the skin in **cats** and occur on the abdomen and medial thigh and are thought to be associated with hypersensitivity reactions. **Lesions** consist of raised erythematous, pruritic, and eroded to ulcerated plaques. **Microscopically,** epidermal lesions include acanthosis, spongiosis, erosion, and ulceration, accompanied by superficial and deep, perivascular to diffuse mainly **eosinophilic dermatitis.**

Eosinophilic granulomas (collagenolytic granulomas) are lesions with **collagen degeneration (collagenolysis)** which occur in **cats, dogs,** and **horses.** The **causes** of these syndromes are poorly understood, but collagen degeneration may develop in any lesion associated with eosinophil degranulation, such as reaction to parasites, foreign bodies (including hair), or in mast cell neoplasms. **Gross lesions** include papules, nodules, plaques, and ulcers in the skin, and nodular or ulcerated lesions in the oral mucosa of **dogs** and **cats,** and footpads of **cats. Microscopically,** nodular dermatitis (or stomatitis) consists of fragmented degenerate collagen fibres bordered by degranulated eosinophils and macrophages.

Multi-systemic eosinophilic epitheliotropic disease in the horse is a generalized, exfoliative dermatitis characterized histologically by a hyperplastic perivascular, eosinophilic to lymphoplasmacytic dermatitis. The dermatitis is accompanied by eosinophilic, lymphoplasmacytic, and sometimes, granulomatous inflammation and fibrosis in other organs including the digestive tract, pancreas, liver, uterus, and bronchial epithelium. **Clinically,** the **horse** loses weight and becomes debilitated. **Cutaneous lesions include** dry scales and serous exudate of the epithelium of the skin of the head, coronets, and oral cavity. The aetiology of the condition is unknown.

Diseases of the Nail Bed

Onychodystrophy refers to abnormal formation of the nail (claw), **onychomadesis** to sloughing of the nails, and **paronychia** to inflammation of the skin of the nail fold. **These conditions are rare.** They **have a variety of causes** including **infections** (e.g., bacterial, fungal), **immune-mediated disorders** (e.g., pemphigus, lupus erythematosus), **systemic disease** (e.g., hyperadrenocorticism, disseminated vascular coagulation), **and disorders of unknown cause** (e.g., idiopathic onychodystrophy). These conditions affect many breeds of **dogs** of varying ages; the **dogs** are healthy otherwise. **History includes sudden loss of nails, eventually**

involving all nails on all feet.

Cutaneous Manifestations of Systemic Disease

Laminitis

Laminitis refers to inflammation of the laminar structures of the hoof. However, **laminitis is a complex disease** in which inflammation is only a part of the disease process. Laminitis may be seen in any hoofed animal, but is **of greatest importance in horses and cattle.** There are **a variety of systemic causes** of laminitis. **Repeated trauma** to the foot may also cause laminitis. **The pathogenesis of laminitis is complex, not completely understood, and controversial.** There are **two basic hypotheses: vascular** and **toxic-metabolic.** The **vascular hypothesis** suggests that digital ischaemia is the main event, whereas the **toxic-metabolic hypothesis** argues that there is direct damage to epithelial cells of the laminae or to the basement membrane, and that the vascular lesions are secondary. The **main clinical sign** of laminitis is **pain** manifested as **lameness,** abnormal posture, or reluctance to move. **Gross findings** of the external foot in acute laminitis may be minimal. Swelling or oedema of the coronary band may be seen. **Chronic lesions** are highly variable. **Common gross lesions include** circumferential hoof rings (ridges), altered foot shape, separation of the wall from the epidermis at the coronet, flattened sole, and in some cases, penetration of the third phalanx through the sole. **Diagnosis** is based mainly on clinical, radiographic, and gross findings. Regardless of whether the initial damage is ischaemic or direct injury to the epithelium or basement membrane, **the lesions of acute laminitis are degeneration and necrosis** of epithelial cells of the laminae, separation of epithelial cells from basement membrane, and loss of the basement membrane.

Cutaneous Neoplasms

The skin is a common site of neoplastic growth in most animals. The neoplasms are of ectodermal, mesodermal, and melanocytic origin. **Most cutaneous neoplasms are primary, as the skin is an uncommon site for metastasis.** However, the skin can be the site of **secondary tumour growth.** Examples include mammary gland neoplasms which invade into adjacent skin, feline pulmonary bronchogenic carcinomas that metastasize to multiple digits of the feet, and canine visceral haemangiosarcomas which metastasize to the skin.

Only some important neoplasms of the skin are considered briefly.

Neoplasms of Epidermis

Papilloma

Papilloma, also called 'wart', is **a benign neoplasm** of stratified squamous epithelium. **Grossly,** papillomas appear as single or multiple, raised, flat, or cauliflower-like growths with a smooth or irregular surface. Common sites are face, neck, and oral mucosa, but they originate anywhere including oesophagus, rumen, and external genitalia.

Microscopically, a papilloma consists of multiple papillary projections of fibrovascular connective tissue covered by a layer of heavily keratinized stratified squamous epithelium. Papillomas do not contain cutaneous adnexal structures or rete ridges. **Rete ridges** are inward projections of epidermis into the dermis. The fibrovascular stroma is not neoplastic, but is an extension of the normal dermis. Most papillomas of **humans** and **animals** are caused by DNA-containing **papillomaviruses**. However, the aetiology of some is not known.

Squamous-Cell Carcinoma

This is **the commonest form of carcinoma of the skin,** and is derived from **stratified squamous epithelium.** The epithelium may or may not cornify. **Pigmentation** and **papillation** (formation of rete ridges) are not features of the squamous-cell carcinoma. However, the neoplastic squamous cells are not restricted to the outer surface of the neoplasm, as with papilloma. Instead, irregular masses and elongate chords of tumour cells extend haphazardly throughout the neoplasm. Cross sections of the chords appear as islands of neoplastic epithelium surrounded by stroma. The basal layer of epithelial cells is often situated at the periphery of such an island. In the case of a cornifying neoplasm, the red-staining keratin of the stratum corneum is produced at the centre of the epithelial mass, becomes compact from the pressure of proliferating cells, and forms a round, concentrically laminated structure known as a 'keratin pearl', 'epithelial pearl' or 'cell nest'. The term 'epidermal' or 'epidermoid carcinoma' is sometimes used as a synonym for these neoplasms derived from the epidermis. The tongue, oesophagus, rumen, ocular surfaces, and vagina are also sites of squamous-cell carcinoma.

The more anaplastic squamous-cell carcinomas lack differentiation into distinct layers. The epithelial cells consist of almost uniform cells, with hyperchromatic nuclei. Sometimes, the epithelial cells of a highly anaplastic carcinoma assume a fusiform shape (tapering at each end, spindle-shaped). It then becomes difficult even to determine if the neoplasm is a **carcinoma** or **sarcoma**. In such cases immunohistochemical staining for specific epithelial (cytokeratin), mesenchymal (desmin, vimentin), and endothelial (factor 8-related antigen) **cell markers** and **electron microscopy** can be extremely useful in differentiation.

Squamous-cell carcinomas originate from the epidermis of the skin, and the stratified squamous epithelium of various mucosal surfaces. They occur in all domestic species. Like other carcinomas, these are prone to **metastasize** to regional lymph nodes and then to visceral organs. The **cause** is not known, but there is a relationship to solar irradiation with the occurrence of squamous-cell carcinoma of the eyelid in **cattle** and the skin of the pinnae of **white cats.**

An unsual form of squamous-cell carcinoma called 'horn cancer' or 'carcinoma of the horn' occurs at the junction of the skin and the horn. Since it is an important neoplasm of Zebu cattle in India, it will be discussed at some length.

Horn Cancer

Horn cancer is a widely prevalent and economically important neoplasm of Indian Zebu cattle. It is a squamous-cell carcinoma of horn, originating from core epithelium in **mainly aged bullocks,** and less commonly in **cows, bull,** and only rarely **buffaloes.** The aetiology is unknown. **The disease is characterized by bending and dropping of affected horn, development of cauliflower-like cancerous growth, cachexia, anaemia, and death after prolonged illness.**

Horn cancer (HC) is seen in Zebu cattle of India and Sumatra. Usually one horn is affected, but sometimes bilateral involvement is also observed. In India, sporadic cases of HC have been reported from most of the states, particularly from Haryana, Uttar Pradesh, Gujarat, Maharasthra, Orrisa, Tamil Nadu, Karnataka, Bihar, Madhya Pradesh, and Assam. HC is more prevalent in long-horned, white-coat coloured breeds of cattle. The neoplasm has not been found in animals less than four years of age. Most cases are seen in eight years old animals. **The 7-10 years age group appears most susceptible to HC.** The neoplasm **affects working bullocks much more than cows.** It is seen only occasionally in **bulls.**

Although various intrinsic factors such as genetic predisposition, sex hormone imbalances in bullocks (iatrogenic), and extrinsic factors such as chronic irritation and trauma, paints, solar radiations, viruses, and combination of some of these factors have been suspected to cause HC, **the aetiology remains unknown.**

Clinical signs include frequent shaking of the head, rubbing of the horn on some hard object, bloody discharge from the nostril or affected horn, and slight bending of the horn. **In the advanced stages,** there is gradual loosening and marked bending of the horn, formation of soft swelling at the base, sloughing of the horn, and development of highly vascular, friable, and foul-smelling, cauliflower-like neoplastic growth. The growth may acquire infections, and bleed. **Affected animals suffer from weakness, anaemia, cachexia, and die.** The neoplasm mostly recurs after surgical removal.

Pathogenesis and pathology

The bulk of the evidence indicates that HC originates from horn core epithelium. The cancerous growth arises from the middle or distal region of the core and as the condition advances fills up the entire core, and progresses towards the frontal sinus. **Microscopically,** HC is a **squamous-cell carcinoma** characterized by the presence of **epithelial pearls.** Generally, the microscopic appearance is of low grade malignancy. The stroma is infiltrated by lymphocytes and polymorphonuclear cells. Ultrastructurally, the neoplasm is composed of pleomorphic epithelial cells.

Metastasis occurs mostly in regional lymph nodes and sometimes visceral organs, such as lungs, heart, and pituitary gland. The metastasis occurs by direct extension, through the lymphatic system, and sometimes haematogenously.

Immunological studies indicate **depression of the cell-mediated immunity in the affected animal.** HC can be **routinely diagnosed on the basis of clinical signs, and confirmed by histopathology. Prognosis** is good if the base is not affected. The **conventional treatment** consists of amputation of the affected horn, removal of the cancerous tissue, and dressing of the wound with antiseptic agents. **An autogenous vaccine** has also been tried with limited success. **Dehorning** of young animals has been suggested as a preventive measure.

Basal Cell Neoplasm

The term **'basal cell neoplasm'** includes a number of morphologically distinct cutaneous neoplasms **which are derived from basal cells of the epidermis and hair follicle,** but differ in their pattern of growth and differentiation. **In humans,** these are known as **'basal cell carcinoma',** but **in animals** this name is considered inappropriate because the neoplasm has a tendency to remain localized.

Basal cell Neoplasm (Basal Cell Carcinoma)

These neoplasms occur in dogs and cats. Most of them behave in a **benign** manner, in that they tend to remain localized, are non-invasive, and rarely recur following excision. **In dogs,** as in humans, the head, neck, shoulders, and thorax are the common sites. **Grossly,** they appear as a well-circumscribed solitary, solid or cystic mass confined to the dermis and subcutis. They vary in size. **Microscopically,** basal-cell neoplasms are composed of solid, or cystic masses of small round to fusiform cells (i.e., spindle-shaped) with an ovoid, deeply basophilic nucleus and eosinophilic cytoplasm.

Melanocytoma and Melanoma

Recently, the term **melanocytoma** has been used to refer to all **benign neoplasms of melanocytes.** The term **melanoma,** with or without adjective malignant, is used to refer to **all malignant neoplasms of melanin-producing cells.** Cells which produce melanin (melanocytes, melanoblasts) originate in neuro-ectoderm.

Melanocytomas and **melanomas of the skin** are **common neoplasms in most species.** Dermal **melanocytomas,** equivalent to dermal naevus (pigmented mole) of humans, **occur in dogs.** They are confined to the superficial dermis. **Microscopically,** the neoplasm is composed of plump fusiform cells arranged in whorls or sheets. There is little stromal collagen between the closely packed neoplastic cells. The neoplastic cells have ovoid, vesicular nuclei with prominent nucleoli. **Mitotic activity is low.**

Melanomas (Malignant Melanoma)

These are **malignant counterpart of melanocytoma**. They **occur in most animals.** Their main characteristic is the great pleomorphism (i.e., occurrence in various forms), and variation in the pattern of growth and degree of pigmentation of the neoplastic cells. The cells may be so filled with the dark brown melanin that nuclei and cytoplasmic morphology are indistinct, or at the other extreme, the cells may contain no melanin at all, in what is known as an **amelanotic melanoma.** The shape of the cells varies from round to polygonal forms,including elongated, fusiform to stellate cells. Spindle-shaped cells dominate. The cells are demarcated by thin fibrous trabeculae. The cytoplasm tends to be basophilic. The nucleoli are large and prominent. The basement membrane is lost. Features which are useful in differentiating melanomas from melanocytomas include the presence of large, hypochromatic nuclei, bizarre (odd, unusual) forms, and **high mitotic activity.** Invasion of lymphatics or small blood vessels is complete evidence of malignancy.

Grossly, melanoma is recognized by its deep black colour. Melanomas occur in many forms and locations. **Actively malignant melanomas are common in old grey horses.** Death may result from metastasis to the spleen, lungs, or other internal organs. **In cattle,** melanomas occur in the skin at various locations. **In pigs,** cutaneous melanomas are more common on the posterior half of the body. **In the dog,** they occur in the lip and oral cavity. Most melanomas arise in the skin. Those arising in the eyes are discussed in chapter 13.

Neoplasms of Adnexa

Adenomas and Adenocarcinomas of Sweat Glands

The benign neoplasms resemble normal gland. **Adenocarcinomas have the usual features of malignancy.** Adenocarcinomas **of anal sacs of dogs** are highly invasive, and are associated with **hypercalcaemia** due to secretion of a parathormone-like substance.

Adenomas and Adenocarcinomas of Sebaceous Glands

These are **common neoplasms of the skin in dogs.** They may be single or multiple. Head is the common site of their occurrence. **Grossly,** they appear as yellow-white, raised, alopecic, nodules. **Microscopically,** adenomas resemble the normal sebaceous gland. Adenocarcinomas are much more anaplastic than adenomas. Many of the neoplastic cells are irregular nodules, with no orderly pattern of growth. Lymphatic invasion and metastasis also occur. **In dogs,** neoplasms of sebaceous glands are most common in the skin of the hind quarters, abdomen, and thorax.

Adenomas and Adenocarcinomas of Perianal Glands

The perianal (circumanal) glands of the skin in dogs are modified sebaceous glands.

Adenomas of perianal glands are common, particularly in intact (not castrated) **male dogs,** and are usually spherical masses of varying size. **Microscopically,** the adenoma closely resembles the normal glands.

Adenocarcinomas are much less common. Surprisingly, they may occur in **aged spayed** (varies removed) **females,** in which the benign form is rare. Adenocarcinoma may metastasize to the iliac lymph nodes, and from there to other lymph nodes, and eventually reach general circulation. **Microscopically,** the neoplasms are characterized by the presence of **small nests of invasive neoplastic cells** in the dermal connective tissue surrounding the neoplasm.

Hair Matrix Neoplasm (Pilomatrixoma)

This is a benign, usually cystic neoplasm derived from the germinative cells of the follicular matrix, or hair bulb. The **neoplasm is common in dogs,** but **rare in cats.** It is composed of multiple solid masses, or cystic masses lined by an outer rim of cells which resemble hair matrix.

Neoplasms of the Dermis and Subcutis

Fibroma and Fibrosarcoma

Fibromas and **fibrosarcomas** are the **most common** mesenchymal neoplasms of **skin in most species, except the dogs. In the dog,** histiocytoma and mast cell neoplasms are more common In general, fibrosarcomas are more common than fibromas. The neoplasms originate from fibrous connective tissue, and resemble it in appearance. The cells with their collagenous fibrils proliferate in a variety of patterns. **Long interlacing bundles of neoplastic cells is a common pattern.** This is useful in differentiating the fibrosarcoma from nerve sheath neoplasms and haemangiopericytoma, in which this is not a feature.

In fibromas, the neoplstic cells make significant amounts of collagen, which separates neoplastic cells from each other. Mitotic activity is extremely low in fibromas in contrast to fibrosarcomas. Fibromas, in some species, are caused by papillomaviruses. **Fibrosarcomas are more cellular than fibromas, make less collagen, have a high mitotic index and usually invade tissues.** The cells are spindle-shaped with ovoid nuclei and mitotic figures. Other criteria of malignancy include cellular and nuclear pleomorphism, hyperchromasia, and the presence of **tumour giant cells.** Fibrosarcomas of the skin in **cats** have been associated with feline sarcoma virus.

Equine Sarcoid

First recognized in 1936 by Jackson, it was so named by him because of the histological appearance, which resembled that of a sarcoma of moderate malignancy. The lesion is often multiple. It is perhaps more **common in mules,**

and donkeys, than in the horse. The growth may reach the size of a softball, and bulge from under the skin. The skin sooner or later becomes ulcerated and infected.

Microscopically, the growth is made up mainly of interlacing bundles of spindle-shaped cells which may form whorls and bundles suggestive of a neurofibrosarcoma. The neoplasm does not metastasize. The neoplasm is believed to be caused by the bovine papillomavirus.

Lipoma and Liposarcoma

Lipomas occur in many locations as masses of adipose tissues of various sizes and shapes. They are often multiple, and occur mostly in the subcutis. The fat may be yellowish. **Grossly,** they form lumps or masses. **Microscopically,** there is a great variation in the size and shape of the fat cells from the normal adipose tissue. **The liposarcoma is rare.** It is characterized by areas of anaplastic fibrous tissue along with adipose tissue, and an intermediate tissue, in which only rudimentary fat cells with small vacuoles are present.

Myxoma and Myxosarcoma

These neoplasms are composed of connective tissue that forms mucin, that is, connective tissue of embryonal type. The nuclei tend to be round or stellate, and the intercellular fibrils are **bluish** (H & E stain). The neoplasms are always more or less malignant. They should be differentiated from a fibrosarcoma with myxomatous degeneration.

Mast Cell Neoplasm

This is **the most common cutaneous neoplasm of the dog.** It originates in the dermis. It also occurs in the skin of **cats,** but is less common. It occurs rarely in **pigs** and **cattle.**

In dogs, the flank and scrotum are the common sites. The neoplasm appears as a bulging cutaneous mass 2-5 cm in diameter. **Clinical signs** include pruritus, erythema, oedema, and ulceration, and are because of the release of histamine from the neoplastic cells. These neoplasms are diffusely infiltrative. Metastasis can also occur. **Microscopically,** the cells form diffuse chords of round to somewhat polygonal cells with a round, centrally placed nucleus and a moderate amount of basophilic cytoplasm. The cords of cells are separated by bundles of collagen. Scattered throughout are esosinophils, in response to eosinophil chemotactic factor, a normal product of mast cell granules. Based on differentiation, pleomorphism, and mitotic index of the cells, the neoplasm has been classified for prognostic purposes into three grades. **In grade I,** the cells are most differentiated, uniform in size and shape, and have prominent basophilic cytoplasmic granules. Mitotic figures are very rare, and neoplasm has the best prognosis. **Grade III is the least differentiated and has the worst prognosis.** The cells have very few or no basophilic granules in their cytoplasm. Nuclei vary in size and shape, and may contain binucleated tumour cells. The few granules require staining with metachromatic stains, such as Giemsa or toluidine blue, to find them. **Grade II neoplasms** have features intermediate between grade I and III.

In the cat, mast cell neoplasms occur in **two forms: a primary cutaneous mast cell neoplasm**, and **a visceral mast cell neoplasm**. The **cuatneous neoplasms** usually occur on head and neck, and **visceral neoplasms** usually in the spleen, and less commonly, in other organs. The spleen is markedly enlarged.

Canine Cutaneous Histiocytoma

This is **the most common cutaneous neoplasm of dogs,** and occurs in dogs of all ages. **Common sites** of its occurrence are face, pinnae, neck, distal extremities, and scrotum. **Grossly,** the neoplasm appears as a solitary or multiple, raised 1.0-3.0 cm alopecic plaque or mass, often with ulceration. Because of this appearance, it is also referred to as **'button tumour'. Microscopically,** histiocytomas are composed of nodular infiltrates or round to polygonal cells arranged in chords or sheets. The infiltrate destroys most adnexal structures. Older neoplasms contain infiltrates of lymphocytes and have areas of coagulative necrosis.

Histiocytomas, if left alone, eventually undergo **spontaneous regression** after several weeks or months. The regression is mediated by CD8[+] cytotoxic T-lymphocytes which infiltrate neoplasm's deepest margins. Neutrophils may be present, if the lesion is ulcerated and secondarily infected. Until recently the exact source of the neoplastic cells was not known. Using a wide range of monoclonal antibodies, it has now been demonstrated that the neoplastic cells express a variety of leukocyte antigens characteristic of activated **Langerhans' cells'.** These are the antigen-presenting cells of the epidermis. Therefore, now this neoplasm has been characterized as a **localized form of self-limiting histiocytosis.** Thus, this neoplasm may not be a neoplasm at all, but instead a localized reactive proliferation of Langerhans' cells due to some unknown cause, and may resemble Langerhans' cell histiocytoma of humans.

Benign Cutaneous and Systemic Histiocytosis

Three forms of histiocytosis have been described in dogs. Two of these involve the skin. **Histiocytosis is different from cutaneous histiocytoma.** (1) **The first is** called **benign cutaneous histiocytosis.** This is characterized by the development of multiple erythematous plaques and nodules in the panniculus (subcutaneous fat) of the face, neck, back, and trunk. **Microscopically,** the lesion is characterized by infiltrates in the dermis and panniculus of **large histiocytic cells** along with other inflammatory cells. (2) **The second form** is called **systemic histiocytosis.** It is a rare, familial disease, and has been described only in male dogs. (3) **The third is** the lethal form, termed **malignant histiocytosis.** The skin is spared, and lesions occur mostly in lungs, visceral lymph nodes, spleen, and central nervous system. The proliferating histiocytes are extremely pleomorphic, often forming multinucleated giant cells, and bizarre mitotic figures.

Fibrous Histiocytoma

Malignant Fibrous Histiocytoma

These are **rare neoplasms** of the skin of **dogs** and **cats** characterized by a mixture of neoplastic cells having features of **fibroblasts** and **histiocytes.**

Cutaneous (Extra-medullary) Plasmacytoma

These are **benign neoplasms of plasma cells** which occur on the skin of the digits, lips, pinnae, and ear canals of **middle-aged dogs of both sexes.** They appear as solitary (single), spherical, alopecic nodules. **Microscopically,** neoplastic cells range from those which resemble normal plasma cells to those which are poorly differentiated, with pleomorphic nuclei. Multinucleate giant cells are found in most neoplasms. Most neoplasms do not recur following excision.

Cutaneous Lymphomas

These are **of two basic types**: (1) non-epitheliotropic, and epitheliotropic. The **non-epitheliotropic** forms are of B-lymphocyte origin. The **epitheliotropic** are derived from T-lymphocytes. **Although visceral lymphomas** occur with some frequency in most domestic animals, **cutaneous lymphoma is rare.** It has been reported in **cattle, dogs,** and **cats.**

Haemangiopericytoma

Haemangiopericytoma is a subcutaneous neoplasm of dogs, and is rare in other species. It is thought to **originate from the pericytes** which surround small blood vessels. **Grossly,** these neoplasms appear as solitary, firm masses in the subcutis. The neoplasm is composed of spindle-shaped cells with ovoid or elongated nuclei and considerable cytoplasm. **A characteristic feature of this neoplasm is the presence of numerous small capillaries,** closely encircled by pleomorphic 'spindle' cells. The neoplasm is always sub-cutaneous. Metastasis is extremely rare.

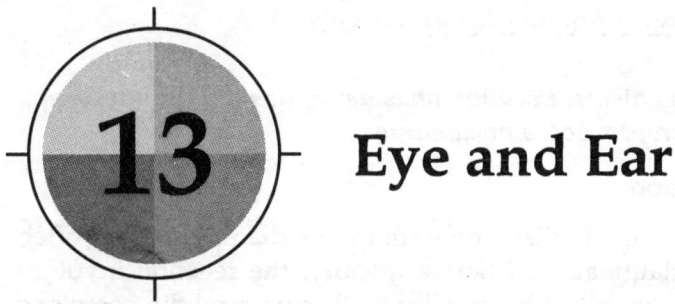

13 Eye and Ear

Eye

The **ocular apparatus includes the eyeball (globe), optic nerve, and accessory structures,** including the eyelids, lachrymal apparatus, orbital fasciae, and oculomotor muscles. The eyeball contains three refractive media – the **aqueous humour, lens,** and **vitreous body.**

Anomalies of the Globe

These have been **described especially in the dog,** but are rare in other species.

Anophthalmia is the absence of globe.

Cyclopia is a developmental anomaly characterized by the presence of a single median (middle) eye in a single median orbital fossa.

Synophthalmia is either partial separation or fusion of the globes.

Microphthalmia is an abnormally small globe, either unilateral or bilateral. The highest incidence has been described in **pigs** and **dogs.**

Coloboma is a congenital absence of an ocular tissue, such as portions of various layers.

Ocular Inflammation

Inflammation of the globe can be suppurative, non-suppurative, or granulomatous. **Panophthalmitis** is an inflammation which is widespread in the globe, and also involves the outer coat. In **endophthalmitis,** the inflammation involves only the ocular cavities, and their adjacent structures.

Suppurative Inflammation

Panophthalmitis and **endophthalmitis** are **acute suppurative processes,** and cause variable degrees of destruction of the retina and uvea, abscess formation in the vitreous, and exudate in the anterior chamber. **In panophthalmitis,** extension of inflammation through the sclera produces tenonitis (inflammation of tendon's capsule), and orbital cellulitis. Suppurative inflammation is often due to the introduction of bacteria through lacerated wounds, ulcers and perforation, and also from septicaemia with bacterial metastasis to the choroid and retina. Bacteria involved include coliform organisms, *Pseudomonas aeruginosa*, **Salmonella** sp., *Haemophilus somnus*, **and** *Streptococcus pneumoniae.*

Non-Suppurative Inflammation

Surgical and other traumas, foreign bodies, and immune-mediated reactions often produce non-suppurative inflammation. **Microscopically,** the reaction involves mainly lymphocytes and plasma cells. Mononuclear cells surround the vessels of the sclera, ciliary body, and choroid diffusely, and form thick cuffs around retinal vessels.

Granulomatous Inflammation

This may follow trauma with introduction of foreign bodies, perforation of the lens and subsequent auto-sensitization to lenticular protein, fungal infections, microfilaria and larvae of parasites, and certain bacterial diseases, such as tuberculosis. **The reaction is characterized by the presence of epthelioid and giant cells, lymphocytes and plasma cells,** and some fibrosis.

Complications of Ocular Inflammation

These include **glaucoma, cataract, retinal detachment,** and **atrophy of the uvea.**

Bacterial Causes of Ocular Disease

Many species of bacteria produce ocular disease when carried to the eyeball by the bloodstream, and when introduced into the eyeball by traumatic penetrating wounds, by foreign bodies and by surgery. Diseases in which ocular inflammation has been described include colibacillosis in **calves, pigs,** and **birds**; streptococcosis in **calves** with meningitis; salmonellosis in **pigs, calves,** and **chicks**; erysipelas in **pigs**; listeriosis in **lambs** and **calves**; brucellosis in **dogs**; and tuberculosis in **several species.**

Viral Causes of Ocular Disease

Bovine Malignant Catarrhal Fever

Cattle with malignant catarrhal fever clinically have mucopurulent kerato-conjunctivitis, and corneal oedema and ulceration.

Feline Infectious Peritonitis

Cats with infectious peritonitis may have unilateral or bilateral ocular lesions. These include oedema of the cornea and detachment of the retina. The **pyogranulomatous inflammation** involves iris, ciliary body, choroid, retina, optic nerve, and blood vessels. The reaction is more intense in the uvea.

Marek's Disease

Ocular lesions occur in several tissues of the **eyeball of chickens** infected with the **herpesvirus of Marek's disease**. The retina may get detached due to nodular accumulations of lymphoid cells in the choroid and sub-retinal space.

Parasitic Causes of Ocular Disease

Onchocerciasis

In horses, microfilariae of *Onchocerca cervicalis* are found in the eyelids, with and without ocular lesions.

Ocular Larval Migrans

Larval granulomatosis of the retina and choroid occurs **in dogs due to larvae of** *Toxocara canis*. **Lesions** include raised nodules in the fundus, retinal detachment, and retinal haemorrhages. Parasites are found within granulomas composed of mononuclear cells, fibroblasts, a few giant cells, and eosinophils.

Ocular Leishmaniasis

Ocular leishmaniasis (*Leishmania donovani*) **is rare.** Ocular lesions include pannus (newly formed fibrovascular tissue involving cornea), and exudate in the anterior chamber, over iris, and in the vitreous.

Fungal Causes of Ocular Disease

Aspergillosis

Ocular infection with *Aspergillus fumigatus* is commonly seen **in birds,** in which it occurs as part of the systemic disease. It may occur as a pure **keratitis,** or as **granulomatous endophthalmitis.** Branching fungal hyphae are present in several ocular structures.

Blastomycosis

Ocular lesions due to infection with *Blastomyces dermatitidis* occur mostly in **dogs,** but are also described in **cats.** Lesions include exophthalmos, scleritis (inflammation of sclera), corneal oedema, conjunctivitis, purulent ocular discharge, and even blindness in affected dogs. The **basic lesion is pyogranulomatous endophthalmitis, or panophthalmitis.** Fungal organisms are numerous in areas of granulomatous inflammation.

Coccidioidomycosis

Ocular infection with the fungus *Coccidioides immitis* is **rare**, and has been described in **dogs.** The **lesion** is a granulomatous endophthalmitis involving cornea, iris, and retina.

Cryptococcosis

Intra-ocular infection with the fungus *Cryptococcus neoformans* has been reported in **dogs** and **cats**. The lesions include solid retinal and sub-retinal granulomas resulting in retinal detachment.

Histoplasmosis

Ocular histoplasmosis in **dogs** and **cats** is usually a granulomatous endophthalmitis. Mononuclear cells in various ocular compartments include macrophages containing blastospores of *Histoplasma capsulatum*.

Cornea

Anomalies

Anomalies of the cornea include variation in size (**megalocornea, microcornea**), congenital opacities, congenital anterior synechiae (**synechia** is fibrous adhesion of iris to lens and cornea), and dermoids (see 'dermoid' below). In **megalocornea**, cornea is excessively large, but otherwise normal. **It is rare in domestic animals.**

Dermoid

A **dermoid** is a congenital **choristoma** characterized by the **presence of a piece of skin on cornea, conjunctiva, or both.** (The term **choristoma** has been applied to microscopically normal cells or tissues which are present in abnormal locations). The **lesion** has been described in several species, but is **most common in cattle.** Microscopically, dermoids have the structure of skin.

Degenerations

Keratoconjunctivitis Sicca

This disease, also known as **'dry eye'** (L. sicca = dry) and **'xerophthalmia'** (G. xero = dry) is **common in dogs, but rare in other domestic animals.** It is a chronic disease of the cornea and conjunctiva due to inadequate tear production. It can be primary or secondary. **Primary type** results from congenital lack of lachrymal secretion. **Secondary type** follows canine distemper, traumatic and toxic damage to the lachrymal glands, and occlusion of the lachrymal ducts. As the disease progresses, the cornea becomes opaque, is ulcerated, and eventually becomes vascularized. **Corneal ulceration may extend to perforation.** Cellular infiltration is present in vascularized areas, containing a large number of plasma cells and lymphocytes.

Corneal Lipidosis

Fatty change in the cornea occurs in **adult dogs.** It is associated with inflammation and with hyperlipoproteinaemia resulting from thyroid atrophy, thyroiditis, and thyroidal carcinoma. **Lesions** consist of deposits of neutral fat, fat laden macrophages, and crystals of cholesterol.

Pigmentary Keratitis

Keratitis is inflammation of cornea. Corneal pigmentation is not common in domestic animals. Only **melanosis** is of significance. Melanosis is a common cause of blindness. The pigment may be accompanied by vascularization and scarring of the cornea. The condition has been reported in **dogs.**

Pannus

Pannus refers to the **lesion of the cornea in which a vascular granulation tissue invades the cornea** beneath the epithelium. **The fibrovascular tissue is called pannus.** Pannus occurs in lesions characterized by corneal oedema and corneal inflammation (**inflammatory pannus**). **In 'degenerative pannus'** masses of the hyaline material accumulate and replace fluid. Eventually, a thick hyaline plaque raises the epithelium. It differs from the inflammatory pannus in having much less lymphocyte and plasma cell infiltration, and in having the accumulated hyaline material.

Band Keratopathy

Band keratopathy is **calcification of the cornea.** It represents a degenerative process following intraocular inflammation and hypercalcaemia in hyperparathyroidism and vitamin D toxicity. It consists of deposition of calcium salts in the superficial layer of the cornea.

Dystrophies

Corneal dystrophy is a primary, inherited, bilateral corneal disorder unassociated either with a systemic disease, or with pre-existing corneal vascularization and inflammation. Corneal diseases of animals which qualify as dystrophies include primary corneal lipidosis, oedema, and crystalline deposits. The opacity in corneal dystrophy is due to oedema. The cornea is thickened by oedema. **Corneal dystrophies** have been **described mostly in dogs and cats.**

Inflammation of the Cornea (Keratitis)

Cornea lacks vessels. This modifies the early lesions of inflammation and the development of pathological changes. Oedema of the corneal epithelium and stroma accompanies corneal inflammation. The fluid may originate from absorption of tears and aqueous humour, due to damage to the corneal epithelium. Neutrophils migrate into areas of corneal injury. Macrophages from the limbal (on the edge of the cornea) vessels appear at the injury site and phagocytose bacteria, dead neutrophils, and damaged corneal tissue. With healing, cellular exudate contains many lymphocytes and plasma cells. Keratitis may be accompanied by pain, photophobia (intolerance of light), blepharospasm (spasmodic contraction of the eyelid), and lachrymation.

Non-ulcerative corneal inflammation can be epithelial, sub-epithelial, and deep stromal. However, epithelial keratitis without ulceration is uncommon, but may occur in certain viral diseases.

Corneal Vascularization

The cause of corneal vascularization remains unknown. It may follow trauma to the cornea, especially any injury resulting in ulceration of the corneal epithelium. It can also occur from dietary deficiency of certain vitamins (riboflavin), or amino acids (tryptophan).

Capillaries which extend into the cornea toward an ulcer originate from the vessels in the limbus (corneo-scleral junction). **Superficial vascularization,** that is, formation of new capillaries in the stroma adjacent to the epithelium, occurs first. Proliferation of blood vessels deeper in the stroma, that is, **deep vascularization,** usually occurs after more prolonged effects on cornea. Vascularization of nutritional deficiency is characterized by proliferation of new capillaries from the corneo-scleral junction (limbus), all around the circumference of the cornea. **Grossly,** newly formed vessels in the cornea appear as vascular arborizations (tree-like branching appearance). **Microscopically,** each vessel forms a capillary loop through which the blood can return to the venules at the limbus. Vascularization is associated with neutrophilic infiltration. Recently it has been suggested that neutrophils increase neovascularization (formation of new blood vessels) by the release of vasoproliferative factors.

Corneal Ulceration

Corneal ulceration (ulcerative keratitis) may be due to bacterial, viral, and fungal infections. It may occur in acute or chronic keratitis, suppurative ophthalmitis, trauma, and caustic damage. Most infectious ulcerative lesions are due to **bacteria.** Almost all virulent pyogenic organisms can cause corneal ulcers, but streptococci, staphylococci, coliform organisms, and **Pseudomonas** sp. **(horses)** are the most frequently involved.

Sequelae of Corneal Ulceration

Scars

These are common sequelae after corneal ulceration, and result in opacification (formation of opacities). **Corneal opacities** are classified according to the degree of density: (1) **nebula-faint,** clouding, (2) **macula,** definite grey opacity, and (3) **leukoma,** dense white opacity. Neovascularization and fibrosis of the corneal stroma cause scarring.

Glaucoma and Phthisis Bulbi

Glaucoma is sustained increase in intraocular pressure. Phthisis bulbi is atrophy of eyeball following intraocular inflammation. The cornea is shrunken, flattened, and opaque. The contents of the eyeball are replaced by scar tissue. Both glaucoma and phthisis bulbi may follow corneal ulceration, especially if the ulceration is followed by perforation.

Acquired Corneal Inflammations

Chronic Superficial Keratitis (Inflammatory Pannus)

This is a chronic progressive disease of the **canine cornea**. It is associated with an inflammatory reaction characterized by the formation of granulation tissue in the cornea (**inflammatory pannus**), and deposition of melanin pigment. **The cause is unknown**. An immunological mechanism, involving cellular hypersensitivity against corneal protein, has been proposed. The disease has been observed in **dogs**, of all ages. There is no sex predilection.

Superficial Indolent Corneal Ulcers

Superficial indolent (non-healing) corneal ulcers are observed most frequently in **dogs**. The cause of the ulceration is not known. Recently it has been suggested that they may be associated with endocrine or senile disturbances.

Feline Chronic Ulcerative Keratitis

This is a distinct corneal disease of **cats** characterized by **chronicity**, and by unilateral or bilateral formation of **brown to black corneal plaques.** The cause is not known. **Lesions** include corneal vascularization, corneal opacity, and corneal ulceration. Pigmentation does not appear to be due to melanin or haemosiderin, but to desiccation of the corneal stroma and pigment absorbed from tears.

Infectious Keratoconjunctivitis of Cattle (Bovine Pink Eye)

This **disease of cattle** is caused by the bacterium *Moraxella bovis*, an aerobic, Gram-negative, coccobacillus. The disease is highly contagious. Transmission can be by direct contact as well as by mechanical vectors, such as flies. **Clinical signs** include marked lachrymation, conjunctivitis, photophobia, and oedematous swelling and hyperaemia of the lower lid. **Lesions include** keratitis, corneal opacity, and corneal ulceration. If central ulceration extends deep, the cornea may perforate with development of panophthalmitis, and loss of sight.

Keratoconjunctivitis in Sheep (Ovine Pink Eye)

The disease is considered highly contagious, but the cause remains obscure. A number of organisms have been proposed. The disease begins as a simple conjunctivitis. The whole of the conjunctiva is reddened due to hyperaemia, congestion, and petechiae. Excessive lachrymation is accompanied by photophobia. Keratitis often develops and may lead to corneal opacity.

Keratoconjunctivitis in Goats

The aetiology appears to be **mycoplasma organisms**, possibly a species of **Acholeplasma**. The earliest signs are excessive lachrymation. **Lesions** include conjunctivitis, corneal opacity with vascularization, ulceration, pannus, and iritis.

Infectious Bovine Rhinotracheitis

This **viral disease of cattle** is manifested by various syndromes, including respiratory disease, pustular vulvovaginitis, and **keratoconjunctivitis**. In some outbreaks, **keratoconjunctivitis** has been observed to be the only presenting sign. Common ocular lesions include ocular exudate (serous to mucopurulent), corneal opacity, and white plaques of the conjunctivae.

Uvea

Uvea is the second or vascular coat of the eye, lying immediately beneath the sclera. It consists of **iris, ciliary body**, and **choroid**, forming pigmented layer.

Anomalies of the Uvea

Congenital anomalies of the uvea are uncommon in domestic animals.

Aniridia

Aniridia is **complete absence of the iris**, and is rare in all species.

Coloboma of the Iris, Ciliary Body, and Choroid

Coloboma is a Greek word and means a mutilation. With reference to eye, it refers to **a congenital absence of a portion of an ocular tissue**, or a defect in the continuity of one of the tunics of the eye, usually the iris. **The defect appears as a cleft in the iris.** It is believed to be the result of incomplete fusion of parts of the optic vesicle during embryonic life.

The absence of a sector of the iris produces variations in papillary size and shape. Coloboma may be either unilateral or bilateral, and may involve whole sections of the iris. Coloboma of the ciliary body and choroid is an uncommon defect.

Persistent Pupillary Membrane

The persistence of the vascular pupillary membrane is common in **dogs**, but has also been described in **cattle, horses,** and **cats**.

Cysts of the Iris and Ciliary Body

These occur on the posterior surface of the iris and the ciliary body. They result from separation of the two neuro-ectodermal layers, and have been described in **dogs** and **horses**.

Uveitis

As mentioned earlier, uvea is composed of iris, ciliary body, and choroids. Inflammation may involve the anterior uvea (**iritis, cyclitis**, i.e. inflammation of ciliary body), **iridocyclitis** (i.e. inflammation of the iris and ciliary body), the posterior uvea (**choroiditis**), or the entire uveal tract (**panuveitis**).

Suppurative Uveitis

Pyogenic inflammation of the uvea follows accidental and surgical wounds, ulcerations of the cornea and sclera, and haematogenous spread of systemic bacterial infections. Purulent uveitis is a part of suppurative endophthalmitis. In purulent anterior uveitis, exudate in the anterior chamber consists of neutrophils and fibrin. Pus in anterior chamber of the eye in front of iris, but behind cornea, is called '**hypopyon**'.

Non-Suppurative Uveitis

This inflammatory reaction is milder than purulent and granulomatous uveal inflammations. Diffuse and focal infiltrations of lymphocytes, monocytes, and plasma cells are present in the uvea.

Granulomatous Uveitis

Organisms causing tuberculosis, actinomycosis, coccidioidomycosis, blastomycosis, and cryptococcosis, and certain parasitic forms are found in uveal granulomas. The **microscopic findings** are similar in granulomatous uveitis, regardless of aetiology. Granulomatous inflammation occurs as small nodules, and also as diffuse involvement of the iris, ciliary body, and choroid accompanied by necrosis. **The nodules consist of lymphocytes, plasma cells, epithelioid cells, and multinucleated giant cells.**

Sequelae to Uveal Inflammation

These include posterior and anterior synechiae. **Synechia** is adhesion of the iris to the lens and cornea. **Anterior synechia** is adhesion between the anterior of the iris and the posterior corneal surface. **Posterior synechia** is adhesion between the posterior surface of the iris and the anterior lens capsule. Fibrinous adhesion of the iris to the lens is followed by **fibrovascular organization**. Synechiae occur in all type of uveal inflammation. Blockage of the filtration meshwork by synechia can result in **glaucoma**.

547

Cyclitic membrane is a band of fibrovascular tissue which extends across the eyeball from one portion of the ciliary body along the posterior surface of the lens. Contraction of the cyclitic membrane results in partial detachment of the retina. Eventually, as the vitreous shrinks, **the retina becomes totally detached.**

Atrophy and **fibrosis** of the uvea follow inflammation. **Detachment of the retina** follows choroiditis due to the formation of an exudate beneath the neural retina.

Acquired Uveal Inflammation

Equine Recurrent Uveitis

Equine recurrent uveitis, also known as **'equine periodic ophthalmia'**, is an inflammatory disease of the eyes of **horses** and **mules**. (Ophthalmia is inflammation of the eye). It is the most common cause of **blindness** in these species. The disease begins as an **iridocyclitis** (inflammation of the iris and ciliary body), but later lesions develop in other tissues. These lesions eventually lead to impaired vision or blindness. Cataracts and posterior and anterior synechiae are common. The retina usually gets detached. Leptospirosis has been considered a cause of recurrent uveitis. *Leptospira interrogans* serovar *pomona* has been isolated from **horses**.

Lens-Induced Uveitis

Ocular inflammation due to leakage of lenticular proteins (**phacolytic uveitis**: G. phaco = lens) is a mild lymphocytic-plasmacytic anterior uveitis. A severe uveitis (**phacoclastic uveitis**) can occur following release of lenticular material after trauma to the lens and other causes. **Lens-induced uveitis** appears to be an immunological disease. It represents an autoimmune response to lenticular protein liberated through a ruptured capsule.

Infectious Canine Hepatitis

Corneal opacity, usually unilateral, sometimes occurs during the convalescent stage (period of recovery) of infectious canine hepatitis.

Avian Encephalomyelitis

Chickens infected with the enterovirus of avian encephalomyelitis have, besides lesions of the central nervous system, ocular changes of lens (**cataract**), and **non-suppurative anterior uveitis.**

Injuries of the Uvea

These include contusion of the iris, ciliary body and choroid, and haemorrhage. Secondary glaucoma may follow severe contusion. Perforation injuries include mechanical and surgical lacerations and penetration by foreign bodies.

Lens

Anomalies

Abnormalities of the lens may either be associated with, or result from anomalies of the surrounding tissues. The lens may be absent **'aphakia'**, which is a rare anomaly

Cataract

Lesions of the lens are relatively few. The **most common and important is lenticular** (of lens) opacity, known as **cataract.** Cataract is opacity of the crystalline lens and its capsule. Cataract can be either **congenital** or **acquired. Congenital cataracts** are often **bilateral. Acquired cataracts** are due to trauma, intraocular inflammation, glaucoma, and toxins. Cataracts can either be cortical or nuclear or involve anterior or posterior pole of the lens.

The cortical lenticular fibres, when traumatized and subjected to toxic or adverse nutritional influences, may suffer rapid necrosis followed by liquefaction. The fibres lose fluid and shrink, and the fluid collects in the resulting clefts and vacuoles. Cell membranes disintegrate, vacuoles form, and eventually the fibres fragment into globules.

Primary cataracts with a heritable basis have been reported in **dogs.** In **cattle,** cataracts have been reported as a primary entity, and in association with other ocular anomalies. Congenital cataracts are not uncommon in **foals.**

Luxation of the Lens

Congenital dislocation (luxation) **of the lens** occurs in **dogs, calves,** and **horses** as a part of multiple ocular anomalies. **Acquired luxations** are most common in **dogs.**

Vitreous Body

The vitreous (hyaloid = hyaline) is a transparent avascular gel filling the eyeball (globe) posterior to the lens. **About 99% of its weight is water.** It is a thin structure formed by a network of fine fibrous proteins permeated by the vitreous humour. It functions to retain the retina and prevent rapid spread of large molecules while allowing small molecules to diffuse within it. In humans, the vitreous is attached to the retina and the ciliary body. **In domestic animals, there is no attachment of the vitreous to the retina.**

Anomalies of the Vitreous Body

Persistence of Primary Vitreous

Complete or partial persistence of the hyaloid vascular system may occur in postnatal life.

Persistent Hyperplastic Primary Vitreous

This uncommon lesion in domestic animals has been described in **dogs.** Lesions include fibrous plaques located on the posterior capsule of the lens. **Microscopically,** the plaques consist of fibrous connective tissue.

Reactions of the Vitreous Body

These are usually characterized by liquefaction and opacification. Its avascularity and relative acellularity accounts for its susceptibility to infection. **Liquefaction is the most common degenerative change of the vitreous.**

Asteroid Hyalosis

This is the occurrence of spherical or disc-shaped white bodies in the vitreous. These bodies consist chiefly of calcium-containing lipids.

Retina

The retina is composed of the retinal pigment epithelium and the sensory retina. The **retinal pigment epithelium**, a single layer of rectangular cells, is normally non-pigmented over the tapetum (a covering structure), but over most of the fundus, the cells contain pigment granules. The **sensory retina** is composed of **nine layers.**

Anomalies

Retinal Dysplasia

Dysplasia means abnormal development. Retinal dysplasia has been described in most species, but **especially in dogs.** It is characterized microscopically by a series of branching tubes. The tubes represent elements which have failed to form the rod and cone layer, external limiting membrane, and other outer layer.

Hereditary Retinal Atrophy: Dog

The hereditary retinal degeneration in the **dog**, also called **'progressive retinal atrophy'** can be generalized, or central. It is characterized by rod dysplasia, and rod-cone dysplasia and degeneration.

Rod Dysplasia: Dog

In this progressive **retinal** disease, the rods are involved early and never reach functional maturity. **Young dogs** have impaired vision in dim light. **Adults are both day and night blind.** Vascular thinning in the retina becomes prominent after 2 years of age, and the end result is an avascular retina.

Cone Dysplasia: Dog

The **affected dogs** suffer from **day blindness** up to 8 to 10 weeks of age. Night vision is not impaired. The microscopic changes include presence of degenerated cones. The rods and the inner retinal layers are normal.

Central Progressive Retinal Atrophy: Dog

This is a specific pigment epithelial atrophy of **dogs**, and is uncommon. The pigment epithelial cells become hypertrophied and hyperplastic. These changes cause a secondary retinal degeneration.

Senile Retinal Degeneration: Dog

Changes in the eyeballs of senile (aged) **dogs** include the common cystic degeneration of the peripheral retina, and retinal breaks. Retinal breaks may be complete without retinal detachment, and comprise holes, ruptured peripheral retinal cysts, and breaks. **The most common type of defect is the atrophic hole.**

Inflammatory Retinal Degeneration

Degeneration followed by atrophy can occur in the retina of various species due to inflammatory changes. These changes are produced by several infectious agents, which include bacteria, viruses, fungi, and parasites.

Canine Distemper

Retinal atrophy in the **dog** can occur in infection with the virus of canine distemper. The **lesions include** degenerative changes in the retinal ganglion cells, perivascular cuffing, and the presence of eosinophilic intracellular inclusion bodies.

Pseudorabies

Ocular lesions occur in some **pigs** infected with the herpesvirus of pseudorabies. The lesions include perineuritis of the optic nerve, optic neuritis, and focal retinal gliosis.

Toxoplasmosis

Lesions in animals affected with the protozoan parasite *Toxoplasma gondii* include anterior uveitis and reticulo-choroiditis (retinal haemorrhage and detachment). **Microscopic lesions** comprise multifocal necrosis of the retina with little inflammatory reaction, retinitis, papillitis (inflammation of optic papilla), and non-suppurative uveitis. Toxoplasma are usually found in active ocular lesions.

Toxic Retinal Degeneration

This has been observed as a **progressive retinal degeneration in sheep,** also known as **bright blindness.** The disease is confined to those flocks grazing bracken fern. **Clinically,** affected sheep become permanently blind. **Lesions** are bilateral and confined to the retina.

Nutritional Retinal Degeneration

This has been observed as **'feline nutritional retinal degeneration'** in **cats** fed semipurified diet with casein as the protein source. The disease is characterized by **retinal degeneration.**

Diabetic Retinal Degeneration

Only a few cases of diabetic retinopathy have been described, and these are in **dogs**. The retina of **diabetic dogs** contains several saccular capillary micro-aneurysms and exudate, similar to those observed in human diabetic retinopthy.

Retinal Degeneration by Visible Light

The retina of various species can be damaged by light, both fluorescent and incandescent (visible) illumination, which is not intense enough to burn or cause thermal injury. **Several types of lasers can produce retinal damage.** The extent of damage to the retina is modified by wavelength of light, intensity of the source, duration of exposure, body temperature, and age. **Microscopically,** the outer segments of the photoreceptor cells developa stratified appearance, separate from the retinal pigment epithelium, and later, become fragmented and are removed by phagocytes.

Retinal Detachment

Retina is firmly attached only at the optic nerve head, and at the ora ciliaris retinae. Thus there exists a **potential space** between retina and the retinal pigment epithelium. Accumulation of fluid, exudate, blood, or neoplastic cells within this **potential space** constitutes **detachment of retina.** Retinal detachment (or non-attachment) can occur in congenital ocular anomalies. The results of detachment are degeneration and necrosis of the retina. Degenerative changes occur in the outer segments of the photoreceptor cells. Atrophy of the retina is slow but progressive.

Optic Nerve

The optic nerve consists of the ganglion cells of the retina. It is a white fibre tract of the central nervous system, extending from the eyeball to the optic chiasma. It consists of ocular, orbital, and intracranial portions. In most species, the optic fibres within the eyeball are unmyelinated and take on myelin sheath as they leave the eyeball. The nerves vary in size.

In cross section, the axis cylinder of the nerve fibres appears as small, faintly stained eosinophilic dots surrounded by clear halos - **the myelin sheath.** The normal nerve is rather pale, with a somewhat spongy appearance. **Microscopically** glial cells are neither large nor numerous, and the nerve is normally **hypocellular.** In diseases of the optic nerve myelin may be lost and collagenous tissue increased. The nerve is then less spongy, more compact, and more eosinophilic because the nerve tissue contains increased numbers of glial and mesenchymal cells.

Anomalies

Aplasia

In aplasia, the optic disc, optic nerve, and optic tracts are absent. **Aplasia of the optic nerve is rare in animals.**

Hypoplasia

Hypoplasia of the optic nerve is a rare lesion, and has been reported as an isolated defect in several species.

Coloboma

Coloboma (congenital absence of a portion) of the optic nerve may occur alone, but it is often associated with microphthalmia, mainly in **dogs.** True optic colobomas are confined to the optic disc and nerve.

Papilloedema

Papilloedema (disc oedema) is oedema with swelling of the nerve head, from any cause. Lesions which alter the pressure gradient such that flow of tissue fluid is outward (from optic nerve into eyeball) result in papilloedema. The **microscopic changes** are similar, regardless of the cause. The vessels of the papilla may be congested, and the nerve head is swollen. Papilloedema, if present for a long time, results in degenerative changes.

Inflammation

Optic neuritis is involvement of any part of the nerve by inflammatory, vascular, or degenerative disease. The term **'papillitis'** is used when the nerve head is involved, and the term **'neuro-retinitis'** when there are associated changes in the retina. Optic papillitis is part of retinitis and ophthalmitis. It is characterized by oedema, perivascular cuffing and gliosis.

The optic meninges and meningeal spaces are continuous with those of the brain, and **perineuritis** can occur as a complication of primary (especially bacterial) cerebral leptomeningitis. It results from an extension of inflammation along the meninges of the optic nerve, or may develop as a direct extension of localized inflammation in the sinuses, orbital space, or eyeball.

Degeneration

The optic nerve is a special white-matter tract of the central nervous system. It is composed of axons of the ganglion cells of the retina, **and reacts to injury differently than do peripheral nerves.** Since the optic nerve is part of the CNS, the nerve fibres have no Schwann cells, and no capacity for regeneration. Glial, meningeal, and connective tissue components of the optic nerve respond to injury by proliferation. Optic nerve degeneration may be ascending when lesions affect the ganglion cells of the retina and nerve fibre layers. The process may be either focal or general, depending on the extent of the lesions in the retina.

Secondary Optic Nerve Degeneration

These lesions in the optic nerves are due to inflammation, or vascular disease near the eyeball. Optic atrophy can be related to retinal degeneration, inflammation, papilloedema, glaucoma, and destructive lesions of the optic nerves and tracts.

Optic Neuropathy

This occurs in **calves fed vitamin A-deficient diets.** These calves are blind and have changes of oedema of the optic papilla, distorted retinal vessels, and constriction of the optic nerve and raised cerebrospinal fluid pressure.

Calves deficient in vitamin A have gross changes in the bones of the skull. The size of the optic foramen is reduced due to encroaching bone. The nerves are swollen, and have zones of haemorrhage. The optic nerve near constriction is necrotic and atrophic. **Microscopically,** areas of necrosis and gitter cell (large foamy macrophage) accumulation are present in the region of greatest constriction.

Proliferative Optic Neuropathy

This has been described in **horses.** The lesion varies from a whitish-grey, oval, elevated to a round, protuberant, whitish mass at the optic disc. The mass is composed of large, round to ovoid cells with small, dense nuclei, and eosinophilic, foamy to vacuolated cytoplasm.

Storage Diseases

Storage diseases in animals have ocular lesions. Many different cells of the eyeball and optic nerve, especially neurons of the retina, accumulate materials within lysosomes due to enzyme deficiency and faulty degradation.

Gangliosidosis

Gangliosidosis with **retinal lesions** has been described in the **dog, cat,** and **calf. Corneal opacities** occur due to polysaccharide (GM_1 ganglioside) accumulation within the corneal endothelium and in stromal fibroblasts. **Microscopically,** retinal ganglion cells are enlarged, swollen, and have granular cytoplasm.

Mannosidosis

Ocular lesions have been described in animals (**cattle, cats, goats, dogs**) with alpha and beta-mannosidosis. **Goats** affected with beta-mannosidosis have a paucity of myelin in the optic nerves, and the presence of numerous, spherical intracytoplasmic vacuoles in retinal ganglion cells, retinal pigment epithelium, and other retinal cells. **Similar lesions have been observed in cattle.**

Mucopolysaccharidoses

These storage diseases are characterized by biochemical derangements in metabolism of **glycosaminoglycans. Ocular lesions** have been described in **cats.**

Glaucoma

Glaucoma is not a specific disease entity, but a composite of the clinical and pathological manifestations which result **from a sustained (persistent) increase in intraocular pressure.** The increased pressure is due to tissue changes which reduce the outflow of aqueous humour. Many different causes and processes may be responsible for this. Thus, glaucoma results from a complex of ocular diseases. They all raise intraocular pressure as a result of obstruction to aqueous outflow. The most important aspects of the pathology of glaucoma are the changes induced by the continued elevated intraocular pressure.

When the obstruction in aqueous outflow is due to an ocular disease, the glaucoma is called **secondary**. If the increased pressure occurs without prior ocular disease, the glaucoma is classified as **primary**. Glaucoma which appears at, or soon after birth, as a result of some developmental error is called **congenital glaucoma.**

Primary Glaucoma

Primary glaucoma has been described in **dogs.**

Secondary Glaucoma

Most cases of glaucoma in animals are of the secondary type, and the complications of a large number of intraocular diseases, including inflammatory, traumatic, neoplastic and degenerative lesions. Most cases are unilateral and occur in eyeball with causative lesions. Glaucoma usually develops in animals having an intraocular neoplasm. In the late stages, it is not always possible to differentiate primary from secondary forms.

Light-Induced Avian Glaucoma

In chicks reared under continuous light, the developing glaucoma has such features as increased intraocular pressure, eyeball enlargement, retinal damage, and eventually blindness. The retina is detached.

Ocular Effects of Glaucoma

In chronic cases of glaucoma, the eyeball is enlarged, its tunics are thinned, the uvea is atrophied, and the iris is displaced forward. Eyeball enlargement is common in the **dog** and **cat**, but is uncommon in other domestic animals, which have a thicker sclera. **Changes in the retina** include atrophy of the nerve fibre and ganglion cell layers, which may progress to complete absence of these tissues. The iris stroma, the ciliary body and ciliary processes become atrophic and fibrotic. The choroid may be thinned, and the vessels are sclerosed.

Conjunctiva

Conjunctivitis

Bacterial conjunctivitis is common in domestic animals, especially in **dogs** and **cattle**. Several organisms are responsible. These include staphylococci, streptococci, *Pseudomonas aeruginosa, E. coli,* and *Moraxella bovis.* The conjunctiva is very sensitive to bacterial infection. Some organisms, such as those of brucellosis, listeriosis, and tularaemia, **penetrate the intact conjunctiva. Epiphora** (abnormal overflow of tears) is the main clinical sign. At first serous, later it becomes mucoid or mucopurulent. The ocular discharge is accompanied by congested, swollen, and oedematous conjunctiva.

The **microscopic changes** include oedema, hyperaemia, necrosis, and neutrophilic infiltration of the epithelium and underlying stroma. The epithelium of the conjunctiva is not keratinized normally, but readily becomes keratinized when chronically irritated. The global cells and the small lymphoid aggregates, normally present in the conjunctival propria, undergo hyperplasia. Lymphoid hyperplasia can produce large, increased number of follicles – **follicular conjunctivitis.**

In cats, chlamydia (*Chlamydia psittaci,* feline pneumonitis) and mycoplasma together produce conjunctivitis. Clinical signs are lachrymation, conjunctival oedema, and purulent exudate. In severe cases, a pseudomembrane forms on the membrana nictitans.

Feline Infectious Conjunctivitis

Ocular lesions in cats with feline herpesvirus occur in **kittens,** and consist of conjunctivitis, keratitis, corneal ulceration, and perforation of the eyeball.

Episclera

Episclera is the well-vascularized connective tissue between the bulbar conjunctiva and the sclera. Few lesions involve this structure. An important lesion is the **nodular episcleritis.** It is a benign nodular lesion of connective tissue, and has been described in the **dog.**

Eyelids

Lesions peculiar to the skin of the eyelids include trichiasis, districhiasis, entropion, and ectropion. **Trichiasis** is inversion of eyelashes. Eyelashes then rub against the cornea, causing continued irritation of the eyeball. **Districhiasis** is double row of eyelashes. **Entropion** is congenital inward turning of the eyelids. **Ectropion** is an outward eversion of the eyelid. These lesions result in conjunctivitis and keratitis. Other lesions include epidermoid and dermoid cysts, and cyst of the membrana nictitans. Inflammation of the gland of the membrana nictitans, and hyperplasia of lymphoid follicles are lesions which enlarge the third eyelid, and cause it to protrude.

Inflammation

Inflammatory lesions include blepharitis, hordeolum, internal hordeolum, and chalazion. **Blepharitis** is inflammation of the edges of the eyelids. **Hordeolum** is a follicular (inflammation of a hair follicle) due to pyogenic infection of the perifollicular tissue. In other words, it is abscess formation in a hair follicle, or glands of cilium of the eyelid. **Internal hordeolum** is pyogenic infection of meibomian (tarsal) glands. This results in occlusion of the duct and abscess formation. **Chalazion** is chronic inflammation of meibomian or Zeis glands. It is a granulomatous inflammatory lesion. **Microscopically**, granulomatous inflammation contains lymphocytes, macrophages, plasma cells, and giant cells. (**Meibomian gland** is also known as **tarsal gland**. It is one of the sebaceous glands between the tarsi and conjunctiva of the eyelid. **Zeis gland** is one of the sebaceous glands at free edge of eyelids).

Lachrymal Apparatus

Inflammation of the **lachrymal gland** (**dacryoadenitis**) can be primary, or secondary due to the spread of disease processes from the conjunctiva and from the orbit.

Orbit

Orbit is the bony cavity of the skull which holds the eyeball. Space-occupying lesions of the orbit result in deviation or protrusion of the eyeball (**exophthalmos**). **Causes** include retrobulbar abscess, salivary gland cysts, orbital parasites, sinus neoplasms such as lymphosarcoma. **Retrobulbar abscess is common in the dog.** Exophthalmos, if prolonged, can result in exposure keratitis and excessive drying of the cornea.

Inflammation of the orbit is called **orbital cellulitis**. It is an acute inflammation and is characterized by congestion and oedema, **but is not common in domestic animals.** Orbital cellulitis can be caused by parasites and fungi, penetrating foreign bodies, and spread of infection from paranasal sinuses, infected teeth, and suppurative panophthalmitis, through the sclera. Most of the orbital inflammations are suppurative.

Neoplasms of the Eyeball and Ocular Adnexa

Neoplasms of the Eyelids

Neoplasms of the eyelids are the same which occur in the skin. They are found in all domestic animals, but are more common in **cattle and **dogs**. Sebaceous gland neoplasms are most numerous in **dogs,** and squamous-cell carcinoma in **cattle**.

Neoplasms of the Conjunctiva and Cornea

Epithelial neoplasms of the conjunctiva and cornea include squamous-cell papilloma (**cattle, horses, dogs**) and squamous-cell carcinoma (**cattle, horses**). **Squamous-cell papillomas are most common in cattle.** They are either soft or hard, pigmented masses. **Microscopically,** they consist of proliferated squamous prickle-cells around a connective tissue core. Squamous-cell carcinomas in **horses** involve the cornea and conjunctiva. The neoplasms vary in size, and appear as ulcerated pink to white, irregular masses. **Microscopic features** are like those of this neoplasm at other sites.

Bovine Ocular Squamaous-Cell Carcinoma

Ocular squamous-cell carcinoma of **cattle** has a marked predilection for the medial and lateral aspects of the eyeball, portions not usually covered by the eyelids. This indicates that **exposure to sunlight is a factor in the development of the lesions.** Lesions develop when pigment is lacking from some areas of the corneo-scleral junction. The incidence of benign and carcinomatous lesions is greatest on the eyeball, and least frequent on the nictitating membrane. **The corneo-scleral junction is the most common site.** About 75% are either at the limbus (corneo-scleral junction), or on the cornea proper.

The lesions are plaque, squamous-cell papilloma, early squamous-cell carcinoma, and invasive squamous-cell carcinoma. Plaque and squamous-cell papilloma represent early stages. Most of the lesions are squamous-cell carcinomas.

Vascular Lesions

Haemangiomatous lesions occur in the conjunctiva in **dogs**. Most lesions begin as small haemorrhages. Lesions are composed of endothelial, blood-containing spaces.

Lachrymal Gland Neoplasms

Neoplasms of the lachrymal glands, including the gland of third eyelid of animals, **are rare.** They are either adenomas or adenocarcinomas. The adenoma and adenocarinoma cause **exophalmos** and deviation of the eyeball.

Harderian Gland Neoplasms

In most species (except the dog) an accessory lachrymal gland exists at the base of the third eyelid. This is called the **Harderian gland.** This tubulo-alveolar gland has alveoli lined by columnar epithelial cells with round, pale-staining nuclei. Spontaneous neoplasms, usually adenomas, occur in mice and hamsters, but are rare in rats. **They have not been described in domestic animals.**

Neuro-Ectodermal Neoplasms

These are **classified morphologically** into adenoma and adenocarcinoma if they originate from **mature** neuroepithelium, and into retinoblastoma, medulloepithelioma, and teratoid medulloepithelioma if they originate from the **primitive** medullary epithelium. Retinoblastoma is an extremely rare neoplasm in domestic animals.

Adenoma and Adenocarcinoma

Adenoma and adenocarcinoma of the irido-ciliary epithelium **are uncommon in animals**. Most cases have been observed in the **dog** and **cat**. Grossly, the mass may be solid and occupy the intraocular space. **Microscopically**, the cells are composed of cuboidal to columnar cells. Mitotic figures may be either numerous, or rare. Adenocarcinoma has features of the cellular anaplasia. Metastasis of adenocarcinoma of irido-ciliary epithelium is rare, but the neoplasm can penetrate the eyeball and invade the orbit.

Medulloepithelioma and Teratoid Medulloepithelioma

The **medulloepithelioma** contains poorly differentiated normal tissue which resembles embryonic retina. In **teratoid medulloepithelioma**, areas of neuroglia and foci of cartilage occur, as well as ganglion cells, and striated muscle.

Mesenchymal Neoplasms of Eyeball

Primary mesenchymal neoplasms of the eyeball are **extremely rare**. A few cases have been reported. These are haemangioma, leiomyoma, leiomyosarcoma, and chondrosarcoma.

Feline Trauma-Associated Sarcomas

Sarcomas and osteosarcomas have been observed in the eyeballs of **cats, years after trauma to the eyeball**. The neoplasms are composed of anaplastic spindle cells with deposits of osteoid. The osteoid is considered metaplastic.

Melanogenic Neoplasms

These (both benign and malignant) involve the conjunctiva and skin of the eyelids. They are common only in the **dog**. **Microscopically**, spindle or epithelioid cells may contain abundant or scant melanin pigment.

Epibulbar (Limbal) Melanomas

These neoplasms originate in the sclera and subconjunctival tissue at the limbus (corneal-scleral junction), and appear as raised, firm, pigmented masses at the corneal-scleral junction.

Uveal Melanomas

These are the most common primary intraocular neoplasms in domestic animals, but have been recorded mainly in **dog** and **cat**. Nearly all the animal cases have involved the anterior uvea, but a few choroidal melanomas have been recorded in the **dog**.

Orbital Neoplasms

Orbital and retrobulbar neoplasms originate from mesenchymal and epithelial tissues of the eyeball and orbit, and also by direct extension from adjacent tissues, and from the nasal cavity and sinuses.

Metastatic Intraocular Neoplasms

Secondary intraocular neoplasms may arrive at the interior of the eyeball by extension of an orbital, or adnexal neoplasm, or haematogenously in cases of disseminated neoplasia. The haematogenous route accounts for most of the reported cases. Metastatic intraocular neoplasms are rare in domestic animals, except lymphosarcoma in the **dog**.

Lymphosarcoma

These have been recorded only in the **dog**. Most cases of ocular lymphosarcoma are bilateral. Although all segments of the globe can be involved by neoplastic lymphoid cells, the anterior uvea is the primary site of metastasis.

Ear

The ear is a sensory organ. It is composed of the **external ear, middle ear,** and the **inner ear (labyrinth)**. The labyrinth is divided into anatomical and functional divisions: the **cochlea** for hearing and the **vestibular system** equilibrium. Sensory information from these two structures is transmitted to the brain through the eighth cranial nerve, and then through the central auditory pathway. **Any portion of the ear may be involved in the disease.**

External Ear

The external ear is composed of the **auricle (pinna)** and the **external auditory meatus**. The pinna is composed of a flat sheet of cartilage covered by skin. The external auditory meatus is lined by epidermis containing sebaceous glands, as well as sudoriferous (sweat) and modified sweat glands (ceruminous glands).

Congenital Anomalies

At birth, the pinna may be abnormally large (**macrotia**) or abnormally small (**microtia**). Absence of pinna (**anotia**) is an inherited defect in **sheep**. Extra pinnae (**polyotia**) have been reported in the **cat**. **Deafness** may occur from an absence of the external auditory meatus (**atresia**), or failure of the meatal plug to be shed (persistent meatal plug). This has been reported in the **dog. Goats,** affected with beta-mannosidosis are born with abnormally shaped pinnae.

Ear-Tip Necrosis and Fissures

Necrosis of the tip of the pinna may be due to frostbite (**pigs, calves**), ergot poisoning (**cattle**), septicaemia (**pigs**), and trauma. It is associated with inflammation of the external ear (**otitis externa**). Fissures may develop on the digital edge of canine pinnae from trauma.

Auricular Haematoma

This may result from an intrachondral fracture of the pinnal cartilage. They appear as fluctuant, blood-filled swellings on the canine pinna near the apex. With maturation, it is replaced by granulation tissue. Contraction of the granulation tissue can result in distortion of the pinna.

Dermatological Diseases

The external ear may be involved in generalized or regional dermatological diseases. Regional diseases include idiopathic pinnal alopecia and feline solar dermatitis in **cats,** and **equine aural plaques. Feline solar dermatitis** is a chronic actinic disorder of the margin of the pinna characterized by erythema, necrosis, ulceration, and superficial perivascular dermatitis.

Parasitic Otitis Externa

A variety of parasites (**mites, ticks**) can infest the external ear. Transmission of mites among animals occurs readily. Otitis externa from parasitic infestation can have an allergic basis. **Many ticks have a predilection for the external ear.** The **mites** commonly involved are *Demodex canis* (**dog**), *Ixodes cati* (**cat**), and *Sarcoptes scabiei* (**dog, pig**), and ticks are Boophilus sp. (**cattle, other ruminants, horses**), and **Rhipicephalus** sp. (**dog, horse, ruminants**). Since pinnae have less hair, they are sites for sand fly bites. These can cause auricular nodules in **dogs** due to **Leishmania** infections.

Mycotic Otitis Externa

Dermatomycosis of the external ear (**otomycosis**) is usually caused by fungi of the genera **Microsporum, Candida, Trichophyton,** and **Aspergillus.**

Bacterial Otitis Externa

This has been usually reported in the **dogs, cats,** and **pigs** and mycoplasmas have been isolated from the external ears of **goats.** In the **dog** and **cat,** *Staphylococcus aureus,* beta haemolytic **Sreptococcus** sp., **Proteus** sp., **Pseudomonas** sp., and *E. coli* may infect the external ear. *Actinomyces bovis* produces granulomatous

561

inflammation in the external ears of **pigs.**

Non-Infectious Otitis Externa

Non-infectious causes of otitis externa include **foreign bodies** and **hormonal imbalances.** Hypothyroidism, ovarian imbalances, and Sertoli cell tumours have been associated with ceruminous externa.

Lesions of Otitis Externa

The external auditory meatus may contain dry, brown cerumen. If the cause is parasitic, ova and parasites may be present within the exudate, or epidermis. **Chronic lesions include** epidermal hyperplasia with acanthosis, folliculitis, and glandular atrophy. Scabs often form due to epidermal burrowing of mites. The meatus may become narrowed due to the inflammatory changes.

Neoplasms of the External Ear

These originate from the auricular skin, auricular cartilage, and the ceruminous glands. Squamous-cell carcinoma has been reported in the pinnae of **white cats** exposed to sunlight for prolonged periods. Other reported neoplasms include canine histiocytoma, basal-cell epithelioma, plasmacytoma, equine sarcoid, chondroma and chondrosarcoma. **Adenomas and adenocarcinomas of ceruminous glands occur in old cats and dogs.**

Middle Ear

The middle ear is lined by a two-layered, ciliated or non ciliated, secretory or non-secretory mucosa containing goblet cells. This mucosa also forms the inner layer of the tympanic membrane, which is in contact with the manubrium (handle) of the **malleus,** one of the three tympanic ossicles. The malleus articulates with the **incus,** which articulates with the **stapes.** The footplate of the stapes articulates with the membrane of the vestibular window of the chochlea. The middle ear, through the ossicles, communicates sound-induced vibrations of the tympanic membrane in the inner ear.

Otitis Media

The main lesion which occurs in the middle ear is **inflammation - otitis media.** However, middle ear can be the site of metastatic and primary neoplasms. **Otitis media is usually due to bacterial infection.** The bacteria involved are *Actinomyces pyogenes* (**pig, calf,** and **sheep**), *Corynebacterium pseudotuberculosis* (**cattle**), *Escherichia coli* (**dog**), *Pasteurella haemolytica* (**sheep, cattle**), *Pasteurella multocida* (**cat, cattle,** and **pig**), *Pseudomonas aeruginosa* (**pig**), **Staphylococcus** sp. (**dog**), and **Streptococcus** sp. (**pig, dog**). **In dogs,** infections are due to **Candida** sp. and **Aspergillus** sp. Infection may occur through the auditory tube, and from an otitis externa with inflammation of the tympanic membrane (**myringitis**). A possible sequel to otitis media is the otitis interna which may lead to meningo-encephalitis. Pharyngitis could follow otitis media and develop into pneumonia.

Nasopharyngeal Polyps

In response to inflammation, **in cats**, there is formation of **nasopharyngeal polyps** from the mucosa of the tympanic cavity, middle ear, and auditory tube. The polypoid masses may fill the tympanic cavity, and are composed of well-vascularized, fibrous to myxomatous connective tissue diffusely infiltrated by lymphocytes. The masses may contain mucous glands and lymphoid nodules.

Beta-Mannosidosis

This storage disease has been described in **goat kids** and **calves**. Deafness was reported in affected **goats**. The cavity of the middle ear is narrowed in **goats**, and numerous mucosal folds are present.

Eustachitis

Eustachitis is inflammation of the auditory tube. It is common, and can occur in association with otitis media in **pigs,** and usually involves the guttural pouches of **horses.** Changes in the auditory tube include empyema (accumulation of pus), tympany in **young horses,** foreign bodies, abscesses, and rarely neoplasms. In mycotic eustachitis of the guttural pouches, inflammation is fibro-necrotic. Empyema is the accumulation of a suppurative exudate (pus), occurring as a sequel to an upper respiratory infection. The causative agents are **Streptococcus** sp. in **horses,** and *Pasteurella multocida* and *Actinomyces pyogenes* in **pigs**. Changes in chronic eustachitis include mucosal swelling and formation of granulation tissue.

Inner Ear

Inner ear (labyrinth) consists of membranous channels (**membranous labyrinth**) lining cavities within the temporal bone (**bony labyrinth**). Portions of the membranous labyrinth are separated from the bony labyrinth by a fluid (perilymph). The bony labyrinth is divided into **three parts:** the **cochlea, semicircular canals,** and the **vestibule**. The cochlea and semicircular canals each contain a portion of the membranous labyrinth, with cochlea containing the cochlear duct. The vestibule contains the endolymphatic duct, the utricle, and the saccule of the membranous labyrinth. The sensory organ of hearing is the **organ of Corti,** a portion of the cochlear duct. Axons of bipolar neurons that have their cell bodies in the ganglion (cochlear) constitute the auditory portion of the eighth cranial nerve.

Dysplasia and degeneration of the cochlear duct result in deafness. This has been reported in **cats and dogs**. Inflammation of the inner ear (**otitis interna, labyrinthitis**) and metastatic neoplasia, such as lymphosarcoma, result in destruction and loss of the cochlear duct, along with destruction of the structures of the vestibular labyrinth. Infections may be due to viral, bacterial, and fungal agents.

Vestibular Disorders

Congenital vestibular disorders have been reported in **dogs** and **cats**.

Neoplasms of the Middle and Inner Ear

Neoplasms are rarely found in the tissues of the middle and inner ear of domestic animals. The described cases include squamous-cell carcinoma in the middle and inner ear of **cats**, and adenoma of the middle ear of **dogs**. Adenomas fill the tympanic cavity. They are solid or papillary, and are composed of small tubular formations of cuboidal to columnar ciliated epithelial cells.

Index

(Page numbers in bold type indicate main discussion)